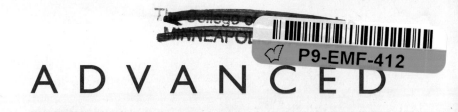

ADVANCED

RESPIRATORY THERAPIST

WITHDRAWN

EXAM GUIDE

The Complete Resource for the Written Registry and Clinical Simulation Exams

ADVANCED

RESPIRATORY THERAPIST

EXAM GUIDE

The Complete Resource for the Written Registry and Clinical Simulation Exams

JAMES R. SILLS, MEd, CPFT, RRT
Director, Respiratory Care Program
Rock Valley College
Rockford, Illinois

Original illustrations by

SANDRA HOGAN
Rock Valley College
Rockford, Illinois

Second Edition
with 518 illustrations

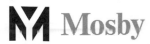 Mosby

A Harcourt Health Sciences Company

St. Louis   London   Philadelphia   Sydney   Toronto

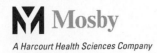

Acquisitions Editor: Karen Fabiano
Developmental Editor: Mindy Copeland
Project Manager: John Rogers
Designer: Kathi Gosche

SECOND EDITION

NOTICE

Pharmacology is an ever-changing field. Standard safety precautions must be followed, but as new research and clinical experience broaden our knowledge, changes in treatment and drug therapy may become necessary or appropriate. Readers are advised to check the most current product information provided by the manufacturer of each drug to be administered to verify the recommended dose, the method and duration of administration, and contraindications. It is the responsibility of the treating physician, relying on experience and knowledge of the patient, to determine dosages and the best treatment for each individual patient. Neither the publisher nor the editor assumes any liability for any injury and/or damage to persons or property arising from this publication.

Mosby, Inc.
A Harcourt Health Sciences Company
11830 Westline Industrial Drive
St. Louis, Missouri 63146

Printed in USA

Library of Congress Cataloging in Publication Data
Sills, James R.
    Advanced respiratory therapist exam guide : the complete resource for the written registry and clinical simulations exams / James R. Sills ; original illustrations by Sandra Hogan.—2nd ed.
       p. ; cm.
    Rev. ed. of: Respiratory care registry guide. c1995.
    "Complement and supplement Entry level respiratory therapist exam guide. ed. 3"—Pref.
    Includes bibliographical references and index.
    ISBN 0-323-00784-8
    1. Respiratory therapy—Examinations, questions, etc.   I. Sills, James R. Respiratory care registry guide.   II. Sills, James. R. Entry level respiratory therapist exam guide.   III. Title.
    [DNLM: 1. Respiratory Therapy—methods.   2. Respiratory Therapy—Examination Questions.   WB 342 S584a 2002]
    RC735.I5 S574 2002
    616.2'0046'076—dc21

                                    2001045247

01 02 03 04 05 GW/MV 9 8 7 6 5 4 3 2 1

REVIEWERS

JEFF ANDERSON, MA, RRT
Associate Professor, Director of Clinical Education
Department of Respiratory Therapy
Boise State University
Boise, Idaho

STEVEN BISHOP, PhD, RRT
Program Director, Respiratory Care Department
Ozark Technical Community College
Springfield, Missouri

NANCY COLLETTI, MS, RRT, RCVT, CPFT
Clinical Assistant Professor
Respiratory Care Program
School of Health Technology & Management
Stony Brook, New York

MICHAEL W. COOK, MA, RRT
Director, Respiratory Care Program
Mountain Empire Community College
Big Stone Gap, Virginia

KEN DRECHNY, RRT, RCP
Clinical Technical Supervisor
University of Chicago-Mitchell Hospital
Chicago, Illinois

JOHN EVANS, RRT, BS
Program Director, Respiratory Care Department
Florence-Darlington Technical College
Florence, South Carolina

MARIE A. FENSKE, EDD, RRT
Department Chair, Respiratory Care
GateWay Community College
Phoenix, Arizona

JOHN GIETZEN, BS, RRCP
Coordinator of Clinical Education
Respiratory Therapy School
North Dakota State University
Fargo, North Dakota

CHRISTINE HAMILTON, BA, RRT
Respiratory Care Program Director
Nebraska Methodist College
Omaha, Nebraska

CHRIS KALLUS, MEd, RRT
Program Director, Respiratory Care Program
The Victoria College
Victoria, Texas

SINDEE KARPEL, MA, RRT
Assistant Professor, Allied Health Sciences
Borough of Manhattan Community College
New York, New York

KEVIN KELLMAN, MS, RRT
Respiratory Therapy Department
Fredrick Memorial Hospital
Fredrick, Maryland

NANCY LORANCE, BS, RRT, RPFT
Program Director, Respiratory Therapist Program
Rose State College
Midwest City, Oklahoma

ANN MOORE, MS, RRT, CPFT
Department of Respiratory Care
Trident Technical College
Charleston, North Carolina

JOSEPH L. RAU, PhD, RRT
School of Allied Health Professions
Department of Cardiopulmonary Care Services
Georgia State University
Atlanta, Georgia

CANDACE SCHLADENHAUFFEN, BS, RRT, RPFT
Department of Respiratory Care
Ivy Tech State College
Fort Wayne, Indiana

ROBERT E. ST. JOHN, MSN, RN, RRT, CCRN, CS
Mallinckrodt, Inc.
St. Louis, Missouri

STEPHEN F. WEHRMAN, RRT, RPFT
Associate Professor/Program Director
Respiratory Care Program, Health Sciences
Kapi'olani Community College
Honolulu, Hawaii

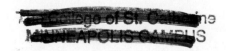

This book is dedicated to my wife
Deb
and our children **Rachael** *and* **David**
who make my life full and complete;
the memory of our dog **Amber,**
who always kept me company when I worked at home;
my **mom** *and the memory of my* **dad;**
and
Carl Hammond,
who taught me respiratory care.

Words to live by:

The journey of 1000 miles begins with a single step.

Confucius

Hope for the best but plan for the worst.

FOREWORD

Advanced Respiratory Therapist Exam Guide, Second Edition, is, in this writer's opinion, the definitive textbook and resource guide to the successful completion of the National Board for Respiratory Care (NBRC) Written Registry Examination and Clinical Simulation Examination. This textbook clearly—and quickly—presents the essential knowledge, skills, and professional attributes required by the NBRC examination board. There are six new—and very important—features included in the Second Edition. They are the following:

- Every item that appears on the most recent **NBRC Detailed Content Outline for the Written Registry Exam** has been covered and updated. No other resource presents every testable item.
- Every chapter provides the reader with **Exam Hints** that discuss the various concepts associated with frequently asked questions. The material presented in the Exam Hints will very likely appear in every Written Registry Exam.
- Every chapter has more **self-assessment questions.** In addition, every question now has a rationale and explanation for the correct answer and the incorrect answers.
- A **sample Written Registry Exam** provides 100 questions with (1) the same question styles, (2) areas of emphasis, and (3) level of difficulty. Every question has a rationale and explanation for the correct answer and the incorrect answers.
- A **CD-ROM** provides a 100-question, computer-based Written Registry Examination like the actual NBRC computer-based exam. This computer software package

is also designed to use the same question styles, emphasis of content areas, and question difficulties presented by the NBRC. Every question has a rationale and explanation for the correct answer and the incorrect answers.

- To complete this new edition, the CD-ROM includes a **practice Clinical Simulation Examination** designed to run like the actual NBRC exam. The ten simulations match the same patient scenarios used by the NBRC—two adult COPD patients, two adult cardiovascular patients, two adult trauma patients, two adult neurologic patients, one pediatric patient, and one neonatal patient. Also, every tested item has a rationale and explanation for the correct answer and the incorrect answers.

Without a doubt, the *Advanced Respiratory Therapist Exam Guide, Second Edition,* is an excellent resource for both the student and the respiratory care educator. It provides a precise and clear review of the essential components required by the NBRC advanced practitioners examinations. This latest edition can truly serve to enhance the reader's ability to master the knowledge, skills, and professional attributes needed to pass the NBRC Written Registry Exam and Clinical Simulation Exam. Again, Jim Sills provides us with a very useful and wonderful resource. Thank you, Jim. The profession of respiratory care continues to reap what you sow.

Terry DesJardins, MEd, RRT
Department of Respiratory Care
Parkland College
Champaign, Illinois

PREFACE

The *Advanced Respiratory Therapist Exam Guide, Second Edition* has been extensively redesigned—new title, new format, exam hints that focus on commonly tested concepts, and CD-ROM–based practice exams. It is my sincere hope that these revisions help the exam taker to better focus on the key factors that will lead to successfully passing the National Board for Respiratory Care (NBRC) Written Registry Examination and Clinical Simulation Examination. By passing these two examinations the advanced practitioner will earn the Registered Respiratory Therapist (RRT) credential.

This book is designed to complement and supplement *Entry Level Respiratory Therapist Exam Guide, Third Edition,* which was written for anyone preparing for the entry level examination to earn the Certified Respiratory Therapist (CRT) credential. In this book I have attempted to write a standard textbook that covers every testable item listed by the NBRC in its 1998 examination content outline for the Written Registry Examination. When preparing for the Clinical Simulation Examination, this book and *Entry Level Respiratory Therapist Exam Guide* should both be studied. This is because some NBRC listed items are tested only on the Entry Level Exam and the Clinical Simulation Exam. Therefore they are not presented in this book.

James R. Sills, MEd, CPFT, RRT

INTRODUCTION

Introduction and Recommendations for Exam Success

Every item listed on the National Board for Respiratory Care (NBRC) Written Registry Examination Detailed Content Outline released in August 1998 is discussed in this text. A program graduate preparing for this exam and the Clinical Simulation Examination can use this text to help focus on what needs to be studied. Exam Hints within the chapters point out commonly tested items. Self-assessment questions are included at the end of each chapter. The pretest and posttest will help you analyze your strengths and weaknesses. It is recommended that the pretest be taken and analyzed before beginning the text and studying. After studying, take the computer-based Written Registry Examination posttest and Clinical Simulation Examination on the enclosed CD-ROM. Both Written Registry Examination sample tests are designed to follow the format, question styles, difficulty levels, and the relative weight of tested areas as the real exam. The ten Clinical Simulation Examination problems are the same mix of patient scenarios as seen on the actual exam.

The text includes bold headings followed by two codes. The first (in parentheses) is the NBRC code for that subject found in the previously listed August 1998 Written Registry Examination detailed content outline. My choice of words is a paraphrasing of theirs. Occasionally a heading appears without an NBRC code after it. These headings are added in because they will help you understand what the NBRC is testing for. Some discussion of pathologic processes is included in the general discussion of each chapter as they relate to the treatment or procedure that the respiratory therapist performs. It is recommended that you study the major types of adult and infant disease states and abnormal conditions.

The second code [in brackets] is the NBRC code for the difficulty level of the questions that will be used to test your understanding of the material. *R* stands for Recall, *Ap* stands for Application, and *An* stands for Analysis. You will find that the NBRC asks questions at these three different levels of difficulty.

WRITTEN REGISTRY EXAMINATION

The Written Registry Examination is made up of 100 questions. (The NBRC also includes 15 extra questions that are being pretested for future versions of the examination. Therefore the exam totals 115 questions in length. These pretested questions are not scored as part of your exam. However, because you will not know which questions are real and which are being pretested, answer all questions to the best of your ability.) The examination is offered in a computer-based testing format. You cannot bring a calculator or any other type of test aid device with you. A pencil and blank piece of paper is provided for making notes and calculations.

Make sure that you follow all commands listed on the computer screens so that you do not make any mistakes. You will have 2 hours to complete the examination. Pace yourself to be at about question 60 after 1 hour and question 115 after 2 hours. If you have difficulty with a question, make a note of it and move on. Go back to these near the end of the second hour. Do not leave any questions unanswered. A passing score is listed as 70% or greater (at least 70 correct questions). However, you can get less than 70 correct and still pass. This is because the Application and Analysis questions are weighted more heavily than the Recall questions (see the following). Those who pass the exam (and the Clinical Simulation Examination) are awarded the Registered Respiratory Therapist (RRT) credential by the National Board for Respiratory Care.

The actual content of a given examination is a closely guarded secret. Several exams are usually maintained at a given time by the NBRC with others in production. Old exams are retired. Not everyone will be taking the same exam even at the same test site. The best way to prepare is to know the types of things that may be tested and how the test is constructed. There are three difficulty levels to the questions:

Recall [R]

Recall refers to remembering factual information that was previously learned. "Identify" is a commonly used action verb in these types of questions. You may be asked to identify specific facts, terms, methods, procedures, principles, or concepts. Prepare for these types of questions by studying the full range of factual information, equations, and so on that are seen in respiratory care practice. These types of questions are on the lowest order of difficulty. You either know the answer or you do not; there is little to ponder more deeply. It is very important to have a solid understanding of the factual basis of respiratory care to do well in this and the next two categories of questions.

Application [Ap]

Application refers to being able to use factual type information in real clinical situations that may be new to you. *Apply, classify,* and *calculate* are commonly used action verbs in these types of questions. You may be asked to apply laws, theories, concepts, and/or principles to new, practical clinical situations. Calculations may have to be performed. Charts and graphs, such as seen in pulmonary function testing, may need to be used. These types of questions are on a higher order of difficulty than the Recall

[R] types. Critical thinking must be applied to the factual information to answer these questions.

Analysis [An]

Analysis refers to being able to separate a patient care problem into its component parts or elements to evaluate the relationship of the parts or elements to the whole problem. *Evaluate, compare, contrast, revise,* and *select* are commonly used action verbs in these types of questions. You may be questioned about revising a patient care plan or evaluating therapy. These types of questions require the highest level of critical thinking. You may have to recall previously learned information, apply it to a patient care situation, and make a judgment as to the best way to care for the patient.

You will find that the NBRC uses two different types of questions on the exam in the following three ways.

One Best Answer

This type of question has a stem (the question) followed by four possible answers coded A, B, C, and D. You must select the *best* answer from among those presented. Only one is clearly best even though other possible answers may be good. Carefully read the stem to make sure that you do not misunderstand the clear intent of the question. Controversial issues may be questioned. The use of *should* in the stem will clue you in to the need to select the answer that would be selected by the majority of practitioners.

Some questions may be worded in such a way that you will need to exclude a false answer. In other words, three answers are correct and one is incorrect. The use of *except* will clue you in to this type of question. Other phrases to pay attention to include the following: "What is the *first* thing . . .," "What is the *most* important thing . . .," and "What is the *least* important thing. . . ."

Multiple True-False

This type of question has a stem (the question) followed by four or five possible answers coded with Roman numerals I, II, III, IV, and V; four combinations of the answers coded by letters A, B, C, and D follow. The stem may ask you to include all true statements or all false statements in the final answer. You must select the letter that represents the correct combination of answers.

No controversial answers should be offered. They are all either clearly correct or incorrect. That is the key to selecting the best answer. Read each possible answer as separate from the others. It is suggested that you mark each possible answer as true or false. Even if you are not sure of every option you should be able to determine the best answer.

Situational Sets

These are seen on the Entry Level Examination only. They have been replaced with the Clinical Simulation Examination for advanced practitioners.

Suggestions for Preparing for the Written Registry Examination

1. Pace yourself so that you have enough time to get through the 115 total questions before the 2-hour time limit is reached. You should be at about question 60 in 1 hour. Make a note on your blank paper on any difficult questions that you skip or want to go back to. The computer based test will prompt you if any questions have been skipped. Come back to them at the end of the test time. Do not leave any blank questions. You will not be penalized for guessing on the last few questions if you are running out of time.

2. Completely read each question. Determine what it is that you are really being asked. Look for qualifying words such as *not, except, most, least desirable, undesirable,* and so forth.

3. Separate the important information from that which is not important. Many questions contain patient information and data on blood gases, pulmonary function, hemodynamics, ventilator settings, and so forth. Disregard what does not pertain to the question being asked. Interpret the important data.

4. Do not read beyond the question. Resist the temptation to "psych out" what you think the question writer wants. Use only what is given to you.

5. Carefully read every answer that is offered.

6. In one best answer (multiple choice) questions, pick the best answer that is offered. The answer that you might like best may not be offered. Regardless, you must pick from among those that are offered.

7. In multiple true-false (multiple-multiple choice) questions, use the following strategy: (a) Find an option that you know to be incorrect and cross off any of the answers that contain it; (b) find an option that you know to be correct and cross off any answers that do *not* contain it; (c) find the remaining answer, which must be correct.

8. Again, answer every question. There is no penalty for guessing incorrectly.

9. Take a practice Written Registry Examination under actual testing conditions. Evaluate your strengths and weaknesses and spend more time studying your weak areas. A printable paper-and-pencil exam is offered on the CD-ROM along with a computer-based posttest formatted like the actual examination. A practice exam is offered on the enclosed CD-ROM. Other exams are

available from Applied Measurement Professionals. Their address is included at the end of this Introduction.

Relative Weights of the Various Tested Areas on the Written Registry Exam

I have attempted to analyze the content of each of the 100 questions on the available Written Registry Examinations covering the content of the 1998 examination content outline. Each question has been matched to one of the chapters in this book and listed in Table 1. The numbers of questions and percentages are averages and may not be followed exactly on all versions of the examination. However, the relative weights can offer solid guidance as to what content is relatively more important or less important. Study time can be spent accordingly.

The content of Sections 1, 3, 4, and 5 must be thoroughly understood. This information is questioned directly and also incorporated into questions covering all the other chapters. The content in Chapter 14, "Mechanical Ventilation of the Adult," is the most heavily questioned of all the chapters. You *must* understand

mechanical ventilation to do well on the Written Registry Exam and the Clinical Simulation Exam.

CLINICAL SIMULATION EXAMINATION

The Clinical Simulation Examination (CSE) is composed of ten broad-based problems. They are designed to evaluate how well the exam taker is able to gather information, evaluate it, and make clinical decisions that relate to simulated real patient situations. This test does *not* look at the recollection of simple facts. Box 1 lists the types of patient care problems that will be seen.

The computer-based examination process is unique. Each clinical simulation problem is designed to flow in the same manner that actual patient data is delivered. Therefore the problems are designed in a branching logic format. This means that there is more than one way to solve them. To some extent, you choose your own path; however, there is only one answer that is best. There may be one or two that are acceptable. There may be another one or two that are unacceptable. The exam taker is allowed

---

TABLE 1	Examination Content Found in Each Chapter	

Chapters	Question numbers/ percentage of the examination content
1. Patient Assessment	7
2. Infection Control	2
3. Blood Gas Analysis and Monitoring	6
4. Pulmonary Function Testing	5
5. Advanced Cardiopulmonary Monitoring	13
6. Oxygen and Medical Gas Therapy	6
7. Humidity and Aerosol Therapy	2
8. Pharmacology	3
9. Bronchopulmonary Hygiene Therapy	3
10. Cardiac Monitoring and Cardiopulmonary Resuscitation	9
11. Airway Management	6
12. Suctioning the Airway	2
13. Intermittent Positive Pressure Breathing (IPPB)	1
14. Mechanical Ventilation of the Adult	21
15. Mechanical Ventilation of the Neonate	3
16. Home Care and Pulmonary Rehabilitation	4
17. Special Procedures	7
TOTAL	100

BOX 1	The Mix of Ten Problems Found on the Clinical Simulation Examination

1. Two adult patients with chronic obstructive pulmonary disease (COPD). These patients could have chronic bronchitis, emphysema, and/or asthma. Areas of focus on the simulation include, but are not limited to, pre/postoperative evaluation, critical care management, mechanical ventilation, pulmonary function testing, home care, rehabilitation, and infection control.
2. One or two adult patients with trauma. These patients could have chest/head/skeletal injuries, surface burns, smoke inhalation, carbon monoxide poisoning, or hypothermia.
3. One or two adult patients with cardiovascular disease. These patients could have congestive heart failure, coronary artery disease, myocardial infarction, valvular heart disease, or cardiac surgery.
4. One or two adult patients with neurologic or neuromuscular diseases. These patients could have myasthenia gravis, Guillain-Barré syndrome, tetanus, muscular dystrophy, cerebrovascular accident (stroke), or drug overdosage.
5. One pediatric patient. This patient could have epiglottitis, laryngotracheobronchitis (croup), bronchiolitis, asthma, cystic fibrosis, foreign body aspiration, toxic substance ingestion, or bronchopulmonary dysplasia.
6. One neonatal patient. This patient could require care in the delivery room, need resuscitation, have infant apnea, meconium aspiration, respiratory distress syndrome, or a congenital heart defect.
7. The *possible* miscellaneous category could involve one adult patient with a medical or surgical problem. This could include head/neck/thoracic surgery, obesity-hypoventilation syndrome, or acquired immunodeficiency syndrome (AIDS).

4 hours to complete the exam, which works out to 24 minutes per problem.

There are three components to the clinical simulation problem: (a) the scenario, (b) information-gathering sections, and (c) decision-making sections. Each is discussed in turn.

Scenario

The scenario establishes the setting for the patient and for you as the respiratory therapist. Typically, it includes the type of hospital, where the patient is within the hospital, and the time of day. General information about the patient is given such as his or her name, age, sex, some general presenting conditions, and a brief history of the illness or event. Your role as a respiratory therapist is described. You may have to gather more information or may need to make a clinical decision. Determine if the situation is an emergency. If it is, you will have to take immediate steps to help the patient. (The exam taker should assume that any and all services needed to give optimal care are available in any of the patient scenarios.)

Information-Gathering Sections

Usually the respiratory therapist is directed to gather more information. A list of about 15 to 20 parameters will be available from which to choose, for example, vital signs, blood gases, pulmonary function tests, various laboratory studies, and so forth. You will be instructed to select as many as you believe are important based on what you know at that point in time. Obviously, do not select information that is unnecessarily risky, irrelevant, or delays important care. Select the desired information. The computer screen will then reveal the data. Interpret the data that you find to make the proper decisions in the next section. When you have finished gathering and interpreting the data you will be directed to go to a decision-making section. Typically there are between 2 and 4 information-gathering steps in each clinical simulation problem.

Decision-Making Sections

It is now required that you make a decision on the best care for the patient based on the information that you have at this point in time. Usually you are instructed to "choose only one" from about 4 to 8 options. One of the choices is best, one or two may be acceptable, and the others are not acceptable. Select the option and the computer will reveal the answer. Usually it will say "Physician agrees. Done" or something to that effect. One or more of the available answers will reveal "Physician disagrees. Make another selection in this section" when it is exposed. This may or may not mean that a bad choice was made. It is possible that the author of the scenario simply does not want to follow that particular course of action.

TABLE 2	Scoring of the Clinical Simulation Problem and Examination

All the options selected on each problem are scored on the following scale. The score is based on how appropriate it is to the condition of the patient at the time it was selected.

Score	Score rationale
+3	Critically important for good patient care. It is necessary for prompt, proper care. Omitting it would result in the patient being seriously harmed from delays in care, pain, cost, and increased chance of morbidity and/or mortality.
+2	Very important for good patient care.
+1	Helpful for good patient care.
0	Neither helpful nor harmful to patient care.
−1	Somewhat counterproductive to good patient care.
−2	Quite counterproductive to good patient care.
−3	Extremely counterproductive to good patient care. Detrimental to prompt, proper care. Its inclusion will result in the patient being seriously harmed from delays in care, pain, cost, and increased chance of morbidity and/or mortality.

Occasionally, you will be directed to "select as many as indicated" for the situation with which you are dealing. This involves a scenario in which proper care includes several procedures being done simultaneously with a patient. Again, select the option and the computer will reveal the answer.

Whether you are directed to make one or several decisions, when finished you will be instructed to go to a new area. This usually takes you to another information-gathering section. You will now need to evaluate how the patient responded to your earlier decision(s). You will then need to make one or more patient care decisions. Typically, there are 8 to 10 decision-making steps in each clinical simulation pattern. This pattern of information gathering and decision making repeats itself until the problem is ended. You will then go on to the next problem until all ten have been completed. See Table 2 for how this unique examination is scored.

Each problem is individually scored for information gathering and decision making based on the judgment of the problem author and the examination committee. The scores in these two areas on all ten problems are totaled to give two final scores. Both the information-gathering and decision-making areas must be passed to pass the examination. The examination committee determines the two required scores to pass the Clinical Simulation Examination. These scores may vary from exam to exam, but a score of at least 65% on both exam areas is needed to pass the Clinical Simulation Examination.

Suggestions for Preparing for the Clinical Simulation Examination

Things you should do:

1. Carefully follow all directions. If instructed to make only one choice, make only one.

2. Read the scenario to understand the patient's situation and what you are required to do. Is this an emergency? If it is, you will want to gather only the most vital information needed to make a patient care decision. Quick action will be required to decide on the best care to give. If it is not an emergency, a more thorough gathering of data is called for. Then a more well-considered decision for patient care can be made.

3. Know the rules for the initiation and changing of mechanical ventilation parameters. Use 10 mL/kg of ideal body weight for the initial tidal volume setting. Make adjustments from there based on arterial blood gas results.

4. Thoroughly read all options. For information-gathering sections, make a list of each desirable option on your paper before making your choices. Choose all the options that will give you important information. You will be penalized for skipping over important data and also for making dangerous or wasteful choices. When sure of your selections, reveal them all and then review and interpret them. Avoid the temptation to reveal and interpret one piece of data at a time. You may mistakenly decide not to gather some important information later.

5. Try to visualize yourself in the real situation as described. Do what you would do on the job. Make the best choice(s) that you can based on what you know at this point. This is true for both information-gathering and decision-making sections. It may be necessary to go back over past information or choices.

6. It is recommended that you make a map on your paper of where you have been for each of the ten problems. This will help you to keep track of past choices.

7. Pace yourself to get through all ten problems in the 4-hour time limit. That gives you 24 minutes per problem. For example, you should be finishing your third problem after 1 hour. Unlike the Written Registry Exam, you should *not* rush ahead at the end and pick just anything. You will be penalized for incorrect choices.

8. Take a practice Clinical Simulation Examination. Ten practice patient simulations are offered on the CD-ROM. Others are available, for a fee, from Applied Measurement Professionals.

Things you should avoid:

1. Do not try to jump ahead in the problem or guess what it is that the author is leading to. With the branching logic format, there are several possible pathways. Work only with what you know now and from the past.

2. Try not to become flustered if you are faced with a scenario you have never experienced at work. Imagine what you would do if faced with this problem and go from there. Also, do not become frustrated if the choice that you prefer is not available. There is more than one way to take care of a patient's problems. Make your next best choice and move on.

3. Do not make changes in patient care unless they are needed. If a patient is stable with acceptable arterial blood gas values and vital signs, be content to leave the patient as he or she is.

4. Do not get flustered by patient complications or equipment problems. They do not mean that you did anything wrong! They are meant to test your ability to solve problems.

5. Do not select everything in the information-gathering section. You will lose points by choosing unimportant, time-consuming, unnecessarily expensive, or dangerous procedures.

6. Avoid selecting new or unusual procedures that you are not familiar with, for example, jet ventilation. You will lower your score if you do not know how to operate the equipment properly.

7. Do not misinterpret the data you are given. Avoid assumptions about things that are not printed out for you.

Summary—General Suggestions for Either Examination

1. Take the Written Registry Exam pretest included in the CD-ROM that accompanies this book. Evaluate your results to find your strengths and weaknesses.

2. Begin studying about 2 months before the exam. Pace yourself so that everything can be covered in the time that you have. Avoid "cramming" a few days before the examination; these tests demand more than the simple recall of facts.

3. Study the most important and heavily tested areas first. Work down to the less important ones.

4. Focus on the areas where you are weakest, especially if they are heavily tested.

5. Take the Written Registry Exam posttest and Clinical Simulation Exam included on the CD-ROM.

6. If it is necessary to travel out of your home town to take the exam, arrive at the city where the test will be given the evening before the exam. Make a practice drive from your motel to the test site and see where you will park. Check the time required and add more for the morning traffic.

7. Get a good dinner. Avoid alcohol, even if nervous, to give you a clear head in the morning.

8. Do not cram for the exam back at the motel. Unfortunately, if you are not prepared by now, a few more hours will not really help. If necessary, brush up on only a few test areas.

9. Set the alarm to get you up in plenty of time to be ready. Get a good night's sleep. Avoid sleeping pills.

10. Eat a good breakfast to get you through to lunch. Minimize caffeine. You will have plenty of adrenaline running through your system to keep you awake while taking the test!

11. Attempt to relax with the self-confidence that comes from knowing that you are well prepared.

IMPORTANT ADDRESSES AND PHONE NUMBERS

For information on the examination process and to get a copy of the Candidate Handbook and Applications booklet (containing a CD-ROM with sample exams), contact:
National Board for Respiratory Care
8310 Nieman Road
Lenexa, KS 66214-1579
(913) 599-4200
Fax: (913) 541-0156
E-mail: nbrc-info@nbrc.org
Internet address: http://www.nbrc.org

For information on examination sites and purchasing self-assessment examinations, contact:
Applied Measurement Professionals
8310 Nieman Road
Lenexa, KS 66214-1579
(913) 541-0400
Fax: (913) 541-0156
Internet address: http://www.goAMP.com

For information on accredited respiratory care educational programs, contact:
Committee on Accreditation for Respiratory Care
1248 Harwood Road
Bedford, TX 76021-4244
800-874-5615 or (817) 283-2835
Fax: (817) 252-0773
Internet address: http://www.coarc.org

For information on state credentialing requirements, contact:
American Association for Respiratory Care
11030 Ables Lane
Dallas, TX 75229
(214) 234-AARC (2272)
Fax: (972) 484-2720
E-mail: info@aarc.org
Internet address: http://www.aarc.org

CONTENTS

1 Patient Assessment

A review of the most recent Written Registry Exams has shown an average of five questions (5% of the exam) on patient assessment.

MODULE A	Review the patient's chart for the following data and recommend the following diagnostic procedures based on current information

Note: The following discussion involves noninvasive, bedside activities that apply to adults in most respiratory care settings. Some assessment items have been placed in later chapters because they are procedure specific. Topics that relate to neonates and children are included in Module H.

1. **Review the patient's history: present illness, admission notes, respiratory care orders, and progress notes (Code: IA1a) [Difficulty: Ap, An]**
   a. **Patient history**
   Review the complete initial patient history and note the following:
   1. Date of history taking
   2. Patient data: name, age, sex, race, and occupation
   3. Primary complaints
   4. Secondary complaints
   5. Present illness history and symptoms
   6. Family history
   7. Medical history of cardiopulmonary disease(s)

   After the medical history is completed, the patient should be placed into one of the following four categories. Refer to Table 1-1 for examples of each category.
   1. Crisis/acute onset of illness
   2. Intermittent but repeated illness
   3. Progressive worsening
   4. Mixed patterns/multiple problems

   It is important to obtain a *brief* history before beginning therapeutic procedures. Determine how the patient has been doing since the last treatment. Has there been a change in dyspnea, cough and secretions, chest pain, and so on? This will help guide therapy as effectively as possible.

   b. **Current respiratory care orders**
   Physician orders must have the patient's name, date, time, complete and proper orders for each therapeutic procedure, and the physician's signature. Verbal orders from the physician to the nurse or respiratory therapist must follow hospital guidelines and include the preceding information. Incomplete, improper, or questionable orders must be confirmed by calling the physician for clarification or correction.

   c. **Progress notes**
   Review the physician's, nurse's, and respiratory therapist's patient progress notes before seeing the patient and beginning the therapeutic procedure. Look for any cardiopulmonary or other organ system changes that will have an impact on the patient's ability to take the treatment. You may need to revise the therapy, get different equipment, or seek help. Check for new patient care orders if the physician notes a change in the patient's care plan.

2. **Review electroencephalogram results (Code: IA1i) [Difficulty: R, Ap, An]**
   An electroencephalogram (EEG) is a graphic recording of the electrical activity of the brain. The procedure involves pasting 16 or more electrodes to specific locations on the patient's scalp to receive electrical activity from the brain. An EEG is performed to help determine several neurologic conditions including seizure disorders (epilepsy), cerebral lesions (tumors or infarctions), brain abscess, and intracranial hemorrhage. Any of these conditions are identified by a characteristic change from normal brain wave activity. In addition, an isoelectric (flat) EEG is found in a patient who is brain dead.

   There are a number of interfering factors that lead to misinterpretation of EEG results. These include body or eye movements by the patient while the test is being performed, hypoglycemia, and drugs such as caffeine and sedatives.

3. **Review intracranial pressure monitoring results (Code: IA1i) [Difficulty: R, Ap, An]**
   The intracranial pressure (ICP) is the pressure that occurs within the cranium. Normal intracranial pressure is less than 10 mm Hg. A catheter must be placed through the patient's cranium into either the subarachnoid space or within a ventricle of the brain to measure the ICP. When a patient has suffered head trauma that results in brain edema or intracranial hemorrhage, the ICP is increased. This higher than normal pressure within the cranium results in increased pressure on the patient's brain. Because this increased pressure can cause further brain injury, every attempt is made to decrease the pressure toward normal. It is a general clinical goal to keep the ICP less than 20 mm Hg

TABLE 1-1	Patient Illness Categories
Category	**Examples**
Crisis/acute onset of illness	Trauma, heart attack, allergic reaction, aspiration of a foreign body, pneumothorax, pulmonary embolism, and some pneumonias
Intermittent but repeated illness	Asthma, chronic bronchitis, congestive heart failure, angina pectoris, myasthenia gravis, and some pneumonias
Progressive worsening	Congestive heart failure, chronic bronchitis, emphysema, and upper respiratory tract infection leading to bronchitis or pneumonia
Mixed patterns/ multiple problems	Chronic obstructive pulmonary disease and cystic fibrosis complicated by multiple problems, mucous plugging, or infection; mixes of congestive heart failure and chronic lung disease; mixes of neuromuscular and lung disease; mixes of renal failure and congestive heart failure with chronic lung disease

if possible. Several procedures can be performed to accomplish this goal. One of these is placing the patient on a mechanical ventilator and hyperventilating him or her to a $PaCO_2$ of 25 to 30 torr while maintaining normal oxygenation.

4. Review ultrasonography results (Code: IA1i) [Difficulty: R, Ap, An]

Ultrasonography involves directing high-frequency sound waves (ultrasonic waves) at internal body structures. These sound waves bounce (echo) off solid and cystic structures differently, which provides an image of the various organs. This widely-used diagnostic test provides important information on fetal development, the heart (echocardiogram) and venous structures, and the status of tumors. In addition, it is used to guide the needle-directed biopsy of a tumor.

5. Review fluid balance (intake and output) results (Code: IA1f1) [Difficulty: R, Ap, An]

Fluid intake and output (I and O) should be approximately equal in a normal person with a properly functioning heart and kidneys. Fluid intake includes liquids that the patient drinks or is given by nasogastric tube and intravenous fluids. Output includes urine output and fluid loss from vomiting or the nasogastric tube. Insensible loss from sweating and breathing cannot be measured. Often a patient with heart or kidney failure will have a decreased output compared with input. This can

lead to fluid overload problems with peripheral or pulmonary edema and heart failure. If a patient is given a diuretic medication, the urine output greatly increases to exceed the intake.

6. Review the results of the patient's physical examination and vital signs (Code: IA1b) [Difficulty: Ap, An]

Review the results of the physical examinations performed by physicians, nurses, and respiratory therapists. Review the following organ systems:

1. Pulmonary
2. Cardiovascular
3. Neuromuscular
4. Renal

a. Current vital signs

Review the current vital signs in the patient's chart. Compare them with the admission vital signs and what you observe in the patient now. Look for a change in pattern that suggests either a worsening or an improvement in the patient.

b. Temperature

The textbook "normal" oral body temperature is 98.6° F (37° C). It is normal for there to be some range from 96.5° to 99.5° F (35.8 to 37.4° C). Make sure the patient has not eaten any hot or cold foods recently or has been smoking before taking an oral temperature.

A rectal or core temperature is commonly taken in very sick patients because it is more accurate and reliable. The normal rectal temperature is 97.5° to 100.4° F (36.4° to 38° C). It is normal to see some variance here, but less so than orally. Axillary temperatures are used as a last resort in stable patients. These run 1° F less than oral temperatures and are less accurate and reliable.

The variations in temperature noted depend on the time of day, activity level, and, in women, menstrual cycle. For example, it is normal to see a lower body temperature when a person is in a deep sleep. An oral temperature of more than 99.4° F or 37.4° C in a patient with a history of respiratory disease indicates a fever. Typically, it can be caused by atelectasis or a pulmonary or systemic infection. Patients are commonly treated to keep the fever below 103° F, if possible. In general, a rectal temperature below 97° F (36° C) is considered hypothermic. There are some procedures, such as open-heart surgery, during which a patient's temperature is lowered to reduce metabolism and oxygen needs. The rectal temperature must be kept above 90° F (32° C) to prevent cardiac dysrhythmias from occurring because of the cold.

c. Respiratory rate

The respiratory rate (f for frequency) is the number of breaths the patient takes in a minute. The number is counted by looking at or feeling the chest and/or

TABLE 1-2	Normal Resting Respiratory Rates	
Age (years)	Male	Female
0-1	31 ± 8	30 ± 6
1-2	26 ± 4	27 ± 4
2-3	25 ± 4	25 ± 3
5-6	22 ± 2	21 ± 2
9-10	19 ± 2	19 ± 2
13-14	19 ± 2	18 ± 2
15-16	17 ± 3	18 ± 3
17-18	16 ± 3	17 ± 3
Older	16 ± 3	17 ± 3

From Eubanks DH, Bone RC: *Comprehensive respiratory care*, ed 2, St Louis, 1990, Mosby.

TABLE 1-3	Normal Pulse Rates According to Age
Age	Beats/min
Birth	70-170
Neonate	120-140
1 year	80-140
2 year	80-130
3 year	80-120
4 year	70-115
Adult	60-100

From Eubanks DH, Bone RC: *Comprehensive respiratory care*, ed 2, St Louis, 1990, Mosby.

abdominal movements. The normal rate varies with age (Table 1-2). It is assumed that the patient is resting but awake and has a normal temperature and metabolic rate. A respiratory rate that is above or below normal should be a cause for alarm.

Hyperthermia (fever), acidemia, hypoxemia, fear, anxiety, and pain causes a patient to breathe more rapidly. Hypothermia, alkalemia, hyperoxia in the patient breathing on hypoxic drive, sedation, and coma causes a patient to breathe more slowly.

It must be remembered that even in healthy people, there is considerable variation in the respiratory rate. It is best to consider the respiratory rate and the patient's tidal volume and minute volume to have a more complete impression of how the patient is breathing. Carefully measure the respiratory rate of any patient with cardiopulmonary disease or with a respiratory rate outside of the normal range. The rate should be checked as often as needed to monitor the patient's condition.

d. Blood pressure (Code: IA1g1) [Difficulty: An]

The blood pressure (BP) is the result of the pumping ability of the left ventricle (made up of the heart rate [HR] and stroke volume), arterial resistance, and blood volume. Normal blood pressure is caused by all three factors being in balance with each other. If one factor is abnormal, the other two have some ability to compensate. For example, if the patient has lost a lot of blood, the body attempts to maintain blood pressure by increasing the arterial resistance and increasing the heart rate.

Normal blood pressures

Adults: 120/80 mm Hg

Infants and children less than 10 years: 60–100/20–70 mm Hg

As with the other vital signs, there is some variation of blood pressure among individuals. It is important to know what the patient's normal blood pressure is to compare it with the current value. Carefully measure the blood pressure in any patient who has cardiopulmonary disease or a history of hypotension or hypertension.

Hypotension in the adult is a systolic blood pressure of less than 80 mm Hg. Recommend a blood pressure measurement in any patient who has a history of hypotension, appears to be in shock, has lost a lot of blood, has a weak pulse, shows mental confusion, is unconscious, or has low urine output.

Hypertension in the adult is a systolic blood pressure of 140 mm Hg or greater and/or a diastolic blood pressure of 90 mm Hg or greater. Carefully measure the blood pressure of any patient with a history of hypertension, bounding pulse, or symptoms of a stroke (mental confusion, headache, and sudden weakness or partial paralysis). Fear, anxiety, and pain also cause the patient's blood pressure to temporarily rise.

e. Heart/pulse rate (Code: IA1g1) [Difficulty: An]

The heart/pulse rate (HR) is the number of heartbeats per minute. It can be counted by listening to the heart tones with a stethoscope or by feeling any of the common sites where an artery is easy to locate. Table 1-3 shows the normal pulse rates based on age. It is assumed that the patient is alert but resting when the pulse is counted. Carefully measure the heart/pulse rate in any patient with cardiopulmonary disease or any of the aforementioned conditions for hypotension or hypertension.

7. Electrolytes

a. Recommend an electrolyte or other blood chemistry study be done (Code: IA2a) [Difficulty: R, Ap, An]

The serum (blood) electrolytes are commonly measured in most patients as they are being admitted to the hospital and as needed after that. This is to determine if they are within the normal ranges listed in Box 1-1.

b. Review the results of the patient's serum electrolyte levels and other blood chemistries (Code: IA1c) [Difficulty: An]

Any abnormality should be promptly corrected so that the patient's nervous system, muscle function, and cellular

BOX 1-1	Normal Serum Electrolyte and Glucose Levels

NORMAL ELECTROLYTE VALUES*

Chloride (Cl⁻)	95-106 mEq/L
Potassium (K⁺)	3.5-5.5 mEq/L
Sodium (Na⁺)	135-145 mEq/L
Calcium (Ca⁺⁺)	4.5-5.5 mEq/L
Bicarbonate (HCO₃⁻)	22-25 mEq/L

NORMAL GLUCOSE VALUES*

Serum or plasma	70-110 mg/100 mL (dl)
Whole blood	60-100 mg/100 mL (dl)

*These values may vary somewhat among references.

processes can be optimized. Diet and a number of medications have effects on the various electrolytes. Most abnormalities can be corrected by dietary adjustments or, if necessary, by oral or intravenous supplement.

1. Potassium (K⁺)

Potassium is the most important electrolyte to follow because of its effect on general nerve function and cardiac function. Hyperkalemia is a high blood level of potassium that causes the following electrocardiographic (ECG) changes: high, peaked T waves and depressed S-T segments, widening QRS complex, and bradycardia. Hypokalemia is a low blood level and will cause the following ECG changes: flat or inverted T waves, depression of the S-T segments, premature ventricular contractions (PVC), and ventricular fibrillation (if severe enough). Chapter 10 offers a more complete discussion of ECG interpretation.

EXAM HINT

Hypokalemia may be caused by the use of diuretic medications such as furosemide (Lasix). Signs of hypokalemia include cardiac rhythm disturbances noted previously and muscle weakness. In addition, a metabolic alkalosis is found when interpreting the results of an arterial blood gas analysis. Be prepared to recommend the administration of potassium if the serum level is low.

2. Chloride (Cl⁻)

Hyperchloremia is a high blood level of chloride that causes a significant prolongation of the S-T segment and the Q-T interval on the ECG. Hypochloremia is a low blood level that causes the Q-T interval to be shortened and perhaps widen and round off the T waves on the ECG.

3. Sodium (Na⁺)

Hypernatremia is a high blood level of sodium that might be seen in a patient who is dehydrated or

has been given excessive amounts of sodium intravenously. Hyponatremia is a low blood level that might be seen in a patient who has lost a lot of gastrointestinal secretions because of vomiting, nasogastric tube drainage, or diarrhea.

4. Bicarbonate (HCO₃⁻)

Altered bicarbonate levels are commonly seen in patients with pulmonary conditions. The kidneys of patients with a chronically elevated $PaCO_2$ typically retain bicarbonate to moderate the respiratory acidosis caused by the elevated carbon dioxide level. Conversely, the kidneys of patients with a chronically decreased $PaCO_2$ level excrete bicarbonate to moderate the respiratory alkalosis caused by the decreased $PaCO_2$ level.

5. Calcium (Ca⁺⁺)

Hypercalcemia is an elevated level of calcium that may be associated with patients taking diuretics. ECG changes associated with an increased calcium level include a shortened Q-T interval and widened and rounded T waves. Hypocalcemia is a decreased level of calcium. ECG changes include a lengthening of the S-T segment and the Q-T interval.

6. Glucose

The blood glucose level is important to follow because it directly relates to how much sugar is available to the patient for energy for daily activities. The normal values are listed in Box 1-1. Hypoglycemia is a low blood level of glucose; it can mean that the patient is malnourished. Hyperglycemia is a high blood level that can indicate the patient has diabetes mellitus, has Cushing's disease, or is being treated with corticosteroids. More specific testing must be done to prove the diagnosis.

8. Review the patient's urinalysis (Code: IA1c) [Difficulty: An]

A urine sample is routinely taken from every patient admitted to the hospital, pregnant women, and presurgical patients. Much information about the functioning of the kidneys and other metabolic processes can be gathered from the urinalysis results. A urinalysis is also done for diagnostic purposes in patients with abdominal or back pain, hematuria, and chronic renal disease. Table 1-4 lists the normal findings found in a urinalysis. Any abnormal findings should be further investigated to discover the cause.

9. Complete blood count
a. Recommend a complete blood count study be done (Code: IA2a) [Difficulty: R, Ap, An]

A complete blood count (CBC) is routinely done on all hospitalized patients and patients being seen for a variety of illnesses and for routine physical examinations.

TABLE 1-4	Normal Urinalysis Results

Test item	Normal value
Appearance	Clear
Color	Amber yellow
pH	4.6-8.0 (average 6.0)
Specific gravity	Adult: 1.005-1.030 (usually 1.010-1.025)
	Newborn: 1.001-1.020
White blood cells	0-4
Red blood cells	0-2

The red blood cell (RBC or erythrocyte) count, white blood cell (WBC or leukocyte) count, and differential (Diff) provide a great deal of information about the hematologic system and many other organ systems.

b. Review the results of the patient's complete blood count (Code: IA1c) [Difficulty: An]

The key normal RBC count values are listed in Table 1-5. The hemoglobin and hematocrit values are important because they directly relate to the patient's oxygen-carrying capacity. Decreased hemoglobin and hematocrit values indicate that the patient is anemic. An anemic patient has less oxygen-carrying capacity, which places more stress on the heart during exercise. Hypoxemia resulting from a cardiopulmonary abnormality places this patient at great risk. A transfusion is indicated if the hematocrit is below what the physician considers to be a clinically safe level.

Increased numbers of circulating erythrocytes indicate that the patient has polycythemia. When this is seen as a response to chronic hypoxemia from chronic obstructive pulmonary disease (COPD), cyanotic congenital heart disease, or another disorder, it is labeled as secondary polycythemia. This patient is at added risk because the thickened blood causes an increased afterload against which the heart must pump. These patients are also more prone to blood clots. Supplemental oxygen or other clinical treatment to raise the PaO_2 to at least 55 to 60 torr will, over time, result in the erythrocyte and hematocrit levels returning to normal.

The key normal leukocyte count and differential are listed in Table 1-6. A normal leukocyte count and differential count reveals two things about the patient. First, there is no active bacterial infection. Second, the patient has the ability to produce the normal number and variety of WBCs to combat an infection.

A mild to moderate increase in the leukocyte count is called leukocytosis. It is seen as a WBC count of 11,000 to 17,000 per cubic millimeter (mm^3). Usually the higher the count, the more severe the infection. A WBC count of more than 17,000/mm^3 is seen in patients with severe sepsis, miliary tuberculosis, and other overwhelming infections. An extreme shift to the left in the differential count means that there is a significant increase in the

TABLE 1-5	Normal Hemoglobin, Hematocrit, and Red Blood Cell Counts for Adults and Children

	Adult*	Infant*	Child*
HEMOGLOBIN (in g/100 mL [g/dl])			
Female	12.0-16.0	12.2-20.0	11.2-13.4
Male	13.5-18.0	Same	Same
HEMATOCRIT (in mL/100 mL [mL/dl])			
Female	38%-47%		
Male	40%-54%		
RED BLOOD CELL COUNT (in millions/mL)			
Female	4.2-5.4	5.0-5.1	4.6-4.8
Male	4.6-6.2	Same	Same

*These values may vary somewhat among references.

TABLE 1-6	White Blood Cell and Differential Counts

WHITE BLOOD CELL COUNT (mm^3)*	
Adult	4500-11,000
Infant and child	9000-33,000
DIFFERENTIAL COUNT*	
Segmented neutrophil	40%-75%
Lymphocytes	20%-45%
Monocytes	2%-10%
Eosinophils	0%-6%
Bands	0%-6%
Basophils	0%-1%

*These values may vary somewhat among references.

number of neutrophils. This is usually seen when a patient has an acute, severe bacterial infection. Exceptions to this are patients who are elderly, have acquired immunodeficiency syndrome (AIDS), or have other immunodeficiencies. They may have an infection but show only a mildly elevated WBC count.

Leukopenia is a low absolute WBC count of 3,000 to 5,000/mm^3 or less. An acute viral infection can cause a mild to moderate decrease in the neutrophil count. The patient who has a low WBC count is at great risk of bacterial or other infections.

10. Review the patient's coagulation study results (Code: IA1c) [Difficulty: An]

Coagulation studies are routinely done on many hospitalized patients, those who are to have surgery, or if a blood clotting disorder is known or suspected. Additionally, many medications speed up or slow down clotting time (so-called blood thinners). It is important to review a patient's coagulation studies before drawing a blood

TABLE 1-7	Normal Coagulation Study Results	
Test name	Normal value	Critical value
Bleeding time	1-9 min	>15 min
Prothrombin time (PT or Pro-time)	11.0-12.5 sec; 85%-100%	>20 sec
Partial thromboplastin time (PTT)	60-70 sec	>100 sec
Activated partial thromboplastin time (APTT)	30-40 sec	>70 sec

sample or performing a procedure that may lead to bleeding. Table 1-7 lists normal coagulation study results. It the patient's clotting time is increased, he or she is at risk of bleeding. Be prepared to apply pressure to a blood-sampling site (especially if arterial) longer than expected.

11. **Gram stain results, culture results, and antibiotic sensitivity results**
    a. **Recommend a Gram's stain and culture and sensitivity study (Code: IA2c) [Difficulty: An]**

Whenever an infection is suspected, it is important to get a sample of fluid or tissue from the site in question. This patient material is tested for possible bacterial infection by a Gram's stain and culture and sensitivity (C & S) study. Whenever bronchitis or pneumonia are suspected, it is important to get a mucous or sputum sample for evaluation. A sample of mucus suctioned from the lungs should show only pulmonary organisms. Sputum is the mix of mucus from the lungs and saliva from the mouth; therefore the organisms that are found in it may have come from either place. If the patient has pleural fluid, that must also be sampled. Often a blood sample is also taken to look for evidence of a septicemia.

b. **Review the patient's Gram's stain results, culture results, and antibiotic sensitivity results (Code:IA1c) [Difficulty: An]**

The first step in the microbial analysis of sputum, mucus, and so on is a Gram's stain. It is a special staining process to colorize bacteria into one of two groups. Gram$^+$ (g$^+$) bacteria are stained violet. The most common types of bacteria that cause bronchitis and pneumonia are g$^+$. In general, penicillin or related drugs and sulfa-type antibiotics kill these bacteria. Gram$^-$ (g$^-$) bacteria are stained pink. These organisms, unfortunately, are found in many of the sickest and weakest patients. Often the only way to kill these bacteria is with a specific antibiotic to which they have been proven sensitive. So-called *broad spectrum* antibiotics, such as tetracycline, may also be used.

After the sample of fluid or tissue is Gram stained, a culture and sensitivity test is performed. Culturing involves actively growing the organism(s) to determine what they are. A sensitivity test is the act of exposing the cultured organisms to a variety of antimicrobial drugs. The goal is to find which drug(s) kill the pathogen most effectively. The patient is then treated with that antibiotic. It may take 1 to 3 days to get the C & S results back.

Viruses cannot be identified by Gram's stain. The Ziehl-Neelsen stain has been widely used to identify the *Mycobacterium tuberculosis* (TB) organism. Other pathogens, such as protozoa and fungi, need specialized stains for identification. Fungi and *M. tuberculosis* may take 6 to 8 weeks to culture.

MODULE B **Radiographic imaging**

1. **Review the patient's radiologic findings (Code: IA1e) [Difficulty: An]**

Look for the results of radiographs of the chest or upper airway, computed tomography (CT) scan results, or magnetic resonant image (MRI) study results. If possible, view the radiographs and other studies to gain a better understanding of the patient's condition.

2. **Recommend a chest radiograph, upper airway radiograph, computed tomography (CT) scan, or barium swallow to get additional information on the patient (Code: IA2b) [Difficulty: An]**

A chest radiograph should be recommended in the following situations:
   a. After an endotracheal or tracheostomy tube has been placed or repositioned
   b. After the jugular/subclavian route has been used to insert a central venous pressure (CVP) or pulmonary artery (Swan-Ganz) catheter
   c. After a chest tube has been placed in the pleural space to remove air or fluids
   d. Hemoptysis (bloody sputum)
   e. There is a sudden deleterious change in the patient's cardiopulmonary condition
   f. The balloon on the pulmonary artery (Swan-Ganz) catheter has been inflated for a prolonged period, and a pulmonary infarct is suspected
   g. A pneumothorax is suspected

If possible, the patient should be moved to the radiography department and the chest radiograph should be taken from the anteroposterior (A-P) position. Because x rays penetrate from back to front, the size of the heart is viewed as normal on an A-P film. If a portable chest radiograph must be taken because the patient is too sick to be moved, the posteroanterior (P-A) position must be used. This should be noted in the chart because the heart's size appears abnormally enlarged on a P-A radiograph. A lateral radiograph position is used to see behind the heart and hemidiaphragms. It can be combined with an A-P or a P-A view to localize lesions within the chest. This view is also

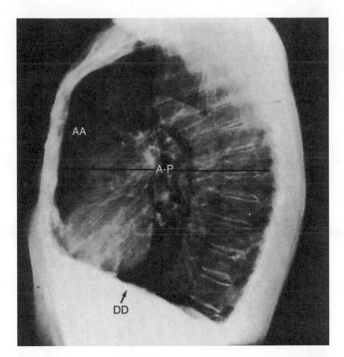

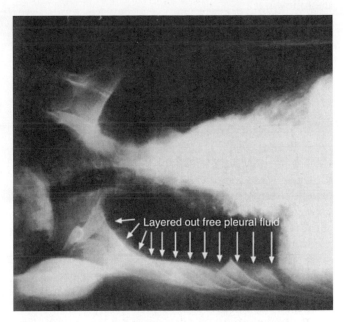

Fig. 1-1 Lateral radiograph of an adult with advanced COPD. Note the characteristic shape of a "barrel chest" from the overinflated lungs. The anteroposterior (A-P) diameter of the chest is increased. *AA* marks an increased anterior airspace between the heart and sternum. The angle of the manubrium and body of the sternum is more obtuse than normal. *DD* marks depressed hemidiaphragms that are flattened. (From Sheldon RL, Wilkins RL: Clinical application of the chest radiograph. In Wilkins RL, Sheldon RL, Krider SJ, editors: *Clinical assessment in respiratory care,* ed 2, St Louis, 1990, Mosby.)

Fig. 1-2 Lateral decubitus radiograph of an adult showing the shift of a small pleural effusion to the now-dependent part of the pleural space. The layer of fluid is marked by arrows. (From Sheldon RL, Wilkins RL: Clinical application of the chest radiograph. In Wilkins RL, Sheldon RL, Krider SJ, editors: *Clinical assessment in respiratory care,* ed 2, St Louis, 1990, Mosby.)

used to measure the patient's anterior to posterior chest diameter. This is often enlarged in patients with air trapping (Fig. 1-1). The lateral decubitus position enables any fluid within the pleural space to be viewed (Fig. 1-2). The patient must be told to take in a deep breath and hold it while the chest radiograph is taken. If the patient is on a mechanical ventilator, a sigh breath should be delivered and held by the respiratory therapist to fully inflate the lungs.

> ### 📖 EXAM HINT
>
> Questions pertaining to recommendation of a chest radiographic examination to rule out or confirm a pneumothorax have regularly appeared on the Written Registry Examination. Signs and symptoms that the patient may have a pneumothorax include the following: sudden chest pain with an increase in dyspnea and shortness of breath (SOB), absent breath sounds over a lung field, tracheal deviation, asymmetrical chest movement, sudden increase in peak pressure and/or plateau pressure on the patient's ventilator, and/or air in the soft tissues. Also be prepared for questions related to recommendation of a chest radiograph to

check the placement of an endotracheal tube or to check for a foreign body obstructing the upper airway or a bronchus.

An upper-airway radiograph (anterior and/or lateral) should be recommended in a patient who presents with symptoms of upper airway obstruction. This can include:

a. Aspirated foreign body
b. Laryngeal edema
c. Laryngeal tumor
d. Epiglottitis (see Module H for more information)

A CT scan provides a more detailed image than a conventional radiograph. It is able to identify abnormalities of the lungs and mediastinum. Indications include, but are not limited to, the following:

a. Tumor
b. Hematoma
c. Abscess and cyst
d. Pleural effusion
e. Aortic or other vascular abnormalities (after intravenous contrast material is given)

A barium shallow enables a radiographic image to be

taken of the esophagus and stomach. Indications include the following:

   a. Dysphagia

   b. Noncardiac chest pain

   c. Painful swallowing and swallowing abnormalities

   d. Gastroesophageal reflux

3. Recommend and review the patient's chest radiograph film to evaluate and monitor the patient's response to respiratory care procedures (Code: IIIA1a) [Difficulty: An]

See the previous discussion. A chest radiograph should be taken whenever there is a significant change in the patient's cardiopulmonary condition or whenever an invasive thoracic procedure (chest tube insertion, endotracheal intubation, pulmonary artery catheter placement) is performed.

4. Look for the presence of, or any changes in, pneumothorax, subcutaneous emphysema, or any other extrapulmonary air (Code: IB7a) [Difficulty: An]

Free air that leaks into the interstitial spaces of the lung or body cavities is abnormal in any patient. Causes for an air leak include barotrauma/volutrauma (alveolar rupture related to the use of a mechanical ventilator), a ruptured bleb (congenital or acquired blister on the visceral pleura), puncture wound through the chest wall, and needle puncture through the pleural space during the insertion of a CVP or pulmonary artery catheter via the subclavian or jugular vein. Once air under pressure is forced through a bronchial or alveolar tear into the interstitial tissues, it tends to follow the path of least resistance. This may result in air being found in any of the following areas singly or in combination.

Pneumothorax is air in the pleural space. The lung tends to collapse toward the hilum. A pneumothorax is identified on the chest radiograph as an area of black, indicating air that surrounds the collapsed lung. No lung markings are visible in the air-filled space, and the edge of the lung can be seen (Fig. 1-3). If the air is under sufficient pressure to shift the lung and mediastinal structures to the opposite side, it is called a *tension pneumothorax*. This is a serious condition that can lead to the death of the patient if it is not quickly identified and treated. A pleural chest tube is always placed into the affected side to remove the air so that the lung can reexpand.

Subcutaneous emphysema is air found in the soft tissues such as the skin, axilla, shoulder, neck, or breast of the affected side. In extreme cases, the air forces its way into skin and soft tissues throughout the body. Scattered dark areas (air pockets) appear in the various soft tissues on the chest radiograph (Fig. 1-4).

The following are other locations where free air can be found: *Pneumomediastinum* is air in the mediastinal space (Fig. 1-4). *Pneumopericardium* is air in the pericardial space

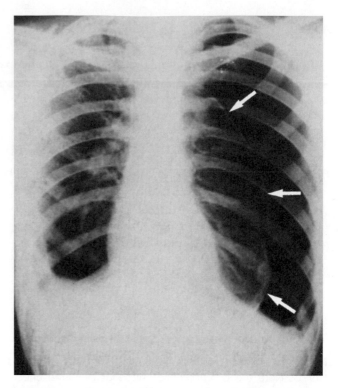

Fig. 1-3 Frontal radiograph of an adult male with a left-sided tension pneumothorax. The edge of the collapsed lung is shown by the arrows. Note how the mediastinum is shifted to the right, the right lung is compressed, and the left hemidiaphragm is depressed. (From Des Jardins TR: *Clinical manifestations of respiratory disease,* ed 2, St Louis, 1990, Mosby.)

(Fig. 1-5). Both of these conditions can be very serious. A cardiac tamponade is created if the pressure around the heart is great enough to interfere with its function. *Pneumoperitoneum* is air in the peritoneal space. This condition can be dangerous in an infant if a large enough volume of air is below the diaphragm and its movement is limited. *Pulmonary interstitial emphysema (PIE)* is air that has disseminated throughout the interstitial spaces of the injured lung(s). The lungs appear "bubbly" on the chest radiograph image (Fig. 1-5). The air may further leak into any of the previously listed locations. PIE is most commonly seen in infants with infant respiratory distress syndrome (RDS) who require mechanical ventilation (MV).

5. Look for the presence of, or any changes in, mediastinal shift (Code: IB7e) [Difficulty: An]

The mediastinum is the area between the lungs that contains the heart and great vessels, trachea, hilar structures, and esophagus. In the neonate, the heart and other mediastinal structures should be approximately in the center of the chest with the left ventricle to the left of center. In the adult, the majority of the heart and mediastinal structures should be left of center in the chest. A shift of the mediastinum (and heart) is abnormal, as

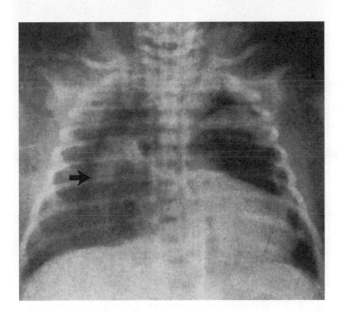

Fig. 1-4 Frontal radiograph of a neonate showing subcutaneous emphysema in the shoulders and neck area. Other abnormal air in the patient's chest includes a pneumomediastinum, which outlines the right lobe of the thymus gland *(arrow),* and a left anterior pneumothorax. (From Carlo, C: *Neonatal respiratory care,* St Louis, 1988, Mosby.)

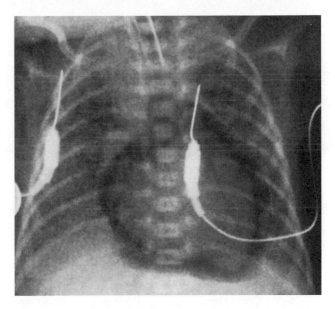

Fig. 1-5 Frontal radiograph of a neonate showing a pneumopericardium that resulted from pulmonary interstitial emphysema. Note the dark outline of air around the heart. Chest tubes have been placed to remove air from around the heart and the right pleural space from an earlier pneumothorax. An endotracheal tube is also seen. (From Koff PB, Eitzman DV, Neu J: *Neonatal and pediatric respiratory care,* St Louis, 1988, Mosby.)

shown by several conditions in Fig. 1-6. Either atelectasis or pulmonary fibrosis, if unilateral and great enough, will result in a shift *toward* the problem area. Tension pneumothorax will result in a shift *away* from the problem area. Fluid in the pleural space, if great enough, will result in a shift *away* from the problem area.

6. **Look for the position of any chest tubes, nasogastric and/or feeding tubes, pacemakers, pulmonary artery catheter, central venous pressure catheters, or other catheters (Code: IB7d) [Difficulty: Ap, An]**

All medical devices placed into the body are made of radio opaque material. They can be seen on a chest radiograph as a white object or line.

Chest tubes are placed to remove any abnormal collection of air or fluid from the thoracic cavity so that the function of the heart and lungs will return to normal. A pleural chest tube is placed to remove air or fluid from the pleural space (see Fig. 1-5). The insertion site and depth of insertion of the tube depend on the patient's disorder. (See Chapter 17 for more discussion on the placement of pleural chest tubes.)

A mediastinal or pericardial chest tube is placed to

remove air or fluid from either of these spaces (see Figs. 1-5 and 1-7). Cardiac tamponade can result from either the pressure of air or fluid compressing the heart. Most postoperative open-heart surgery patients have one or more mediastinal chest tubes in place for several days to remove any blood from around the heart. The insertion site is below the sternum, and the tube(s) are placed posterior to the heart in the pericardial and/or mediastinal space.

A nasogastric tube appears as a white line on the chest radiograph from the patient's nose or mouth through the esophagus and into the stomach (on the left side below the diaphragm). A feeding tube may be placed as a nasogastric tube or surgically placed through the abdominal wall and into the stomach or small intestine. A white line on the radiograph shows its position.

A cardiac pacemaker is placed in two ways. An external pacemaker is identified on the chest radiograph by the long electrode leads that run through a vein in the right arm, through the superior vena cava, and into the right ventricle. The battery and control unit of an internal pacemaker is placed under the skin below a clavicle. The electrode leads run through the superior vena cava into the right ventricle.

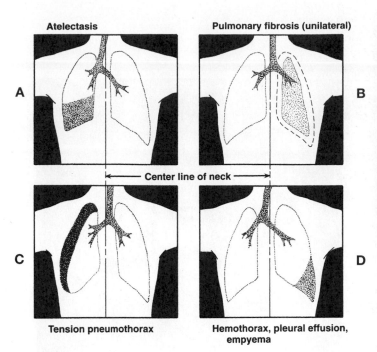

Atelectasis

Pulmonary fibrosis (unilateral)

Center line of neck

Tension pneumothorax

Hemothorax, pleural effusion, empyema

Fig. 1-6 Conditions causing tracheal deviation and mediastinal shift (simulated chest radiograph findings). **A,** Unilateral atelectasis with tracheal deviation *toward* the affected lung. **B,** Unilateral pulmonary fibrosis with tracheal deviation *toward* the affected lung. **C,** Tension pneumothorax with tracheal deviation *away* from the affected lung. **D,** Pleural fluid with tracheal deviation *away* from the affected lung. The normal lung expands more than the abnormal lung during inspiration. (From Sills JR: *Respiratory care certification guide,* St Louis, 1991, Mosby.)

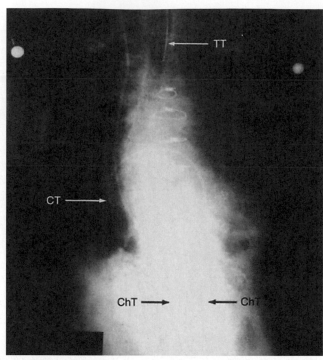

Fig. 1-7 Frontal radiograph of an adult postoperative open-heart surgery patient with several medically necessary devices. A properly placed pulmonary artery (Swan-Ganz) catheter is noted to loop through the right side of the heart and out into the right pulmonary artery. The catheter tip is marked at *CT.* Other foreign bodies include a properly placed endotracheal tube marked at *TT,* sternal wire sutures, ECG chest leads on each shoulder, and pericardial chest tubes marked by *ChT.* (From Sheldon RL, Wilkins RL: Clinical application of the chest radiograph. In Wilkins RL, Sheldon RL, Krider SJ, editors: *Clinical assessment in respiratory care,* ed 2, St Louis, 1990, Mosby.)

The various venous catheters (pulmonary artery catheter, CVP catheter, umbilical artery catheter [UAC], and umbilical vein catheter [UVC]) should be seen on the chest radiograph from their insertion point to their end point. See Figs. 1-7 and 1-8 for the placement of several catheters.

7. Look for the presence of, or any changes in, pulmonary infiltrates or consolidation (Code: IB7a) [Difficulty: An]

A pulmonary infiltrate occurs when blood plasma (water) passes from the pulmonary vascular bed into the lung tissues. Usually this fluid moves into the lung because the alveolar capillary membrane is damaged. On a chest radiograph, an infiltrate often appears as a faint white blurring of the lung and other associated structures.

A consolidation is a filling of the alveoli with fluid from an infiltrate, aspirated vomitus, blood, or water. It is often segmental or lobar. Consolidation is noticed on the chest radiograph as a dense white shadow because fluid has replaced the air. The mediastinum and heart will be seen in their normal location. Fig. 1-9 shows the P-A and lateral chest radiograph showing consolidation in each of the segments of both lungs. Air bronchograms may also be noticed on a radiograph film that reveals consolidation.

8. Look for the presence of, or any changes in, atelectasis (Code: IB7a) [Difficulty: An]

Atelectasis is the collapse of alveoli; no air is found in them. This problem is commonly seen postoperatively in the lower lobes of patients who have had abdominal or thoracic surgery and do not breathe deeply because of pain. The radiograph of atelectasis shows an increase in lung markings and a decrease in the lung volumes. If one sided, the mediastinum may shift toward the affected side. (see

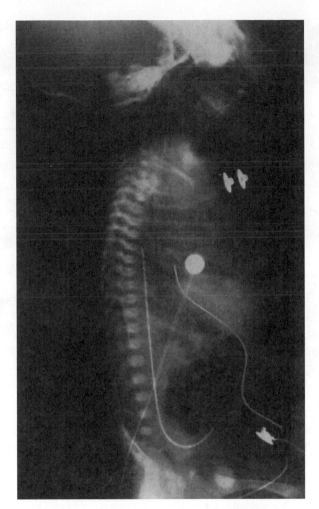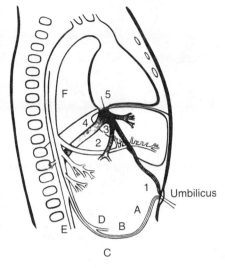

Fig. 1-8   Lateral radiograph and drawing of the internal vascular structures of an infant with an umbilical artery catheter (UAC) and umbilical vein catheter (UVC) in place. The UAC passes through the umbilicus, umbilical artery (*A*), hypogastric artery (*B*), internal iliac artery (*C*), common iliac artery (*D*), abdominal aorta (*E*), to the thoracic aorta (*F*). The umbilical vein catheter passes through the umbilicus, umbilical vein (*1*), portal vein (*2*), ductus venosus (*3*), inferior vena cava (*4*), to the right atrium (*5*). Other medical devices include an endotracheal tube and ECG leads. (From Sheldon RL, Wilkins RL: Clinical application of the chest radiograph. In Wilkins RL, Sheldon RL, Krider SJ: *Clinical assessment in respiratory care,* ed 2, St Louis, 1990, Mosby.)

Fig. 1-6, *A*). If bilateral, the mediastinum will be properly located. If severe enough, the lungs will appear a uniform white (see Fig. 1-10).

9. Look for the positions of, or any changes in, the hemidiaphragms (Code: IB7e) [Difficulty: An]

The normal infant's and adult's A-P or P-A chest radiograph reveals a domed shape to the hemidiaphragms with the edges turning down to acute costophrenic angles. A lateral chest radiograph reveals the same domed shape with the edges turning down to acute costophrenic angles. The edges of the hemidiaphragms should be smooth without any unusual dips or peaks. The following

conditions result in one hemidiaphragm being positioned abnormally: unilateral atelectasis, pleural fluid, tension pneumothorax, or check-valve bronchial obstruction (see Figs. 1-3 and 1-6). Asthma and COPD result in both hemidiaphragms being depressed (see Figs. 1-1 and 1-11). An improvement in the patient's condition should result in a return of the hemidiaphragm(s) to a closer to normal position.

10. Look for the presence of, or any changes in, hyperinflation (Code: IB7e) [Difficulty: An]

Hyperinflation is an excessive amount of air in one or both lungs. The specific chest radiograph findings, to some

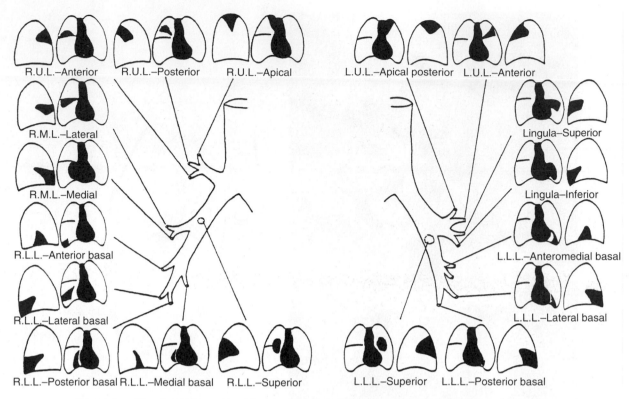

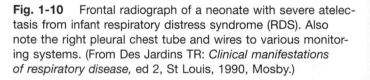

Fig. 1-9   Simulated frontal and lateral radiograph findings for consolidation in the various segments of both lungs. L.L.L., Left lower lobe; L.U.L., left upper lobe; R.L.L., right lower lobe; R.M.L., right middle lobe; R.U.L., right upper lobe. (From Cherniack RM, Cherniack L: *Respiration in health and disease,* ed 3, Philadelphia, 1983, WB Saunders.)

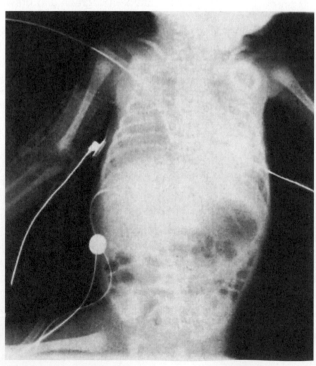

Fig. 1-10   Frontal radiograph of a neonate with severe atelectasis from infant respiratory distress syndrome (RDS). Also note the right pleural chest tube and wires to various monitoring systems. (From Des Jardins TR: *Clinical manifestations of respiratory disease,* ed 2, St Louis, 1990, Mosby.)

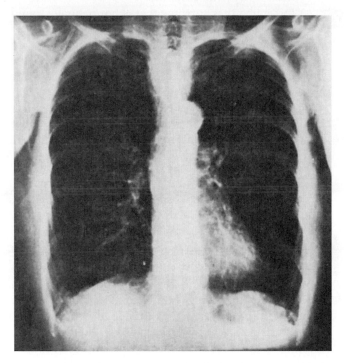

Fig. 1-11   Frontal radiograph of an adult with advanced chronic obstructive pulmonary disease (COPD). Both lungs are overinflated and hyperlucent. The ribs are spread more widely than normal. Often these patients have a cardiothoracic ratio that is smaller than normal because the heart is elongated and the lateral chest diameter is increased. (From Sheldon RL, Wilkins RL: Clinical application of the chest radiograph. In Wilkins RL, Sheldon RL, Krider SJ, editors: *Clinical assessment in respiratory care,* ed 2, St Louis, 1990, Mosby.)

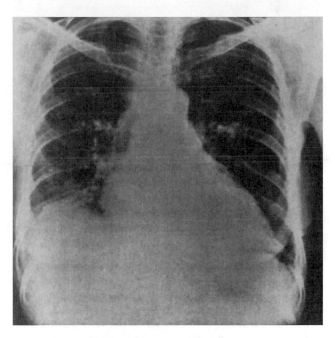

Fig. 1-12   Frontal radiograph of an adult showing a small pleural effusion in the right chest. Note how the costophrenic angle and hemidiaphragm are obscured by the white shadow of fluid. (From Sheldon RL, Wilkins RL: Clinical application of the chest radiograph. In Wilkins RL, Sheldon RL, Krider SJ, editors: *Clinical assessment in respiratory care,* ed 2, St Louis, 1990, Mosby.)

degree, depend on the underlying condition that causes the hyperinflation. Unilateral hyperinflation is caused by a check-valve obstruction from a foreign body or airway tumor. At first glance, a tension pneumothorax appears as unilateral lung hyperinflation. Remember that with this condition the chest is hyperinflated and the lung is collapsed (see Fig. 1-3).

In the adult with asthma, bronchitis, and emphysema (COPD) or newborn with meconium aspiration, both lungs are overinflated and both hemidiaphragms are depressed (see Figs. 1-1 and 1-11). Other radiograph findings include widened intercostal spaces; hyperlucent lung fields; a small, vertical heart; a small cardiothoracic diameter; and decreased vascularity of peripheral areas of the lungs with enlarged hilar vessels. The lateral chest radiograph findings in the COPD patient are the same and they include anterior bowing of the sternum, increased retrosternal air space, and kyphosis.

11. Look for the presence of, or any changes in, pleural fluid (Code: IB7e) [Difficulty: An]

Pleural fluid is typically shown on a P-A or A-P film as obscuring the costophrenic angle. This is because gravity tends to draw the fluid to the lowest level. Often this results in an obscuring or blunting of the costophrenic angle of the affected side (Fig. 1-12). In some cases an air/fluid level is seen within the intrapleural space. The term *meniscus* is used to describe the upward curve seen in the fluid part of this intrapleural air/fluid level. Small amounts of fluid can sometimes be better visualized by taking a lateral decubitus radiograph. If the fluid is able to freely move in the pleural space, it will shift in a few minutes to the lower side (see Fig. 1-2). An empyema that is loculated (fixed) by adhesions will not move when the patient lies on his or her side. If large amounts of fluid are removed by a thoracentesis procedure, a chest radiograph should be taken to confirm

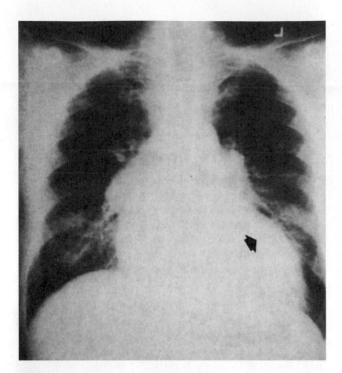

Fig. 1-13 Frontal radiograph of an adult showing pulmonary edema, increased pulmonary vascular markings, and enlarged left ventricle. The cardiothoracic diameter is increased, with the arrow showing where the border of the left ventricle should normally be seen. (From Des Jardins TR: *Clinical manifestations of respiratory disease,* ed 2, St Louis, 1990, Mosby.)

the removal of fluid, the reexpansion of the lung, and that a pneumothorax did not result.

12. Look for the presence of, or any changes in, pulmonary edema (Code: IB7e) [Difficulty: An]

Pulmonary edema is watery fluid (plasma) that has leaked out of the pulmonary capillary bed into the interstitial spaces and alveoli. It is most commonly caused by left ventricular failure (also known as congestive heart failure), but can also be the result of fluid overload, pulmonary capillary damage, or decreased osmotic pressure in the blood from a low level of protein.

Pulmonary edema appears on a P-A or A-P chest radiograph as fluffy, white infiltrates in either or both lung fields. These tend to be seen more extensively in the lower lobes as a result of gravity pulling the fluid to the basilar vessels where it leaks out. If the root cause is left ventricular failure, the vessels in the hila will also be engorged and the left ventricle enlarged (Fig. 1-13). A worsening problem will result in more fluid leaking into the lungs and the appearance of more white infiltrates on succeeding chest radiographs. Once the problem is corrected, the lungs will return to normal as the fluid is reabsorbed and removed.

13. Look for the presence and position of any foreign bodies (Code: IB7d) [Difficulty: An]

A foreign body is anything that is not naturally found in the chest. Metallic objects (e.g., bullets or swallowed or aspirated coins or metal buttons) are easily noticed because they completely block any x-ray penetration through the chest and are clearly outlined on the film as solid, white shadows (Fig. 1-14). Nonmetallic foreign objects (such as plastic pieces from toys and foods such as peanuts) are much more difficult to identify because they have about the same densities as normal body tissues. Determining the exact location of a foreign body may require taking P-A, lateral, and oblique chest radiographs. Lung volumes can be compared by taking inspiratory and expiratory films. A CT scan may be the most successful method of finding a nonmetallic foreign body.

14. Check the chest radiograph for the size and patency of the patient's major airways (Code: IB7e) [Difficulty: An]

The trachea and both the right and left mainstem bronchi should be seen on a properly-taken chest radiograph film. They appear as straight, dark air columns in contrast with the white shadows of the various surrounding tissues. A white shadow within the airway may be a foreign body or tumor. A lung tumor that presses on an airway causes the airway to narrow or be occluded.

15. Check the chest radiograph for the position of the patient's endotracheal or tracheostomy tube (Code: IB7c) [Difficulty: An]

The distal end of all these tubes should be seen within the lumen of the trachea and about midway between the larynx and the tracheal bifurcation to the right and left mainstem bronchi (see Figs. 1-5 and 1-7 for endotracheal tube placement). The proximal end of the tracheostomy tube (or transtracheal oxygen catheter) is seen on the film coming out of the surgical insertion site in the suprasternal notch. The distal end should be centered within the trachea above the carina (see Fig. 17-14). Most of these tubes are made of a radio opaque material or have a line of radio opaque material imbedded into them so that they can be easily seen on the radiograph.

Care must be taken not to push the endotracheal tube deeper into a bronchus, usually the right, or to pull it out. The tracheostomy tube and transtracheal oxygen catheter are less likely to be displaced if they are properly cared for. Take another radiograph to check the position of any of these tubes if there is clinical evidence that a position may have changed.

16. Check the chest radiograph for a sign that the cuff on the endotracheal or tracheostomy tube is overinflated (Code: IB7c) [Difficulty: An]

A properly inflated cuff fills the space between the tube and the patient's trachea so that an airtight seal is made. If

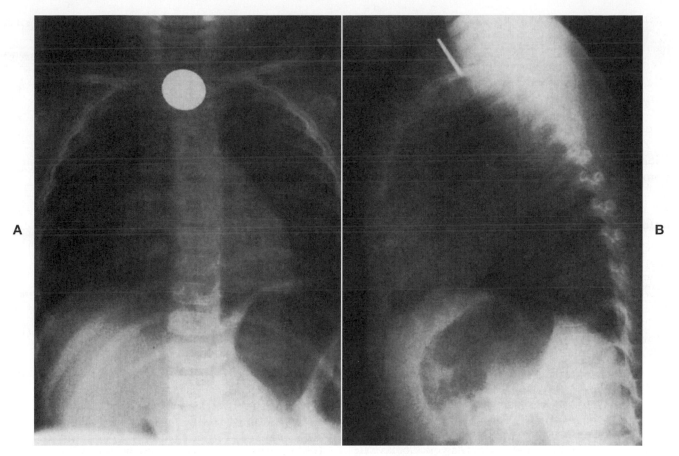

Fig. 1-14 Foreign body obstruction in an 18-month-old girl. **A** shows a frontal radiograph with the solid white disk of a coin clearly seen in the hypopharynx. **B** shows a lateral view of the chest with the edge of the coin seen as a solid white line. (From Hunter TB, Bragg DG: *Radiologic guide to medical devices and foreign bodies,* St Louis, 1994, Mosby.)

the cuff is overinflated, it places excessive pressure on the trachea. This can cause it to dilate and be seen as a wider dark area than the rest of the tracheal air column. If this is noticed, the cuff pressure should be measured. Excessive pressure should be reduced to a safer level.

EXAM HINT

Past exams have had at least one question that requires the identification of the cause of an abnormal chest x-ray. Typically the question refers to a patient who has a pneumothorax or pleural effusion. The National Board for Respiratory Care (NBRC) sometimes uses the term *radiograph* in examination questions rather than *x-ray*.

MODULE C   Interview the patient

1. What is the patient's level of consciousness? (Code: IB6a) [Difficulty: An]

One common way to evaluate a patient's level of consciousness is to categorize him or her as alert, stuporous, semicomatose, or comatose as follows:

a. Alert

This is the normal mental state. The patient is conscious or can be fully awakened from sleep by calling his or her name. The patient can voluntarily ask logical questions and answer questions logically. The conversation is relevant to the topic under discussion. The patient's movements and actions are willful and purposeful.

b. Stuporous/very lethargic

The patient is sleepy or seems to be in a trance. He or she can be aroused to respond with willful, purposeful movements and actions, but the patient may be slow. The patient may not respond to questions in a totally appropriate way.

c. Semicomatose

The patient does not perform requested movements or actions. The patient will not answer questions in an appropriate way. He or she will respond defensively to pain. For example, if the right arm is pinched, it will be withdrawn. Posturing of semicomatose patients includes the following:

1. Decerebrate: legs are extended; arms are extended and rotated either inward or outward.
2. Decorticate: legs are extended; arms are flexed, and the forearms may be rotated either inward or outward.
3. Opisthotonic: legs, arms, and neck are extended, and the body is arched forward.

d. Comatose/coma

The patient has no spontaneous, oriented responses to the environment. Pain causes no defensive movement, but there may be an increase in the heart and respiratory rates.

Another common way to evaluate a patient's level of consciousness is to make use of the Glasgow Coma Scale (GCS). With this scale of 3 to 15, the larger the total number, the more normal the patient. A score of 15 is achieved in a patient normally awake and alert; a score of 3 is found in an unresponsive patient. See Table 1-8 for details of the scale.

2. **Is the patient oriented to time, place, and person? (Code: IB6a) [Difficulty: An]**

Time refers to the patient knowing the calendar date, the day of the week, and the time of day. Ask the patient, "Do you know what day of the week it is? Do you know what the date is?" (The patient must be able to see a calendar.) "Do you know what time it is?" (The patient must be able to see a clock.) If the patient can answer these questions, he or she is oriented to time. If not, inform and show him or her. Tell the patient that you will return at a certain time. Ask the same questions when you return.

Place refers to the patient knowing where he or she is located (hospital, nursing care unit, extended care facility, home, etc.). Ask the patient, "Do you know where you are?" If the patient knows, he or she is oriented to place. If not, inform the patient of the location. Tell the patient that you will return at a certain time. Ask the same question when you return.

Person refers to the patient knowing his or her own name, address, and telephone number. The patient should also know the names of obviously important people. Ask

TABLE 1-8	Glasgow Coma Scale	
Test parameter	**Response**	**Score***
EYES		
Open	Spontaneously	4
	To verbal command	3
	To pain	2
	No response	1
BEST MOTOR RESPONSE		
To verbal command	Obeys command	6
Moves arms to painful stimulus of knuckles against sternum	Localizes pain	5
	Flexion–withdrawal	4
	Flexion–abnormal movement (decorticate rigidity)	3
	Extension–abnormal movement (decerebrate rigidity)	2
	No response	1
BEST VERBAL RESPONSE (MAY AROUSE BY PAINFUL STIMULUS IF NECESSARY)		
	Oriented and converses	5
	Disoriented and converses	4
	Inappropriate words used	3
	Incomprehensible sounds	2
	No response	1

From *Apache II: A severity of disease classification system*, ICU Research Unit, Washington, DC; product information from Upjohn, Kalamazoo, Mich.
*The total is obtained by adding the scores in all three areas. The range is 3 to 15.

the patient, "Do you know who the President (or the physician) is?" If not, inform the patient. Tell the patient who you are and what your job is. When you return for your next treatment ask the patient if he remembers who you are and what you do. If the patient remembers who the President (or the physician) is and your name or job, he or she is oriented to person.

Orienting the stuporous/very lethargic patient to person, place, and time may encourage him or her to cooperate more in his or her care. Pain-relieving and sedative drugs, stroke, injury to or edema of the brain, and other illnesses may cause disorientation to person, place, or time.

3. **What is the patient's emotional state? (Code: IB6a) [Difficulty: An]**

Acute illness or injury with great pain may result in some patients feeling fear, anxiety, or panic. Because of these feelings, the patient may be unable to concentrate closely on what you are telling him or her. This can result in directions not being understood or followed. It is important to tell the patient that you are there to help and need the patient to calm down so that you can help.

TABLE 1-9	Teaching-Learning Process in Adaptation to Chronic Illness		
Stages of adaptation	Patient's behavior	Nurse's behavior	Nurse's facilitation of the teaching-learning process
Disbelief	Denies threatening condition to protect self and conserve energy; refuses to accept diagnosis; may claim to have something else; may behave so as to avoid the issue; may seem to accept diagnosis but avoids feelings about it	Allows patient to deny illness as he or she needs to; functions as noncritical listener; accepts patient's statements of how he or she feels; helps clarify patient's statements; does not point out reality	Orients all teaching to the present, not to tomorrow or next week; teaches as he or she does other nursing activities; assesses patient's level of anxiety; assures patient that he or she is safe and being observed carefully; explains all procedures and activities to the patient; gives clear, concise explanations; coordinates activities to include rest periods
Developing awareness	Uses anger as a defense against being dependent and against guilt about being sick	Listens to patient's expressions of anger and recognizes them for what they are; explores own feelings about illness and helplessness; does not argue with patient; gives dependable care with an attitude that it is necessary	Does not give anxious patient long lists of facts; continues development of trust and rapport through good physical care; orients teaching to present; explains symptoms, care, and treatment in terms of the fact that they are necessary now; does not mention long-range care needs
Reorganization	Accepts increased dependence and reorganizes relationships with significant others; members of patient's family may also use denial while they adapt to what patient's illness means to them	Establishes climate in which family and friends can express feelings about patient's illness; does not solve patient's problems but helps build communication so that patient and family can work together to solve problems	Assures family that patient is all right and safe; uses clear, concise explanations; does not argue about need for care
Resolution	Acknowledges changes seen in self; identifies with others with same problem	Encourages expression of feelings, including crying; understands own feelings of loss	Brings groups of patients with same illness together for group discussions; has a recovered person visit patient; teaches patient what he or she wants to learn (or perceives he or she needs to learn) first
Identity change	Defines self as an individual who has undergone change and is now different; "There are limits to my life because I have a disease"	Understands own feelings about patient becoming independent again	Realizes that as patient's own perceived needs are met, more mature (more progressive) needs will surface; is prepared to answer patient's questions as they arise
Successful adaptation	Can live comfortably or resignedly with himself as a person who has a specific condition	Initiates closure of nurse-patient relationship	Has helped develop a relationship with the patient in which the nurse is a guide with whom the patient can consult when he or she wishes

From Kenner CV, Guzzetta CE, Dossey BM: *Critical care nursing: body—mind—spirit,* Boston, 1981, Little, Brown.

Chronic illness has been approached by a number of authors from varying points of view. Table 1-9 represents a presentation of a patient's reaction to chronic illness. Substitute "respiratory therapists" for "nurses" as needed.

A patient's statements and actions that indicate the *disbelief* stage of adaptation include the following:

    a. "I don't have (fill in the disease or condition)."
    b. "There is nothing really wrong with me."
    c. "The laboratory results are wrong."
    d. "The equipment is faulty."
    e. "The doctor/nurse/therapist is incompetent."
    f. Refusal to take medications.
    g. Refusal to take treatments or follow other physician orders.

| TABLE 1-10 | Severity of Dyspnea in Evaluating Permanent Impairment |

Class I	Class II	Class III	Class IV	Class V
Dyspnea only on severe exertion ("appropriate" dyspnea)	Can keep pace with person of same age and body build on the level without breathlessness but not on hills or stairs	Can walk a mile at own pace without dyspnea but cannot keep pace on the level with a normal person	Dyspnea present after walking about 100 yd on the level or on climbing one flight of stairs	Dyspnea on even less activity or at rest

From Burton GG: Practical physical diagnosis in respiratory care. In Burton GG, Hodgkin JE, editors: *Respiratory care: a guide to clinical practice,* ed 2, Philadelphia, 1984, Lippincott.

A patient's statements and actions that indicate the *developing awareness* state of adaptation include the following:

a. "The doctor/nurse/therapist doesn't know what he or she is doing."
b. "It's all their fault."
c. "Why is this happening to me?"
d. The patient is angry about his or her illness.
e. The patient may strike out verbally or physically at staff members.
f. Some patients who do not get angry will withdraw into a depression and wish to be left alone.

A patient's statements and actions that indicate that he or she is progressing from the *reorganization* to the *successful adaptation* stage include the following:

a. "I'll never be able to do that again." (Fill in the activity.)
b. "I have to get on with my life."
c. "At least I'm still alive and can do this for myself."
d. The patient may be sad and cry often.
e. The patient may invent a nickname for his or her defect or diseased body part.
f. The patient accepts the disability and focuses on his or her abilities.
g. The patient works with family and others in planning for the future.

4. What is the patient's ability to cooperate? (Code: IB6a) [Difficulty: An]

You should be able to judge the patient's ability to cooperate. It should be based on his or her responses to your questions on level of consciousness; orientation to time, place, and person; and emotional state. An alert patient should be able to understand and follow directions. He or she should be able to take an effective treatment or cooperate in a procedure. On the other hand, if the patient truly refuses the treatment or procedure, it should not be forced. Contact the patient's nurse or physician about the refusal. The physician must then decide what to do.

An alert but panicked, fearful, or anxious patient may be unable to fully cooperate until he or she is calmed by understanding who you are, what you are there to do, and why the treatment or procedure is important. Try to reassure the patient to improve cooperation.

If the patient appears alert but does not follow what you are saying, check to see whether he or she is deaf or does not speak English. An effective way to communicate must be found. Writing materials, a picture board, or a sign language interpreter is needed to communicate with a deaf patient. A native language translator will be needed to communicate with a patient who does not speak English.

The stuporous/very lethargic patient may be aroused by talking more loudly or by gentle shaking. He or she may or may not be able to cooperate fully. The practitioner may have to modify the treatment plan or how it is administered to compensate for the patient's lack of cooperation.

Pain relievers and sedatives may make a normally alert patient seem stuporous. If the patient has not been medicated, check with the nurse or physician to see what may have recently changed in the patient's condition.

A semicomatose patient may present the greatest problems in providing treatment or performing a procedure. These patients do not cooperate in any way but are unlikely to fight treatment either. In addition, some of their involuntary body posturings make correct positioning impossible. You must modify your equipment or procedure to accommodate the patient's inability to cooperate.

5. Does the patient complain of dyspnea and/or orthopnea? (Code: IB6b) [Difficulty: An]

Dyspnea is the patient's subjective feeling of SOB or labored breathing. This is normal after vigorous exercise but abnormal in a resting patient. Orthopnea is the condition in which a patient must sit erect or stand to breathe comfortably. Lying flat causes dyspnea.

Table 1-10 classifies the degrees of dyspnea and Table 1-11 lists different kinds of dyspnea, including orthopnea. Only class I is normal dyspnea (on severe exertion). Classes II to V are progressively severe and limiting for the patient.

TABLE 1-11 Causes of Dyspnea Related to Preferred Body Position

Kind of dyspnea	Clinical correlations
Orthopnea (must sit up to breathe; often occurs at night as paroxysmal nocturnal dyspnea)	Congestive heart failure
Obstructive sleep apnea (periodically stops breathing, particularly when lying on back)	Obesity; obstructive sleep apnea syndromes
Emphysematous habitus	COPD
Platypnea	Pleural effusion; dyspnea associated with various body positions
Orthodeoxia	Pulmonary fibrosis; dyspnea improved when patient is lying flat

COPD, Chronic obstructive pulmonary disease.
From Burton GG: Patient assessment procedures. In Barnes TA, editor: *Respiratory care practice*, Chicago, 1990, Mosby.

Any orthopnea is abnormal, and the more the patient must sit up to breathe, the more limited the patient.

The following are examples of questions to ask in evaluating dyspnea:

a. "How far can you walk before you feel short of breath (SOB)?"
b. "How many flights of stairs can you climb before you become SOB?"
c. "How far can you walk when walking as fast as your spouse?"
d. "Is there anything you do that makes the SOB *worse*?"
e. "Is there anything you do that makes the SOB *better*?"
f. "How long does the SOB last after you stop to rest?"
g. "Is the SOB worse at any particular time of the *day*?"
h. "Is the SOB worse at any particular time of the *year*?"

The following are examples of questions to ask in evaluating orthopnea:

a. "Do you wake up at night with SOB?"
b. "Does your nighttime SOB get better after you sit up on the side of your bed or in a chair?"
c. "Do you get SOB when lying down to take a nap?"
d. "Do you use extra pillows behind your head and back to help you not get SOB at night or during a nap?"
e. "How many pillows do you need to keep you from getting SOB at night or when taking a nap?"

6. What is the patient's sputum production like? (Code: IB6b) [Difficulty: An]

a. Time of maximal and minimal expectoration

Interview the patient to determine the following:

1. Time of maximum expectoration. Ask the patient, "When do you cough up the most? For example, is it in the morning; after eating spicy foods; after a breathing treatment; after smoking, work, or other exposure to dusts; etc."
2. Time of minimum expectoration. Ask the patient, "When do you cough up the least? For example, during certain nonallergic seasons of the year, after a breathing treatment, after consuming milk or milk products, etc."

b. Quantity

Some practitioners prefer to know of a specific amount such as a teaspoon, tablespoon, 10 mL, and so on. Others prefer to use subjective measures such as "a little" or "a lot." Interview the patient to determine the following:

1. How does the quantity of sputum relate to the times of maximum and minimum expectoration and the patient's lifestyle? Ask the patient, "Is there anything that you do that increases or decreases the amount you cough out?" For example, the patient states that he coughs up 20 mL after breathing treatments but can cough up nothing after eating a bowl of ice cream.
2. Does the amount coughed up change in a cyclical way? Ask the patient, "Do you cough up the most in the mornings or at night? Is there a work or lifestyle habit that changes how much you cough up? Is there a seasonal allergic condition that influences your asthma and sputum production?"

c. Adhesiveness of the sputum

Interview the patient to determine the following:

1. "Are there times of the day or things that you do in the day that seem to result in your secretions becoming thicker or thinner?"
2. "Do your medications (like acetylcysteine [Mucomyst]) make the secretions easier to cough out?"
3. "Are there foods that make your secretions easier to cough out?"

7. What is the patient's work of breathing? (Code: IB6b) [Difficulty: An]

Work of breathing (WOB) refers to the patient's subjective feeling of how easy or difficult it is to breathe. A person at rest should feel no difficulty in breathing. During vigorous exercise a person should be aware that he or she is working harder than normal to breathe. This is to be expected. After recovering from exercise, the work of breathing should again be easy.

Patients with acute or chronic lung disease feel that they are breathing with some difficulty. Because this is a subjective feeling of the patient, it is helpful to have the patient quantify it. Ask the patient to rate his or her WOB on a 1-to-10 scale with 1 being easy breathing and 10 being extremely difficult.

If bronchospasm or secretions have increased, the patient will tell you that his or her work of breathing has worsened. If medications such as bronchodilators or mucolytics are effective, the patient should feel that his or her breathing is easier.

8. Assess the patient's learning needs (Code: IB5) [Difficulty: An]

Based on the previously gathered information, the respiratory therapist should be able to determine what the patient understands of his or her condition and what the patient needs to be taught. Assess the following and teach so that the patient will learn:

a. Age-appropriate teaching

The patient is taught based on his or her age and ability to understand. This is most important with small children. They commonly have these fears when hospitalized:

1. Fear of abandonment (separation anxiety). Small children are afraid of being abandoned in the hospital by their parents.
2. Fear of the unknown. Equipment and procedures must be explained so that the child will not be left to use his or her imagination.
3. Fear of punishment. Children may imagine that their illness is a punishment for doing something wrong.
4. Fear of bodily harm. Explain a procedure so that the child understands what is going to happen.
5. Fear of death. Children who are sick but expected to recover need to understand that they will get better. It is all right for children to feel afraid. Talking about those feelings or fear of death should be encouraged.

b. Language-appropriate teaching

Use nonmedical terms whenever possible. The patient's native language must be used so that he or she will understand the situation. A translator may be needed.

c. Education level

Patients should be taught in a manner and at a level that is matched to their education and knowledge of their medical condition.

d. Prior disease knowledge

The patient should be taught, as needed, about his or her condition.

e. Medication knowledge

The patient should be taught, as needed, about his or her medication(s), including how the medication is to be taken (e.g., metered dose inhaler with spacer).

MODULE D	Use *observation* to determine the patient's complete respiratory condition

1. Evaluate the patient's general appearance (Code: IB1a) [Difficulty: An]

Start by quickly inspecting the patient from head to toe, including how he or she is dressed and found in the room. Ideally, this is done without the patient knowing that he or she is being observed. The patient who is not suffering from cardiopulmonary disease should be able to lie flat in bed or on either side without any breathing difficulty. The patient with one-sided lung disease may prefer to lie with the good side down. This might be the case with lobar pneumonia, pleurisy, or broken ribs. The patient with severe airway obstruction, as seen with asthma, bronchitis, or emphysema, tends to sit up in a chair or on the edge of the bed and use locked arms and shoulders for support. This enables the patient to use accessory muscles (Fig. 1-15). The patient with orthopnea will not want to lie down flat because of the resulting SOB. This is commonly seen in patients with congestive heart failure and pulmonary edema.

2. Determine if the patient is cyanotic (Code: IB1a) [Difficulty: An]

Cyanosis is an abnormal blue or ashen gray coloration of the skin and mucous membranes. It is most easily seen in white persons by looking at the lips and nailbeds. It can be seen in darker-pigmented people by looking at the inner portion of the lip, the inner portion of the lower eyelid, and the nailbeds. Commonly, cyanosis is said to be caused by hypoxemia and that the more bluish a patient's color, the more hypoxemic he or she is. This is often the case, but cyanosis is not an accurate measurement of a patient's oxygenation. To be safe, a patient with cyanosis should have an arterial blood gas sample drawn for PaO_2 measurement or pulse oximetry performed for SpO_2 measurement to evaluate oxygenation.

3. Determine if the patient is diaphoretic (Code: IB1a) [Difficulty: An]

Diaphoresis is profuse sweating. It is normally seen after vigorous exercise. A patient is expected to sweat after a

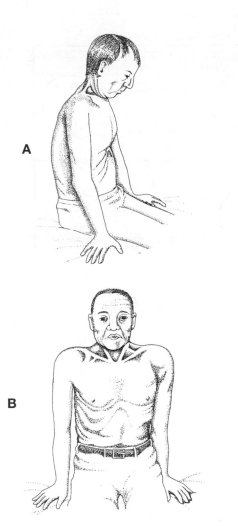

A

B

Fig. 1-15 Typical posture seen in patients using accessory muscles of respiration. The shoulders are locked so that the accessory muscles can be used more effectively. (**A,** from Burton GG: Practical physical diagnosis in respiratory care. In Burton GG, Hodgkin JE, editors: *Respiratory care,* ed 2. Philadelphia, 1984, Lippincott,. **B,** from Barriascout JR: Chest physical therapy and related procedures. In Burton GG, Hodgkin JE, editors: *Respiratory care,* ed 2.)

stress test or even an oxygen-assisted walk. Diaphoresis in a patient who is resting in bed should be investigated. When the body is severely stressed, it releases adrenaline into the blood stream. Diaphoresis is one of many bodily effects caused by the release of the hormone adrenaline. Similar sweating may be seen if a large enough dose of the drug epinephrine is given.

Diaphoresis is a nonspecific sign of serious cardiopulmonary difficulties. It may be seen any time the patient is in shock or hypoxemic. Patients suffering from a myocardial infarct are commonly diaphoretic. The practitioner should promptly evaluate the diaphoretic patient's pulse, respiratory rate, blood pressure, and arterial blood gases.

4. Determine if the patient has nasal flaring (Code: IB1b) [Difficulty: An]

Nasal flaring is a dilation of the nares on inspiration. A person breathing comfortably should have little or no nasal flaring. A person who is exercising vigorously may exhibit nasal flaring. It is abnormal to see nasal flaring in a patient who is resting in bed, and it is a sign of increased work of breathing. The patient is attempting to reduce airway resistance by dilating the nares. Patients of any age have nasal flaring when experiencing increased WOB, but it is most commonly seen in the premature newborn (Fig. 1-16).

Nasal flaring is not specific to any disease or condition. Examples of conditions during which nasal flaring is seen include infant respiratory distress syndrome, acute respiratory distress syndrome, or any condition in which pulmonary compliance is decreased or airway resistance is increased.

5. Determine if the patient has clubbing of the fingers (Code: IB1a) [Difficulty: An]

Clubbing of the fingers (also known as digital clubbing) is an abnormal thickening of the ends of the fingers. It can also occur in the toes. The key finding is an angle of more than 160 degrees between the top of the finger and the nail when seen from the side. Clinically, you will notice both a lateral and an A-P thickening of the ends of the fingers. See Fig. 1-17 for a comparison of normal fingers with clubbed fingers. The finger and toenail beds may be cyanotic.

The underlying cause is not completely understood but at least in part seems to be chronic hypoxemia. This results in arteriovenous anastomosis with thickening of the tissues. The list of diseases in which clubbing is seen includes chronic obstructive pulmonary disease (COPD), bronchogenic carcinoma, bronchiectasis, sarcoidosis, and infective endocarditis.

6. Determine if the patient has peripheral edema (Code: IB1a) [Difficulty: An]

Peripheral edema is seen when fluid leaks from the capillary bed into the tissues. It is most commonly seen in the ankles and feet or along the back when the patient is lying supine in bed. The extent of the edema is measured by pressing a finger into the tissues. Normal skin springs back, whereas edematous skin is pitted or depressed. The pitting edema is graded as 1+ for less than ¼-inch (mild), 2+ for ¼- to ½-inch (moderate), and 3+ for ½- to 1-inch (severe) indentation. Obviously, the deeper the pitting, the more peripheral edema the patient has.

Peripheral edema is most commonly seen in patients

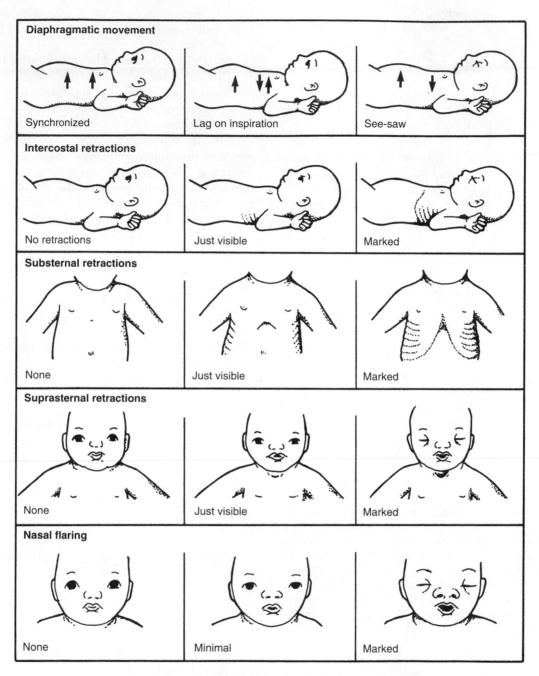

Fig. 1-16   Physical indications of labored breathing.

with congestive heart failure or those who are fluid overloaded. Patients with septicemia often have peripheral edema because the blood-borne pathogen (usually *Staphylococcus*) causes abnormal capillary leakage.

7. Determine the shape (configuration) of the patient's chest (Code: IB1b) [Difficulty: An]

The patient should be sitting up straight or standing erect when being examined for chest configuration. Look at the patient from the front, back, and both sides to see the symmetry. See Fig. 1-18 for the appearance of a normal infant's and adult's chest, barrel chest, funnel chest, pigeon chest, and thoracic kyphoscoliosis. There are several variations on curvature of the spine. Kyphosis is an exaggerated A-P curvature of the upper portion of the spine. Lordosis is an exaggerated A-P curvature of the lower portion of the spine. Scoliosis is either a right or left lateral curvature of the spine. Kyphoscoliosis is either a right or left lateral curvature combined with an A-P curvature of the spine.

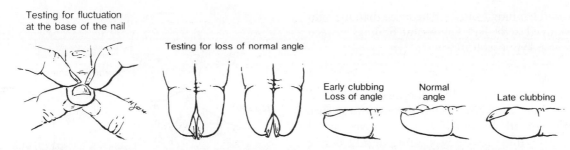

Testing for fluctuation
at the base of the nail

Testing for loss of normal angle

Early clubbing
Loss of angle

Normal
angle

Late clubbing

Fig. 1-17 Signs of and test for clubbing. (From Lehrer S: *Understanding lung sounds,*
Philadelphia, 1984, WB Saunders.)

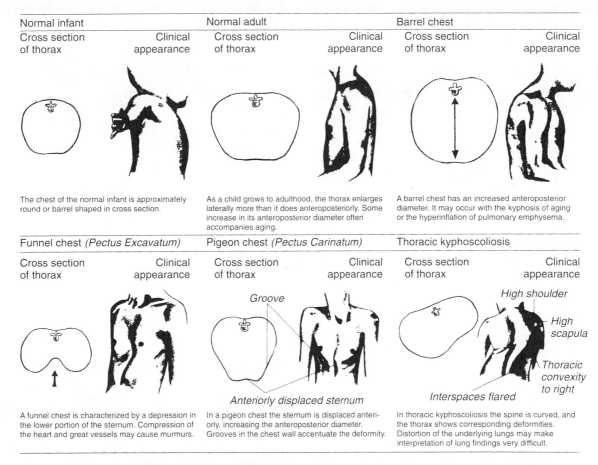

Normal infant

Cross section of thorax	Clinical appearance

The chest of the normal infant is approximately round or barrel shaped in cross section.

Normal adult

Cross section of thorax	Clinical appearance

As a child grows to adulthood, the thorax enlarges laterally more than it does anteroposteriorly. Some increase in its anteroposterior diameter often accompanies aging.

Barrel chest

Cross section of thorax	Clinical appearance

A barrel chest has an increased anteroposterior diameter. It may occur with the kyphosis of aging or the hyperinflation of pulmonary emphysema.

Funnel chest *(Pectus Excavatum)*

Cross section of thorax	Clinical appearance

A funnel chest is characterized by a depression in the lower portion of the sternum. Compression of the heart and great vessels may cause murmurs.

Pigeon chest *(Pectus Carinatum)*

Groove

Anteriorly displaced sternum

Cross section of thorax	Clinical appearance

In a pigeon chest the sternum is displaced anteriorly, increasing the anteroposterior diameter. Grooves in the chest wall accentuate the deformity.

Thoracic kyphoscoliosis

High shoulder

High scapula

Thoracic convexity to right

Interspaces flared

Cross section of thorax	Clinical appearance

In thoracic kyphoscoliosis the spine is curved, and the thorax shows corresponding deformities. Distortion of the underlying lungs may make interpretation of lung findings very difficult.

Fig. 1-18 Deformities of the thorax. (From Bates B: *A guide to physical examination and history taking,* ed 4, Philadelphia, 1987, JB Lippincott.)

8. Determine if the patient has asymmetrical chest movement when breathing (Code: IB1b) [Difficulty: An]

Normal infants and adults have symmetrical chest movement when breathing at rest or during exercise. All breathing efforts are best observed when the patient is shirtless. In females, it may be necessary to observe only the uncovered back to judge chest movement. Any kind of asymmetrical chest movement is abnormal. The asymmetrical movement may result from an abnormality of the chest wall or abdomen or from a pulmonary disorder.

a. Thoracic scoliosis or kyphoscoliosis

(Refer to Fig. 1-18 for the back view of a patient with thoracic scoliosis or kyphoscoliosis.) The scoliosis patient in Fig. 1-18 tends to have more chest movement on the right side because of the right spinal curvature. The left side of the chest and left lung would inflate more than the right if the spine curved to the left. These same findings are seen in a patient with kyphoscoliosis.

b. Flail chest

The flail segment moves in the opposite direction from the rest of the chest (also known as paradoxical movement). That is, with inspiration, the flail segment moves inward while the rest of the chest moves outward, and during expiration the flail segment moves outward as the rest of the chest moves inward. As the ribs heal, the segment stabilizes and moves with the rest of the chest.

c. Pneumothorax

The side with the collapsed lung does not move as much as the chest wall over the normal lung (see Fig. 1-3).

d. Atelectasis/pneumonia

The side with the atelectasis or pneumonia does not move as much as the chest wall over the normal lung (see Fig. 1-6).

9. Determine if the patient has intercostal or sternal retractions when breathing (Code: IB1b) [Difficulty: An]

Intercostal retractions are noticed when the soft tissues between the ribs are drawn inward during inspiration as the chest wall moves outward. Suprasternal retractions are noticed when the soft tissues *above* the sternum are drawn inward during an inspiration as the chest wall moves outward. Substernal retractions are noticed when the soft tissues *below* the sternum are drawn inward during an inspiration as the chest wall moves outward (Fig. 1-16).

A person who is breathing at rest should not have any retractions. That same person may have some minor retractions during vigorous exercise. Retractions of any kind are abnormal in any patient of any age who is resting in bed. Retractions are commonly seen in conditions in which airway resistance is increased or lung compliance is decreased. Both increase a patient's WOB. The patient must generate a more negative intrathoracic pressure to breathe, and as a result the various soft tissues are drawn inward during inspiration. Conditions in which this is seen include infant respiratory distress syndrome, acute respiratory distress syndrome, pulmonary edema, pneumonia, asthma, bronchitis, and emphysema.

10. Determine if the patient uses accessory muscles when breathing (Code: IB1b) [Difficulty: An]

Accessory muscles of respiration should not be needed during passive, resting breathing. They may be used when breathing vigorously during exercise. A dyspneic patient will likely use them even when resting. The accessory muscles of inspiration are the intercostal, scalene, sternocleidomastoid, trapezius, and rhomboid. The abdominal

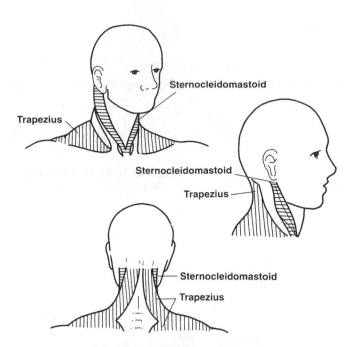

Fig. 1-19 The sternocleidomastoid and trapezius accessory muscles of respiration.

muscles are used during active expiration. The easiest accessory muscles of inspiration to observe in action are the sternocleidomastoids from the front and side of the patient and the trapezius from the back of the patient (Fig. 1-19).

Accessory muscle use in a patient who is resting should make it obvious that the WOB is greatly increased. The finding is not specific for any one condition but is commonly seen in a patient with emphysema (see Fig. 1-15).

11. Determine if the patient has diaphragmatic movement when breathing (Code: IB1b) [Difficulty: An]

Normally, an adult's diaphragm moves downward several centimeters toward the abdomen during inspiration as the chest wall moves outward. This is seen when the abdomen protrudes as its contents are forced forward. The chest and abdomen should rise and fall together during quiet and vigorous breathing efforts. There are two conditions in which this normal chest and abdominal movement does not occur.

First, patients with emphysema, severe air trapping, and a barrel chest have a diaphragm that is depressed and flat rather than domed because of the air that is trapped in the lungs. On inspiration, the diaphragm still contracts, but is unable to displace the abdominal contents down to permit air to be drawn into the lungs. These patients do not have the expected abdominal movement during inspiration. These patients use the accessory muscles of inspiration to assist breathing.

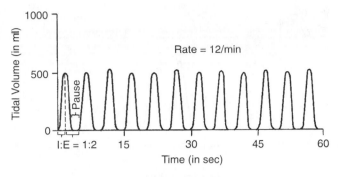

Fig. 1-20   Eupnea.

Second is any condition in which the airway resistance is increased or lung compliance is decreased. The greater negative intrathoracic pressure needed to draw the tidal volume into the lungs can cause the chest wall to collapse inward as the abdominal contents are displaced outward. The result is a kind of "seesaw" or paradoxical movement relationship between the chest wall and abdomen. On inspiration the chest wall may move inward as the abdomen moves outward. Patients with RDS typically demonstrate this because the premature neonate's rib cage is relatively compliant when compared with stiff lungs (see Fig. 1-16).

12. Determine the patient's breathing pattern (Code: IB1b) [Difficulty: An]

The various respiratory patterns can be identified by their characteristic respiratory rate, respiratory cycle, and tidal volume.

a. Eupnea (normal breathing) (Fig. 1-20)
1. Normal respiratory rate for the age of the patient (see Table 1-1).
2. Normal respiratory cycle. When timing the flow of air into and out of the lungs, the inspiratory/expiratory (I:E) ratio is 1:1.5 to 1:2. A pause of variable time follows exhalation of the tidal volume. This will change the true I:E ratio from 1:2 to 1:4.
3. Tidal volume normal for the size of the patient. (Fig. 1-20 relates to an average adult. The following abnormal breathing patterns can be compared with it.) Inspiration is achieved without the use of accessory muscles of inspiration; exhalation is passive.

b. Hypopnea (shallow breathing)
1. Respiratory rate usually somewhat slower than normal.
2. Normal respiratory cycle.
3. Tidal volume decreased for the size of the patient.

4. Possible causes: deep sleep, sedation, coma, hypothermia, alkalemia, restrictive lung disease.
5. May be combined with bradypnea.

c. Hyperpnea (deep breathing)
1. Respiratory rate may be normal or somewhat faster.
2. Normal respiratory cycle.
3. Tidal volume increased for the size of the patient.
4. Possible causes: acidemia, fever, pain, fear, anxiety, increased intracranial pressure.
5. May be combined with tachypnea.

d. Bradypnea (slow breathing)
1. Slower-than-normal respiratory rate.
2. Expiration may be longer than normal as a result of a longer pause.
3. Tidal volume may be decreased for the size of the patient.
4. Possible causes: deep sleep, sedation, coma, hypothermia, alkalemia.
5. May be combined with hypopnea.

e. Tachypnea (rapid breathing)
1. Faster than the normal respiratory rate.
2. Inspiration may be faster than normal with the help of inspiratory accessory muscles. Expiration may be shorter than normal, and expiratory accessory muscles may be used to force the air out faster. The pause seen in eupnea is absent. The I:E ratio may be 1:2 or less.
3. Tidal volume may be increased for the size of the patient.
4. Possible causes: acidemia, fever, pain, anxiety, increased intracranial pressure.
5. May be combined with hyperpnea.

f. Obstructed inspiration
1. Normal to slower respiratory rate.
2. Inspiratory time is equal to or longer than expiratory time. Inspiration is aided by use of the inspiratory accessory muscles. Expiration is passive.
3. Tidal volume may be normal, larger, or smaller than normal depending on how the patient adapts to the increased WOB. It is most common to see a slower rate with a larger tidal volume.
4. Possible causes: croup, epiglottitis, foreign body aspiration with partial airway obstruction, postextubation laryngeal edema, airway tumor, or airway trauma.

g. Obstructed expiration
1. Normal to slower respiratory rate.
2. Expiratory time is longer than normal. Accessory muscles of inspiration and expiration may be used.

3. Tidal volume may be normal or decreased for the size of the patient.
4. Possible causes: asthma, emphysema, bronchitis, cystic fibrosis, bronchiectasis, airway tumor, or airway trauma.

h. Kussmaul's respiration (rapid, large breaths)
1. Faster-than-normal rate.
2. I:E ratio approaches 1:1. Both inspiratory and expiratory accessory muscles may be used.
3. Tidal volume is increased for the size of the patient.
4. Probable cause: acidemia (pH 7.2 to 6.95) from diabetic ketoacidosis.

i. Cheyne-Stokes respiration (waxing and waning tidal volumes) (Fig. 1-21)
1. The respiratory rate varies from normal to faster and may have short periods of apnea.
2. The respiratory cycle is normal or approximates it except if the patient has periods of apnea.
3. The tidal volumes increase and decrease over a variable time cycle. A 20-second cycle is fairly common. There may be periods of apnea between the decreased tidal volumes.
4. Possible causes: head injury, stroke, increased intracranial pressure, or congestive heart failure.

j. Biot's respiration (unpredictably variable)
1. The respiratory rate varies from rapid to short periods of apnea.
2. The respiratory cycle varies considerably.
3. Tidal volume varies from shallow to large.
4. Possible causes: head injury, brain tumor, increased intracranial pressure.

k. Apnea (cessation of breathing at the end of exhalation)
1. Apnea that lasts long enough to result in hypoxemia, bradycardia, and hypotension must be treated aggressively. Artificial respiration, with or without supplemental oxygen, must be started immediately.
2. It is important to evaluate the patient's previous breathing pattern to determine the cause of the apnea. Normal breathing followed by apnea might lead to consideration of causes of heart attack, stroke, or upper airway obstruction. An abnormal breathing pattern followed by apnea might lead to consideration of the cause(s) of the original abnormal breathing.
3. Evaluate the previous tidal volume variation for the reasons previously listed.
4. Possible causes: airway obstruction, heart attack, stroke, or head injury.

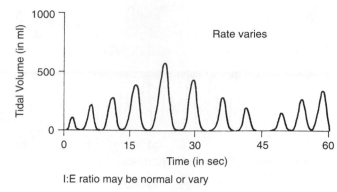

Fig. 1-21 Cheyne-Stokes.

13. Determine the kind of cough the patient has (Code: IB1b) [Difficulty: An]

a. Normal cough
A normal cough has four parts:
1. A person takes a deep breath.
2. The epiglottis and vocal cords close to keep the air trapped within the lungs.
3. The abdominal and other expiratory muscles contract to raise the air pressure in the lungs.
4. The epiglottis and vocal cords open to allow the compressed air to explosively escape and remove any mucus or foreign matter.

All components must work individually and in a coordinated manner for the patient to have an effective cough. The following are possible variations used by patients who for some reason cannot cough normally.

b. Serial cough
All actions of a normal cough take place except that the patient performs a series of smaller coughs rather than a single large one. This method of coughing may be used by postoperative patients who have too much abdominal or thoracic pain to cough normally. As the pain lessens, the patient should be able to cough normally.

c. Midinspiratory cough
All actions of a normal cough take place except that the patient does not take as deep a breath. Patients with emphysema and chronic bronchitis (COPD) sometimes use this to help prevent airway collapse when they cough.

d. Huff cough
Patients with artificial airways use this method. They cannot close their epiglottis and vocal cords, so they can take only a large breath and blow out with as much force as possible. It is still an effective way to remove watery secretions.

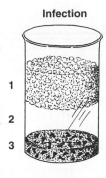
Infection

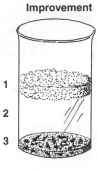
Improvement

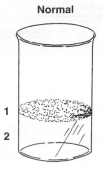
Normal

1. Gel layer:
   thicker than normal

2. Sol layer: thinner
   in ratio to gel
   layer than normal

3. Cellular debris:
   dead bacteria, WBCs,
   other cells

NOTE: The total volume of
sputum is greatly increased

1. Gel layer:
   reducing toward
   normal

2. Sol layer: returning
   to normal ratio with
   gel layer

3. Cellular debris:
   thinning out as fewer
   dead cells are being
   coughed out

1. Gel layer:
   normal volume

2. Sol layer: normal
   volume and ratio
   with the gel layer

NOTE: The total volume
of sputum is reduced
to normal; also, there
is no third layer of
cellular debris

Fig. 1-22   Evaluation of the homogeneity of sputum in the infected patient.

e. Assisted cough

This patient needs direct help from the therapist. The patient is given a deep breath by means of intermittent positive pressure breathing (IPPB) machine or manual ventilator. Then the therapist helps the patient blow the air out quickly by pushing on the abdominal area to move the diaphragm up. This procedure is limited to conscious patients with neuromuscular defects who cannot cough effectively on their own.

14. Determine the quantity and characteristics of the patient's sputum (Code: IB1b) [Difficulty: An]

a. Quantity

Normally a person is not aware of mucous production. The mucociliary escalator moves mucus toward the throat where it is unconsciously swallowed. Normally mucus is uninfected and clear or white in color.

Typically, infections causing bronchitis or pneumonia result in the production of large amounts of mucus. The patient will report coughing and spitting it up. This mix of mucus from the lungs and saliva from the mouth is sputum. Any increase in mucus or sputum production, to the extent that the patient is aware of it, is abnormal.

As mentioned earlier, some practitioners prefer to use subjective measurements of sputum production such as "a little," "medium amount," or "copious."

Objective measurements such as teaspoon, tablespoon, or 5, 10, or 15 mL, for example, are preferred to quantify production. A marked measuring cup is needed to do this.

Note any changes in the amount of sputum that the patient is producing. This is best done in a timed manner such as production per hour or per shift. It is also wise to correlate sputum production with breathing treatments or other procedures that may increase or decrease its production or clearance.

b. Characteristics

Homogeneity is best determined by letting a sputum sample stand in a test tube for several hours so that it stratifies. This is an important test to perform in the patient with a pulmonary infection. Normal sputum separates into a relatively thin surface layer of gel that floats on a lower layer of water (sol). The patient with a pulmonary infection has more viscous sputum because it contains dead bacterial cells, dead white blood cells, and cellular debris from the infected lung tissues. These cells settle over time to the bottom of a sputum sample and create a third layer of sediment.

See Fig. 1-22 for an example of how this layering looks in the sputum from a patient who has a pulmonary infection that eventually clears up. Table 1-12 explains other details on sputum characteristics.

TABLE 1-12	Sputum Characteristics			
Sputum type	**Color**	**Contents**	**Illnesses**	**Odor**
Bloody (hemoptysis)	Red	Blood	Bronchogenic carcinoma; pulmonary hemorrhage; lung abscess; tuberculosis; pulmonary infarction	Typically none
Frothy or bubbly	Clear or pink	Water; plasma proteins; red blood cells	Pulmonary edema	Typically none
Mucoid	Clear or white	Water; complex sugars; glycoproteins; some cellular debris	Asthma; chronic bronchitis	Typically none
Mucopurulent	Light to medium yellow	Decreased water and complex sugars; increased cellular debris and causative organisms (if applicable); organisms are usually aerobes	Chronic and acute bronchitis	Typically none, but may exist depending on organism
Purulent	Dark yellow or green	Decreased water; greatly increased cellular debris and causative organisms that are usually aerobes; complex sugars	Bronchiectasis; lung abscess; pneumonia	Depending on organism, along with clearance of mucus; also may be foul tasting to the patient; odor usually not offensive
Purulent (fetid)	Dark yellow or green	Decreased water; may contain some blood; greatly exaggerated cellular debris and causative organisms that frequently are anaerobes; complex sugars	Bronchiectasis; lung abscess; cystic fibrosis	Offensive odor

From DiPietro JS: *Clinical guide for respiratory care and cardiopulmonary disease,* Acton, Mass., 1998, Copley Custom Publishing.

 EXAM HINT

There is usually one question that requires the therapist to evaluate the patient's sputum. For example, a change from white or yellow to green indicates pneumonia. Or, a lung abscess is likely because the sputum is now green and foul smelling.

15. Determine if the patient has excessive venous distension (Code: IB1a) [Difficulty: An]

The internal jugular vein and external/anterior jugular vein are observed in the normal patient by having him or her lie supine with the head elevated 30 degrees. The crest of the vein column should be seen just above the border of the midclavicle. Make a rough measure of the intravascular volume and CVP by pressing on the veins at the base of the neck. The returning blood should fill the veins and make them distend (Fig. 1-23). When the pressure is released, the veins should return to their previous level of distension just above the level of the midclavicle. Increased venous distension is noted when the veins stand out at a level above the clavicle. This is seen in patients with right heart failure (cor pulmonale), cardiac tamponade, fluid overload, COPD, and when high airway pressures and positive end-expiratory pressure (PEEP) are needed for mechanical ventilation. The higher the veins are distended, the more the patient is compromised.

It is not normal for the veins to collapse below the clavicle when the obstructing finger is removed. If seen, this patient should then have his or her head laid flat. Normally, when flat, the external jugular vein should be seen as partially distended. If the vein collapses on inspiration, low venous pressure is confirmed and the patient is probably hypovolemic. This is commonly seen in dehydration, hemorrhage, or increased urine output following the use of diuretics.

16. Determine the patient's capillary refill (Code: IB1a) [Difficulty: An]

Capillary refill is the time needed for blood to refill the capillary bed after it has been forced out. The procedure is to pinch the finger or toenail until it blanches, then release the pressure. The pink color of the nailbed should return in less than 3 seconds. Any delay in the return to pink color indicates reduced blood flow to the extremities. Cyanotic nailbeds are also seen with reduced blood flow. Examples of conditions that result in a decreased capillary refill

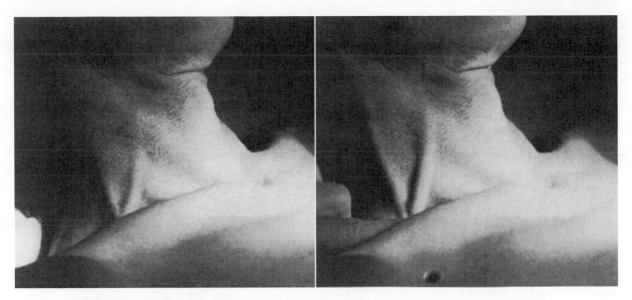

Fig. 1-23   Evaluating distension of the external jugular vein. These photographs show a patient with right-sided heart failure. Note that the left photograph shows the external jugular vein distended above the level of the clavicle. The right photograph shows how pressing a finger over the external jugular vein results in its further filling with blood and distending. In a normal person, when the pressure is released the vein should collapse to just above the superior border of the midclavicle. See the text for further discussion. (From Daily EK, Schroder JS: *Techniques in bedside hemodynamic monitoring,* ed 4, St Louis, 1989, Mosby.)

include decreased cardiac output, low blood pressure from any cause, and the use of vasopressor medications.

17. Determine if the patient has muscle wasting (Code: IB1a) [Difficulty: An]

Muscle wasting is an abnormal condition of decreased muscle mass. Muscle wasting can be generalized or localized depending on the underlying cause. Examples of conditions in which muscle wasting is seen include the following:

a. COPD

COPD (emphysema and bronchitis) often results in muscle wasting because the patient is consuming an unusually large number of calories through the act of breathing. In addition, these patients often do not eat well because a full stomach restricts the movement of the diaphragm and worsens their WOB and SOB. Because of this, they are frequently malnourished or undernourished. Their arms and legs are thin; their shoulder, elbow, and knee joints are prominent; and their ribs are clearly outlined by deep intercostal spaces.

b. Lung cancer

Lung cancer or other cancers usually result in a loss of muscle mass. This is because the growing tumor consumes many calories that are then not available to the normal body tissues. These patients usually also have thin arms and legs with prominent joints during advanced disease.

c. Neurologic injuries

Neurologic injuries, such as transsection of the spinal cord, result in atrophy of the affected muscles. Atrophy of the muscles is a decrease in size resulting from lack of use. This is an unavoidable consequence of the permanent loss of nerve input to the affected muscles. For example, transsection of the spinal cord at the first lumbar vertebrae (L1) results in loss of nerve input to the legs. The patient is a paraplegic. In time, the muscles of the legs atrophy; however, if the arms are exercised, they retain normal muscle mass. If the patient has a spinal transsection that results in the loss of nerve input to both the arms and legs (quadriplegia), all of the limbs atrophy.

MODULE E	Use *palpation* to determine the patient's complete respiratory condition

1. Determine the patient's pulse rate, rhythm, and force (Code: IB2a) [Difficulty: An]

The heart rate is most commonly counted by palpating the following locations: carotid, femoral, radial, and brachial arteries and apical pulse of the heart (see Fig. 1-24). The apical pulse is normally located in the area of the left

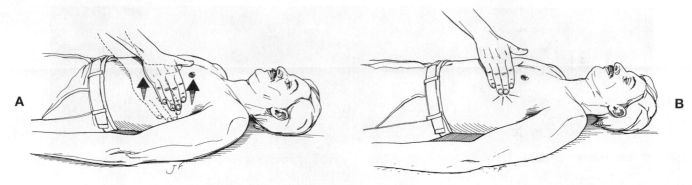

Fig. 1-24 Determining the position of the apical pulse. **A,** Technique for locating the apical pulse by palpation. **B,** Location of the apical pulse. (From Eubanks DH, Bone RC: *Comprehensive respiratory care,* ed. 2, St Louis, 1990, Mosby.)

midclavicular line in the fifth intercostal space. The apical pulse is also known as the point of maximal impulse (PMI). The location indicates the apex of the heart (left ventricle). Other arterial sites such as the temporal, dorsalis pedis, and posterior tibial can be used but are more difficult to find. The pulse should be counted for a minimum of 30 seconds; counting for 1 minute provides the most accurate measure of heart rate.

Palpating a pulse at any of the aforementioned sites reveals the timing between the heartbeats. This rhythm is normally regular in people who are at rest or exercising at a steady level. The rhythm is felt and mentally timed as the pulse rate is counted. The period between beats should be about the same.

The respiratory effort may have some influence on the rhythm. Fairly common in children and sometimes in adults, the heart rhythm and rate increase on inspiration and decrease on expiration. This sinus arrhythmia is not really abnormal. It is caused when the negative intrathoracic pressure during inspiration draws blood more quickly into the thorax and heart. The opposite may be true during mechanical ventilation with a high peak pressure or mean airway pressure. Then the heart rhythm and rate may slow down during inspiration and speed up during expiration. In any other case, an irregular rhythm indicates some sort of cardiac problem. An electrocardiogram is needed to help determine the specific cause.

The force of the pulse is an indicator of the strength of the heart's contraction and blood pressure. Normally each heartbeat should be felt with the same amount of force. A "thready" or variable force felt with each heartbeat is usually a sign of heart disease. Atrial fibrillation is an example of an irregular heart rhythm that results in an irregular force. The irregular rate and rhythm cause variable volumes of blood to be pumped with each contraction. A large volume of blood is felt as a strong pulse, whereas a small volume of blood is felt as a weak pulse.

A "bounding" or greater-than-normal force felt with

each beat is usually a sign of hypertension. In either case, for safety's sake, blood pressure should be measured and compared with the patient's previous blood pressure to see if there has been a change.

2. Determine if the patient has asymmetrical chest movements when breathing (Code: IB2b) [Difficulty:An]

Normally the lungs and chest move together in symmetry throughout the respiratory cycle. Asymmetrical chest wall movement during inspiration indicates a lung or chest wall problem. If the patient does not have an abnormal chest wall configuration, the problem has to be in the lungs. Less air is getting into the affected lung area(s), so the chest wall does not move out as far as the chest wall over the normal lung. This is a nonspecific finding of lung disease but is also seen in pneumonia, bronchial or lung tumor, and pneumothorax.

The therapist's hands should be placed over the patient's chest to assess for asymmetrical chest movement (Fig. 1-25). The thumbs should touch at the end of expiration. The patient is then instructed to breathe in deeply as asymmetrical movement is looked and felt for. In Fig. 1-25, *A* and *B* show the movement of the anterior apical lobes, *C* and *D* show the movement of the anterior middle and lower lobes, *E* and *F* show the movement in the posterior lower lobes, and *G* and *H* show the movement of the costal margins.

3. Determine if the patient has tactile fremitus (Code: IB2b) [Difficulty: An]

Tactile fremitus is a vibration felt through the chest wall when the patient speaks. Normally, when a sound is created in the larynx, its vibration is carried throughout the tracheobronchial tree to the lung parenchyma and to the chest wall. The intensity of the vibration or its absence gives the practitioner important information on the patient's condition.

Fig. 1-26 shows different methods of detecting tactile

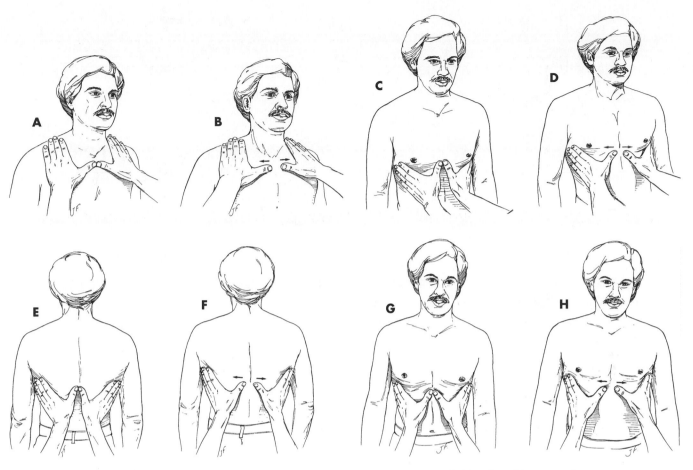

Fig. 1-25 Palpation to access symmetrical chest movements. **A,** Hand position over the apical lobes during expiration. **B,** Apical movement during inspiration. **C,** Hand position over middle and lower lobes during expiration. **D,** Middle and lower lobe movement during inspiration. **E,** Hand position over the posterior middle lobes during expiration. **F,** Movement of the posterior middle lobes during inspiration. **G,** Hand position to check for movement of the costal margins during expiration. **H,** Costal movement during inspiration. (From Eubanks DH, Bone RC: *Comprehensive respiratory care,* ed. 2, St Louis, 1990, Mosby.)

fremitus. Some practitioners may prefer to use their fingertips as in *A* and *B*, whereas others prefer the ulnar edge of the open or closed hand as in *C* and *D*. The practitioner should feel all areas of the patient's chest for tactile fremitus to detect any variations and should touch the chest over both lung fields to compare their symmetry as well as anterior and posterior differences (Fig. 1-26, *E* and *F*). Fig. 1-27 shows the posterior and anterior locations for the evaluation of tactile fremitus. Start with the supraclavicular fossae and proceed to alternate intercostal spaces. An attempt must be made to preserve the adult female patient's modesty when evaluating the anterior locations. The patient may be asked to lift the breast to palpate beneath it.

The procedure for evaluating tactile fremitus is to have the patient say "99" in a normal voice as the practitioner's fingers or hand are moved from location to location. This procedure is also called *palpation for bronchophony*. The "99" should be spoken at least once for each location to determine any variations. Having the patient speak more loudly or deeply should increase the intensity of the vibrations felt. The intensity of the vibrations directly relates to the density of the underlying lung and chest cavity. Conditions that increase density result in more intense vibrations. Conversely, conditions that decrease density result in less intense vibrations. Vibrations are also reduced when they are blocked from penetrating through to the surface. See Table 1-13 for conditions that alter tactile fremitus.

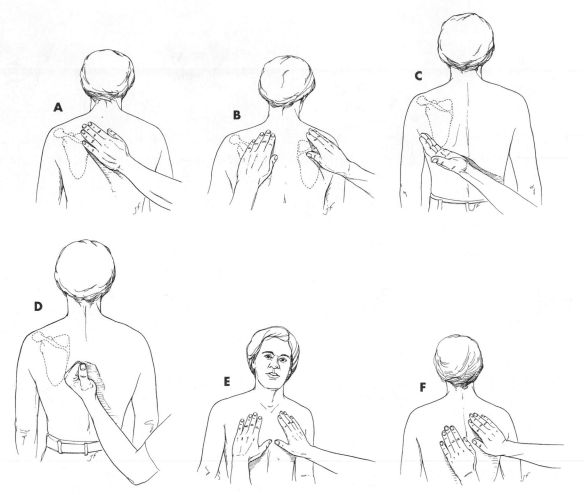

Fig. 1-26   A-D, Techniques for feeling tactile fremitus. **E** and **F,** Anterior and posterior placement of the hands to detect tactile fremitus. (From Eubanks DH, Bone RC: *Comprehensive respiratory care,* ed 2, St Louis, 1990, Mosby.)

4. Determine if the patient has rhonchial fremitus indicating secretions in the airway (Code: IB2b) [Difficulty: An]

Rhonchial fremitus, also known as palpable rhonchi, are a type of tactile fremitus noticed when vibrations from airway secretions can be felt through the chest wall as the patient breathes. They are abnormal because they indicate that the patient has a significant secretion problem. Palpable rhonchi is not detected in a patient with clear airways. Having the patient cough or suctioning the airway to remove secretions results in the reduction or complete elimination of palpable rhonchi. Remember that an airway that is completely occluded by a mucous plug or foreign body will *not* reveal palpable rhonchi because there is no airflow. Breath sounds are also absent in this area.

There are different methods of detecting palpable rhonchi. Some therapists may prefer to use their fingertips whereas others prefer to the edge of the open or closed hand. It is important to assess all areas of the patient's chest to detect the exact location(s) of the secretions.

5. Determine if the patient has crepitus (Code: IB2b) [Difficulty: An]

Crepitus (or crepitation) is the sound heard when an area with subcutaneous emphysema is gently pressed. The dry crackling-like sound resembles that of Rice Krispies in milk. A stethoscope can be used to help focus the sound to the exact location. In extreme instances, the unaided ear detects the sound. As the fingers of one hand are sequentially pressed into the affected area, the subcutaneous air is felt to move away from the pressure points.

Subcutaneous emphysema is air under the skin that has leaked from a damaged lung. The skin appears puffy or edematous and is most commonly seen in the tissues on the side of the leaking lung. The pressurized air dissects through the tissues following the path of least resistance and is most likely found under the skin in the axilla, neck, chest wall, and breast. In extreme cases, air is found under the skin throughout the body.

Although not dangerous, crepitus is a serious finding because it indicates that the patient has a pulmonary air

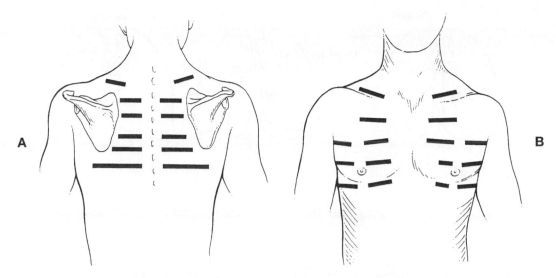

Fig. 1-27 **A,** Locations on the posterior chest for feeling tactile fremitus and performing percussion. **B,** Locations on the anterior chest for feeling tactile fremitus and performing percussion. (From Swartz MH: *Textbook of physical diagnosis,* Philadelphia, 1989, WB Saunders.)

TABLE 1-13	Abnormal Tactile Fremitus	

Increased	Decreased
UNILATERAL	**UNILATERAL**
Pneumonia	Pneumothorax
Atelectasis	Pleural effusion
Consolidation	Bronchial obstruction
BILATERAL	**BILATERAL**
Pulmonary edema	Thick chest wall (fat or muscle)
Acute respiratory distress syndrome	Chronic obstructive pulmonary disease

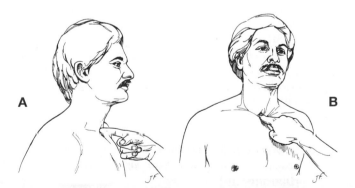

Fig. 1-28 **A** and **B,** Detecting the position of the trachea by pressing the index finger into the suprasternal notch. (From Eubanks DH, Bone RC: *Comprehensive respiratory care,* ed 2, St Louis, 1990, Mosby.)

leak. It may be accompanied by pneumothorax, pneumomediastinum, or pulmonary interstitial emphysema. A chest radiograph examination should be done immediately if the crepitation is a new finding.

6. **Determine if the patient has any tracheal deviation (Code: IB2b) [Difficulty: An]**

Normally the trachea is in a midline position within the neck and thorax. The location of the trachea is found by having the patient look straight ahead and gently inserting the index finger into the suprasternal notch of an upright or supine patient (see Fig. 1-28). The trachea should be detected in midline with soft tissues on both sides. A trachea that is shifted off to one side is abnormal and can be caused by the following (see Fig. 1-6):

   a. Atelectasis, which causes the trachea to be pulled *toward* the affected side
   b. Pulmonary fibrosis, which causes the trachea to be pulled *toward* the most affected side
   c. Tension pneumothorax, which causes the trachea to be pushed *away* from the affected side
   d. Hemothorax, pleural effusion, and empyema, which push the trachea *away* from the affected side

Correction of the underlying pulmonary problem results in the trachea returning to its normal midline position.

7. **Determine if the patient has any tenderness (Code: IB2b) [Difficulty: An]**

Tenderness is an increased local sensation of pain when the chest is gently hit with the ulnar area of the fist.

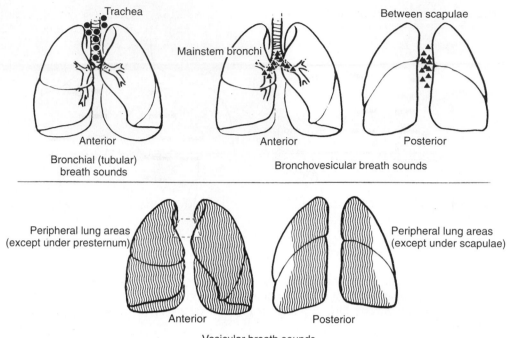

Fig. 1-29 Breath sounds heard over the normal chest. (From Lehrer S: *Understanding lung sounds.* Philadelphia, 1984, WB Saunders Company.)

This tapping is done in a symmetrical pattern over the posterior and anterior lung areas and normally should not cause any pain. Intercostal tenderness is felt at the site of an inflamed pleura. Local tenderness and a history of trauma to an area of the chest leads to the conclusion of musculoskeletal pain. A chest radiograph might be indicated to determine if any ribs have been fractured. The absence of chest wall tenderness should lead to a further investigation as to the cause of the chest pain. Consider angina pectoris (hypoxic heart pain).

MODULE F	Use *auscultation* to determine the patient's complete respiratory condition

1. Breath sounds

a. Determine if the patient has bilaterally normal breath sounds (Code: IB4a) [Difficulty: An]

There are three types of normal breath sounds (Fig. 1-29):

1. *Normal* breath sounds are also called *vesicular.* These normal breath sounds are heard over all areas of normally-ventilated lungs. Normal breath sounds have been variously described as "leaves rustling" or "like a gentle breeze." These faint sounds are made as air is moved through the small airways of the lungs during the breathing cycle. The inspiratory to expiratory (I:E) ratio is about 3:1. The inspiratory sound is louder than the expiratory sound, and there is no pause between inspiration and expiration.

2. *Bronchial* breath sounds are also called *tracheal.* These normal breath sounds are heard over the trachea and main bronchi. Bronchial breath sounds have been described as being louder, harsher, and higher-pitched than normal. They have a fairly uniform pitch on inspiration and expiration with a distinct pause in the transition of flow. The I:E ratio is about 1:1.5.

3. *Bronchovesicular* sounds are a cross between bronchial and vesicular. Bronchovesicular sounds are more muffled than bronchial but louder than vesicular, and it has the same pitch throughout inspiration and expiration. The I:E ratio is about 1:1.

Bronchial and bronchovesicular breath sounds are abnormal if heard in any other areas except those mentioned here. When these sounds are heard over areas that should be normal vesicular, it is a sign of consolidation or atelectasis with a patent airway.

b. Determine if the patient has increased, decreased, absent, or unequal breath sounds (Code: IB4a) [Difficulty: An]

This discussion is limited to variations in normal vesicular breath sounds. The abnormal appearance of bronchial and bronchovesicular breath sounds was discussed earlier.

1. Increased normal vesicular breath sounds

a. Found most often in children and in debilitated adults because their thinner chest walls transmit the sounds better.

b. Increased breath sounds are commonly described as *harsh.*

2. Decreased normal vesicular breath sounds

a. Most commonly caused by a pleural effusion, hemothorax, or empyema because of fluid between the lung and the stethoscope (see Fig. 1-6, *D*).

b. Pulmonary fibrosis resulting from decreased airflow (see Fig. 1-6, *B*).

c. Emphysema resulting from decreased airflow.

d. Pleural thickening resulting from dampening from the thicker pleural tissues.

3. Absent normal vesicular breath sounds

a. Pneumothorax caused by the lung being forced away from the chest wall (see Fig. 1-6, *C*).

b. Atelectasis (see Fig. 1-6, *A*) or severe bronchospasm results because no air is moving into the alveoli.

c. Endotracheal tube placed into a bronchus instead of the trachea. In this case, the right bronchus is most commonly intubated so that the breath sounds are absent over the left lung.

d. Large pleural effusion.

e. Obese patient.

4. Unequal normal vesicular breath sounds

a. Pneumonia, consolidation, or atelectasis that decreases airflow into a segment or lobe.

b. Foreign body or tumor in a bronchus that decreases airflow to the distal lung.

c. Spinal or thoracic deformity that reduces airflow to the underlying lung.

c. Determine if the patient has wheezing (rhonchi) or crackles (rales) (Code: IB4a) [Difficulty: An]

The term *adventitious* is used to collectively describe all types of abnormal breath sounds.

1. Wheezing

Wheezing (also known as wheeze and rhonchi) has the following features or characteristics:

a. They are continuous sounds.

b. They are more commonly heard on expiration than inspiration.

c. Low-pitched, polyphonic expiratory wheezing is commonly associated with secretions in the airways. A common term for these sounds is *rhonchi.* Common pulmonary conditions include bronchitis, pneumonia, or any other secretion-causing problem. Coughing or tracheal suctioning often causes these sounds to be modified or eliminated.

d. High-pitched, *monophonic* expiratory sounds are commonly associated with closure of one large airway. This is commonly found with an airway tumor.

e. High-pitched, *polyphonic* expiratory sounds are commonly associated with closure of many small airways. The term *wheeze* is commonly used to describe these sounds caused by bronchospasm in an asthmatic patient. Coughing or tracheal suctioning is unlikely to eliminate these high-pitched sounds. Effective treatment with bronchodilating medications should make the wheezing diminish and vesicular sounds return.

2. Crackles (rales)

Crackles have the following features or characteristics:

a. They are discontinuous sounds.

b. They are more commonly heard on inspiration than expiration.

c. They may be caused by the sudden opening of collapsed airways. Early inspiratory crackles are heard in patients with obstructive lung diseases such as chronic bronchitis, bronchiectasis, asthma, and emphysema. Late inspiratory crackles are heard in patients with atelectasis, pneumonia, pulmonary edema, or fibrosis.

d. They may be caused by air passing through secretions and are heard as a repeated sound during the same phase of the respiratory cycle.

d. Determine if the patient has any stridor (Code: IB4a) [Difficulty: An]

Stridor is heard as a harsh, monophonic, high-pitched inspiratory sound over the larynx. (It is not the normal tracheal sound.) It has these features or characteristics:

1. Stridor can often be heard without a stethoscope.

2. Common pediatric conditions include acute epiglottitis, laryngotracheobronchitis (croup), and laryngomalacia (congenital stridor).

3. Common adult conditions include postextubation laryngeal edema and a laryngeal tumor.

4. When stridor is heard on inspiration and expiration, it is commonly caused by an aspirated foreign body, tracheal stenosis, or a laryngeal tumor.

🔲 EXAM HINT

There is usually one question on the interpretation of breath sounds or identifying a situation that might cause an abnormal breath sound, for example, absent breath sounds over an area of pneumothorax or an endotracheal tube misplaced into the right mainstem bronchus with no breath sounds heard over the left lung field. Remember that severe stridor is a respiratory emergency because the airway may rapidly close completely. The patient is usually intubated to provide a secure airway.

e. Determine if the patient has a friction rub (Code: IB4a) [Difficulty: An]

A friction rub (also known as a *pleural* friction rub) is the sound caused by the rubbing together of the inflamed and adherent visceral and parietal pleura as seen in pleurisy. It is heard through a stethoscope and is described as loud and grating, clicking, or the creaking of old leather. The inspiratory sound frequently is reversed from the expiratory sound as the pleural tissues rub against each other in the opposite direction.

A friction rub is heard most commonly over the lower lung areas. Commonly, the sound is found at the site where the patient complains of pleural pain on breathing. Coughing and suctioning do not affect it. The causes include pulmonary infarct or any pneumonia that leads to an abscess or empyema.

2. Heart sounds

a. Determine if the patient has heart sounds (Code: IB4b) [Difficulty: An]

The patient's heart rate and rhythm can be easily determined by listening at the point of the apical pulse (see Fig. 1-24). Obviously, if a heart sound cannot be detected, the patient should be assessed for cardiac arrest. Begin cardiopulmonary resuscitation (CPR) if needed.

b. Determine if the patient has dysrhythmias (Code: IB4b) [Difficulty: An]

A steady rhythm has approximately equal amounts of time between ventricular contractions. It is considered normal to have a slight increase in the heart rate and faster rhythm during an inspiration than during an expiration. This is caused by the increase in blood brought into the chest during the inspiration when the intrathoracic pressure is more negative. The opposite pattern might be seen when a patient is being mechanically ventilated with high peak airway pressures. This indicates that the venous return to the heart is decreased during a mechanically delivered inspiration.

Any sudden variations in rate and rhythm not related to the respiratory cycle are abnormal. It is difficult to determine the origin of most dysrhythmias solely on the basis of their sound patterns; an ECG is indicated. A premature ventricular contraction (PVC) can be noted by the following rhythm characteristics: (1) the heartbeat is premature, and (2) there is a complete compensatory pause between the PVC and the following normal beat. The complete compensatory pause is the time interval of two normal heartbeats. (See the representative rhythm strip [Fig. 10-22] in Chapter 10.)

c. Determine the presence of murmurs (Code: IB4b) [Difficulty: An]

Heart sounds are caused by the closing of the four heart valves during a cardiac cycle. The first heart sound, S_1, is heard when the mitral (bicuspid) and tricuspid valves close when the ventricles contract during systole. This has been described as a "lub" sound. The second heart sound, S_2, is heard when the pulmonary semilunar and aortic valves close when the ventricles relax during diastole. This has been described as a "dup" or "dub" sound. Occasionally, a third heart sound (S_3) or fourth heart sound (S_4) is heard. When a patient has these extra sounds, the patient is described as having a "gallop" rhythm. This is a pathologic finding and is usually found in patients with congestive heart failure.

A murmur is an abnormal fluttering or humming sound heard during the cardiac cycle. The murmur indicates that blood is flowing through one or more heart valves when it should not. The valve(s) can be either incompetent (not closing properly, causing blood to leak) or stenotic (narrowed, preventing normal blood flow). Fig. 1-30 shows the areas where a stethoscope should be placed to listen for a murmur from each of the four valves. The bell should be held lightly on the chest to hear low-frequency sounds. The diaphragm should be held firmly on the chest to hear high-frequency sounds. It may be helpful when listening to have the patient lie on the left side. A systolic murmur is heard after the S_1 sound but before the S_2 sound. The sound sequence is "lub-murmur-dup, lub-murmur-dup." A diastolic murmur is heard after the S_2 sound but before the S_1 sound. The sound sequence is "lub-dup-murmur, lub-dup-murmur". It is beyond the scope of this text to fully describe all of the possible types of murmurs and their causes. However, understand that the presence of a murmur indicates a defect in a cardiac valve.

d. Determine the presence of bruits (Code: IB4b) [Difficulty: An]

A bruit is a murmur (fluttering or humming) sound originating from an artery. A carotid bruit should be listened for in a patient with cardiovascular disease. Place the bell of the stethoscope over each carotid artery to listen. A murmur heard during systole indicates a bruit. It can be caused by increased blood flow or stenosis (narrowing) of the artery from plaque deposits. It is more commonly found in patients of advanced age. If the bruit is caused by atherosclerosis, the patient has an increased risk of stroke.

3. Determine the patient's blood pressure (Code: IB4c) [Difficulty: An]

Measure a blood pressure (BP) on any patient to establish a baseline normal value and whenever you think there might be a significant increase or decrease in the blood pressure. The BP should be the same on any arm or

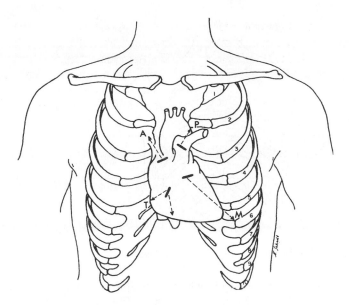

Fig. 1-30 Areas to listen for heart murmurs. The solid bars show the approximate location of the valves within the heart. The arrows indicate where each valve sound is best heard. *A,* Aortic valve. *P,* Pulmonary semilunar valve. *M,* Mitral valve. *T,* Tricuspid valve.

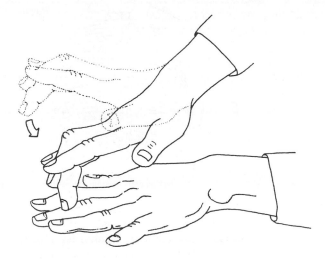

Fig. 1-31 Technique for performing mediate chest percussion. (From Shapiro BA, Kacmarek RM, Cane RD, Peruzzi WT, Hauptman D: *Clinical application of respiratory care,* ed 4, St Louis, 1991, Mosby.)

leg. However, an arm is typically used. Place the proper cuff around the arm and inflate the cuff pressure above the patient's normal value. Place the diaphragm of the stethoscope over the brachial artery and slowly let the air out of the cuff. The first distinct sound heard as the blood flows through the artery is the systolic pressure. The last distinct sound heard is the diastolic pressure. Clinical practice is needed to accurately determine blood pressure.

MODULE G	Use *percussion* to determine the patient's complete respiratory condition

Percussion of the chest is performed to determine normal and abnormal densities of the lungs and related structures. It must be performed properly to be a reliable diagnostic tool. There are two generally accepted methods of performing percussion. Both must be performed with equal force and speed or the resulting sound will reflect the technique rather than the condition of the lungs. Avoid percussing over a woman's breast tissue.

Immediate percussion involves striking the tip of the middle finger of one hand directly onto the chest wall in a symmetrical pattern. This is useful for finding large general differences in density and for finding landmarks such as the sternum and other bony structures, the liver, and the heart. Mediate percussion involves striking the tip of the middle finger of one hand onto the central section of the middle finger of the other hand (Fig. 1-31). The finger to be struck is fitted firmly between the ribs in a symmetrical pattern

shown in Fig. 1-27. Mediate percussion is better for precisely locating an abnormal area and will be used in the following discussions.

1. **Determine the patient's diaphragmatic excursion (Code: IB3) [Difficulty: An]**

It is helpful to determine the patient's diaphragmatic excursion during both normal tidal volume breathing and during maximal inspiration and expiration. Both hemidiaphragms should move the same amount during both the normal and maximal efforts. It should be remembered that, because of the liver, the right hemidiaphragm is usually found to be about 1 cm higher than the left.

The following procedure determines diaphragmatic excursion during tidal volume breathing:
   a. The patient should be sitting up straight, exhale passively, and hold.
   b. Percuss down the posterior chest to find the level of both hemidiaphragms. The air-filled lungs will have a resonant sound, whereas the more solid tissues below the lungs will have a dull sound.
   c. Have the patient inhale a normal tidal volume and hold.
   d. Percuss down the posterior chest to find the level of both hemidiaphragms.
   e. Note the range of movement on both sides by the intercostal space when the dull sound was heard at the end of expiration and at the end of inspiration. During a quiet tidal volume breath, the adult's hemidiaphragms moves down about 1.5 cm on

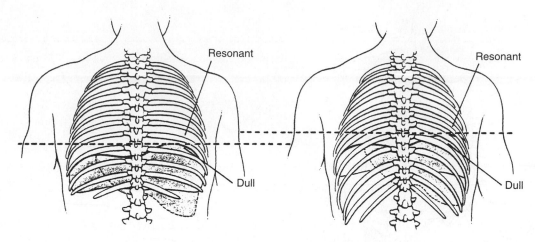

Fig. 1-32 The excursion of the hemidiaphragms can be determined by percussing the patient's posterior chest. This should be done at the end of inspiration, as shown on the left, and expiration, as shown on the right. The change from a resonant (lung) sound to a dull (abdominal) sound indicates the border of the hemidiaphragm on each side. (From Swartz MH: *Textbook of physical diagnosis,* Philadelphia, 1989, WB Saunders.)

BOX 1-2   Conditions That Affect the Position of the Hemidiaphragms

ELEVATED
Unilateral
Atelectasis (on the affected side)
Paralysis of the hemidiaphragm (on the affected side)
Enlarged liver (right side only)
Bilateral
Third trimester of pregnancy
Obesity
Ascites
Atelectasis (if bilateral)

DEPRESSED
Unilateral
Pneumothorax (on the affected side)
Check-valve obstruction to exhalation (on the affected side)
Pleural effusion (on the affected side)
Bilateral
Emphysema
Asthma

---

both sides. For example, the dull sound was heard at the 9th intercostal space at the end of exhalation and the 10th intercostal space at the end of inspiration.

The following procedure determines diaphragmatic excursion during maximal expiratory and inspiratory (vital capacity) breathing:

a. The patient should be sitting up straight, exhale as completely as possible, and hold.

b. Percuss down the posterior chest to find the level of both hemidiaphragms. The air-filled lungs will have a resonant sound, whereas the more solid tissues below the lungs will have a dull sound.

c. Have the patient inhale as completely as possible and hold.

d. Percuss down the posterior chest to find the level of both hemidiaphragms.

e. Note the range of movement on both sides by the intercostal space when the dull sound was heard at the end of expiration and at the end of inspiration. During the vital capacity effort, the adult's hemidiaphragms move down about 5 cm on both sides. (For example, the dull sound was heard at the 7th intercostal space at the end of exhalation and the 11th intercostal space at the end of inspiration [Fig. 1-32]).

Box 1-2 shows conditions that can affect the position of one or both hemidiaphragms.

2. Determine if the patient has areas of altered resonance (Code: IB3) [Difficulty: An]

Mediate percussion with proper technique should be performed over the posterior and anterior areas of the chest while avoiding breast tissue (see Fig. 1-27). The usual pattern is to proceed from the top down and side to side to compare for symmetrical sounds. The shoulders should be rolled forward when percussing the posterior chest to move the scapulae as much out of the way as possible. Table 1-14 shows the different types of percussion notes, their common characteristics, and example locations. See Fig. 1-33 for the location of the normal percussion sounds over the anterior chest.

Sounds such as hyperresonance are always abnormal when found over lung areas. They indicate that more

TABLE 1-14	Percussion Notes and Characteristics			
Percussion notes	**Relative intensity**	**Relative pitch**	**Relative duration**	**Example locations**
Resonant/resonance	Loud	Low	Long	Normal lung
Flat/flatness	Soft	High	Short	Sternum, spine, scapula
Dull/dullness	Medium	Medium	Medium	Liver, heart
Tympanic/tympany	Loud	High	Longer	Stomach air
Hyperresonant/hyperresonance	Very loud	Low	Long	Bilateral: emphysema, asthma Unilateral: pneumothorax, bleb

air than normal is present. Be careful not to confuse hyperresonance with the normal sound of tympany found over an air-filled stomach. An increase in the density of the underlying lung or related structures results in a dull sound at an abnormal location. This sound is associated with pneumonia, consolidation, or atelectasis when the alveoli are fluid filled or airless; with tumor; and with pleural fluid such as effusion, blood, pus, or chyle. It is normal to hear dullness over the heart and liver.

MODULE H   Neonatal Assessment

1. Review the perinatal/neonatal patient's chart for the following data

a. Review the maternal and perinatal/neonatal history and data (Code: IA1h) [Difficulty: Ap, An]

Perinatal refers to the period toward the end of a pregnancy and for up to 4 weeks after the neonate is born.

1. Antenatal assessment (assessment during the pregnancy)

The medical and personal history of the mother is obviously important because it directly relates to the health of the fetus she is carrying. The mother's age is important because women younger than 16 years and older than 40 years are more likely to have a high-risk pregnancy. This is especially true if a woman older than 40 is having her first child. *Gravida* is the term that refers to pregnancy; *primigravida* refers to a woman's first pregnancy. *Para* is the term that refers to the woman delivering a potentially live infant; *primipara/primiparous* refer to a woman's first delivery of an infant. Box 1-3 lists a number of maternal and other factors that can result in the anticipation of a high-risk infant being born. It must be noted that about 25% of high-risk infants are born with no indication from the history of there being any problem.

2. Intrapartum assessment (assessment during labor)

Some of the labor and delivery/obstetric factors that can adversely affect the delivery process include premature labor (less than 38 weeks' gestation), postmature labor (greater than 42 weeks' gestation), prolapsed umbilical cord, and cesarean section. Fetal heart rate (FHR, or fetal heart tones) is usually monitored to determine how the fetus is tolerating the stress of labor and delivery.

FHR should range between 120 and 160 beats/min and is normally variable with the fetus's waking and sleeping periods. The FHR can be measured externally through the mother's abdominal wall. During a contraction of the uterus, the heart rate commonly slows to near or less than 120 beats/min. This is because of vagus nerve stimulation during the compression of the head into the birth canal (see Fig. 1-34, *A*). The heart rate returns to normal when the contraction is over. This normal decrease and increase in FHR that is related to uterine contractions is called early deceleration or type I dips.

Late deceleration or type II dips are seen when the fetal heart rate slows sometime after the contraction begins and does not return to normal until sometime after the contraction is over (see Fig. 1-34, *B*). This is often caused by uteroplacental insufficiency from compression of the vessels in the placenta. It is frequently associated with low Apgar scores and fetal asphyxia and acidosis.

Variable deceleration is seen when the fetal heart rate slows and increases in an unpredictable pattern in comparison with the contractions (see Fig. 1-34, *C*). This pattern is more commonly seen than late deceleration and is believed to be caused by compression of the umbilical cord by a body part. During the compression, little or no blood reaches the fetus. It is also often associated with low Apgar scores and fetal asphyxia and acidosis.

With late and variable deceleration, the mother's heart rate and blood pressure should be monitored. Treatment includes giving the mother supplemental oxygen and placing her in a head-down, left lateral position. If the fetus is felt to be at risk of asphyxia, a cesarean section must be performed.

Other heartbeat irregularities are not related to labor and delivery. Tachycardia of greater than 160 beats/min can be associated with infection, fetal immaturity, congenital heart malformations, and the effects of maternal drugs.

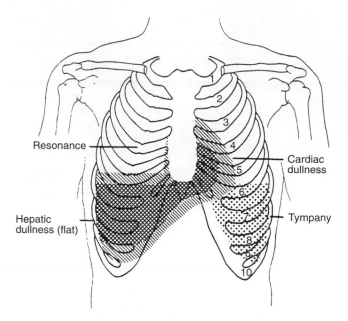

Fig. 1-33 Areas over the normal anterior thorax where resonance, dullness, tympany, and flatness can be heard during percussion. (From Prior JA, Silberstein JS, Stang JM: *Physical diagnosis,* ed 6, St Louis, 1981, Mosby.)

Bradycardia of less than 120 beats/min and decreased beat-to-beat variability (fixed heart rate) are seen with fetal asphyxia and distress.

3. Postpartum or neonatal assessment

Some of the fetal factors that can adversely affect the newborn include multiple births, meconium in the amniotic fluid, abnormal fetal heart rate or rhythm, prematurity or postmaturity, small or large for gestational age, congenital malformation, and birth trauma.

4. Resuscitation and vital signs

All newborns require some level of resuscitation. This is usually limited to suctioning amniotic fluid out of the nose and mouth, drying the skin, providing warmth, and the tactile stimulation that comes from these procedures. Newborns with moderate Apgar scores may need to breathe in some supplemental oxygen until they are more vigorous and ventilating better. The newborn with a low Apgar score requires cardiopulmonary resuscitation. Table 1-15 lists the vital signs seen in a normal newborn.

5. Weight

The relationship between birth weight and gestational age is important to evaluate. In general, if an infant is between the 10th and 90th percentile of normal weight for

gestational age, the infant is within normal limits. Any infant who is either large or small for gestational age is at increased risk of complications during and after delivery. Large postterm infants and small preterm infants are especially at risk.

BOX 1-3 Some Factors Associated with a High-Risk Newborn Infant

MATERNAL FACTORS:
Maternal age of less than 16 or greater than 40 years
Low socioeconomic status
Poor nutrition
Lack of medical care during pregnancy
Smoking, drug, or alcohol abuse
Underweight or overweight
Abnormal fetal growth
Hereditary anomalies
Vaginal bleeding early in pregnancy
Low maternal urinary estriol
Polyhydramnios or oligohydramnios
Toxemia of pregnancy/preeclampsia
Previous history of infant(s) with jaundice, respiratory distress, or previous premature delivery
Chronic disease:
  Hypertension unrelated to pregnancy
  Diabetes mellitus
  Cardiovascular
  Pulmonary
  Anemia
  Renal

LABOR AND DELIVERY/OBSTETRIC FACTORS:
Premature rupture of the membranes
Prolonged rupture of the membranes over 24 hours
Premature labor (less than 38 weeks' gestation)
Postmature labor (greater than 42 weeks' gestation)
Rapid or prolonged labor
Prolapsed umbilical cord
Previous or primary cesarean section
Breech or other abnormal presentation
Analgesia and anesthesia

FETAL FACTORS:
Multiple births
Meconium in amniotic fluid
Abnormal fetal heart rate or rhythm
Fetal acidosis
Prematurity or postmaturity
Small or large for gestational age
Rh factor sensitization
Congenital malformation
Immature lecithin/sphingomyelin (L/S) ratio or negative phosphatidylglycerol (PG) test
Birth trauma

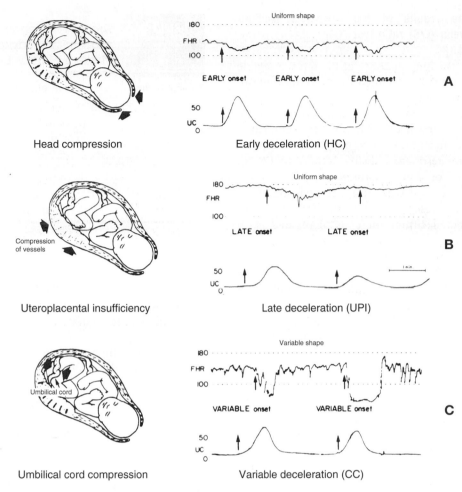

Fig. 1-34 Fetal heart rate patterns showing normal early deceleration and abnormal late deceleration and variable deceleration. (From Avery GB: *Neonatology: pathophysiology and management of the newborn,* ed 2, Philadelphia, 1981, JB Lippincott.)

TABLE 1-15	Normal Newborn Vital Signs

Characteristic	Normal range	
Heart rate	>120 beats/min	
	<160 beats/min	
Blood pressure	*Systolic*	*Diastolic*
1000-2000 g birth weight	55 mm Hg	30 mm Hg
>3000 g birth weight	65 mm Hg	40 mm Hg
Respiratory rate	30-60 breaths/min	
	Periodic breathing with apneic spells of <10 sec common; should not be associated with bradycardia or cyanosis	
Temperature	Keep abdominal skin temperature at 36.5° C	
	Keep rectal (core) temperature between 35.5° and 37.5° C	

b. Review the results of the neonate's lecithin/sphingomyelin (L/S) ratio test (Code: IA1h) [Difficulty: Ap, An]

To determine the lung maturity of the fetus, a sample of amniotic fluid must be obtained by an amniocentesis. The maturity of the fetus's lungs can be determined by evaluating three components of surfactant released by the developing alveolar type II cells. Recall that a premature neonate without sufficient surfactant in its lungs will probably develop infant respiratory distress syndrome (RDS).

The first test of lung maturity is the lecithin/sphingomyelin (L/S) ratio. The test is a comparison of the relative amounts of these two surfactant components. In general, the more lecithin there is compared with sphingomyelin, the more mature the lungs. There is usually a significant increase in the lecithin level at about 35 weeks of gestation. A weakness of the L/S ratio test is that borderline values are difficult to interpret, and false-positive values are sometimes found.

The second test is determining the presence of phosphatidylglycerol (PG) in the amniotic fluid. It appears at about 36 weeks of gestation and increases through the duration of the pregnancy. The laboratory reports PG as either present or absent from the sample of amniotic fluid. Its presence always indicates lung maturity. Table 1-16 gives more information on the interpretation of these two tests.

c. Review the patient's APGAR scores (Code: IA1h) [Difficulty: Ap, An]

The Apgar scoring system is used in the delivery room to give a general evaluation of how a newborn infant is responding. The following five parameters are judged: heart rate, respiratory effort, muscle tone, reflex response, and color. Table 1-17 shows how the five parameters are scored on a scale of 0, 1, and 2. The newborn is evaluated soon after birth to calculate a 1-minute Apgar score. A 5-minute evaluation and Apgar score are also calculated. The infant is rated as good if the score is 7 to 10, fair if the score is 4 to 6, and poor if the score is 0 to 3. If the 5-minute score is less than 7, the newborn is rescored every 5 minutes up to 20 minutes after the delivery.

d. Review information on the patient's gestational age (Dubowitz score) (Code: IA1h) [Difficulty: Ap, An]

The Dubowitz score is made up of 11 physical and 10 neurologic criteria that develop at a set rate during gestation. Ballard and coworkers modified the scoring system by simplifying it to six physical and six neurologic criteria. Fig. 1-34 shows the criteria, scoring system, and scale for rating the maturity of the newborn. A score of between 35 and 45 indicates that the infant was born between 38 and 42 weeks of gestation; this is a normal score for a term infant. A premature infant has a score of less than 35 and a postterm infant has a score of greater than 45.

TABLE 1-16 Lecithin/Sphingomyelin (L/S) Ratio and Phosphatidylglycerol (PG) as Markers of Fetal Lung Maturity

Clinical finding	Interpretation
L/S ratio 2:1 (2.0) or greater	Mature lungs; less than 5% chance of RDS
L/S ratio 1.5:1 (1.5)	Transitional lungs; about a 50% chance of RDS
L/S ratio 1:1 (1.0) or less	Immature lungs; about a 90% chance of RDS
PG present	Mature lungs
PG absent	Immature lungs

RDS, Infant respiratory distress syndrome.

The maturity rating scale can be used to give an estimation of gestational age accurate within 2 weeks.

e. Review information on the patient's preductal and postductal oxygenation studies (Code: IA1h) [Difficulty: Ap, An]

In a normal neonate, the ductus arteriosus closes shortly after birth causing equal oxygenation of all arterial blood to the body. With persistent pulmonary hypertension of the newborn (PPHN) the ductus arteriosus does not properly close. A diagnostic test for PPHN involves measuring the PO_2 in preductal blood and postductal blood. Preductal blood PO_2 is measured by a right radial artery sample, pulse oximetry on the right hand, or transcutaneous probe placed on the right arm or right upper chest. Postductal blood PO_2 is measured by an umbilical artery sample, pulse oximetry of the left hand or either foot, or transcutaneous probe on the abdomen or either thigh.

A right-to-left shunt indicating PPHN is shown by either: (1) a drop in SpO_2 of greater than 10% from preductal to postductal blood or (2) a drop in PO_2 of greater than 15 to 20 torr from preductal to postductal blood. However, it is important to understand that a normal test result does not rule out PPHN.

2. Determine the perinatal or neonatal patient's complete respiratory condition in the following ways by *observation*

a. Determine the patient's Apgar scores (Code: IB1c) [Difficulty: An]

Review the previous information and Table 1-17 as needed. The 1-minute Apgar score is a good index of how the newborn tolerated the delivery process. The 5-minute Apgar score is a good index of how the newborn's cardiopulmonary system is adjusting from fetal to adult conditions. A low 5-minute Apgar score is associated with

TABLE 1-17	Apgar Scoring Chart		
Sign	**0**	**1**	**2**
Heart rate	Absent	Slow (<100 beats/min)	Over 100
Respiratory effort	Absent	Weak cry, hypoventilation	Good strong cry
Muscle tone	Limp	Some flexion of extremities	Well flexed
Reflex response	No response	Grimace	Cough, sneeze, or cry
Response to catheter in nostril or to other cutaneous stimulation			
Color	Blue, pale	Body pink, extremities blue	Completely pink

From Lough MD, Doershuk CF, Stern RC: *Pediatric respiratory therapy,* ed 3, St Louis, 1985, Mosby.

increased mortality in the first month of life. Survivors have a high risk of mental impairment and cerebral palsy.

b. Determine the patient's gestational age (Dubowitz score) (Code: IB1c) [Difficulty: An]

The descriptions of gestational development for the criteria of physical maturity are listed in Fig. 1-35. As can be seen, more points are earned for each step of gestational development. A term infant will score 3 or 4 points for each of the 12 criteria. The illustrations of gestational development for the criteria of neurologic/neuromuscular maturity can be seen in the figure; however, because the infant must be manipulated to perform the rating, the following descriptions will be helpful.

Posture. The infant should be supine and quiet. Simply observe how the infant positions its arms and legs. The more mature infant will fully flex its elbows, hips, and knees.

Square Window. Flex the hand at the wrist. Exert gentle pressure to have the wrist flex as much as possible. The more mature infant will have full flexibility of the hand against the forearm.

Arm Recoil. With the infant supine, fully flex the forearms for 5 seconds. Then, fully extend the forearms by pulling on the hands. When released, the more mature infant will quickly return its forearms to full flexion.

Popliteal Angle. The infant must lie supine with the pelvis flat on the examining surface. The lower leg is flexed onto the thigh and the thigh fully flexed to the abdomen. One hand is used to hold the thigh in the flexed position and the other hand is used to extend the lower leg. The angle between the thigh and lower leg is then measured. The more mature infant will have less joint flexion and a smaller angle.

Scarf Sign. With the infant supine, take one of the infant's hands and extend it as far as possible across the neck toward the opposite shoulder. The infant is scored as follows:

0 = The elbow reaches the opposite anterior axillary line.

1 = The elbow reaches closer to the opposite anterior axillary line than the midline of the chest.

2 = The elbow reaches midway between the opposite anterior axillary line and the midline of the chest.

3 = The elbow reaches the midline of the chest.

4 = The elbow does not reach the midline of the chest.

Heel-to-Ear Maneuver. The infant should be supine on the examining table with the pelvis flat. Take the infant's foot in one hand and move it as near to the head as possible. Do not force it! The more-mature infant will have less joint flexibility and will not be as able to move the foot as near the head as a less-mature infant.

c. Assess the patient's cardiopulmonary condition by viewing the results of transillumination of the chest (Code: IB1c) [Difficulty: An]

Transillumination of the chest is a test performed on a neonate to identify the presence of a pneumothorax. To perform a test for a pneumothorax, the room is darkened and a bright light from a flashlight is placed against the patient's chest. When free air is around the collapsed lung, the light will create a "halo" effect through the thin chest wall of the neonate. This confirms the pneumothorax.

3. Inspect a lateral neck radiograph to evaluate the following:

Note: The following discussion usually applies to a child but can also apply to an adult.

a. Look for the presence of epiglottitis (Code: IB8a) [Difficulty: An]

Epiglottitis is an inflammation of the epiglottis and surrounding supraglottic structures. It is a medical emergency and is usually diagnosed on the basis of the history and physical examination and results in the child being intubated. If a lateral neck radiograph is taken of an epiglottitis, it will show a white haziness in the supraglottic area. This is the swollen epiglottis and is sometimes obvious enough to be called the "thumb sign." This is seen when the usually thin epiglottis is swollen and looks like the end of the thumb. It must be emphasized that under no circumstances should the child be laid supine for the neck radiograph. This can result in the swollen epiglottis fatally

Neuromuscular maturity

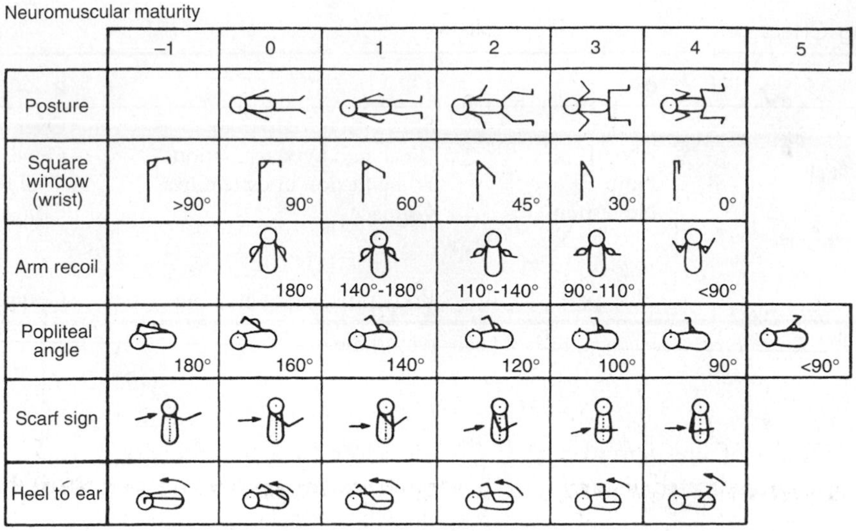

	−1	0	1	2	3	4	5
Posture							
Square window (wrist)	>90°	90°	60°	45°	30°	0°	
Arm recoil		180°	140°-180°	110°-140°	90°-110°	<90°	
Popliteal angle	180°	160°	140°	120°	100°	90°	<90°
Scarf sign							
Heel to ear							

Physical maturity

Skin	Sticky, friable, transparent	Gelatinous red, translucent	Smooth, pink, visible veins	Superficial peeling and/or rash, few veins	Cracking, pale areas, rare veins	Parchment, deep cracking, no vessels	Leathery, cracked, wrinkled
Lanugo	None	Sparse	Abundant	Thinning	Bald areas	Mostly bald	
Plantar surface	Heel-toe 40-50 mm:−1 <40 mm:−2	>50 mm No crease	Faint red marks	Anterior transverse crease only	Creases ant. 2/3	Creases over entire sole	
Breast	Imperceptible	Barely perceptible	Flat areola, no bud	Stippled areola, 1-2 mm bud	Raised areola, 3-4 mm bud	Full areola, 5-10 mm bud	
Eye/Ear	Lids fused loosely: −1 tightly: −2	Lids open; pinna flat; stays folded	Slightly curved pinna; soft; slow recoil	Well-curved pinna; soft but ready recoil	Formed and firm instant recoil	Thick cartilage ear stiff	
Genitals male	Scrotum flat, smooth	Scrotum empty; faint rugae	Testes in upper canal; rare rugae	Testes descending; few rugae	Testes down; good rugae	Testes pendulous; deep rugae	
Genitals female	Clitoris prominent; labia flat	Prominent clitoris; small labia minora	Prominent clitoris; enlarging minora	Majora and minora equally prominent	Majora large; minora small	Majora cover clitoris and minora	

Maturity rating

score	weeks
−10	20
−5	22
0	24
5	26
10	28
15	30
20	32
25	34
30	36
35	38
40	40
45	42
50	44

Fig. 1-35 The Ballard modification of Dubowitz Gestational Age Assessment. (From Ballard JL, Khoury JC, Wedig K: *J Pediatr* 119:417, 1991.)

closing over the opening to the trachea. Allow the child to sit upright in the most comfortable position. (Fig. 1-36 shows the epiglottis and Fig. 1-37 shows a lateral neck radiograph of the epiglottis. Table 1-18 lists the general history and physical findings for distinguishing between epiglottitis and laryngotracheobronchitis.)

b. Look for the presence of subglottic edema (Code: IB8a) [Difficulty: An]

Subglottic edema is an inflammation of the subglottic mucous membranes of the larynx, trachea, and bronchi. This condition is also known as laryngotracheobronchitis (LTB) and croup. Subglottic edema is usually treated by the inhalation of a cool aerosol in a mist tent and racemic epinephrine for mucosal vasoconstriction. If a lateral neck radiograph of subglottic edema is taken, it will show a white haziness in the subglottic area. This is the swollen laryngeal and tracheal tissue and is sometimes obvious enough to be called the "pencil sign" or "steeple sign." This is seen when the usually blunt end of the trachea at the vocal cords is thinned to a narrow point by the swollen mucous membrane. (Fig. 1-36 shows subglottic edema and Fig. 1-37 shows a lateral neck radiograph image of this problem.)

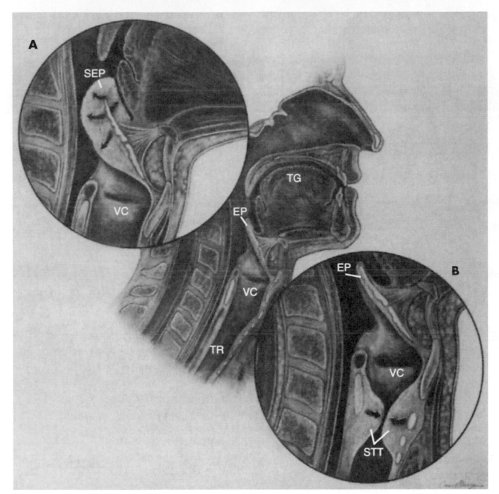

Fig. 1-36 A drawing of the normal upper airway is shown in the middle. Contrast it with: **A,** epiglottitis and **B,** laryngotracheobronchitis (croup). *TG,* tongue; *EP,* epiglottis; *VC,* vocal chords; *TR,* trachea; *SEP,* swollen epiglottis; *STT,* swollen trachea tissue. (From Des Jardins TR: *Clinical manifestations of respiratory disease,* ed 2, St Louis, 1990, Mosby.)

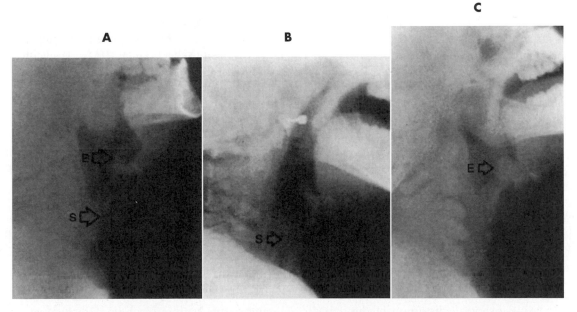

Fig. 1-37 Lateral neck radiographs on children showing: **A,** normal upper airway during an inspiration; **B,** laryngotracheobronchitis (croup) showing haziness of the subglottic trachea from mucosal edema; **C,** epiglottitis with a swollen, rounded epiglottis. Areas marked *E* show the epiglottis; areas marked *S* show the subglottic trachea. (From Williams JL: Radiographic evaluations. In Koff PB, Eitzman DV, Neu J, editors: *Neonatal and pediatric respiratory care,* St. Louis, 1988, Mosby.)

TABLE 1-18	General History and Physical Findings of Laryngotracheobronchitis (LTB) and Epiglottitis	
Clinical finding	LTB	Epiglottitis
Age	3-36 mo	2-4 yr
Onset	Slow (24-48 hr)	Abrupt (2-4 hr)
Fever	Absent	Present
Drooling	Absent	Present
Lateral neck radiograph	Haziness in subglottic area	Haziness in supraglottic area
Inspiratory stridor	High pitched and loud	Low pitched and muffled
Hoarseness	Present	Absent
Swallowing difficulty	Absent	Present
White blood cell count	Normal (viral)	Elevated (bacterial)

From Des Jardins TR: *Clinical manifestations of respiratory disease*, ed 2, St Louis, 1990, Mosby-Year Book.

 EXAM HINT

A past version of the Clinical Simulation Examination included a problem with a pediatric patient in which the differential diagnosis between croup and epiglottitis had to be made. The care of the patient was then tested.

c. Look for the presence and position of any foreign bodies (Code: IB8b) [Difficulty: An]

The history of sudden breathing difficulty, cough, and inspiratory stridor combined with a physical examination of the patient usually points to aspiration. A lateral neck radiograph and/or P-A or A-P chest and neck radiograph often helps to confirm the presence and position of a foreign body. See Fig. 1-14 for an A-P chest and neck radiograph image. The clearly seen solid white shape of the foreign body indicates that the object is metallic (a coin).

d. Look for any airway narrowing (Code: IB8c) [Difficulty: An]

Plastic toy pieces and foods such as peanuts are much harder to see on a neck radiograph than metallic objects because their densities are closer to those found in the body. It is easier to identify obstructing plastic toys or food by looking for a narrowing or distortion of the dark air column of the upper airway and trachea.

Airway narrowing can also be caused by a tumor. This can be either a growth within the lumen of the airway or a growth from outside of the trachea or bronchi that forces it to collapse.

 EXAM HINT

The Written Registry Exam has usually included one question that tested some aspect of fetal, neonatal, or pediatric patient assessment.

MODULE I	Determine and continue to monitor how the patient responds to the treatment or procedure

1. **Determine the patient's vital signs (Code: IIIA1d) [Difficulty: An]**

2. **Monitor the patient's heart rhythm (Code: IIIA1d [Difficulty: An]**

3. **Auscultate the patient's breath sounds and interpret any changes (Code: IIIA1k) [Difficulty: An]**

4. **Recommend and review a chest radiograph, as needed, to help determine the patient's condition (Code: IIIA1a) [Difficulty: An]**

5. **Perform bedside spirometry (Code: IIIA1e) [Difficulty: An]**

6. **Look for changes in the patient's sputum production or consistency (Code: IIIA1c) [Difficulty: An]**

7. **Recommend the measurement of the patient's electrolytes, hemoglobin, complete blood count, and/or other chemistry values (Code: IIIA1g) [Difficulty: R, Ap, An]**

All of the preceding topics have been discussed earlier in this chapter. Review them as necessary. They will need to be applied to all respiratory care procedures as presented in the following chapters.

8. **Evaluate the patient's fluid balance (intake and output)**
   a. Perform and/or measure intake and output (Code: IB9e and IC1d)[Difficulty: R, Ap, An]

Intake and output (I and O) should be approximately equal in the normal person with a properly functioning heart and kidneys. Insensible water loss through perspiration and breathing are usually ignored in adults because the amount lost is relatively small and can only be estimated. Insensible water loss is a risk in the low birth weight infant. Prevent this by keeping the infant's environmental temperature within 1° of its body temperature (neutral thermal environment or NTE). Oxygen should be humidified.

Any patient who has a history of heart or kidney problems or who has a current serious cardiopulmonary disorder should have intake and output monitored closely.

Do this by adding all the patient's intake (oral, intravenous, etc.) and output (urine, blood work, etc.) for each 8-hour shift. See Box 1-4 for the normal adult's values for fluid intake and urine output and Table 1-4 for urine specific gravity and other urinalysis information.

b. Interpret the results of intake and output (Code: IC2d) [Difficulty: R, Ap, An]

The dehydrated patient will likely show some or all of the following signs and symptoms: tachycardia, hypotension, high urine specific gravity, oliguria (low urine output), low central venous pressure (CVP) and pulmonary capillary wedge (PCWP) pressure readings, tenting of the skin when pinched, and mental confusion. This patient needs more fluid.

The fluid overloaded patient will likely show some or all of the following signs and symptoms: tachycardia, hypertension, low urine specific gravity, increased urine output, increased CVP and PCWP readings, peripheral edema in the dependent parts of the body, and pulmonary edema with crackles/rales. This patient needs to be fluid- and sodium-restricted. In addition, diuretics help to rapidly increase urine output. Remember that the loss of one liter of fluid results in the patient losing one kilogram (2.2 pounds) of weight.

MODULE J	Respiratory care plan

1. Review the interdisciplinary patient and family care plan (Code: IC3c)[Difficulty: An]

It is beyond the scope of the text to discuss the various cardiopulmonary conditions and disorders for which respiratory therapists provide care. However, the NBRC is known to ask questions on cardiopulmonary pathologic findings. It is recommended that time be taken to study care plans that relate to the most common disorders such as asthma, COPD, pneumonia, pneumothorax, and heart disease.

2. Participate in the development of the respiratory care plan (e.g., case management, develop and apply protocols, disease management education) (Code: IC4) [Difficulty: An]

The respiratory therapist should be a member of the patient care team of the physician, nurse, and others in deciding how to best care for the patient. Be prepared to use the information contained in this section and the rest of the text to help you make decisions on how to care for your patients. The NBRC will ask questions that relate to the best recommendations for care. The following steps are necessary in the respiratory care plan for any patient:

1. Determine an expected outcome or goal(s).
2. Develop a plan to achieve success.

BOX 1-4	Fluid Intake and Urine Output for Normal Adults

Normal, minimal daily water requirement for an adult patient is about 1500-2000 mL
Average urine output is 0.5-1 mL/kg/hr
Polyuria is a urine output of more than 1500 mL/hr
Oliguria is a urine output of less than 400 mL in 24 hr
Anuria is a urine output of less than 100 mL in 24 hr

---

3. Decide how to measure the patient's achievement of the goal.
4. Plan a timeline to measure the patient's progress.
5. Document the patient's response to care and the final outcome.

3. Communicate results of therapy to members of the patient care team and adjust therapy based on respiratory care protocol(s) (Code: IIIA2d) [Difficulty: An]

MODULE K	Record any treatment(s) and/or procedure(s) on the patient's chart and communicate with the other members of the health-care team

1. Record in conventional terminology, as needed, any treatment(s) and procedure(s) performed, including the date, time, frequency of therapy, medication, and ventilatory data (Code: IIIA2a) [Difficulty: An]

2. Apply computer technology to patient management (electronic charting and patient care algorithms) (Code: IIIA2c) [Difficulty: An]

3. Record and evaluate the patient's response to the treatment(s) and procedure(s), including:

a. Record heart rate and rhythm, respiratory rate, blood pressure, and body temperature (Code: IIIA2a3 and IIIA2a4) [Difficulty: An]

b. Record the patient's breath sounds (Code: IIIA2a2) [Difficulty: An]

c. Record the type of cough the patient has and the nature of the sputum (Code: IIIA2a2) [Difficulty: An]

d. Record any adverse reactions the patient had to the treatment(s) and procedure(s) (Code: IIIA2a1) [Difficulty: An]

e. Record and evaluate the patient's subjective feelings and reaction to the treatment(s) and/or procedure(s) (Code: IIIA1c and IIIA2a1) [Difficulty: An]

These topics were discussed previously in this chapter and will be covered again in later chapters.

4. Recheck any math work and make note of incorrect data (Code: IIIA2b) [Difficulty: An]

Errors made in charting must be corrected by drawing a single mark through the error and writing in the correct information. Some prefer that the error be further clarified by writing in "error" next to it and adding your initials. *Never* erase or use any covering material over an error.

BIBLIOGRAPHY

Aloan CA, Hill TV, editors: *Respiratory care of the newborn and child*, ed 2, Philadelphia, 1997, Lippincott-Raven.

Barkauskas VH, Stoltenberg-Allen K, Baumann LC, Darling-Fisher C: *Health & physical assessment*, St Louis, 1994, Mosby.

Barnes TA, editor: *Core textbook of respiratory care practice*, ed 2, St Louis, 1994, Mosby.

Barnhart SL, Czervinske MP: *Perinatal and pediatric respiratory care*. Philadelphia, 1995, WB Saunders.

Burton GC, Hodgkin JE, Ward JJ, editors: *Respiratory care: a guide to clinical practice*, ed 4, Philadelphia, 1997, Lippincott-Raven.

Carlo, C: *Neonatal respiratory care*, St Louis, 1988, Mosby.

Cherniack RM, Cherniack L: *Respiration in health and disease*, ed 3, Philadelphia, 1983, WB Saunders.

Clochesy JM, Breu C, Cardin S, Whittaker AA, Rudy EB, editors: *Critical care nursing*, ed 2, Philadelphia, 1996, WB Saunders.

Daily EK, Schroeder JS: *Techniques in bedside hemodynamic monitoring*, ed 4, St Louis, 1989, Mosby.

Des Jardins TR: *Clinical manifestations of respiratory disease*, ed 2, St Louis, 1990, Mosby.

DiPietro JS, Mustard MN: *Clinical guide for respiratory care practitioners*, Norwalk, CN, 1987, Appleton & Lange.

Erickson B: *Heart sounds and murmurs—a practical guide*, ed 3. St Louis, 1997, Mosby.

Eubanks DH, Bone RC: *Comprehensive respiratory care*. St Louis, 1985, Mosby.

Fink JB, Hunt GE, editors: *Clinical practice in respiratory care*. Philadelphia, 1999, Lippincott-Raven.

Hess DR, Kacmarek RM: *Essentials of mechanical ventilation*. New York, 1996, McGraw-Hill.

Kacmarek RM, Mack CW, Dimas S: *The essentials of respiratory therapy*, ed 3, St Louis, 1990, Mosby.

Kenner CV, Guzzetta CE, Dossey BM: *Critical care nursing: body-mind-spirit*. Boston, 1981, Little, Brown.

Koff PB, Eitzman DV, Neu J, editors: *Neonatal and pediatric respiratory care*, ed 2, St Louis, 1993, Mosby.

Lehrer S: *Understanding lung sounds*, Philadelphia, 1984, WB Saunders.

Levitsky MG, Cairo JM, Hall SM: *Introduction to respiratory care*, Philadelphia, 1990, WB Saunders.

Oblouk DG: *Hemodynamic monitoring: invasive and noninvasive clinical monitoring*, Philadelphia, 1987, WB Saunders.

Pagana KD, Pagana TJ: *Manual of diagnostic and laboratory tests*. St Louis, 1998, Mosby.

Peters RM: Chest trauma. In Moser KM, Spragg RG, editors: *Respiratory emergencies*, ed 2, St Louis, 1982, Mosby.

Rau JL, Pearce DJ: *Understanding chest radiographs*, Denver, 1984, Multi-Media Publishing.

Scanlan CL, Wilkins RL, Stoller JK, editors: *Egan's fundamentals of respiratory care*, ed 7, St Louis, 1999, Mosby.

Shapiro BA, Kacmarek RM, Cane RD, et al, editors: *Clinical Application of Respiratory Care*, ed 4, St Louis, 1991, Mosby.

Stillwell SB, McCarter RE: *Pocket guide to cardiovascular care*, ed 2, St Louis, 1994, Mosby.

Tilkian AG, Boudreau CM: *Understanding heart sounds and murmurs*, ed 2, Philadelphia, 1984, WB Saunders.

Whitaker K: *Comprehensive perinatal & pediatric respiratory care*, ed 2, Albany, NY, 1997, Delmar.

Wilkins RL, Hodgkin JE, Lopez B: *Lung sounds: a practical guide*, St Louis, 1988, Mosby.

Wilkins RL, Krider SJ, Sheldon RL: *Clinical assessment in respiratory care*, ed 3, St Louis, 1995, Mosby.

SELF-STUDY QUESTIONS

1. An adult patient with a smoking history has shown an increased anteroposterior diameter and depressed hemidiaphragms on a P-A chest radiograph. It is most likely that the patient:
   A. Has pulmonary fibrosis.
   B. Has emphysema.
   C. Would have normal findings if an A-P chest radiograph were taken.
   D. Has left ventricular failure.

2. Following 2 days of vomiting and diarrhea caused by the flu, a 50-year-old patient is admitted. Her ECG shows five PVCs in 1 minute and flat T waves. What laboratory test would you recommend?
   A. Urinalysis
   B. Arterial blood gas analysis
   C. Electrolytes
   D. Complete blood count

3. A 48-year-old patient with an extensive smoking history usually coughs out about 20 mL of sputum every day. He developed a "chest cold" 4 days ago and has noticed increased shortness of breath and thicker secretions. What should be done at this time?
   A. Have him increase the flow on his home oxygen concentrator.
   B. Get a sputum sample for a culture and sensitivity study.
   C. Have him perform a 6-minute walk test.
   D. Perform percussion to determine the hemidiaphragm positions.

4. A recently home-delivered baby is brought in to the Emergency Department by the paramedics. The physician asks you to help evaluate its condition. Normal vital signs for a term newborn include all of the following *except*:
   A. Heart rate of 130/min.
   B. Rectal temperature of 36.5° C.
   C. Blood pressure of 64/40 mm Hg.
   D. Respiratory rate of 20/min.

5. You are assisting with the delivery of a high-risk infant. After evaluating the infant, you give him a 1-minute APGAR score of 8 and recommend that the assisting nurse and physician:
   A. Give the infant supplemental oxygen.
   B. Give the mother supplemental oxygen.
   C. Begin bag-mask rescue breathing on the infant.
   D. Give the infant to the mother as soon as possible for bonding.

6. You are called to the Pediatrics Department to help in the evaluation and care of a 4-year-old girl who has been sick with a bad cold for the last 2 days. The nurse shows you a lateral neck radiograph of the child and asks for your opinion. You notice a clear air column through the upper airway but a pointed narrowing of the tracheal air column below the larynx. You tell the nurse that you suspect the child has:
   A. Laryngotracheobronchitis.
   B. Aspirated a coin.
   C. Epiglottitis.
   D. Bilateral upper lobe pneumonia.

7. A young adult who had surgery for a deviated nasal septum was accidentally given 2 liters of intravenous fluid in 1 hour. Which of the following signs cause you suspect that the patient is fluid overloaded?
   I. Tachycardia
   II. Bradycardia
   III. High urine specific gravity
   IV. Peripheral edema in the dependent parts of the body
   V. Low urine specific gravity
   A. I, IV, and V only
   B. III and IV only
   C. I and III only
   D. II and V only

8. Patients with heart or lung disease commonly have shifting of mediastinal structures. In evaluating cardiopulmonary disease patients, which of the following could result in a mediastinal shift being seen on a chest radiograph?
   I. Right hemothorax
   II. Bilateral lower lobe pneumonia
   III. Left tension pneumothorax
   IV. Right lower lobe atelectasis
   V. Fibrosis of the left lung
   A. III only
   B. IV and V only
   C. I, II, and III only
   D. I, III, IV, and V only

9. The radiologist remarks to you during the viewing of a 65-year-old patient's posteroanterior (P-A) chest radiograph film that the patient has an enlarged left side of the heart. This indicates to you that:
   A. The patient has an athletic heart.
   B. The patient has a left pleural effusion.
   C. The patient has an abnormal heart.
   D. The patient has a left middle lobe infiltrate.

10. A patient is suffering from acute respiratory distress syndrome (ARDS) and is significantly hypoxemic. It is likely that the patient will exhibit all the following *except*:
    A. A normal respiratory rate.
    B. Nasal flaring.
    C. Intercostal retractions.
    D. Use of accessory muscles of inspiration.

11. An adult patient with a history of COPD and left ventricular failure has been hospitalized. A series of diagnostic procedures are being performed. The preferred radiographic position to minimize distortion of the heart is:
    A. Anteroposterior.
    B. Posteroanterior.
    C. Lateral.
    D. Oblique.

12. An intubated patient has been moved from the Operating Room to the Intensive Care Unit. There is a concern that the endotracheal tube has been moved. What is the best way to determine its location?
    A. Palpate the larynx
    B. Listen to breath sounds
    C. Percuss the patient's chest
    D. Get a chest radiograph

13. A 65-year-old patient with repeated episodes of congestive heart failure has a chest radiograph taken. It shows the left costophrenic angle to be blunted and an air/fluid level with a meniscus around the left lower lung area. How should this be interpreted?
    A. Pleural effusion of the left lung
    B. Pulmonary edema of the left lung
    C. Pneumonia of the left lung
    D. Pulmonary embolism of the left lung

Answer Key

1. **B.** Rationale: Patients with emphysema will usually have chest radiograph findings of increased anteroposterior diameter, depressed hemidiaphragms, and widened intercostal spaces that result from enlarged lungs caused by air trapping. If the patient had pulmonary fibrosis, the lungs would be small rather than enlarged. If the patient had an A-P chest radiograph (rather than P-A) the lung finding would not be significantly changed. However, the heart size would be enlarged. The reported radiograph findings relate to lung problems, not heart problems. There is no report of the heart being enlarged or out of position.

2. **C.** Rationale: Severe vomiting and diarrhea can result in the significant loss of fluids and electrolytes. Her cardiac problems are likely the result of this. If an electrolyte abnormality is found, it needs to be promptly corrected by intravenous replacement. A urinalysis will be helpful for the evaluation of the patient's kidneys but is not needed at this time. An arterial blood gas analysis will be helpful to determine if the patient's acid-base balance is altered. However, it is not needed at this time because it will not guide the patient's clinical management. A complete blood count will not reveal any information that will guide the patient's care related to her cardiac arrhythmia.

3. **B.** Rationale: The patient's history plus recent illness and worsening symptoms indicate a pulmonary infection. It is important to get a sputum sample for a culture and sensitivity study to determine the infectious organism and the antibiotic to fight it. Although the patient's illness may make him hypoxic, there is no information that he has a home oxygen concentrator. A 6-minute walk test would cause unnecessary stress on the patient at this time. It will surely make him feel more short of breath. Although it may be interesting to know the position of the patient's hemidiaphragms, this will not help him with the current problem. This procedure can be done later if indicated.

4. **D.** Rationale: A normal term newborn should have a respiratory rate of 30 to 60/min. All of the other listed vital signs are normal for a term newborn. Review Table 1-11 if needed.

5. **D.** Rationale: An APGAR score of 8 (out of a maximum of 10) indicates that the newborn is in good condition and can be given to its mother. Review Table 1-17 for the scoring of the five Apgar signs. Because the newborn is in good condition, there is no need to give it or the mother oxygen or begin bag-mask rescue breathing.

6. **A.** Rationale: Laryngotracheobronchitis (croup) is a swelling of the mucous membrane below the vocal cords (subglottic area). This is often identified by a narrowing of the dark air column below the vocal cords. This pointed narrowing is sometimes referred to as the steeple sign or pencil sign. See Fig. 1-37. If the patient had aspirated a coin, a solid shape would be seen. See Fig. 1-14. In addition, the patient with an aspiration problem has a history of a sudden problem, not being sick for two days. Epiglottitis is a swelling of the airway above the vocal cords (supraglottic area). The upper airway radiograph will show haziness in the throat area with a normal tracheal air column. See Fig. 1-37. Bilateral upper lobe pneumonia will present on a chest radiograph as white shadows over both upper lung fields. The airway should show a normal, dark air column.

7. **A.** Rationale: The young, healthy heart usually responds to a fluid overload situation by increasing its rate (tachycardia). The excessive intravenous fluid tends to leak out of the capillaries into the tissues in the dependent parts of the body such as the feet and lower legs. The kidneys quickly put out the extra fluids, and a low urine specific gravity is found. It is highly unlikely that the heart will slow down (bradycardia) in a fluid overload situation. Rather than a high urine specific gravity indicating low urine output, the kidneys put out extra fluid resulting in a low urine specific gravity.

8. **D.** Rationale: A right hemothorax pushes the mediastinum to the opposite side. A left tension pneumothorax pushes the mediastinum to the opposite side. Right lower lobe atelectasis pulls the mediastinum to the affected side. Fibrosis of the left lung pulls the mediastinum to the affected side. Review Fig. 1-6 if needed. If a patient has bilateral lower lobe pneumonia, both lungs are affected. Therefore, there will be no shifting of the lungs or the mediastinum.

9. **C.** Rationale: An enlarged left side of the heart on a 65-year-old patient is abnormal. The patient should be evaluated for left ventricular failure. An athletic heart is not significantly enlarged compared with a normal-sized heart. What makes it "athletic" is that it can pump more effectively with a higher-than-normal stroke volume. A left pleural

effusion is identified by an obscured left costophrenic angle; there may also be a pleural air-fluid level. A left middle lobe infiltrate will have a distinctive shadow over the affected lung area, not the heart. See Fig. 1-9.

10. **A.** Rationale: It is highly unlikely that a patient with ARDS, which results in small and stiff lungs, and significant hypoxemia would be breathing with a normal respiratory rate. A patient with these serious problems will likely show nasal flaring (to reduce airway resistance), intercostal retractions (because of the stiff lungs), and use of accessory muscles of inspiration (to assist the diaphragm in breathing).

11. **B.** Rationale: The posteroanterior (P-A) position has the radiographs penetrating from the back to the front of the patient. Because the heart is located behind the sternum, there is less distortion of its actual size on the radiograph. With the anteroposterior (A-P) position, the radiographs penetrate from the front to the back of the patient. This results in the heart's shadow being abnormally enlarged on the film. The lateral and oblique chest radiograph views are indicated to help find the location of a tumor or other lung lesion. These views are not that useful in evaluating a patient with COPD and left ventricular failure.

12. **D.** Rationale: It is best to get a chest radiograph because the film will show whether the endotracheal tube is within the trachea (or esophagus or a mainstem bronchus) and where the tip of the tube is located within the trachea. Listening to breath sounds (or their absence) is the next best method to determine the tube's location. However, breath sounds alone will not reveal where the tip of the tube is located within the trachea. Palpation of the larynx can be used during the initial intubation to confirm that the endotracheal tube has entered the trachea. It cannot be used to determine tube tip location within the trachea. Percussion of the patient's chest will not help determine endotracheal tube location. Abnormal sounds can be from a variety of problems. See Table 1-14 if needed.

13. **A.** Rationale: Both the blunting of the left costophrenic angle and the air/fluid level with a meniscus are consistent with a left pleural effusion (fluid in the intrapleural space). The patient's history also confirms this problem. Pulmonary edema or pneumonia of the left lung is seen on the radiograph film as a distinctive shadow within the lung field, not around it. Occasionally a pulmonary embolism results in a fluid leak within the lung and a localized shadow within the lung field, not around it.

2 | Infection Control

A review of the most recent Written Registry Exams has shown an average of one or two questions (1% to 2% of the exam) covering infection control issues.

MODULE A   Decontaminate respiratory care equipment

Decontamination is the process of disassembling, washing to remove debris, rinsing, and disinfecting or sterilizing used patient care equipment. The process frees the equipment of any pathogens so that it can be used with another patient. Obviously, once disinfected, the equipment must be aseptically reassembled and stored for future use.

1. Choose the appropriate agent and method for disinfection and sterilization (Code: IIA2) [Difficulty: An]

EXAM HINT

Typically, one question asks about the best disinfectant agent to use in a patient's home. In every question variation, the best answer was either acetic acid, 0.45 acetic acid, or white vinegar. Remember that white vinegar contains 0.45% acetic acid. Or, a question might deal with disinfecting or sterilizing respiratory care equipment in a hospital, or monitoring the effectiveness of these procedures.

a. Disinfection

Disinfection is a procedure that significantly reduces the microbial contamination of the equipment that has been processed. All disinfection processes destroy the vegetative form (the cell) of pathogenic organisms. This includes the vast majority of respiratory system pathogens. However, a few *Bacillus*-type bacteria are difficult to kill because they have a particularly tough cell wall or have spores for reproduction. Spores are analogous to seeds in that they grow into bacteria under the right conditions and are resistant to drying, heat, and many chemicals that are used to kill the bacterial cell. Therefore a spore-forming organism may be able to reproduce itself after the cells have been killed. Obviously, disinfection can be used only on equipment that is *not* contaminated by spore-forming bacteria. It is important, if possible, to know what pathogen has infected the patient so that the appropriate disinfection (or sterilization) method can be used on the contaminated equipment. As will be noted, some disinfecting agents kill different kinds of organisms, depending on the length of time that they are exposed.

Another consideration in selecting the appropriate disinfection method is how the equipment will be used in patient care. Equipment or instruments that do not directly touch the patient (for example, an electrocardiograph machine) are classified as *noncritical* (low risk of spreading infection) and can undergo low-level disinfection. Low-level disinfectants are agents that are capable of killing some vegetative bacteria, fungi, and lipophilic viruses. Equipment or instruments that touch surface mucous membranes and the skin but do not penetrate them (for example, laryngoscope blades and a bronchoscope) are listed as *semicritical* and must undergo high-level disinfection. Agents that kill all microorganisms except bacterial spores are classified as *high-level* disinfectants.

A third consideration in choosing the best disinfection method is the type of equipment that needs to be decontaminated. Certain processes and agents can be used only on certain types of equipment. Table 2-1 lists the various ways to disinfect reusable patient care equipment decontaminated in the hospital.

b. Sterilization

Sterilization is a procedure that destroys all living microbial organisms and renders them unable to reproduce. All sterilization procedures destroy the vegetative forms and spores of all microscopic organisms. Examples of spore-forming bacteria include *Bacillus anthracis* (anthrax), *Clostridium botulinum* (botulism), *Clostridium tetani* (tetanus), and *Clostridium perfringens* (gas gangrene). Any equipment or instruments that penetrate body tissue are listed as "critical" (high risk of spreading infection) and must be sterilized before use on another patient (for example, a surgical scalpel). As discussed, the method of sterilization depends on the type of equipment under consideration. Table 2-2 lists the various methods of sterilization for reusable supplies and patient care equipment that are decontaminated in the hospital.

1. Disinfect or sterilize respiratory care equipment (Code: IIA2) [Difficulty: An]

As discussed, the choice of whether to disinfect or sterilize equipment depends on how it is used clinically, the type of pathogen involved, and from what the equipment is made. Most respiratory pathogens are not spore-formers, so low-level or high-level disinfection is acceptable. Either a glutaraldehyde solution or pasteurization is used in most departments for disinfecting plastic masks, hoses, and so forth.

Any department that processes its own equipment

TABLE 2-1	Methods of Disinfection

| Method | Conditions | Microbes effective against | | | | | Comments |
		Bacteria	TB	Spores	Viruses	Fungi	
Pasteurization	Complete immersion in water heated to 70° C (170° F) for 30 min	Yes	Yes	No	Yes	Yes	Used with rubber and many plastics used in respiratory care, especially those that are sensitive to a high temperature. **Avoid use** with any item that cannot be immersed or will be damaged at this temperature.
GLUTARALDEHYDE SOLUTIONS							
Alkaline glutaraldehyde (Cidex, Cidex 7, Sporicidin)	Complete immersion for 10 min	Yes	Yes	No	Yes	Yes	Used with rubber and many plastics used in respiratory care, especially those that are heat sensitive. Care must be taken to thoroughly rinse items after disinfection. **Avoid use** with any item that cannot be immersed or will absorb the solution.
Acid glutaraldehyde (Sonacide)	Complete immersion for 20 min	Yes	Yes	No	Yes	Yes	Used with rubber and many plastics used in respiratory care, especially those that are heat sensitive. Care must be taken to thoroughly rinse items after being disinfected. **Avoid use** with any item that cannot be immersed or will absorb the solution.
Alcohols (70% ethyl or 90% isopropyl)	Complete immersion for several minutes or pooling of the alcohol on the equipment	Yes	Yes	No	Lipophilic only	Yes	Used with metallic or plastic surfaces of large pieces of equipment that cannot be disinfected by any other means. May also be used with most plastics. **Avoid use** with any item that cannot be immersed or will absorb or be damaged by the alcohol.
Iodines (Iodine or iodophor with 70% ethyl alcohol)	Complete immersion for several minutes or pooling of the solution on the equipment	Yes	Yes	No	Yes	Yes	Used with metallic or plastic surfaces of large pieces of equipment that cannot be disinfected by any other means. May also be used with most plastics. **Avoid use** with any item that cannot be immersed or will absorb or be damaged by the alcohol.

TB, Tuberculosis.

must have adequate facilities to do so. There must be a "dirty" area where contaminated equipment is brought for disassembly, scrubbing of secretions or blood, and rinsing. Then it is either placed into the glutaraldehyde solution or pasteurizing machine. After that, it is taken to a "clean" area to be rinsed, dried, reassembled, and placed into plastic bags for storage. Care must be taken not to recontaminate the equipment during this procedure. Items that must be sterilized are usually processed only through the "dirty" area before being sent to the Central Supply Department. There the equipment is sterilized based on the criteria shown in Table 2-2.

2. Monitor the sterilization process to ensure its effectiveness (Code: IIA2)[Difficulty: An]

The term *surveillance* describes the monitoring of equipment to be sure that the disinfection or sterilization process was successful and that in-use equipment is not a source of patient contamination. Processing (chemical) indicators are used to ensure that disinfection or steriliza-

TABLE 2-2	Methods of Sterilization	
Method	**Conditions**	**Comments**
Steam autoclave	Autoclave chamber with an internal steam pressure of 15 lb per sq in, 121° C (250° F), 15 min	Used with glass, cloth, bandages, unsharpened stainless steel instruments, and reusable ventilator bacteria filters. **Avoid use** with many plastics used in respiratory care, rubber, dextrose solutions, sharpened stainless steel instruments, electrical devices, or machines.
Dry heat	Autoclave chamber at 160°-180° C (320°-356° F), 2 hr use	Used with glass or sharpened stainless steel instruments. **Avoid use** with many plastics used in respiratory care, rubber, dextrose solutions, electric devices, or machines.
Ethylene oxide gas	Specific guidelines vary depending on the manufacturer of the chamber and the supplies or equipment being sterilized. In general a gas concentration of 800-1000 mg/L must be kept for 3-4 hr at 50%-100% relative humidity and 49°-57° C (120°-135° F). Great care must be taken to predry all items before gassing and to properly aerate them after sterilization.	Used with heat-sensitive and moisture-sensitive items like many plastics used in respiratory care. **Avoid use** with supply pouches or plastic films, such as aluminum foil, nylon, thermoplastic resin (Saran), Mylar, cellophane polyamide, polyester, or other films that are not penetrated by the gas, or with PVC that has been previously sterilized by the manufacturer with gamma radiation.
GLUTARALDEHYDE SOLUTIONS		
Alkaline glutaraldehyde (Cidex, Cidex 7, Sporicidin)	Complete immersion. Cidex products for 10 hr; Sporicidin for 6 hr and 45 min	Used with rubber and many plastics in respiratory care, especially those that are heat sensitive. Care must be taken to thoroughly rinse items after being cleaned. **Avoid use** with any item that cannot be immersed or that will absorb the solution.
Acid glutaraldehyde (Sonacide)	Complete immersion for 1 hr at 60° C (140° F)	Used with rubber and many plastics used in respiratory care, especially those that are heat sensitive. Care must be taken to thoroughly rinse items after being cleaned. **Avoid use** with any item that cannot be immersed or will absorb the solution.

PVC, Polyvinyl chloride.

tion was done correctly. Examples of chemical indicators include special tapes used to hold the wrapping around packages of equipment being autoclaved or placed into ethylene oxide. These tapes turn color when the autoclave has reached the proper temperature or the correct concentration of ethylene oxide has been reached. The color change shows the user that the package was processed correctly. The assumption can then be made that the package's contents are sterile.

Another example is a biologic indicator that is placed into the wrapped package before it is sterilized. These biologic indicators are bacterial spores that are killed only if the required conditions are met. For example, the spores of *Bacillus subtilis* are placed onto strips of paper to be killed by ethylene oxide gas. After the equipment and spores have been sent through the sterilization process, the spores are placed into conditions favorable for growth. If no growth

occurs, they are dead. It can then be concluded that no other living organisms survived.

Equipment that is held in storage or is being used in patient care is also randomly sampled for contamination. There are three ways that a sample is taken for culturing of possible organisms. The first involves wiping an equipment surface with a sterile swab. The swab is then rubbed over a plate of growth medium or placed into a tube of liquid broth. The second method, used to check inside lengths of tubing, requires pouring a liquid broth through the tube and into a sterile container. The third involves sampling the aerosol that a nebulizer produces. Usually, a hose is attached to the outlet of the nebulizer. The other end of the hose is connected to a funnel that is attached to a culture plate where the droplets impact. In all three examples, the growth of any organism in the growth medium indicates a form of contamination. The laboratory then determines if the organism is pathogenic. If it is, measures must be taken to improve the disinfection or sterilization process.

BIBLIOGRAPHY

American Respiratory Care Foundation: Guidelines for disinfection of respiratory care equipment used in the home, *Respir Care* 33:801-808, 1988.

Ayerst Laboratories, New York, New York, information on Cidex products.

Bennington JJ: *Saunders dictionary & encyclopedia of laboratory medicine and technology*, Philadelphia, 1984, WB Saunders.

Eubanks DH, Bone RC: *Comprehensive respiratory care*, ed 2, St Louis, 1990, Mosby.

Fink JB: Infection Control and Safety. In Fink JB, Hunt GE, editors: *Clinical practice in respiratory care*, Philadelphia, 1999, Lippincott, Williams & Wilkins.

Guidelines for the prevention of nosocomial infections, *AARTimes*, 49-52, September 1983.

Infection Control Precautions from OSF Saint Anthony Medical Center, Rockford, IL, 1998.

Pagana KD, Pagana TJ: *Mosby's manual of diagnostic and laboratory tests*, St Louis, 1998, Mosby.

Scanlan CL: Principles of infection control. In Scanlan CL, Wilkins RL, Stoller JK, editors: *Egan's fundamentals of respiratory care*, ed 7, St Louis, 1999, Mosby.

The Sporicidin Company, Washington, DC, product information on Sporicidin.

Surgikos, Arlington, Texas, product information on Sonacide.

Washington JA: Infectious disease aspects of respiratory therapy. In Burton GG, Hodgkin JE, Ward JJ, editors: Respiratory care, ed 4, Philadelphia, 1997, Lippincott-Raven Publishers.

SELF-STUDY QUESTIONS

1. A hospitalized patient who recovered from a *Clostridium botulinum* infection received several respiratory care services. How should a nondisposable large-volume nebulizer be sterilized before being reused?
   A. Steam autoclave for 15 minutes
   B. Glutaraldehyde solution soak for 10 hours
   C. Pasteurize for 20 minutes
   D. Soak in an alcohol solution for 15 minutes

2. Select all of the following that can be used in the home to reduce the chance of bacterial growth in a small-volume nebulizer or other respiratory care equipment.
   I. Soak the equipment in white vinegar.
   II. Put the equipment in the oven and turn on the broiler for 10 minutes.
   III. Rinse a nebulizer in sterile, distilled water after each use.
   IV. Wash the equipment in warm, soapy water once a day.
   A. I, III, IV
   B. I, II
   C. III, IV
   D. I, II, III, IV

3. After a mechanical ventilator has been discontinued, what is the best method to sterilize the reusable main-flow bacteria filter?
   A. Wrap it and soak it in acetic acid
   B. Pasteurization
   C. Glutaraldehyde soak
   D. Steam autoclaving

4. A batch of respiratory care equipment has gone through the gas sterilization process with ethylene oxide. Routine surveillance of the equipment shows that spores of *Bacillus subtilis* have survived the process. What should be done next?
   A. Use the equipment, because this organism does not cause illness.
   B. Aerate the gas as usual and put into use.
   C. Resterilize the equipment and check for death of the spores.
   D. Wipe off the equipment with 70% alcohol to remove the spores from the equipment.

5. A retired home-care patient living on a fixed income needs to be able to disinfect her respiratory therapy equipment. Which of the following would be best for her?
   A. Acetic acid
   B. Acid glutaraldehyde
   C. Ethylene oxide system
   D. Warm, soapy water

6. What is the most cost effective way for a respiratory care department to disinfect large amounts of reusable plastic tubing and oxygen masks?
   A. 70% ethyl alcohol
   B. Steam autoclave
   C. Pasteurization
   D. Dry heat

7. A contaminated Bennett PR-II IPPB (intermittent positive-pressure breathing) unit needs to be sterilized before use with another patient. What is the best method?
   A. Pasteurization
   B. Ethylene oxide
   C. 10-hour soak in glutaraldehyde
   D. Steam autoclave

Answer Key

1. **B.** Rationale: A glutaraldehyde solution soak for 10 hours is the only way listed to sterilize plastic equipment without damaging it. Putting plastic equipment into a steam autoclave causes it to melt and be destroyed. Pasteurization or soaking the equipment in an alcohol solution disinfects, but does not sterilize the equipment as needed.

2. **A.** Rationale: The heat generated in an oven under the broiler will melt plastic used in a small-volume nebulizer and other respiratory care equipment. Washing the equipment in warm, soapy water and rinsing in sterile, distilled water helps to remove secretions or other debris. Soaking the equipment in white vinegar kills some of the microorganisms found on it.

3. **D.** Rationale: Steam autoclaving is the only method listed that is acceptable to sterilize a ventilator's bacteria filter. Review Table 2-2 if needed. The other three options involve solutions that will damage the filter medium and make the filter useless.

4. **C.** Rationale: The equipment needs to be resterilized because living spores of *Bacillus subtilis* indicate that the sterilization process was not successful. Other microbes may also have survived. Because of this concern, the equipment should not be used. Aeration of the equipment will not sterilize it, and 70% alcohol will not remove the spores from the equipment or sterilize it.

5. **A.** Rationale: Acetic acid is found in white vinegar. It is inexpensive and available in any grocery store. Realize that acetic acid is not a powerful disinfectant and does not kill most pulmonary pathogens. Acid glutaraldehyde and ethylene oxide system are too expensive to use in a home. Warm, soapy water can be used to clean secretions from equipment but does not disinfect it.

6. **C.** Rationale: Pasteurization is the least expensive way to disinfect large amounts of the plastic equipment used in respiratory care departments. Steam autoclave and dry heat are used to sterilize, not disinfect, equipment. In addition, the high temperatures used with these methods melts the plastic tubing and oxygen masks. Seventy percent ethyl alcohol is used only to wipe off the surfaces of large equipment items for disinfection.

7. **B.** Rationale: Ethylene oxide gas should be used on an IPPB machine because it sterilizes the unit without causing any damage. Pasteurization and glutaraldehyde involve solutions that damage the internal structures of any IPPB machine. The heat of steam autoclaving melts any plastic or rubber components of the unit and seriously damages the machine.

3   Blood Gas Analysis and Monitoring

A review of the most recent Written Registry Examination has shown an average of six questions (6% of the exam) on blood gas analysis and monitoring.

MODULE A   **Make a recommendation to obtain a blood sample for blood gas analysis (Code: IA2e) [Difficulty: An]**

Blood can be sampled from a systemic artery, pulmonary artery, or "arterialized" capillary to determine a patient's oxygen and carbon dioxide pressures, acid-base status (pH), and related values. As is discussed later, a pulmonary artery sample is taken to learn a patient's mixed venous values, and an "arterialized" capillary sample is taken from a neonate when an arterial sample cannot be obtained. Arterial blood gas (ABG) is the term commonly used when discussing drawing a sample of blood from a patient's systemic artery.

There are three broad, general indications for this recommendation:

  a. To check a patient's oxygenation status (PaO_2)
  b. To check a patient's acid-base status (pH)
  c. To check a patient's ventilation status ($PaCO_2$)

Some specific indications follow.

1. Cardiac failure
  a. Congenital defect
  b. Heart attack (myocardial infarct)
  c. Congestive heart failure with or without pulmonary edema
2. Chronic obstructive pulmonary disease
  a. Asthma
  b. Emphysema
  c. Bronchitis
  d. Bronchiectasis
3. Any pneumonia causing hypoxemia
4. Trauma
  a. Broken ribs
  b. Flail chest
  c. Pneumothorax
  d. Hemothorax
  e. Upper airway trauma
5. Ventilatory failure
  a. Overdosage of sedatives or pain relievers
  b. Stroke or head (brain) injury
  c. Spinal cord injury
  d. Neuromuscular diseases such as myasthenia gravis or Guillain-Barré syndrome
6. Airway obstruction
  a. Foreign body aspiration
  b. Laryngotracheobronchitis (croup)
  c. Epiglottitis
7. Miscellaneous
  a. Smoke inhalation
  b. Carbon monoxide poisoning
  c. Near drowning
  d. Infant respiratory distress syndrome (RDS)/hyaline membrane disease
  e. Acute respiratory distress syndrome (ARDS)
  f. The patient does not have an indwelling arterial line
  g. A shunt or $P(A-a)O_2$ calculation must be made
  h. Cardiopulmonary resuscitation

MODULE B   **Obtain a blood sample**

---

1. Blood sampling device

a. Get the appropriate blood gas sampler (Code: IIA1h4) [Difficulty: An]

Obtaining an ABG sample generally involves selecting a prepackaged, sterile blood gas kit that contains the following:

1. Variety of short-bevel needles: 23 or 24 gauge for radial or dorsalis pedis puncture and a 22 gauge for brachial or femoral puncture.
2. 3 mL syringe. Many kits contain a syringe prepared with heparin as an anticoagulant.
3. If needed, liquid sodium or lithium heparin with an appropriate concentration.
4. Alcohol or iodophor (Betadine) wipes to clean the puncture site.

If a blood gas kit is not available, an appropriate individual needle, 3 mL syringe, and liquid sodium or lithium heparin must be obtained. These should be available at any nursing station or from the respiratory care department.

A capillary blood gas (CBG) sample requires the following:

1. Several heparinized glass capillary tubes with a volume of at least 100 µl
2. Metal filing (flea) to place into each capillary tube
3. Plastic caps or clay to seal the tubes
4. Magnet to draw the metal filing back and forth in the tube to mix the blood
5. Lancet to make incision
6. Moist, warm (42° C) cloth or diaper to wrap around the puncture site

7. Sterile cotton balls and bandage to place over the puncture site to aid clotting
8. Seventy percent isopropyl alcohol swabs to clean the puncture site
9. Clean gloves to protect the practitioner's hands from any contact with spilled blood

In addition, an ice-water mix in a cup is needed to chill the blood taken by any method.

b. Put the equipment together, make sure that it works properly, and identify any problems (Code: IIB1h4) [Difficulty: An]

To assemble a blood gas syringe, use sterile technique to screw the selected needle onto the syringe. If the syringe does not contain heparin, it must be added. Do this by aspirating liquid heparin through the needle into the syringe. Coat the inside of the syringe with heparin by tipping the needle up, pulling the plunger back, and pushing the plunger forward to squirt the excess heparin out of the needle. This ensures that the needle and dead space of the needle are filled with heparin, and the inside of the syringe is coated.

c. Perform quality control procedures for a blood gas sampling device (Code: IIB3a) [Difficulty: An]

A properly assembled sampling device should not create any problems with obtaining the blood sample. Quality control (QC) procedures for an arterial sampling device and steps that can be taken to correct a problem follow:

Make sure no air bubbles are in the syringe. Air bubbles result in the oxygen level and the pH being too high and the carbon dioxide level being too low. If an air bubble is found in the syringe, tilt it so that the needle is up. The bubble will rise by itself or may be raised by tapping the syringe. Push the plunger into the syringe to eject the air bubble. Cap off the hub of the syringe or needle to prevent air from entering the syringe.

Use the proper amount of heparin. This is a concern only when liquid heparin is added to a needle and syringe. Aspirate about 1 mL of 10 mg/mL or 1000 units/mL sodium heparin through the needle into the syringe. Pull the plunger back to coat the inside of the syringe. Push the plunger forward to squirt the excess heparin out through the needle. The values of a 2 to 4 mL sample of blood should not be affected by this concentration. Remember that inadequate heparin can cause the blood sample to clot. Excessive heparin can alter the blood gas values by lowering the pH and the carbon dioxide level and raising the oxygen level.

Promptly cool down the blood gas sample. If the sample cannot be analyzed within 10 minutes of being drawn, it should be placed in an ice water bath. Failure to do so results in the living blood consuming the available oxygen and producing carbon dioxide. Obviously, this results in incorrect measured values.

d. Fix any problems with a blood gas sampling device (Code: IIB2h4) [Difficulty: An]

Make sure that the needle is tightly screwed onto the syringe. The plunger should easily slide within the barrel of the syringe. A blood clot or debris within the needle plugs it and prevents this. Replace and safely dispose of a needle that is obstructed.

2. Arterial and umbilical artery line (catheter)

a. Recommend the insertion on an arterial line or umbilical artery line into a patient to obtain additional data (Code: IA2e) [Difficulty: An]

An arterial line is a short, flexible catheter that is placed into a peripheral artery for the purposes of sampling blood and/or continuously monitoring the patient's blood pressure. The procedure is explained in the following discussion. Chapter 5 contains a discussion on blood pressure monitoring and illustrations of how the monitoring system is assembled. The radial artery is the most common site for catheter insertion. Alternate arterial sites may be used if needed.

A newborn with a severe cardiopulmonary problem should have the catheter inserted into either of the umbilical arteries. This long catheter is then advanced into the aorta. If indicated, this should be done as quickly as possible after birth, before arterial spasm prevents the catheter from being advanced. Besides obtaining blood samples and monitoring the blood pressure, the newborn can be given glucose or a blood transfusion through the catheter.

b. Arterial catheters

1. Select the appropriate catheter (Code: IIA1q2) [Difficulty: R, Ap, An]

An adult's radial artery is usually catheterized. To do so, a needle covered with a flexible plastic catheter (an angiocatheter) is selected. Usually the needle is 23 or 24 gauge. After the angiocatheter is inserted into the artery, the needle is removed and the catheter is left in the artery.

A neonatal patient may have the umbilical vein or either umbilical artery catheterized. Usually, a long, flexible umbilical artery catheter (UAC) is placed into the patient. If the patient weighs more than 1250 grams, a 6 French (Fr) catheter is used; a 3.5 Fr catheter is used if the neonate weighs less than 1250 grams.

2. Put the equipment together, make sure that it works properly, and identify any problems (Code: IIB1q2) [Difficulty: R, Ap, An]

3. Fix any problems with the equipment (Code: IIB2q2) [Difficulty: R, Ap, An]

Arterial catheters come as a single unit in sterile packaging. Additional stopcocks, tubing, flush solution, and an automatic solution drip device are needed. These are discussed in Chapter 5 in some detail.

c. Obtain a blood sample from an arterial line (Code: IIIA1b) [Difficulty: An]

The steps for obtaining an arterial blood sample include the following:

1. Tell a conscious adult patient that you are going to take a blood sample from the arterial catheter.
2. Put gloves on both hands.
3. Remove the dead-ender cap from the sample (side) port on the three-way stopcock between the catheter and the intravenous (IV) tubing.
4. Screw a sterile 5 to 10 mL syringe to the sample port for removing the IV solution from the catheter. (A smaller syringe should be used for a neonate.)
5. Turn the stopcock off to the IV tubing. See Fig. 3-1.
6. Pull a waste sample of IV solution and blood into the syringe. (The amount withdrawn and discarded depends on the dead space volume from the tip of the catheter to the side port. Studies indicate that between 2.5 and 6 times this volume should be removed. Typically, this is about 5 mL in an adult, less in a neonate.)
7. Turn the stopcock off to all ports by turning it halfway between any two ports.
8. Attach a preheparinized sterile syringe to the sample port, turn the stopcock open to the syringe, and withdraw about 2 to 3 mL of arterial blood to be analyzed.
9. Turn the stopcock off to all ports by turning it halfway between any two ports.
10. Remove the blood sample syringe and cap off the syringe to seal it.
11. Roll the syringe to mix the heparin and place it into an ice water bath.
12. Turn the stopcock toward the catheter. Fast flush the IV solution so that any blood left in the sample port is forced out onto a sterile gauze pad.
13. Turn the stopcock toward the sample port so that the IV solution runs into the catheter.
14. Fast flush any blood in the catheter back into the patient.
15. Screw the dead-ender cap onto the sample port.
16. Remove and properly dispose of gloves and any other waste materials.

3. Perform an arterial puncture to obtain a blood sample for analysis (Code: IC1e and IIIA1b) [Difficulty: An]

There are a number of possible variations on the technique. The following is a general but thorough listing of the steps and any important related information.

    a. Check for a valid physician order.

    b. Check the patient's chart for pertinent information

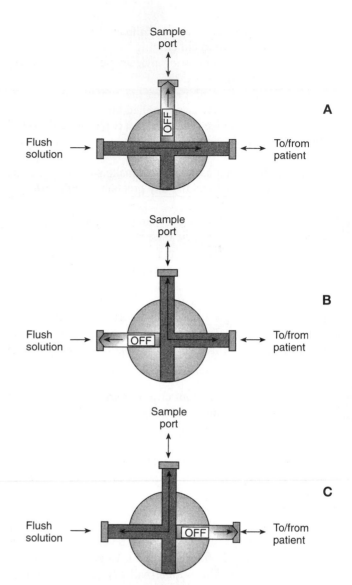

Fig. 3-1 A three-way stopcock for use in an arterial line system. **A,** The normal operating position of the stopcock that allows fluid to flow to the patient (and the blood pressure to be monitored if assembled for continuous blood pressure monitoring). **B,** The stopcock position that allows blood to be withdrawn from the patient through the sample port. The flush solution port is closed. **C,** The stopcock position for flush solution to go to the sample port to clear out any blood. When the stopcock is turned to a 45-degree angle between any two ports, all of the ports are closed. (From Scanlan CL, Analysis and monitoring of gas exchange. In Scanlan CL, Wilkins RL, and Stoller JK, editors: *Egan's fundamentals of respiratory care,* ed 7, St Louis, 1999, Mosby.)

on supplemental oxygen being used, bleeding disorders such as hemophilia, and use of anticoagulant medications. It is important to check the patient's clotting time because a hematoma will result in a patient with a slow clotting time if extra time is not spent holding the puncture site.

c. Collect necessary equipment:
   1. Ice water in a cup
   2. A 3 mL glass or plastic syringe
   3. Appropriate needle(s)
   4. Heparin, if needed
   5. Seventy percent isopropyl alcohol or iodophor swabs to clean the puncture site and a sterile 4 by 4-inch gauze pad to hold over the puncture site to aid clotting
   6. A seal for the needle or syringe to prevent room air contamination
   7. Clean gloves to protect the practitioner's hands from any contact with spilled blood.
   8. Eyeglasses or goggles
d. Introduce yourself and your department to the patient. Identify the patient. Explain what you are there to do. Gain the patient's confidence so that he or she will offer full cooperation.
e. Select the puncture site. The following choices are listed in order from most to least favorable: radial, brachial, dorsalis pedis, and femoral. If the radial site is selected, try to puncture the left wrist if the patient is right-handed or vice versa.
f. If the radial or pedal sites are selected, the modified Allen's test must be performed to ensure that there is adequate collateral flow in case the artery becomes clotted because of the procedure.
   1. Radial artery site. See Fig. 3-2 for the basic procedure. Circulation to the hand is stopped by pressing both the radial and ulnar arteries closed. Releasing the pressure over the ulnar artery should result in the hand flushing within 10 to 15 seconds. This is a positive test result and proves that the ulnar artery has adequate circulation to the hand. If the hand does not flush within 15 seconds of the release of the ulnar artery, the circulation is inadequate, and the radial artery of that wrist must not be punctured. Another site must be evaluated for puncture.
   2. Dorsalis pedis artery site. Press down on the dorsalis pedis artery to occlude it. Press on the nail of the great toe so that it blanches. Release the pressure on the nail and watch for a rapid return of color. This normal test finding confirms that there is good blood flow through the posterior tibial and lateral plantar arteries. It is safe to draw a sample from the site. A slow return of blood flow indicates poor circulation; another site must be chosen.
g. Prepare the equipment and the puncture site by using sterile technique.
   1. If necessary, draw up the heparin solution, flush the syringe with it, and discard the excess.
   2. If a radial or brachial site is selected, the joint

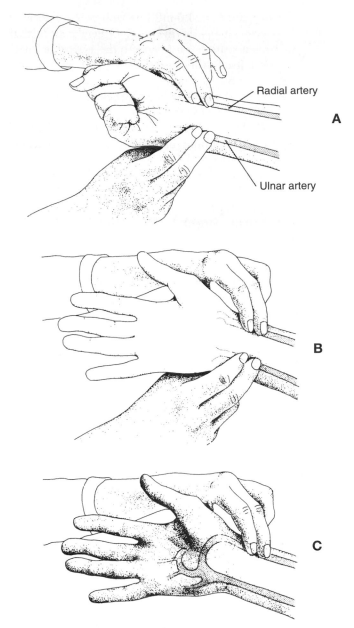

Fig. 3-2 The modified Allen's test. **A,** The hand is clenched into a tight fist and pressure is applied to the radial and ulnar arteries. **B,** The hand is opened (but not fully extended); the palm and fingers are blanched. **C,** Removal of the pressure on the ulnar artery should result in flushing of the entire hand. (From Shapiro BA, Peruzzi WT, Templin R: *Clinical application of blood gases,* ed 5, St Louis, 1994, Mosby.)

should be hyperextended with a folded towel to help stabilize it.
   3. Clean the site by wiping the area with an alcohol or iodophor swab in a widening spiral motion that starts at the desired puncture site.
   4. Put on gloves and goggles.
   5. Some prefer to anesthetize the puncture site

with a 0.8- to 1.0-mL injection of 2% lidocaine (Xylocaine) into the skin. Others believe that this is unnecessary because the lidocaine injection, itself, will cause pain.

h. Draw the blood sample.

1. Hold the syringe like a pencil. The radial and dorsalis pedis arteries should be entered from a 45-degree angle; the brachial and femoral arteries should be entered from a 90-degree angle (Fig. 3-3). Use the first two fingers of your free hand to palpate the pulse and hold the artery still. The bevel of the needle should be up as it enters the skin.
2. Tell the patient that he or she will "feel a stick."

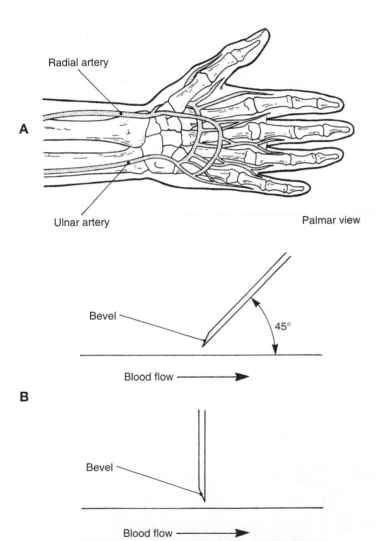

Fig. 3-3 A, Radial arterial position in the lower arm and wrist. B, Bevel and needle positioning for radial arterial puncture and other arterial punctures, respectively. (From Lane EE, Walker JF: *Clinical arterial blood gas analysis.* St Louis, 1987, Mosby.)

3. The needle should enter the skin quickly to minimize pain. Carefully advance the needle into the artery. A pulsatile flow is seen with each heartbeat. If unsuccessful, withdraw the needle to the skin, change the angle as needed, and reinsert into the artery.
4. Withdraw about 1 to 2 mL of blood before removing the needle.
5. Press the sterile gauze onto the puncture site for 2 to 5 minutes. Check the site to ensure that clotting has occurred. Hold longer if necessary. An assistant may help with this.
6. While holding the site, seal the needle.
7. Roll the syringe to mix the heparin, and place the syringe into the ice water. (Failure to put the blood sample in ice water results in a decrease in the Pao_2 value, an increase in the $PaCO_2$ value, and a decrease in the pH value.)
8. Label the syringe with the date, time, patient's name, oxygen percentage, and temperature if abnormal. Some departments may also add the patient's age and position in which he or she was sitting or laying when the sample was drawn because of the effects they may have on oxygenation.
9. Have the sample analyzed as soon as possible.
10. Properly dispose of gloves and waste materials and wash your hands.

4. Perform venipuncture (Code: IIIA1b) [Difficulty: An]

A number of possible variations exist in venipuncture. A general but thorough list of the steps and important related information follows:

a. Check for a valid physician order including the blood tests needed.
b. Collect necessary equipment:
   1. Needle(s) and syringe, butterfly needle, or evacuated tube (VACUTAINER) system
   2. Tube(s) for the blood test(s)
   3. Soft rubber tourniquet
   4. Sterile cotton balls and bandage to place over the puncture site to aid clotting
   5. Seventy percent isopropyl alcohol swabs to clean the puncture site
   6. Clean gloves to protect the practitioner's hands from any contact with spilled blood
c. Introduce yourself and your department to the patient. Identify the patient. Explain what you are there to do. Gain the patient's confidence so that there will be full cooperation.
d. Select the puncture site. The following choices in the antecubital area of the arm are listed in order from most to least favorable puncture sites: median cubital vein, cephalic vein, basilic vein. If no arm

veins are suitable, the veins on the dorsal side of the hand or wrist may be used. The areas that are least desirable but possible to draw from are the dorsal veins on the foot or ankle.

e. Prepare the equipment and the puncture site by using sterile technique.
   1. Wash hands
   2. Put on gloves
   3. Clean the site by wiping the area with an alcohol swab in a widening spiral motion that starts at the desired puncture site
   4. Assemble the needle, syringe, or VACUTAINER tube
f. Draw the blood sample.
   1. A tourniquet may be applied if necessary. If used, it should be left on for only 1 minute. The patient may also be told to make a fist to help the vein expand with blood.
   2. Hold the syringe like a pointer. The veins should be entered from a 15-degree angle. Use the first two fingers of your free hand to palpate the vein and hold it still. The bevel of the needle should be up as it enters the skin.
   3. Tell the patient that he or she will "feel a stick."
   4. The needle should enter the skin quickly to minimize pain. Carefully advance the needle into the vein. If unsuccessful, withdraw the needle to the skin, change the angle as needed, and reinsert into the vein.
   5. Withdraw the needed amount of blood or VACUTAINER tubes of blood before removing the needle.
g. Remove the tourniquet.
h. Press the sterile cotton ball onto the puncture site. Apply a bandage.
i. Label the blood sample with the date, time, patient's name, and needed test(s).
j. Have the sample analyzed as soon as possible.
k. Properly dispose of gloves and wash your hands.

5. Perform capillary blood gas (CBG) sampling (Code: IIIA1b) [Difficulty: An]

Occasionally, a sample of capillary blood from a patient must be obtained for blood gas analysis. The usual clinical situation is a neonate who has a pulmonary problem that warrants evaluation. However, because of the neonate's small arteries, a sample cannot be drawn. The steps and key points to keep in mind during the sampling procedure follow:

a. Select a highly vascularized and well-perfused site. Usually the heel is selected, but the great toe, earlobe, or finger are also acceptable.
b. Warm the heel (or other site) with a warm towel or heat lamp for about 5 to 10 minutes; 42° C is ideal.

Warming vasodilates the vessels and "arterializes" the capillary blood supply.
c. After warming, unwrap the site and wipe it with an antiseptic pad.
d. Use a pediatric lance to deeply puncture the outer edge of the heel (see Fig. 3-4). Blood should flow freely without squeezing the area. The blood will be "dearterialized" if it is squeezed out with venous blood, and the sample will be useless for blood gas analysis.
e. Insert a preheparinized capillary tube (.075 to 1.0 mL) deeply into the drop of blood. The blood should easily flow through the tube, and ideally a second sample tube is filled.
f. Seal both ends of the tubes.
g. Use a magnet to draw the metal filing (flea) back and forth in the tubes to mix the blood.
h. Place the sealed tubes immediately into an ice water bath.
i. Send the samples to the laboratory for analysis along with the proper paperwork.

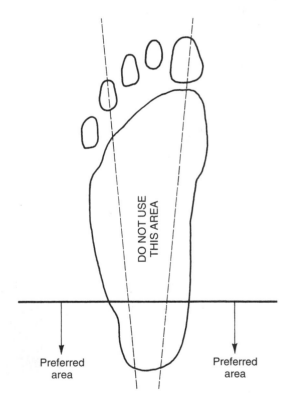

Fig. 3-4 Puncture sites on an infant's heel for obtaining an arterialized capillary blood sample. Avoid the posterior tibial artery that runs through the center of the foot. (From Czervinske MP: Arterial blood gas analysis and other cardiopulmonary monitoring. In Koff PB, Eitzman D, Neu J: *Neonatal and pediatric respiratory care*, ed 2, St Louis, 1993, Mosby.)

j. Apply pressure to stop the bleeding. Complications include infection, bone spurs, and laceration of the posterior tibial artery.

MODULE C **Analyze blood gas values**

1. Standard blood gas analyzer

a. Select the appropriate blood gas analyzer (Code: IIA1h4) [Difficulty: An]

The blood gas values of PaO_2, $PaCO_2$, and pH are typically obtained from a standard blood gas analyzer. These standard units are acceptable for all patient care situations except when carbon monoxide poisoning is known or suspected. A standard blood gas analyzer is unable to measure carboxyhemoglobin (COHb). A

CO-oximeter is needed to measure the patient's level of carboxyhemoglobin in carbon monoxide cases.

b. Put the equipment together, make sure that it works properly, and identify any problems (Code: IIB1h4) [Difficulty: An]

pH electrode. The modern pH electrode has existed since the mid-1950s and is usually referred to as the *Sanz electrode* after its principal inventor. The basic principle behind the pH analyzer is its ability to measure the voltage (potential for electrical flow) between two different solutions. This is based on the different hydrogen ion (H^+) concentrations between the solutions that reflect their relative pHs. The reference electrode is immersed in a solution with a pH of 6.840 that fills a glass or plastic chamber. The blood sample, of unknown pH, is placed in a separate measuring chamber called a *cuvette*. These two

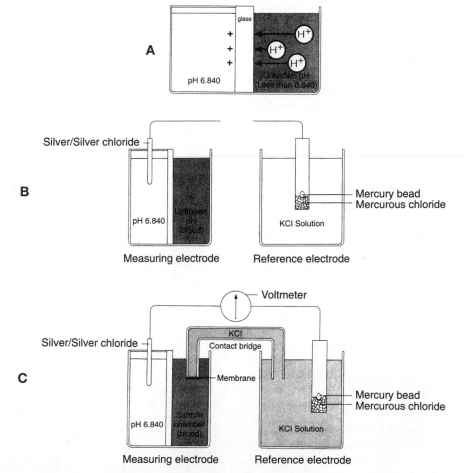

Fig. 3-5 Key components of the pH electrode. **A,** A voltage develops across the pH-sensitive glass when there is a difference in the hydrogen ion concentration between the two solutions. **B,** Two separate half-cells are used for the measuring electrode and the reference electrode. **C,** The addition of a KCl contact bridge and voltmeter completes the electrical circuit and enables the pH of the patient's blood sample to be measured. (From Shapiro BA, Harrison RA, Cane RD et al.: *Clinical application of blood gases,* ed 4, St Louis, 1989, Mosby.)

chambers are separated by a special glass membrane that contains metals and sodium ions (Na^+), thus making it pH sensitive. Both chambers are kept at a stable 37° C temperature. See Fig. 3-5 for a graphic representation of the pH electrode. When blood or a quality control material is introduced into the cuvette, there is the potential for hydrogen ions to replace the sodium ions in the pH-sensitive glass if the two pHs are different. The replacement is proportional to the difference in the two pHs.

PCO_2 electrode. The partial pressure of carbon dioxide (PCO_2) is measured in a modified pH electrode. This was first designed in the mid-1950s by Stowe and further perfected by Severinghaus. Accordingly, these units are now referred to as *Severinghaus,* or sometimes as *Stowe-Severinghaus electrodes.* In Fig. 3-6, the electrode is depicted in cross section. It has a reference half-cell and measuring half-cell that are enclosed within pH-sensitive glass and electrically connected by an electrolyte contact bridge. The blood sample is introduced into a cuvette heated to 37° C.

The principle of operation is based on the amount of CO_2 found in the blood sample that diffuses through the silicon elastic membrane. The CO_2 chemically combines with the bicarbonate solution to change the pH of the solution by the release of H^+. This H^+ change creates a voltage difference between the measuring and reference half-cells that is proportional to the amount of CO_2 found in the patient's blood sample.

PO_2 electrode. This unit is completely different from the others mentioned. It was developed in the late 1950s by Clark and thus is usually called a *Clark electrode.* It is also sometimes known as a *polarographic electrode* because of the basis of its operation. Fig. 3-7 is a drawing of key features of the unit. A phosphate-KCl buffer solution surrounds the silver anode. A thin membrane separates the blood-filled cuvette from direct contact with the electrode, but allows oxygen molecules to slowly diffuse through to contact the platinum wire cathode. The whole unit is heated to 37° C. The term polarographic comes from the addition of about 0.7 volts to the cathode to make it slightly "polarized" or negative compared with the anode. This is needed to ensure that oxygen is rapidly chemically reduced (that it gains electrons) at the cathode. This creates an electrical current directly proportional to the number of reduced oxygen molecules.

It must be understood that the partial pressure of oxygen (PO_2) being measured is derived from oxygen that is dissolved in the plasma. It does not come from the hemoglobin found in the erythrocytes (red blood cells). The reported value for the saturation of oxygen in the hemoglobin (SaO_2) is calculated using a mathematical table. Under normal conditions, the calculated SaO_2 value is the same or close to the true SaO_2 value. Carbon monoxide (CO) poisoning is the only commonly seen clinical situation during which a calculated saturation can be incorrectly high. If carbon monoxide poisoning is suspected or known, the patient's blood sample should be analyzed on a CO-oximeter unit.

c. Perform quality control procedures for a blood gas analyzer (Code: IIB3a) [Difficulty: An]

Quality control (QC). QC refers to creating a measurement and documentation system to confirm the accuracy (precision) and reliability of all blood gas measurements. Accuracy or precision means that the measured physiologic values truly reflect the actual physiologic values. Reliability means that there is a high degree of confidence that the accuracy of the measured values represents the patient's actual physiologic values. Both are critically important if the blood gas results are to be used to make correct clinical decisions.

Quality assurance. Quality assurance refers to the broader concern that the results of the blood gas measurement are not only accurate and reliable but also clinically useful. To help ensure this, the Clinical

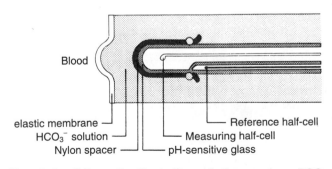

Fig. 3-6 Schematic illustration of the modern PCO_2 electrode. (Note that the space between the silicon membrane and the nylon spacer is greatly enlarged for clarity.) (From Shapiro BA, Harrison RA, Cane RD et al.: *Clinical application of blood gases,* ed 4, St Louis, 1989, Mosby.)

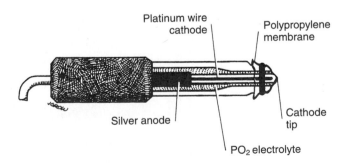

Fig. 3-7 Schematic illustration of the Clark electrode for measuring PO_2. (From Shapiro BA, Harrison RA, Cane RD et al.: *Clinical application of blood gases,* ed 4, St Louis, 1989, Mosby.)

Laboratory Improvement Amendments of 1988 (CLIA '88) require that the department have written policies and procedures on items including record keeping, equipment maintenance, staff training, and the correction of errors.

Calibration. Calibration is the systematic standardization of the graduations of the blood gas analyzer against known values to ensure consistency. Proper calibration of the electrodes is essential to the accuracy of the blood gas values. Some general calibration steps are discussed later. The manufacturer's guidelines must be followed for the specific steps in calibration.

Quality control materials. A variety of quality control materials are available to calibrate the electrodes for PO_2, PCO_2, and pH. Their uses vary. Each of the following materials has its advantages, disadvantages, and limitations. The manufacturer of a particular brand or model of blood gas analyzer may require that a specific type of material be used in its units.

Aqueous buffers are water based and are used to check pH and pCO_2 measurements; they cannot be used to check PO_2 measurements. Commercially prepared gases are used to check PO_2 and PCO_2 measurements; they cannot be used to check pH. The following CO_2 mixes may be used: 0%, 5%, 10%, and 12%. The following O_2 mixes may be used: 0%, 12%, 20%, 20.95% from room air, 21%, and 100%. Tonometered liquids are exposed in the laboratory to known oxygen and carbon dioxide gas mixes until the liquids are saturated and have the same partial pressures as the gases. There are three types of tonometered liquids. The first is human or animal serum or whole blood. This is the most accurate method available and is mainly used to obtain PO_2 and PCO_2 levels. Although whole human blood cannot be used for pH, a bovine blood product can be used to obtain all three values. Second, assayed liquids are non–water-based liquids that are pre-tonometered by the manufacturer and are available in sealed glass vials. They can be used to obtain PO_2, PCO_2, and pH. These are very popular because of the advantages of speed and simplicity. Third, oxygenated fluorocarbon-based emulsions (perfluorinated compounds) can be used to obtain PO_2, PCO_2, and pH measurements. They are considered as accurate as whole blood without its associated risks.

Levey-Jennings charts. The Levey-Jennings charts (also known as Shewhart/Levey-Jennings or Quality Control charts) are used to record the results of each calibration

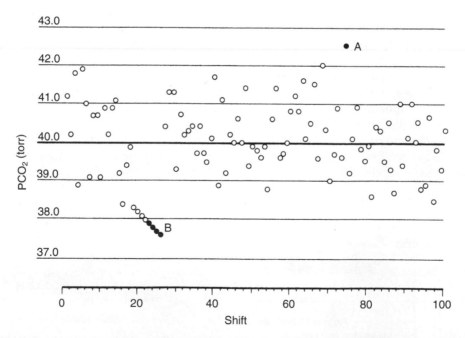

Fig. 3-8 Levey-Jennings quality control chart for $PaCO_2$. The central horizontal line represents the mean value of 40 torr. The next lower and higher horizontal lines show one standard deviation (1 SD) value from the mean. The second-most-distant lower and higher horizontal lines show 2 SD values from the mean. The most distant horizontal lines show 3 SD values from the mean. The bottom number scale represents 8-hour work shifts. Open circles represent calibration values that are within 2 SDs of the mean value. They are considered to be in control. The black circles represent calibration values that are out of control. *A* represents a random error; *B* represents a systematic error. (From Shapiro BA, Peruzzi WT, Templin R: *Clinical application of blood gases*, ed 5, St Louis, 1994, Mosby.)

procedure. They are similarly designed with time plotted on the horizontal scale and the analyte (PO_2, PCO_2, or pH) on the vertical scale. The vertical scale for each analyte has a central value for what is normally expected. On both sides of this normal value are standard deviation (SD) points showing movement away from what is expected. When an analyte electrode is operating within the acceptable limits it is said to be in control. In general, if an analyte is within two standard deviations of the normal value, it is considered to be in control.

An out-of-control situation exists whenever a single calibration value or a series of calibration values are outside established limits. A random error is an unpredictable aberration in precision that occurs when the quality control material is sampled. A systematic error shows an accuracy problem and is much more serious. It must be investigated, corrected, and documented. Fig. 3-8 shows an example of both random error and systematic error. Rules have been established for determining whether the error is random or systematic (Table 3-1).

pH electrode. Note: These and the following guidelines are based on CLIA standards or widely reported industry standards. The various brands and models of blood gas analyzers may have different frequencies of calibration requirements, depending on their Food and Drug Association (FDA) approved manufacturers' studies.

    a. One-point calibration

       1. Should be done before every sample is analyzed

TABLE 3-1	Westgard's Rules for Determining When an Analyzer Is Not Functioning Properly

Rule name	Levey-Jennings chart
RANDOM ERROR	
1-2 SDs	The measurement is more than 2 SDs but not more than 3 SDs from the mean
1-3 SDs	The measurement is more than 3 SDs from the mean
R*-4 SDs	Two consecutive measurements are 4 SDs or more apart
SYSTEMATIC ERROR	
2-2 SDs	Two consecutive measurements are either 2 SDs above or 2 SDs below the mean
4-1 SDs	Four consecutive measurements are either 1 SD above or 1 SD below the mean
7-trend	Seven consecutive measurements are on only one side of the mean; each measurement is progressively more out of control
10-mean	Ten consecutive measurements are on only one side of the mean

* = Repeat.
SDs, Standard deviations.
Modified from Lane EE, Walker JF: *Clinical arterial blood gas analysis,* St Louis, 1987, Mosby.

if one-point calibration is not automatically performed every 30 minutes

       2. Performed with the near-normal quality control material of 7.384 ± .005 pH used to set the balance potentiometer

       3. Recommended every 30 minutes

       4. Should be rechecked after a suspicious pH result; the blood sample should then be rerun

    b. Two-point calibration

       1. Should be done at least once every 8 hours when patient samples are being analyzed

       2. Recommended every 25 patient samples

       3. Performed with the slope potentiometer set with a quality control material of 6.840 ± .005 pH (this is the same pH as the reference electrode solution)

       4. Performed with the balance potentiometer set with a quality control material of 7.384 ± .005 pH

    c. Three-point calibration

       1. Should be done at least every 6 months on existing equipment

       2. Should be done whenever a new electrode is put into use

       3. Covers the physiologic range to confirm linearity: quality control materials of 6.840 ± .005, 7.384 ± .005, and 7.874 ± .005 pH are used

PCO_2 electrode

    a. One-point calibration

       1. Should be done before every sample is analyzed if one-point calibration is not automatically performed every 30 minutes

       2. Performed with 5% ± .03% CO_2 used to set the balance potentiometer

       3. Recommended every 30 minutes

       4. Should be rechecked after a suspicious PCO_2 result; the blood sample should then be rerun

The CO_2 can be directly in contact with the electrode, tonometered with an aqueous material or blood, or premixed in aqueous buffers, assayed liquids, or fluorocarbon-based emulsion.

EXAM HINT

Past examinations have required that the following equation be solved. Remember that more than one carbon dioxide percentage can be used.

The predicted PCO_2 value at a given CO_2% is calculated with this formula:

$$PCO_2 = (P_B - PH_2O) \times \% CO_2$$

In which:

PCO_2 = Predicted PCO_2 in mm Hg torr

P_B = Barometric pressure at the institution where the analysis is being performed

PH_2O = Water vapor pressure based on the patient's temperature; 47 torr at 37° C/98.6° F

% CO_2 = Percentage of CO_2 (also listed as $F CO_2$)

Example for one-point (balance) potentiometer calibration at sea level in which:

PCO_2 = Predicted PCO_2 in torr
P_B = 760 torr
PH_2O = 47 torr
% CO_2 = 5%
1. $PCO_2 = (760 - 47) \times .05$
2. $= (713) \times .05$
3. $= 35.65$ or 36 torr

Therefore set the pCO_2 control at 36 torr

---

  a. Two-point calibration
    1. Should be done at least once every 8 hours when patient samples are being analyzed
    2. Recommended every 25 patient samples
    3. Performed with 10% ± .03% CO_2 to set the slope potentiometer
    4. Performed with 5% ± .03% CO_2 to set the balance potentiometer
  b. Three-point calibration
    1. Should be done at least every 6 months on existing equipment
    2. Should be done whenever a new electrode is put into use
    3. Covers the physiologic range to confirm linearity; three pCO_2 values between 0 and 80 mm Hg should be determined
    4. Room air or a gas cylinder containing 0%–.03% CO_2 can be used to set the 0 point

PO_2 electrode

a. One-point calibration
  1. Should be done before every sample is analyzed if one-point calibration is not automatically performed every 30 minutes
  2. Performed with 12% ± .03% O_2 used to set the balance potentiometer; some analyzers are designed to use 20% ± .03% O_2 from a gas cylinder or draw room air (20.95% oxygen) into the unit
  3. Recommended every 30 minutes
  4. Should be rechecked after a suspicious Po_2 result; the blood sample should then be rerun

The O_2 can be directly in contact with the electrode, tonometered with an aqueous material or blood, or premixed in aqueous buffers, assayed liquids, or fluorocarbon-based emulsion as discussed.

EXAM HINT

Past examinations have required that the following equation be solved. Remember that more than one oxygen percentage can be used.

The predicted PO_2 value at a given O_2% is calculated with this formula:

$$PO_2 = (P_B - PH_2O) \times \% O_2$$

In which:
PO_2 = Predicted PO_2 in torr
P_B = Barometric pressure at the institution where the analysis is being performed
PH_2O = Water vapor pressure based on the patient's temperature; 47 torr at 37° C/98.6° F
% O_2 = Percentage of O_2 (also listed as $F O_2$)

Example for one-point (balance) potentiometer calibration at sea level in which:

PO_2 = Predicted PO_2 in torr
P_B = 760 torr
PH_2O = 47 torr
% O_2 = 12%
2. $PO_2 = (760 - 47) \times .12$
3. $= (713) \times .12$
4. $= 85.56$ or 86 torr

Therefore set the PO_2 control at 86 torr

---

  b. Two-point calibration
    1. Should be done at least once every 8 hours when patient samples are being analyzed
    2. Should be done whenever readjustment of one-point calibration is greater than 3 torr
    3. Recommended every 25 patient samples
    4. Performed with 0% ± .03% O_2 to set the slope potentiometer
    5. Performed with 12% ± .03% O_2 to set the balance potentiometer; some analyzers are designed to use 20% ± .03% O_2 from a gas cylinder or draw room air (20.95% oxygen) into the unit
  c. Three-point calibration
    1. Should be done at least every 6 months on existing equipment
    2. Should be done whenever a new electrode is put into use
    3. Should be done to confirm linearity whenever the PO_2 value could be more than 150 torr, assuming that the balance point is set on room oxygen content; the third point should be set on 100% ± .03% O_2 from a gas cylinder

Miscellaneous topics

a. Calibration gas cylinders. For economic reasons, the low-percentage oxygen and carbon dioxide gases are placed together in one cylinder and the high-percentage oxygen and carbon dioxide gases are placed together in a second cylinder. Box 3-1 summarizes the normal precision of the electrodes discussed and the gases used in their calibration. A cylinder containing 100% oxygen and 0% carbon dioxide can be used for three-point calibration.
b. Temperature correction. Temperature correction

BOX 3-1   Electrode Precision
                and Calibration Gases

ELECTRODES
  pH ± 0.01 unit
  PCO_2 ± 2% (approximately ± 1 torr at 40 torr)
  PO_2 ± 3% (approximately ± 2.5 torr at 80 torr)
  If the PO_2 is over 150 torr, the precision is approximately
    ± 10% unless three-point calibration is performed

CALIBRATION GASES
  "Low" gas: 0% O_2 (+ 0.03%), 5% CO_2 (± 0.03%), balance N_2
  "High" gas: 12% or 21% O_2, 10% CO_2 (both ± 0.03%),
    balance N_2
  Suggested three-point gases: 100% O_2 (− 0.03%), 0% CO_2
    (+ 0.03%)

N_2, Nitrogen; PCO_2, pressure of carbon dioxide; PO_2, pressure of oxygen.

---

refers to mathematical adjustment of a patient's PaO_2, $PaCO_2$, and pH values if his or her temperature is not 37° C. Remember that blood gas analyzers are calibrated at 37° C because it is normal body temperature. If the patient has a fever, the oxygen and carbon dioxide partial pressures in the blood will be greater than those found during the blood gas analysis. Conversely, the hypothermic patient will have lower oxygen and carbon dioxide partial pressures in the blood than those found during the blood gas analysis. The pH value will shift in the opposite direction as the PCO_2 value. Usually, this small shift in values is ignored. However, because some physicians may specify that their patient's blood gases be temperature corrected, the patient's temperature should be listed on the blood gas slip. It is a simple mathematical process to temperature correct the blood gas results. Most modern analyzers perform temperature correction automatically when programmed to do so.

d. Fix any problems with the equipment (Code: IIB2h4) [Difficulty: An]

Remember to flush the electrode membrane after each use, if possible, to prevent protein buildup. If protein buildup occurs, the response time is longer than normal. Follow the manufacturer's guidelines to change an electrode membrane as needed. Make sure that no air bubbles are under the membrane or within the tubing through which the blood travels. Rerun the calibration for any of the electrodes and reanalyze the sample if you are suspicious of the result. If the electrode does not calibrate close to the reference buffer solutions or gases, it should not be used.

In a random error situation, the practitioner likely made a simple error when introducing the material or running the analyzer. Common problems include an air bubble injected into the unit or incomplete flushing of the previous sample. Usually flushing out any residual blood and then carefully injecting more of the current patient blood sample will correct the problem. Run the analyzer again to obtain new patient values. Also, you can run the same patient sample through another analyzer and compare the two sets of results.

A systematic error usually indicates a problem with the analyzer, quality control materials, or processes. Examples of systematic errors include misanalyzed CO_2 or O_2 standards for calibration; contaminated quality control materials; or deteriorated oxygen, carbon dioxide, or pH electrode function. Each of these must be investigated until the problem is found and corrected. The unit cannot be used again until after it is proven to work properly and to give accurate results.

e. Perform blood gas analysis (Code: IB9c and IC1e) [Difficulty: An]

Modern blood gas analyzers are simple to operate. Follow the manufacturer's guidelines for insertion of the blood sample. Perform the specified steps in analysis. Print out the results. Many current units run a self-diagnosis if there are any problems.

2. CO-oximeter
a. Get the necessary equipment to perform CO-oximetry (Code: IIA1h4) [Difficulty: An]

Most hospitals have a CO-oximeter in addition to a blood gas analyzer. A CO-oximeter should be used to analyze a blood gas sample whenever carbon monoxide poisoning is known or suspected. In addition, a CO-oximeter gives a complete analysis of the relative amounts of the different types of patient hemoglobin.

CO-oximeters are also called *spectrophotometric oximeters* and are the most accurate method available to measure the four different hemoglobin moieties (species or variations in the hemoglobin molecule). These hemoglobin species include the following:

1. Oxyhemoglobin (HbO_2 or O_2Hb), which carries oxygen to the tissues, and reduced hemoglobin (HbR or RHb), which has given up its oxygen and picked up carbon dioxide
2. Carboxyhemoglobin (HbCO or COHb), which is nonfunctional because of the tightness with which carbon monoxide binds to the hemoglobin
3. Methemoglobin (HbMet or MetHb), which is nonfunctional because the Hb molecule is unable to combine reversibly with oxygen
4. Sulfhemoglobin (HbS or SHb), which is similar to the HbMet and is also nonfunctional. In addition, a CO-oximeter can measure the fetal hemoglobin (HbF or FHb) found in a newborn infant instead of adult oxyhemoglobin

Each of these hemoglobin moieties has a spectroscopic "fingerprint" of absorbed lightwave frequencies that is

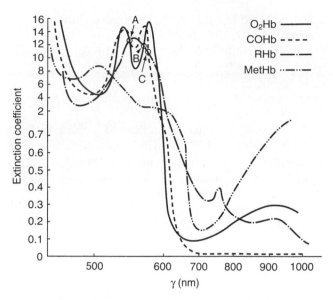

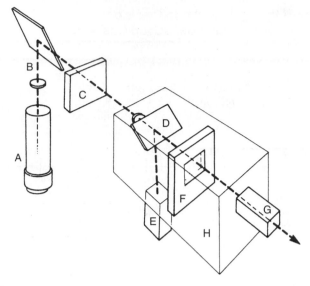

Fig. 3-9 Spectral analysis of the hemoglobin moieties (species). O_2Hb is oxyhemoglobin, COHb is carboxyhemoglobin, RHb is reduced hemoglobin, MetHb (METHb) is methemoglobin. Point A shows the triple isosbestic point at 548 nm for O_2Hb, COHb, and RHb. Point B shows the double isosbestic point at 568 nm for O_2Hb and RHb. Point C shows the double isosbestic point at 578 nm for RHb and COHb. A fourth wavelength at 626.6 nm is used for comparison purposes. (From Shapiro BA, Peruzzi WT, Templin R: *Clinical application of blood gases,* ed 4, St Louis, 1994, Mosby.)

Fig. 3-10 CO-oximeter basic components. A, thallium-neon hollow cathode light source; B, lens and mirror; C, monochromator with four specific wavelength filters; D, light beam splitter that diverts half of the light to the reference detector and half to the cuvette; E, reference wavelength detector; F, patient sample cuvette, G, sample wavelength detector; and H, temperature regulated block set at 37° C. (From Shapiro BA, Peruzzi WT, Templin R: *Clinical application of blood gases,* ed 5, St Louis, 1994, Mosby.)

unique. See Fig. 3-9 for the spectral analysis of the various forms of hemoglobin.

b. Put the CO-oximeter together, make sure that it works properly, and identify any problems with the equipment (Code: IIB1h4) [Difficulty: An]

The unit is preassembled by the manufacturer. Practical experience with a unit is recommended to understand how to add a patient blood sample and perform calibration duties. (See Fig. 3-10 for a schematic drawing of a CO-oximeter.) A thallium-neon hollow cathode lamp emits light in the infrared-visible range. A device called a monochromator contains four filters and rotates through the light beam. Each filter allows only one specific wavelength to pass through it. These four monochromatic wavelengths correspond to the three isosbestic points discussed earlier (shown in Fig. 3-9) and 626.6 nm. This last wavelength is poorly absorbed by all four hemoglobin moieties. It is used to find the maximal difference in absorption so that the relative amounts of the hemoglobin species can be determined.

When a blood sample is placed into the cuvette, the same four wavelengths are passed through it. The amount of absorbance at each wavelength is measured and compared with the absorbance at each wavelength by a reference sample solution (see the following discussion). The computer integrates the data and calculates the total hemoglobin and amounts of the four hemoglobin moieties.

c. Perform quality control procedures on the CO-oximeter (Code: IIB3a) [Difficulty: An]

Total hemoglobin (THb) should be calibrated when the unit is installed, at regular intervals suggested by the manufacturer, after the sample tubing is changed, after the cuvette is disassembled or changed, and whenever there is a suspicious reading. Calibration is done by filling the cuvette with a special dye produced by the manufacturer and analyzing it following the prescribed steps.

Routine calibration is done every 30 minutes. The unit obtains and stores absorbance readings at the four different wavelengths from a "blank" solution in the reference detector. When the same "blank" solution is added to the sample cuvette, the same four wavelengths are measured. Their absorption levels are normally identical. The same procedure is performed after every patient sample is analyzed.

d. Fix any problems with the equipment (Code: IIB2h4) [Difficulty: An]

The following are examples of common problems and their solutions:

1. Incomplete hemolysis of the blood sample causes the light to scatter off cell fragments and lipids. Sickle cells (as in sickle-cell anemia) are difficult to disrupt and may cause false oxyhemoglobin and carboxyhemoglobin readings if extra time is not taken for hemolysis. Follow manufacturer's guidelines on the procedure for hemolyzing the red blood cells.

2. More than 10% methemoglobin may cause errors in the measurement of all hemoglobin moieties. Sulfhemoglobin also causes false readings. The practitioner may need to gather additional information from the chart or laboratory regarding the patient's levels of these abnormal hemoglobin moieties. CO-oximetry should probably not be performed on blood samples with abnormal levels of methemoglobin or sulfhemoglobin.

3. Intravenous dyes such as methylene blue, Evans blue, and indocyanine green used in various cardiac studies can absorb the same wavelengths of light used to identify the various forms of hemoglobin. The presence of these dyes results in a lower measurement of oxyhemoglobin than is actually present. Check the patient's chart for a record of dyes used. CO-oximetry should probably not be used for blood gas analysis on patients who have these dyes in their systems.

4. Failure to reprogram the analyzer for fetal hemoglobin instead of adult hemoglobin may produce false results. Remember to check the chart for the patient's age. Reprogram the analyzer for fetal hemoglobin for any sample taken from an infant who is only a few weeks old.

5. The presence of lipid particles in the blood causes light scattering and results in a reading that is falsely high in total hemoglobin and percent of methemoglobin and falsely low in percent oxyhemoglobin and percent carboxyhemoglobin. Follow the laboratory's guidelines to determine when a patient's blood lipid value is too high for accurate use of the CO-oximeter.

6. Air bubbles or incomplete hemolysis of blood in the cuvette causes an absorbance error. Air bubbles must be flushed out and the blood sample inserted again and reanalyzed. Make sure that all blood samples are hemolyzed according to the manufacturer's guidelines.

7. Blood clots in the sample tubing prevent blood from flowing through to the cuvette. If a sample cannot be inserted into the unit, suspect and check for a blood clot. Remove any clotted tubing, replace it, and confirm that the CO-oximeter is working properly.

e. Perform CO-oximetry (Code: IC1e) [Difficulty: An]

Follow the manufacturer's guidelines on rewarming the blood sample to body temperature, hemolyzing the sample, and inserting it into the measurement cuvette. Failure to do so may result in incorrect patient values.

The principle of operation of a CO-oximeter is the comparison of the relative absorbances of four wavelengths of light by oxyhemoglobin, reduced hemoglobin, and carboxyhemoglobin. This is done by comparing the absorptions at the three isosbestic points (at which the moieties being compared have equal absorption) and a wavelength point (at which there is the greatest difference in absorption between the two moieties). By computer integration of the data, the relative proportions of oxyhemoglobin, reduced hemoglobin, and carboxyhemoglobin are determined. If the total is less than 100% of the hemoglobin present, the difference has to be methemoglobin (or, rarely, sulfhemoglobin). The unit then provides data on total hemoglobin; percentages for oxyhemoglobin, reduced hemoglobin, carboxyhemoglobin, and methemoglobin; and total amounts for them in gm/dl blood. Some units also calculate O_2 content.

MODULE D	Interpret blood gas analysis results to determine how the patient is responding to respiratory care

1. Review the chart for any blood gas results (Code: IA1g2 and IA1d) [Difficulty: An]

Look in the chart for any blood gas results, including arterial, capillary, or mixed venous. Any patient may have had an arterial sample analyzed. A neonate may also have had an arterialized capillary sample analyzed. A patient with a pulmonary artery catheter may have had a mixed venous sample analyzed.

2. Interpret the results of arterial blood gas analysis (Code: IB10c and IC2e) [Difficulty: An]

A number of authors have written extensively on how to interpret arterial blood gases. The system proposed by Shapiro and associates (1994) has been found to be both practical and relatively easy to understand. Most of the following discussion and tables are based on this system. This does not mean that if one has learned another system he or she is at any disadvantage for taking the National Board of Respiratory Care (NBRC) examination.

📋 EXAM HINT

The NBRC examination includes specific questions about blood gas interpretation. The exam also includes blood gas results in other questions that relate to any respiratory care technique or procedure, such as oxygen therapy and mechanical ventilation. The examinee must be proficient in blood gas interpretation to do well on the NBRC examinations.

Assessment of oxygenation. Hypoxemia or hypoxia can rapidly become life threatening. Table 3-2 shows the normal PaO_2 values for the newborn, child to adult, and

TABLE 3-2	Age-Based Acceptable Levels of Partial Pressure of Oxygen in Arterial Blood (PaO$_2$) When Breathing Room Air (21% Oxygen) at Sea Level

Age	PaO$_2$
NEWBORN	
Acceptable range	50 to 70 torr
CHILD TO ADULT	
Normal	97 torr
Acceptable range	>80 torr
Hypoxemia	<80 torr
OLDER ADULT	
60-year-old	>80 torr
70-year-old	>70 torr
80-year-old	>60 torr
90-year-old	>50 torr

Modified from Shapiro BA, Harrison RA, Cane RD, Kozlowski-Templin R: *Clinical application of blood gases*, ed 4, St Louis, 1989, Mosby.

TABLE 3-3	Evaluation of Hypoxemia

CONDITIONS: ROOM AIR IS INSPIRED; THE PATIENT IS LESS THAN 60 YEARS OLD*

Hypoxemia	*PaO$_2$*
Mild	<80 torr
Moderate	<60 torr
Severe	<40 torr

CONDITIONS: SUPPLEMENTAL O$_2$ IS INSPIRED; THE PATIENT IS LESS THAN 60 YEARS OLD

Hypoxemia	*PaO$_2$*
Uncorrected	Less than room air acceptable limit
Corrected	Within room air acceptable limit (<100 torr)
Excessively corrected	>100 torr

*Subtract 1 torr of O$_2$ from limits of mild and moderate hypoxemia for each year over 60. A PaO$_2$ of less than 40 torr indicates severe hypoxemia in any patient at any age.
Modified from Shapiro BA, Harrison RA, Cane RD, Kozlowski-Templin R: *Clinical application of blood gases*, ed 4, St Louis, 1989, Mosby.

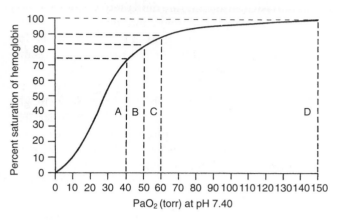

Fig. 3-11 The oxygen (oxyhemoglobin) dissociation curve plots the relationship between hemoglobin saturation (y-axis) and plasma PaO$_2$ (x-axis). A, 75% saturation and a PaO$_2$ of 40 torr are normally seen in venous blood; B, 85% saturation and a PaO$_2$ of 50 torr are the minimal levels that should be allowed in a chronically hypoxemic patient; C, 90% saturation and PaO$_2$ of 60 torr are the minimal levels that should be allowed in an acutely hypoxemic patient; and D, Hemoglobin in the pulmonary capillaries adjacent to normal alveoli will become 100% saturated when the PaO$_2$ reaches 150 torr. (Modified from Lane EE, Walker JF: *Clinical arterial blood gas analysis*, St Louis, 1987, Mosby.)

the elderly when room air (almost 21% oxygen) is inhaled at sea level. These values decrease progressively as altitude increases. However, under most clinical conditions, this is not a factor unless working in a high-altitude setting.

A general rule is that any patient is seriously hypoxemic if the PaO$_2$ is less than 60 torr on room air. See Table 3-3 for guidelines on judging the seriousness of hypoxemia. Once hypoxemia is recognized, it must be corrected. The most obvious way to correct hypoxemia is to give supplemental oxygen. The clinician must realize that oxygen alone will not correct the hypoxemia if the patient is hypoventilating (increased PaCO$_2$), has heart failure, or is unable to carry or make use of the oxygen. In general, try to keep the patient's PaO$_2$ between 60 and 100 torr.

Shapiro and associates (1994) suggested the following formula, in which FIO$_2$ is the fraction of inspired oxygen, for determining whether the patient will be hypoxemic on room air: "If PaO$_2$ is less than FIO$_2 \times 5$, the patient can be assumed to be hypoxemic on room air."

Fig. 3-11 shows a normal oxyhemoglobin dissociation curve. The saturation value is important to know because it shows how much hemoglobin is saturated with oxygen. There are several important points of correlation between the SaO$_2$ and the PaO$_2$. (Calculated saturation values can be misleadingly high if the patient has inhaled carbon monoxide. In this situation it is best to directly measure the saturation on a CO-oximeter type blood gas analyzer.)

Fig. 3-12 shows a number of factors that can influence the oxyhemoglobin dissociation curve and how oxygen loads onto and unloads from hemoglobin. In a patient with normal oxygenation, these factors are not clinically significant. However, when the PaO$_2$ is less than 60 torr and the SaO$_2$ is less than 90%, these factors can become an important consideration. As can be seen, a left-shifted

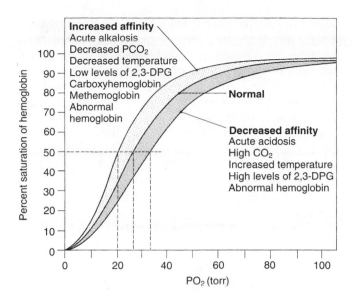

Fig. 3-12 Conditions associated with altered affinity of hemoglobin for O_2. P_{50} is the PaO_2 at which hemoglobin is 50% saturated, normally 26.6 torr. A lower than normal P_{50} represents increased affinity of hemoglobin for O_2; a high P_{50} is seen with decreased affinity. Note that variation from the normal is associated with decreased (low P_{50}) or increased (high P_{50}) availability of O_2 to tissues (dashed lines). The shaded area shows the entire oxyhemoglobin dissociation curve under the same circumstances. (From Lane EE, Walker JF: *Clinical arterial blood gas analysis*, St Louis, 1987, Mosby.)

TABLE 3-4	Normal Laboratory Ranges for Partial Pressure of Carbon Dioxide in Arterial Blood (PaCO₂) and pH		
	Mean	**1 SD**	**2 SDs**
PaCO₂	40.00	38-42 torr	35-45 torr
pH	7.40	7.38-7.42	7.35-7.45

SD, Standard deviation.
Modified from Shapiro BA, Harrison RA, Cane RD, Kozlowski-Templin R: *Clinical application of blood gases*, ed 4, St Louis, 1989, Mosby.

oxyhemoglobin dissociation curve results in a lower PaO_2 at any given saturation. This results in even less oxygen being delivered to the tissues.

Assessment of carbon dioxide and pH. The pH is the next important value to interpret because extreme acidemia/acidosis and alkalemia/alkalosis can be life threatening. The carbon dioxide value is important to interpret because it has a direct effect on the pH and indirectly affects the oxygen level. A high or low $PaCO_2$ level, by itself, is not life threatening.

Table 3-4 shows normal values for pH and $PaCO_2$ and the acceptable ranges around the mean or average. Table

TABLE 3-5	Acceptable Clinical Ranges for Partial Pressure of Carbon Dioxide in Arterial Blood (PaCO₂) and pH
PaCO₂	30-50 torr*
pH	7.30-7.50

*This is the range for patients with an acute change. It does not apply to patients with long-standing disease, such as chronic obstructive pulmonary disease. These patients may have $PaCO_2$ values greater than 50 torr. Modified from Shapiro BA, Harrison RA, Cane RD, Kozlowski-Templin R: *Clinical application of blood gases*, ed 4, St Louis, 1989, Mosby.

TABLE 3-6	Naming Unacceptable Values for Partial Pressure of CO₂ in Arterial Blood (PaCO₂) and pH
PaCO₂ >50 torr	Respiratory acidosis/alveolar hypoventilation/ventilatory failure
pH <7.30	Acidemia
PaCO₂ <30 torr	Respiratory alkalosis/alveolar hyperventilation
pH >7.50	Alkalemia

Modified from Shapiro BA, Harrison RA, Cane RD, Kozlowski-Templin R: *Clinical application of blood gases*, ed 4, St Louis, 1989, Mosby.

3-5 shows the most widely acceptable therapeutic ranges for pH and Paco₂. Values that fall outside of these ranges present a progressively greater risk to the patient.

Table 3-6 shows the definitions of Shapiro and associates for alkalemia and acidemia from a respiratory cause. An acute change in the patient's ventilation causes the following when starting from a $PaCO_2$ of 40 torr:

    a. If the $PaCO_2$ increases by 20 torr, the pH decreases by 0.10 units.

    b. If the $PaCO_2$ decreases by 10 torr, the pH increases by 0.10 units.

Thus the body can be seen as better able to compensate with metabolic buffers for a respiratory acidosis than a respiratory alkalosis.

Metabolic effects are evaluated by interpreting either the bicarbonate (HCO_3^-) value or base excess/base deficit (BE/BD) value. Both reveal whether there is any metabolic effect on the pH. Normal values are as follows:

    a. HCO_3^-: 24 mEq/L.

    b. BE/BD: 0 mEq/L; ± mL mEq/L is often listed as the normal range.

Values indicating metabolic acidosis of a primary or secondary nature are as follows:

    a. Bicarbonate greater than 24 mEq/L.

    b. BE greater than 0 or greater than + 1 mEq/L.

Values indicating metabolic acidosis of a primary or secondary nature are as follows:

    a. Bicarbonate less than 24 mEq/L.

b. BE less than 0 or less than − 1 mEq/L; some laboratories report this as a base deficit (BD) or negative base excess.

EXAM HINT

The NBRC uses BE for base excess (regardless of whether it has a positive or negative value) and HCO_3^- for bicarbonate.

Tables 3-7 through 3-9 show definitions of terms and classifications of the various acid-base states. As stated earlier, there are other systems for interpreting blood gases. All are probably satisfactory for interpretation purposes and preparing for the NBRC examinations.

3. Interpret the results of CO-oximetry blood gas analysis (Code: IC2e and IIIA1b) [Difficulty: An]

The CO-oximeter type blood gas analyzer gives values for oxyhemoglobin (O_2Hb), reduced hemoglobin (RHb), carboxyhemoglobin (COHb), and methemoglobin (MetHb)/sulfhemoglobin (SHb). Each of these hemoglobin moieties can be displayed in terms of grams per deciliter, percentage of the whole, and added together for a total hemoglobin (THb). Table 3-10 shows normal adult hemoglobin values. The amount of carboxyhemoglobin and methemoglobin should be subtracted from the total hemoglobin to find the amount of functional hemoglobin. Any increase in the carboxyhemoglobin or methemoglobin levels above those listed is abnormal and results in even less normal hemoglobin to carry oxygen. The patient who suffers from carbon monoxide poisoning is at greatest risk. A COHb level of 30% saturation or greater can be fatal. By subtraction, the O_2Hb (SaO_2) level can be no greater than 70% with a resulting PaO_2 of less than 40 torr.

The following example shows how to calculate the amount of functional hemoglobin and saturation for a patient with normal COHb and MetHb levels:

$$
\begin{array}{r}
15.0 \text{ gm total Hb} \\
- .225 \text{ gm COHb} \\
\hline
14.775 \text{ gm} \\
- .15 \text{ gm MetHb} \\
\hline
14.625 \text{ gm functional Hb}
\end{array}
$$

$$
\begin{array}{l}
100\% \text{ potential saturation of oxyhemoglobin in arterial blood} \\
- 1.5\% \text{ saturation of COHb} \\
\hline
98.5\% \\
- 1.5\% \text{ saturation of MetHb} \\
\hline
97\% \text{ saturation of arterial blood (} SaO_2 \text{ of 97\%)}
\end{array}
$$

TABLE 3-7 Clinical Terminology for Arterial Blood Gas Measurements

Clinical terminology	Clinical findings
Respiratory acidosis/alveolar hypoventilation/ ventilatory failure	$PaCO_2$ >50 torr
Acute ventilatory failure	$PaCO_2$ >50 torr; pH <7.30
Chronic ventilatory failure	$PaCO_2$ >50 torr; pH 7.30-7.40
Respiratory alkalosis/alveolar hyperventilation	$PaCO_2$ <30 torr
Acute alveolar hyperventilation	$PaCO_2$ <30 torr; pH >7.50
Chronic alveolar hyperventilation	$PaCO_2$ <30 torr; pH 7.40-7.50
Acidemia	pH <7.40*
Acidosis	Pathophysiologic condition in which the patient has a significant base deficit (plasma bicarbonate below normal)
Alkalemia	pH >7.40*
Alkalosis	Pathophysiologic condition in which the patient has a significant base excess (plasma bicarbonate above normal)

*Some authors prefer wider limits, such as acidemia with a pH ≤7.35, and alkalemia with a pH ≥7.45.
Modified from Shapiro BA, Harrison RA, Cane RD, Kozlowski-Templin R: *Clinical application of blood gases,* ed 4, St Louis, 1989, Mosby.

TABLE 3-8 Evaluation of Ventilatory and Metabolic Effects on Acid-Base Status

EVALUATION OF $PaCO_2$

$PaCO_2$ >50 torr	Respiratory acidosis/alveolar hypoventilation/ventilatory failure
$PaCO_2$ 30-50 torr	Acceptable alveolar ventilation
$PaCO_2$ <30 torr	Respiratory alkalosis/alveolar hyperventilation

EVALUATION OF $PaCO_2$ IN CONJUNCTION WITH pH
Acceptable alveolar ventilation ($PaCO_2$ from 30 to 50 torr)

pH >7.50	Metabolic alkalosis
pH 7.30-7.50	Acceptable ventilatory and metabolic pH
pH <7.30	Metabolic acidosis

Alveolar hypoventilation ($PaCO_2$ >50 torr)

pH >7.40	*Partially compensated* metabolic alkalosis
pH 7.30-7.40	*Chronic* ventilatory failure
pH <7.30	*Acute* ventilatory failure

Alveolar hyperventilation ($PaCO_2$ <30 torr)

pH >7.50	*Acute* alveolar hyperventilation
pH 7.40-7.50	*Chronic* alveolar hyperventilation
pH 7.30-7.40	*Compensated* metabolic acidosis
pH <7.30	*Partially compensated* metabolic acidosis

$PaCO_2$, Partial pressure of CO_2 in arterial blood.
Some authors use a narrower pH range for these classifications.
Modified from Shapiro BA, Harrison RA, Cane RD, Kozlowski-Templin R: *Clinical application of blood gases,* ed 4, St Louis, 1989, Mosby.

The following example is for a patient with an elevated COHb and a normal MetHb level:

$$15.0 \text{ gm total Hb}$$
$$\underline{-3.0 \text{ gm COHb}}$$
$$12.0 \text{ gm}$$
$$\underline{- .15 \text{ gm MetHb}}$$
$$11.85 \text{ gm functional Hb}$$

TABLE 3-9	Primary Blood Gas Classifications

	PaCO$_2$	pH	Bicarbonate	BE
VENTILATORY IMBALANCE				
Acute alveolar hypoventilation	I	D	N	N
Chronic alveolar hypoventilation	I	N	I	I
Acute alveolar hyperventilation	D	I	N	N
Chronic alveolar hyperventilation	D	N	D	D
METABOLIC IMBALANCE				
Uncompensated acidosis	N	D	D	D
Partially compensated acidosis	D	D	D	D
Uncompensated alkalosis	N	I	I	I
Partially compensated alkalosis	I	I	I	I
Compensated acidosis or alkalosis	I or D	N	I or D	I or D

D, Decreased; *I,* increased; *N,* normal range; *BE,* base excess; *PaCO$_2$,* partial pressure of CO$_2$ in arterial blood.
Modified from Shapiro BA, Harrison RA, Cane RD, Kozlowski-Templin R: *Clinical application of blood gases,* ed 4, St Louis, 1989, Mosby.

TABLE 3-10	Normal Hemoglobin Values for Adults

Total hemoglobin (THb)	Men: 13.5-18.0 g/dl
	Women: 12.0-16.0 g/dl
	15.0 g/dl is often listed as an average for both
Oxyhemoglobin	94%-100% of THb (reported as SaO$_2$ of 94% to 100%)
Carboxyhemoglobin	Nonsmokers: <1.5% (0.225 g/dl) of THb
	Smokers: 1.5%-10% of THb
Methemoglobin	0.5%-3% (0.075-0.45 g/dl) of THb
Oxygen content (arterial sample)	15-23 g/dl

g/dl, Grams per deciliter (sometimes listed as g/100 mL); *SaO$_2$,* O$_2$ saturation in arterial blood.

100% potential saturation of oxyhemoglobin in arterial blood

$$\underline{-20\% \text{ saturation of COHb}}$$
$$80\%$$
$$\underline{- 1.5\% \text{ saturation of MetHb}}$$
$$78.5\% \text{ saturation of arterial blood (SaO}_2 \text{ of } 78.5\%)$$

4. Mixed venous blood gases

a. Review the patient's chart for mixed venous blood gas results (Code: IA1g2) [Difficulty: An]

A mixed venous blood sample can be taken from the pulmonary artery of any patient who has a pulmonary artery (Swan-Ganz) catheter. This is a true mixed venous sample and should not be confused with a blood sample taken from an arm vein or other venous site. The symbol $P\bar{v}$ is the prefix for venous blood gas values of oxygen and so forth. In general, a typical patient has mixed venous blood gas values of: $S\bar{v}O_2$, 75%; $P\bar{v}O_2$ 40 mm Hg; $P\bar{v}CO_2$ 46 mm Hg; and pH 7.35. (Table 3-11 gives details on normal venous blood gas values and their interpretation in patients with cardiovascular disease.)

b. Interpret the results of mixed venous blood gas analysis to evaluate the patient's response to respiratory care (Code: IB10c and IC2e) [Difficulty: An]

In the critically ill patient, it is just as important to measure the mixed venous blood gases as it is to measure the arterial blood gases. The venous blood gas values reveal what has happened as the arterial blood has passed through the body. Oxygen has been extracted and carbon dioxide has been added to the blood. The difference between the arterial and venous oxygen levels reflects oxygen consumption by the body as well as cardiac output.

TABLE 3-11	Normal and Abnormal Mixed Venous Blood Gas Values

NORMAL VALUES
Average: $S\bar{v}O_2$ 75%; $P\bar{v}O_2$ 40 torr; $P\bar{v}CO_2$ 46 torr; pH 7.35
Range: $S\bar{v}O_2$ 76%-70%; $P\bar{v}O_2$ 43-37 torr; $P\bar{v}CO_2$ 46-44 torr; pH 7.36-7.34

CRITICALLY ILL PATIENT

	P$\bar{v}$O$_2$ (torr)		S$\bar{v}$O$_2$ (%)	
	Average	Range	Average	Range
Excellent cardiovascular reserves	37	40-35	70	75-68
Limited cardiovascular reserves	32	35-30	60	68-56
Failure of cardiovascular reserves	<30	<30	<56	<56

Modified from Shapiro BA, Peruzzi WT, Kozlowski-Templin R: *Clinical application of blood gases,* ed 5, St Louis, 1994, Mosby.

Because of this, the most critical venous blood gas values to measure are the $S\bar{v}O_2$ and $P\bar{v}O_2$. It is generally accepted that a $P\bar{v}O_2$ value of less than 30 torr or $S\bar{v}O_2$ of less than 56% indicates that the patient has tissue hypoxia. Both values can be obtained by analyzing a mixed venous blood sample taken through a pulmonary artery catheter. If the patient has a fiber optic catheter, the $S\bar{v}O_2$ value can be monitored continuously. This is extremely helpful if the patient is unstable or having frequent changes in inspired oxygen or ventilator settings. (Pulmonary artery catheters are discussed in more detail in Chapter 5.)

5. Interpret the results of capillary blood gas analysis to evaluate the patient's response to respiratory care (Code: IB10c and IC2e) [Difficulty: An]

If the infant's sampling site is well perfused and the sample properly obtained, the blood can be analyzed. Because this is not a true arterial blood gas sample, the following limitations are placed on interpreting the results:

a. The capillary pH (c pH) has a good correlation with the arterial pH.
b. The capillary CO_2 ($PcCO_2$) correlates with the $PaCO_2$ about 50% of the time.
c. The capillary O_2 (Pco_2) does not correlate well with the $PaCO_2$.

Based on these limitations, an arterialized capillary blood pH value can be clinically useful. The capillary CO_2 value should be viewed with suspicion. It should not be the only parameter followed to judge the infant's ability to ventilate; however, the combination of a low pH and elevated CO_2 both indicate hypoventilation. Evaluate the infant's vital signs, breathing efforts, chest radiograph, and so on to determine respiratory status.

Unfortunately, the capillary O_2 value is practically useless for judging the infant's oxygenation. Some infants may have a fairly close correlation with the PaO_2, whereas others do not. Unfortunately, there is no way to predetermine those that will match and those that will not. Many practitioners view a low capillary oxygen level as a sign of clinical hypoxemia. The American Association for Respiratory Care (AARC) Clinical Practice Guideline "Oxygen Therapy in the Acute Care Hospital" notes that a Pco_2 of less than 40 torr documents neonatal hypoxemia. An arterial blood gas sample remains the best way to determine the patient's respiratory status.

MODULE E	Alveolar-arterial difference in oxygen pressure [P(A-a)O₂]

1. Perform the P(A-a)O₂ procedure (Code: IB9c, IC1e, and IIIA1m1) [Difficulty: An]

Perform the following for the alveolar-arterial O_2 pressure difference [P(A-a) O_2] procedure:

a. Note the patient's inspired oxygen percentage.

b. Draw and analyze an arterial blood gas sample. Note the patient's PaO_2 and $PaCO_2$.
c. Note the patient's temperature. This is needed to determine the patient's pulmonary water vapor pressure (PH_2O). The value of 47 torr (mm Hg) is used if the patient's temperature is normal. Check published tables for the pulmonary water vapor pressure if the patient's temperature is higher or lower than normal.
d. Measure the local barometric pressure (P_B) in torr (mm Hg).
e. If possible, calculate the patient's respiratory exchange ratio. If this cannot be done, use the standard value of 0.8.
f. Calculate the patient's PAO_2. The formula presented here is the most commonly used of several versions:

$$PAO_2 = [(P_B - PH_2O)\,F_IO_2] - \frac{PaCO_2}{.8}$$

In which:

PAO_2 = Pressure of alveolar oxygen.

P_B = Barometric pressure of air. This is 760 torr (mm Hg) at sea level; it decreases as the altitude increases.

PH_2O = Pressure of water vapor in the lungs. This is 47 torr (mm Hg) at the normal temperature of 98.6° F/37° C. Remember that water vapor pressure increases if the patient has a fever and decreases if the patient is hypothermic.

F_IO_2 = Fractional concentration (percentage) of inspired oxygen. Use whatever percentage of oxygen your patient is breathing in.

$\dfrac{PaCO_2}{.8}$ = Effect of carbon dioxide and the patient's metabolism. The factor of .8 is based on how much oxygen a normal person uses and how much carbon dioxide is produced in 1 minute. The symbols for this metabolic value are R for Respiratory Exchange Ratio and RQ for Respiratory Quotient. The following calculation is based on a normal person's metabolism:

$$R \text{ or } RQ = \frac{VCO_2}{VO_2} = \frac{200\,mL/min}{250\,mL/min} = .8$$

Because many sick patients do not react as expected, the factor has a range of .6 to 1.1 depending on oxygen consumption and carbon dioxide production. Assume the factor is .8 unless you are told otherwise or measure otherwise.

g. Subtract the patient's PaO_2 from the PAO_2 to determine the $P(A-a)O_2$.

2. **Interpret the results of the alveolar-arterial oxygen pressure difference to evaluate the patient's response to respiratory care (Code: IB10c, IC2e, and IIIA1m1) [Difficulty: An]**

The $P(A-a)O_2$ in a normal young person should be no greater than 15 torr, but slowly increases as a normal person ages. Lung disease causes the value to increase significantly. The following are examples of some conditions in which the measurement of the $P(A-a)O_2$ aids in diagnosis or treatment:

1. Patients who are hypoxemic because they are hypoventilating (increased CO_2) have a normal $P(A-a)O_2$ when breathing room air. The hypoxemia can be corrected by increasing ventilation. Supplemental oxygen results in an expected increase in PaO_2.

2. Any condition in which there is a low ventilation to perfusion ratio reveals an elevated $P(A-a)O_2$ when breathing room air. Supplemental oxygen results in an increase in PaO_2; however, the increase is not as dramatic as that seen in the hypoventilating patient. Examples include asthma, bronchitis, emphysema, or any other condition in which there is unequal distribution of air into and out of the lungs but relatively normal perfusion.

3. Any shunt producing disease or condition. Examples include acute respiratory distress syndrome (ARDS) and right to left anatomic shunt such as is seen in a ventricular septal defect. The $P(A-a)O_2$ becomes greater as the oxygen percentage is increased. It is commonly accepted that a $P(A-a)O_2$ of more than 350 torr, when 80% to 100% oxygen is administered, indicates that the patient is experiencing refractory hypoxemia. The patient probably needs to be supported by a mechanical ventilator. Commonly, positive end-expiratory pressure (PEEP) is administered so that the oxygen percentage can be reduced to a safer level.

4. Any disease producing a diffusion defect. Pulmonary fibrosis from any cause results in a wider than normal $P(A-a)O_2$. Supplemental oxygen results in an increase in the PaO_2, but not as great an increase as desired.

The following examples are offered to aid in the calculation of $P(A-a)O_2$ and the interpretation of the results.

Example 1

You are working in a major teaching hospital in Miami. The patient's physician asks you to calculate the $P(A-a)O_2$ on a 30-year-old patient. The following conditions exist:

$P_B = 760$ torr

$PH_2O = 47$ torr because your patient's temperature is 98.6° F/37° C

$F_IO_2 = .21$ because the patient is breathing room air

$PaCO_2 = 40$ torr from ABGs

$PaO_2 = 90$ torr from ABGs

$R = .8$

1. $PAO_2 = [(P_B - PH_2O) F_IO_2] - \dfrac{PaCO_2}{.8}$

2. $PAO_2 = [(760 - 47) .21] - \dfrac{40}{.8}$

3. $PAO_2 = [(713) .21] - 50$

4. $PAO_2 = [150] - 50$

5. $PAO_2 = 100$ torr

6. $P(A-a)O_2 = 100 - 90 = 10$ torr

Interpretation: A $P(A-a)O_2$ of 10 torr is normal for a patient of this age. It is normal to see a difference between the alveolar and arterial oxygen levels that starts out in the range of 4 to 12 torr and slowly increases with age. See Fig. 3-13.

Example 2

You are working in a major teaching hospital in Denver. You are asked to calculate the alveolar-arterial difference in oxygen on a 40-year-old patient. The following conditions exist:

$P_B = 710$ torr

$PH_2O = 50$ torr because your patient's temperature is 100° F/38° C

$F_IO_2 = .35$ because the patient is breathing 35% oxygen by mask

$PaCO_2 = 55$ torr from ABGs

$PaO_2 = 65$ torr from ABGs

$R = .85$

1. $PAO_2 = [(P_B - PH_2O) F_IO_2] - \dfrac{PaCO_2}{.8}$

2. $PAO_2 = [(710 - 50) .35] - \dfrac{55}{.85}$

3. $PAO_2 = [(660) .35] - 65$

4. $PAO_2 = [231] - 65$

5. $PAO_2 = 166$ torr

6. $P(A-a)O_2 = 166 - 65 = 101$ torr

Interpretation: The difference of 101 torr is elevated even though this patient is older than the patient in Example 1.

MODULE F | **Pulse oximetry**

1. **Check the patient's chart for previous pulse oximetry results (Code: IA1f5) [Difficulty: An]**

Pulse oximetry (SpO_2) spectroscopically analyzes arterial blood to noninvasively determine the percent of hemoglobin that is saturated with oxygen. It generally is indicated whenever a patient's oxygenation must be monitored. An SpO_2 of 92% or greater indicates that the patient is adequately oxygenated. Past values should be

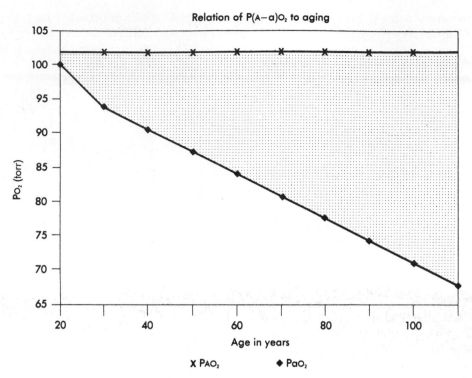

Fig. 3-13 The relationship of P(A-a)O$_2$ to aging. As the PaO$_2$ naturally falls with age, the P(A-a)O$_2$ increases at the rate of approximately 3 torr per decade beyond 20 years. (From Lane EE and Walker JF: *Clinical arterial blood gas analysis.* St Louis, 1987, Mosby.)

compared with current readings to follow the patient's progress or response to treatment.

2. Make a recommendation to perform pulse oximetry (Code: IA2g) [Difficulty: An]

Pulse oximetry is indicated in the following situations: during anesthesia and intraoperative monitoring of oxygenation, postoperatively when the patient is still sedated, when the patient is receiving sedatives or analgesics that can blunt the airway protective reflexes, during bronchoscopy, during a sleep study, and to evaluate the effectiveness of oxygen therapy. An exception to the use of pulse oximetry is when there is known or suspected carbon monoxide poisoning.

3. Get an appropriate pulse oximeter and related equipment (Code: IIA1h4) [Difficulty: An]

Each pulse oximeter reports a percentage of hemoglobin saturation with oxygen on a light-emitting diode (LED) display. Many newer units also display the patient's pulse rate. More expensive units print out a copy of SpO$_2$ percentage and pulse rate to be placed into the patient's chart if it is required. There are a variety of sensors that fit the feet or hands of infants, an adult's fingers, the bridge of the nose, forehead, and ear lobe. Choose a sensor designed to fit the site that is selected.

4. Put the equipment together, make sure that it works properly, and identify any problems (Code: IIB1h4) [Difficulty: An]

Follow the manufacturer's suggestions for setup. The newer pulse oximetry systems visually display the strength of the pulse so that the best place for the probe can be found. (See Fig. 3-14.) Keep bright light out of the patient site and transducer. Fig. 3-15 shows how to properly apply the finger probe.

5. Fix any problems with the equipment (Code: IIB1h4) [Difficulty: An]

The pulse signal will not be strong if the patient has poor circulation at the site of the oximeter probe. This can occur if the patient is hypothermic, hypotensive, or receiving a vasoconstricting medication. If the pulse signal is weak, the pulse oximetry values may not be accurate. See Table 3-12 for common sources of error and their solutions.

6. Perform pulse oximetry on your patient (Code: IB9a, IC1b) [Difficulty: An]

Pulse oximetry has gained wide acceptance because it offers a way to continuously and noninvasively monitor a patient's oxygenation by following the percent of hemoglobin saturated with oxygen. The reported SpO$_2$ % is the percent of oxyhemoglobin.

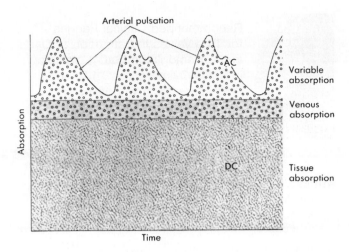

Fig. 3-14 Pulse oximetry signal strength. The strong surge of blood through the artery with each heartbeat results in variable absorption of the light emitted by the pulse oximeter. Venous and tissue absorption of light is stable when the heart is at rest. This absorption difference is used to find the patient's artery and measure the heart rate. (*AC* refers to variable absorption. *DC* refers to stable absorption.) (From Ruppel G: *Manual of pulmonary function testing,* ed 6, St Louis, 1994, Mosby.)

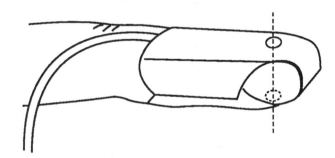

Fig. 3-15 Pulse oximetry transducer properly placed on a finger. (Courtesy Mallinckrodt, Inc.)

Pulse oximetry makes practical use of two physical principles. The first is spectrophotometry, which is used to analyze the transmission of two wavelengths of light through the blood and body tissues. One wavelength is 660 nm and the other is between 920 and 940 nm, depending on the manufacturer. The 660 nm wavelength can be seen as red and is preferentially absorbed by oxyhemoglobin (O_2Hb). The 920 to 940 nm wavelength is not visible, because it is in the infrared range. It is preferentially absorbed by reduced hemoglobin (RHb).

The second principle is plethysmography. It is used to find and then evaluate the amplitude of the arterial pulse waveform. See Fig. 3-14 for the plethysmographic arterial waveform. When the pulse oximeter sensor is placed on a patient site, the fingertip for example, the two wavelengths of light shine through the blood, tissues, and bone within the finger. It is important that the sending LED and

TABLE 3-12   Sources of Error in Pulse Oximetry

Sources of error	Remedy
Light interference: xenon lamp, fluorescent light, infrared (bilirubin) light, probe fell off of patient	Cover the probe with an opaque wrap; put the probe back in place on the patient
Low perfusion: low blood pressure, hypothermia, vasoconstricting drugs	Use earlobe, bridge of nose, or forehead instead of finger or toe; discontinue use if still unreliable
Motion artifact	Secure the probe site; ensure that the SpO_2 reading is synchronized with the heart rate
Darkly pigmented patient	Use lightly pigmented site such as tip of finger or toe; SpO_2 value may overestimate PaO_2; discontinue use if still unreliable
Artificial or painted fingernails	Remove acrylic nails; remove black, blue, green, metallic, or frosted nail polish; use a different site
Venous pulsation being read as an arterial pulsation	Loosen a tight sensor; change the finger sensor site every 2-4 hr; loosen the cause of a tourniquet-like effect
The following vascular dyes will cause low SpO_2 readings: methylene blue, indigo carmine, indocyanine green	Do not use SpO_2

PaO_2, Partial pressure of O_2 in arterial blood; SpO_2, pulse oximeter.

receiving (photodiode) sensors be opposite each other. Most units have a signal strength display that indicates when the photodiode is receiving a strong signal, and the patient's pulse has been detected. The microprocessor is designed to detect a baseline level of light absorption by the tissues and venous blood, containing more RHb, as well as the light absorption of arterial blood, containing more O_2Hb. It can then compare the absorptions of the two wavelengths to determine the level of saturated oxyhemoglobin. This is displayed as saturation by pulse oximetry, or SpO_2.

It must be realized that because pulse oximetry samples only two wavelengths of light, the technology is unable to recognize the presence or quantity of the nonfunctional hemoglobin species of COHb and MetHb. Instead, an ABG should be drawn and sent to the laboratory to be passed through a CO-oximeter for a complete fractional hemoglobin analysis. Even healthy persons have small amounts of COHb and MetHB. For this and other technical reasons, manufacturers report the following SpO$_2$ values for general accuracy at one standard deviation (1 SD) for a general population: ± 2% from 100% to 70% saturation, and ± 3% from 70% to 50% saturation. Because of these limitations, the following clinical guidelines have been created by a number of authors:

a. Do not use pulse oximetry on patients with significant levels of COHb or MetHB.

b. If in doubt about abnormal types of hemoglobin, analyze an ABG through a CO-oximeter and compare the true SaO$_2$ with the SpO$_2$ from pulse oximetry. Pulse oximetry can be used if the correlation of values is within 4%.

c. Question the SpO$_2$ value when the displayed heart rate is different from the actual heart rate.

d. Do not use pulse oximetry when the SpO$_2$ reading is less than 70%.

e. Pulse oximetry can be used on a term neonate or one that is 1500 grams or larger. Smaller neonates should have oxygenation measured by a transcutaneous oxygen monitor. This is because it is too easy to hyperoxygenate a small neonate when small changes in saturation can result in wide swings in PO$_2$. The risk of retinopathy of prematurity (formerly called retrolental fibroplasia) from hyperoxia is too great in the small neonate.

Table 3-13 lists common clinical ranges for SpO$_2$ values. For the aforementioned reasons, the minimum safe values are 2% higher than the corresponding SaO$_2$ value by CO-oximetry. It is important that the patient have good pulsatile blood flow to the measurement site to obtain an accurate reading.

7. Interpret a patient's pulse oximetry value (Code: IB10a, IC2b, and IIIA1b) [Difficulty: An]

The previously healthy patient who has cardiopulmonary failure should have the SpO$_2$ value kept at 92% or greater to ensure adequate oxygenation. The patient with chronic obstructive pulmonary disease can probably tolerate an SpO$_2$ value of as low as 87%. The neonate should have the SpO$_2$ kept between 92% to 96%. Saturations below these values indicate hypoxemia in most patients.

Note the site at which the saturation was measured. This is especially important in neonates who may have congenital heart defects. A higher saturation in the right fingers or right ear lobe compared with the rest of the body is seen with a patent ductus arteriosus. A higher saturation in the fingers and ear lobes as compared with the toes is seen with a coarctation of the aorta.

EXAM HINT

The patient with carbon monoxide poisoning should not be evaluated with a pulse oximeter because the units are unable to distinguish oxyhemoglobin from carboxyhemoglobin. They add

| TABLE 3-13 | Recommended Clinical Ranges for True Values in Saturation of O$_2$ in the Hemoglobin (SaO$_2$), Values in Pulse Oximetry (SpO$_2$),* and Their Correlation with Values in Partial Pressure of O$_2$ in Arterial Blood (PaO$_2$) |

	SaO$_2$	SpO$_2$	Approximate PaO$_2$ (torr)
ADULT			
Acute hypoxemia	90%-95%	92%-95%†	60-95
Chronic hypoxemia	85%-90%	87%-92%	50-60
NEONATE			
<1500 g or in the first week of life	About 97%	92%-96%	60-70
>1500 g or after the first week of life	90%-96%	90%-96%	50-70
>1 month of age with chronic lung disease	85%-90%	87%-92%	50-60

Note: The clinical goal with most neonates is to prevent both hypoxemia, defined as a PaO$_2$ <45 torr, and hyperoxemia, defined as a PaO$_2$ >90 torr.
*Based on the patient having normal carboxyhemoglobin and methemoglobin levels. Elevated level(s) result in an erroneously high SpO$_2$ reading and unsuspected hypoxemia.
†Black patients should have an SpO$_2$ of 95% maintained to ensure adequate oxygenation.

therefore a higher O$_2$Hb saturation will be reported than actually exists. These patients should be evaluated for oxygenation only by an arterial blood gas that is analyzed on a CO-oximeter blood gas analyzer.

MODULE G   Transcutaneous oxygen monitoring

Note: Transcutaneous monitoring (TCM) involves the continuous monitoring of oxygen, carbon dioxide, or both as they diffuse through the skin. Each gas has its own electrode and a combined electrode exists for both gases.

1. Review the patient's chart for a transcutaneous oxygen (PtcO$_2$) value (Code: IA1f5) [Difficulty: An]

Transcutaneous oxygen monitoring (PtcO$_2$, tcPO$_2$, or TcO$_2$) enables any patient's oxygenation status to be followed on a continuous basis. In practice, neonates are monitored much more often than adults. Check the chart for a record of the patient's transcutaneous oxygen values. It is particularly important to compare the PaO$_2$ with the PtcO$_2$. In addition, note what the PtcO$_2$ values are when the inspired oxygen is changed, the patient is suctioned, or changes are made in continuous positive airway pressure (CPAP) or mechanical ventilation. Avoid clinical situations that have previously resulted in hypoxemia.

2. Recommend transcutaneous oxygen monitoring for additional data (Code: IA2g) [Difficulty: An]

$PtcO_2$ monitoring has been used for the following purposes:

a. To monitor oxygenation during transportation of an unstable neonate within the hospital or between two hospitals.

b. To monitor intraoperative and postoperative oxygenation.

c. To monitor oxygenation during changes in the inspired oxygen, during changes in mechanical ventilation, and to detect hypoxemia during an equipment failure.

d. To help detect a right-to-left shunt. When a neonate has a patent ductus arteriosus (PDA), the $PtcO_2$ is higher in the right upper chest than in the left upper chest, abdomen, or thighs.

e. To help detect a coarctation of the aorta. When this defect is present, the $PtcO_2$ is higher in the right and left upper chest than in the abdomen or thighs.

f. To determine the congenital heart disease patient's response to an oxygen challenge test.

3. Obtain the necessary equipment to perform transcutaneous oxygen monitoring (Code: IIA1h4) [Difficulty: An]

The electrode used for monitoring the patient's transcutaneous oxygen level is a miniaturized and modified Clark-type polarographic electrode similar to that used in the blood gas analyzer (see Fig. 3-16). Some authors describe it as a *Huch* or *Hellige* electrode after two researchers who modified the original Clark electrode for their work with pediatric patients.

4. Put the transcutaneous oxygen monitor together, make sure that it works properly, and identify any problems (Code: IIB1h4) [Difficulty: An]

Always follow the manufacturer's recommendations for the assembly and care of the equipment. Select the proper electrode for the monitor based on the physician's order for evaluating transcutaneous oxygen, carbon dioxide, or both together.

5. Perform quality control procedures on a transcutaneous oxygen monitor (Code: IIB3d) [Difficulty: R, Ap, An]

Always follow the manufacturer's recommendations for the assembly and care of the equipment. Select the proper electrode for the monitor based on the physician's order for evaluating transcutaneous oxygen, carbon dioxide, or both together.

Calibration. Two-point calibration must be performed with oxygen percentages that will cause PO_2 values beyond

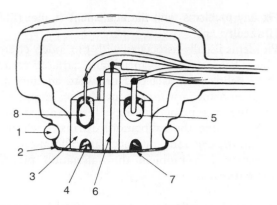

Fig. 3-16 Schematic drawing of the modified Clark electrode used to monitor transcutaneous oxygen tension. 1, O-ring to hold the membrane to the electrode; 2, polypropylene membrane permeable to oxygen; 3, silver anode that surrounds the platinum cathode; 4, electrolyte chamber with solution held in place by the polypropylene membrane; 5, heating element; 6, platinum cathode; 7, electrolyte solution of sodium bicarbonate and sodium chloride held between the membrane and electrode; and 8, negative temperature coefficient (NTC) resistor that serves to regulate the temperature of the sensor. (From Shapiro BA, Peruzzi WT, Templin R: *Clinical application of blood gases,* ed 5, St Louis, 1994, Mosby.)

the clinical range that can be expected. Usually the first calibration point is a "zero" point because the electrode is exposed to 0% oxygen in a nitrogen-filled chamber. This point is usually quite stable. The second calibration point is found when the electrode is exposed to room air (20.95% or 0.2095 oxygen). Always follow the manufacturer's written procedures during the calibration process. Generally, when environmental conditions include a fairly stable room temperature of 25° C and 50% relative humidity, the following equation can be used to predict the room air calibration point:

$$\text{calibration } PtcO_2 = P_B \times 0.2095$$

In which:

P_B = local barometric pressure
0.2095 = oxygen fraction found in room air

Expose the electrode to room air to determine if it matches the calculated calibration value. Adjust the instrument to match the calibration $PtcO_2$ if necessary. It is recommended that the room air calibration point be rechecked every 24 hours when in continuous use, after changing the membrane, or after changing the electrolyte solution. A variation of up to ± 5 torr is acceptable and can be corrected by adjusting the reading on the instrument. If the variation is greater than ± 5 torr, the zero-point and room air calibration procedures should be repeated.

6. **Fix any problems with the equipment (Code: IIB2h4) [Difficulty: An]**

Problems usually associated with too much electrode drift include electrode or membrane surfaces contaminated by debris such as blood or sweat, an improperly applied membrane, a worn-out membrane, an air bubble beneath the membrane, improper gas exposed to the membrane during the calibration, exhausted electrolyte solution in the electrode, or inaccurate calibration values. After correcting a problem the calibration procedure should be repeated.

7. **Perform transcutaneous oxygen ($PtcO_2$) monitoring (Code: IB9a, IC1b, and IIID3) [Difficulty: R, Ap]**

   a. Site selection

Care must be taken to select the best site for the electrode. A bad site will give incorrect information that can lead to mistakes in patient care. See Box 3-2 for a listing of site selection guidelines.

   b. Skin and electrode preparation and application of the skin electrode

An airtight seal between the skin and electrode is necessary for accurate readings. An air leak will result in an increase in the $PtcO_2$ reading (and a fall in the $PtcCO_2$ reading). The following steps should be taken to ensure that the skin site and electrode are prepared and an airtight seal is ensured:

1. Clean the skin. Usually, cleaning with an alcohol swab is enough to remove perspiration. Oily skin should be cleaned with soap and water.
2. Adults may need to have hair shaved from the site.
3. Adults may have dead skin cells removed by placing sticky adhesive tape against the site and pulling it off.
4. Prepare the electrode according to the manufacturer's guidelines. This usually includes placing a drop of the electrolyte solution on the electrode surface and placing a gas permeable membrane with a double adhesive ring over the electrode.
5. The other side of the adhesive ring is pressed against the monitoring site so that there is an airtight seal.
6. As the electrode warms the skin, the patient values will fluctuate. Stabilization usually requires several minutes, after which the patient values should be clinically useful.

   c. Limitations and patient precautions

Because the electrode is heated, it must be rotated to a different skin site on a routine basis. The general manufacturer's guidelines for site rotation are every 4 to 6 hours for neonates weighing between 1000 and 2500 grams; every 3 to 5 hours for neonates weighing between

---

| BOX 3-2 | Optimal Sites and Sites to Avoid with Transcutaneous Gas Monitoring |

OPTIMAL NEONATAL SITES
Upper part of the chest
Right upper chest if a preductal $PtcO_2$ value is desired
Abdomen
Inner aspect of either thigh

OPTIMAL ADULT SITES
Upper part of chest
Inner aspect of the upper arm

SITES TO AVOID
Large fat deposit
Bony prominence
Pressure point
Thick skin
Skin edema
Hands and feet

CONDITIONS WHEN TRANSCUTANEOUS MONITORING SHOULD NOT BE USED
Locally cold skin or general, deep hypothermia
Locally decreased peripheral perfusion or general hypotension
Patient receiving vasoconstricting drugs such as tolazoline or dopamine
Cardiac index less than 1.9 L/min/m² of body surface area
Halothane anesthesia will give erroneously high transcutaneous O_2 values unless a Teflon membrane is used

$PtcO_2$, Transcutaneous monitoring.

2500 and 3500 grams; and 2 to 4 hours for neonates weighing more than 3500 grams, pediatric patients, and adult patients. As a safety precaution, change the electrode on all patients at least every 4 hours, or at least every 3 hours if the patient is hypothermic. The manufacturer's range in times is based on the relative thickness of the patient's skin and the different electrode temperatures. It is important to adjust the site rotation times on an individual patient basis. Some may tolerate longer times, and others will need more frequent rotations.

Care must be taken when removing the adhesive ring and electrode. It is possible to tear the thin, delicate skin of a premature neonate. Loosen the adhesive by running the edge of an alcohol wipe along the side that is being gently pulled up. After the electrode is removed, it is important to examine the skin; it is normal to see a red circle. This warmed, vasodilated area will stay red for some time and will gradually fade away. There will be no scarring or permanent injury. Rarely, the skin will have overheated and a blister is seen; this is a second-degree burn.

Obviously, future site rotations must be made more frequently. Do not use this site again. Treat it as a burn and avoid any further injury that might break the skin and lead to an infection.

8. Interpret transcutaneous oxygen monitoring values to evaluate the patient's response to respiratory care (Code: IB10a and IC2b) [Difficulty: An]

It has been found that heating the electrode speeds up the diffusion of oxygen through the skin. Heating also provides a closer correlation with the patient's PaO_2 value. However, it must be remembered that the $PtcO_2$ value is not the same as the PaO_2 value. Current recommendations are that any unit should give $PtcO_2$ values that are within ± 15% of the PaO_2 over the operating range of the instrument. The values should then correlate within ± 15% as the patient's condition changes. This should always be confirmed.

An arterial blood gas should be drawn for PaO_2 every time transcutaneous oxygen monitoring is started. The PaO_2–$PtcO_2$ gradient can then be calculated as the difference between the two. For example, if the patient's PaO_2 is 100 torr, the $PtcO_2$ should be no less than 85 torr. If the $PtcO_2$ decreases to 70 torr, the PaO_2 should have decreased to no lower than 85 torr. Because of this close correlation, the patient can be trend monitored with some assurance of accuracy. In addition, arterial blood gases do not need to be drawn as frequently for the PaO_2. This trending relationship holds true for changes in the patient's pulmonary condition. It does not, however, hold true when the patient has cardiovascular problems such as hypotension, hypothermia, peripheral vascular disease, or cardiogenic shock with decreased tissue perfusion.

Always follow the manufacturer's recommendations for the proper electrode temperature. In general, the temperature ranges from 42.5° C for a 1000 gm infant to 44° C for a 3500 gm infant. A pediatric patient can tolerate a temperature of 44° C, whereas an adult can have an electrode temperature of 45° C. The higher temperatures are needed in older patients because their skin is thicker. Studies have shown that when the neonate's PaO_2 is greater than 100 torr, the $PtcO_2$ value underestimates it. This can lead to dangerous hyperoxemia. For this reason, it is recommended that the $PtcO_2$ be kept at less than 90 torr. In the adult, there is less correlation between the PaO_2 and $PtcO_2$ because of the thicker skin. $PtcO_2$ can still be used in the adult to follow trends in oxygenation, but the practitioner must realize that a drop in the $PtcO_2$ value can be a result of hypoxemia, a decreased cardiac output, or cutaneous vasoconstriction. An arterial blood gas must be drawn to further evaluate the patient's status.

Correlation of $PtcO_2$ and local power consumption.
As mentioned earlier, the electrode is heated to above body temperature. The amount of electrical current needed to keep the electrode at a constant temperature depends on the temperature of the blood and the speed at which the blood passes beneath the electrode. This is known as local power consumption or simply local power (LP). A change in the LP value and $PtcO_2$ can be used to indicate what is happening to the patient. For example:

a. A normal LP seen with a decreased $PtcO_2$ indicates that the patient's pulmonary problem has worsened.

b. A normal LP seen with an increased $PtcO_2$ indicates that the patient's pulmonary problem has improved.

c. A decreased LP seen with a decreased $PtcO_2$ indicates that the patient's cardiac output has worsened.

d. An increased LP seen with an increased $PtcO_2$ indicates that the patient's cardiac output has improved.

MODULE H	Transcutaneous carbon dioxide monitoring

1. Review the patient's chart for a transcutaneous carbon dioxide value (Code: IA1f5) [Difficulty: An]

Transcutaneous carbon dioxide monitoring ($PtcCO_2$, $tcPCO_2$, or $TcCO_2$) enables any patient's ventilation status to be followed on a continuous basis. In practice, neonates are monitored much more often than adults. Check the chart for a record of the patient's transcutaneous carbon dioxide values. It is particularly important to correlate these values with any arterial blood gas values, which allows comparison between the $PaCO_2$ and the $PtcCO_2$. In addition, note the $PtcCO_2$ values when changes are made in CPAP or mechanical ventilation. Avoid clinical situations that have previously resulted in hypoventilation.

2. Recommend transcutaneous carbon dioxide monitoring for additional data (Code: IA2g) [Difficulty: An]

$PtcCO_2$ monitoring has been used for the following purposes:

a. To monitor ventilation during transportation of an unstable infant within the hospital or between two hospitals.

b. To monitor intraoperative and postoperative ventilation.

c. To monitor ventilation during changes in mechanical ventilation such as tidal volume, rate, minute ventilation, and/or mechanical dead space.

d. To detect hypoventilation during an accidental disconnection from the ventilator.

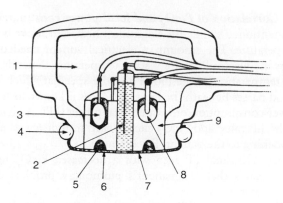

Fig. 3-17 Schematic drawing of the modified Stow-Severinghaus electrode used to monitor transcutaneous carbon dioxide tension. 1, epoxy resin; 2, glass electrode with a chlorinated silver wire, a buffer solution (the inner liquid), and a pH sensitive glass membrane; 3, negative temperature coefficient (NTC) resistor that serves to regulate the temperature of the sensor; 4, O-ring to hold the membrane to the electrode; 5, electrolyte chamber with solution held in place by the polypropylene membrane; 6, electrolyte solution of sodium bicarbonate and sodium chloride held between the membrane and electrode; 7, polypropylene membrane permeable to carbon dioxide; 8, heating element; and 9, silver/silver chloride reference electrode. (From Shapiro BA, Peruzzi WT, Templin R: *Clinical application of blood gases,* ed 5, St Louis, 1994, Mosby.)

3. Obtain the necessary equipment to perform transcutaneous carbon dioxide monitoring (Code: IIA1h4) [Difficulty: An]

The electrode used for monitoring the patient's transcutaneous carbon dioxide level is a miniaturized and modified Stow-Severinghaus type electrode similar to the arterial blood gas electrode (Fig. 3-17).

4. Put the transcutaneous carbon dioxide monitor together, make sure that it works properly, and identify any problems with it (Code: IIB1h4) [Difficulty: An]

Always follow the manufacturer's recommendations for the assembly and care of the equipment. Select the proper electrode for the monitor based on the physician's order for evaluating transcutaneous carbon dioxide, oxygen, or both together.

5. Perform quality control procedures on a transcutaneous carbon dioxide monitor (Code: IIB3d) [Difficulty: R, Ap, An]

Two-point calibration must be performed with carbon dioxide percentages that cause PCO$_2$ values beyond the expected clinical range. Usually, the electrode is exposed to

5% and 10% carbon dioxide from prepared cylinders. Always follow the manufacturer's written procedures during the calibration process. Generally, when environmental conditions include a fairly stable room temperature of 25° C and 50% relative humidity, the following equation can be used to predict the two calibration points:

$$\text{calibration PtcCO}_2 = (P_B \times CO_2\% \text{ used}) - (X\ CO_2 \times \text{electrode temperature factor})$$

In which:
P_B = local barometric pressure
$CO_2\%$ = carbon dioxide fraction exposed to the electrode; either 10% (.10) or 5% (.05)
$X\ CO_2$ = Correction factor to equilibrate the PtcCO$_2$ to PaCO$_2$ (This is discussed later.)

Electrode temperature factor. This is a factor determined by the manufacturer based on the electrode's temperature. It is usually heated to 44° C.

Expose the electrode to 10% carbon dioxide in a sealed chamber to determine if it matches the calculated calibration value. Adjust the instrument to match the calibration PtcCO$_2$ if necessary. Next, expose the electrode to 5% carbon dioxide in the sealed chamber. Again, adjust the instrument to match the calibration PtcCO$_2$ if necessary. It is recommended that the two-point calibration points be rechecked every 24 hours when in continuous use, after changing the membrane, or after changing the electrolyte solution. A variation of up to ± 4 torr is acceptable and can be corrected by adjusting the reading on the instrument. If the variation is greater than ± 4 torr, the two-point calibration procedures should be repeated.

6. Fix any problems with the equipment (Code: IIB2h4) [Difficulty: An]

Problems usually associated with too much electrode drift include electrode or membrane surfaces contaminated by debris such as blood or sweat, an improperly applied membrane, a worn-out membrane, an air bubble beneath the membrane, improper gas exposed to the membrane during the calibration, exhausted electrolyte solution in the electrode, or inaccurate calibration values. After correcting a problem, the calibration procedure should be repeated.

7. Perform transcutaneous oxygen (PtcCO$_2$) monitoring (Code: IB9a and IC1b) [Difficulty: An]

Much of the information on skin site selection and so forth presented in the preceding discussion of transcutaneous oxygen monitors applies here, as well. As with the transcutaneous oxygen electrode, it has been found that heating the PtcCO$_2$ electrode speeds up the diffusion of carbon dioxide through the skin. Always follow the manufacturer's recommendations for the proper electrode temperature. In general, the temperature is 44° C in both neonates and adults. It must be remembered that $PtcCO_2$ value is not the same as the $PaCO_2$ value. An arterial blood gas should be drawn for $PaCO_2$ every time transcutaneous carbon dioxide monitoring is started. Unlike transcutaneous oxygen monitoring, the correlation between $PaCO_2$ and $PtcCO_2$ is equally as good in adult as in neonatal patients. In addition, it is not as easily influenced by changes in the patient's skin blood flow.

8. Interpret transcutaneous carbon dioxide monitoring values to evaluate the patient's response to respiratory care (Code: IB10a, IC2b, and IIIA1b) [Difficulty: An]

The net effect of heating the carbon dioxide electrode and skin results in the $PtcCO_2$ readings being 1.2 to 2 times (120% to 200%) greater than the $PaCO_2$ values. Commonly, an average multiplier of 1.6 is found. The actual value varies among patients and can be found by dividing the $PtcCO_2$ by the $PaCO_2$.

For example, a patient has a $PaCO_2$ of 40 torr and a $PtcCO_2$ of 64 torr. Calculate the gradient between the arterial and transcutaneous values.

$$\text{Gradient} = \frac{PtcCO_2}{PaCO_2} = \frac{64}{40} = 1.6$$

As long as the patient's cardiovascular status is fairly stable, the $PaCO_2$ can be calculated by dividing the $PtcCO_2$ by 1.6. For example, if the patient's $PtcCO_2$ increases to 80 torr, calculate the $PaCO_2$.

$$PaCO_2 = \frac{PtcCO_2}{1.6} = \frac{80}{1.6} = 50 \text{ torr}$$

Rather than perform these calculations every time there is a change in the patient's status, some practitioners divide the CO_2 values found during the calibration procedure by 1.6. This results in "real" $PaCO_2$ values being given continuously on the monitor. This change must be clearly communicated to all staff members to avoid confusion between the original $PtcCO_2$ values and values that have been reduced to "arterialize" them.

MODULE G	Respiratory care plan

1. Participate in the development of the respiratory care plan (e.g., case management, develop and apply protocols, disease management education) (Code: IC4) [Difficulty: An]

As part of the patient care team, you may need to evaluate the patient's blood gas values and other parameters to make a recommendation. For example, a patient with carbon monoxide poisoning is best treated by administering 100% oxygen through a nonrebreather

mask. Pure oxygen reduces the half-life of COHb to 60 to 90 minutes. A pulse oximeter should not be used to measure this patient's saturation of oxyhemoglobin. These units are unable to identify COHb and will give misleadingly high saturation values for O_2Hb.

Arterial blood gas analysis remains the "gold standard" by which all other values are judged. Typically, the arterial sample is analyzed through a standard blood gas analyzer. A CO-oximeter is needed if the patient has carbon monoxide poisoning. Mixed venous and capillary blood sample analysis is limited in clinical application, but very helpful in the right patient situation. However, these offer only momentary insight into the patient's condition.

Pulse oximetry and transcutaneous oxygen monitoring offer continuous information on the patient's oxygenation. Transcutaneous carbon dioxide monitoring allows continuous monitoring of the patient's ventilation. As with all technology, these units have advantages, disadvantages, and limitations. It is up to the practitioner to make the correct choices. Some unstable patients can best be monitored through the combination of periodic evaluation of arterial blood gases and these noninvasive continuous monitoring systems.

Be prepared to make a recommendation regarding adjustment of the patient's inspired oxygen based on the PaO_2 (or related) value. Also be prepared to make a recommendation regarding adjustment of the patient's mechanical ventilation settings for tidal volume, rate, minute volume, and/or mechanical dead space based on the $PaCO_2$ (or related) value.

2. Maintain records and communication on the patient's pulse oximetry values (Code: IIIA2a4) [Difficulty: An]

The discussion on pulse oximetry values and their interpretation was covered earlier.

BIBLIOGRAPHY

American Association for Respiratory Care (AARC) Clinical Practice Guideline: Transcutaneous blood gas monitoring for neonatal and pediatric patients, *Respir Care* 39(12):1176-1179, 1994.

AARC Clinical Practice Guideline: Capillary blood gas sampling for neonatal and pediatric patients, *Respir Care* 39(12):1180-1183, 1994.

AARC Clinical Practice Guideline: Oxygen therapy in the acute care hospital, *Respir Care* 36(12):1410-1413, 1991.

AARC Clinical Practice Guideline: Pulse oximetry, *Respir Care* 36(12):1406-1409, 1991.

AARC Clinical Practice Guideline: Sampling for arterial blood gas analysis. *Respir Care* 37(8):913-917, 1991.

AARC Clinical Practice Guideline: *In-vitro* pH and blood gas analysis and hemoximetry. *Respir Care* 38(5):505-510, 1993.

Aloan CA, Hill TV, editors: *Respiratory care of the newborn and child*, ed 2, Philadelphia, 1997, Lippincott-Raven Publishers.

American Academy of Pediatrics: Task force on transcutaneous oxygen monitors, *Pediatr* 83(1):122-126, 1989.

Barnes TA, editor: *Core textbook of respiratory care practice*, ed 2, St Louis, 1994, Mosby, 1994.

Barnhart SL, Czervinske MP: Perinatal and pediatric respiratory care. Philadelphia, 1995, WB Saunders Company.

Blanchette T, Dziodzio J, Harris K: Pulse oximetry and normoximetry in neonatal intensive care, *Respir Care* 36(1):25-32, 1991.

Bohn DJ: Ask the expert, *The Respiratory Tract*, 9, Feb 1988.

Branson RD, Hess DR, Chatburn RL, editors: *Respiratory care equipment*, ed 2, Philadelphia, 1999, Lippincott Williams & Wilkins.

Burton GC, Hodgkin JE, Ward JJ, editors: *Respiratory care: A guide to clinical practice*, ed 4, Philadelphia, 1997, Lippincott-Raven Publishers.

Cairo JM, Pilbeam SP: *Mosby's respiratory care equipment*, ed 6, St Louis, 1999, Mosby, Inc.

Czervinske MP: Arterial blood gas analysis and other cardiopulmonary monitoring. In Koff PB, Daily KE, Schroeder JS: *Techniques in bedside hemodynamic monitoring*, ed 4, St Louis, 1989, Mosby.

Eitzman D, Neu J, editors: *Neonatal and pediatric respiratory care*, ed 2, St Louis, 1993, Mosby.

Elser RC: Quality control of blood gas analysis: a review, *Respir Care* 31(9):807-815, Sep 1986.

Federal government releases CLIA '88 final regulations, *AARC Times* 16(4):76-86, 1992.

Fell WL: Sampling and measurement of blood gases. In Lane EE, Walker JF, editors: *Clinical arterial blood gas analysis*, St Louis, 1987, Mosby.

Fink JB, Hunt GE, editors: *Clinical practice in respiratory care*. Philadelphia, 1999, Lippincott-Raven Publishers.

Garza D, Becan-McBride K: *Phlebotomy handbook*, ed 4, Stamford, CT, 1996, Appleton & Lange.

Instrumentation Laboratories: Operator's Manual for the IL282 CO-oximeter.

Jubran A, Tobin MJ: Reliability of pulse oximetry in titrating supplemental oxygen therapy in ventilator-dependent patients, *Chest* 97:1420, 1990.

Lane EE, Walker JF: *Clinical arterial blood gas analysis*, St Louis, 1987, Mosby.

Levitzky MG, Cairo JM, Hall SM: *Introduction to respiratory care*, Philadelphia, 1990, WB Saunders.

Martin RJ: Transcutaneous monitoring: instrumentation and clinical applications. *Respir Care* 35(6):577-583, 1990.

Madama VC: *Pulmonary function testing and cardiopulmonary stress testing*, ed 2, Albany, 1998, Delmar Publishers.

Mohler JG, Collier CR, Brandt W, et al: Blood gases. In Clausen JL, editor: *Pulmonary function testing guidelines and controversies*, Orlando, 1984, Grune & Stratton.

Moran RF: Assessment of quality control of blood gas/pH analyzer performance, *Respir Care* 26(6):538-546, 1981.

Moran RF: CLIA regulations. I. The cure might be worse than the disease, *AARC Times* 14(11):41-43, 50-51, 1990.

Moran RF: CLIA regulations. II. An analysis of some technical requirements, *AARC Times* 14(12):25-32, 1990.

Nelson CM, Murphy EM, Bradley JK, et al: Clinical use of pulse oximetry to determine oxygen prescriptions for patients with hypoxemia, *Respir Care* 31(8):673-680, 1986.

Novametrics Medical Systems, Inc.: Product literature on transcutaneous monitoring, Wallingford, CT.

Peters JA, Hodgkin JE, Collier CA: Blood gas analysis and acid-base physiology. In Burton GG, Hodgkin JE, Ward JJ, editors: *Respiratory care: a guide to clinical practice*, ed 3, Philadelphia, 1991, JB Lippincott.

Ruppel G: *Manual of pulmonary function testing*, ed 6, St Louis, 1994, Mosby.

Salyer JW: Pulse oximetry in the neonatal intensive care unit, *Respir Care* 36(1):17-20, 1991.

Scanlan CL, Wilkins RL, Stoller JK, editors: *Egan's fundamentals of respiratory care*, ed 7, St Louis, 1999, Mosby.

Shapiro BA, Kacmarek RM, Cane RD et al., editors: *Clinical application of respiratory care*, ed 4, St Louis, 1991, Mosby.

Shapiro BA, Peruzzi WT, Templin R: *Clinical application of blood gases*, ed 5, St Louis, 1994, Mosby.

Sonnesso G: Are you ready to use pulse oximetry? *Nursing* 60-64, Aug 1991.

Walton JR, Shapiro BA: Value and application of temperature-compensated blood gas data, *Respir Care* 25(2), 1980.

Welch JP, DeCesare R, Hess D: Pulse oximetry: instrumentation and clinical applications, *Respir Care* 35(6):584-601, 1990.

Whitaker K: *Comprehensive perinatal and pediatric respiratory care*, ed 2, Albany, NY, 1997, Delmar.

White GC: *Equipment theory for respiratory care*, ed 3, Albany, NY, 1999, Delmar.

SELF-STUDY QUESTIONS

1. A 35-year-old patient with pneumonia is receiving mechanical ventilation with positive end-expiratory pressure (PEEP). You are ordered to calculate and interpret the patient's $P(A-a)O_2$. The following conditions exist:

   P_B = 750 torr. Normal is 760 torr for sea level.

   PH_2O = 54 torr because your patient's temperature is 104° F/40° C. Normal is 47 torr for a normal temperature.

   F_IO_2 = .5 for 50% inspired oxygen. Normal is .21 for room air.

   $PaCO_2$ = 36 torr

   PaO_2 = 60 torr

   Respiratory Exchange Ratio = .8

   $$PAO_2 = [(P_B - PH_2O)\, F_IO_2] - \frac{PaCO_2}{.8}$$

   Based on the listed conditions, what is the patient's PAO_2?
   A. 312 torr
   B. 303 torr
   C. 101 torr
   D. 95 torr

2. Based on the listed conditions, what is the patient's $P(A-a)O_2$?
   A. 248 torr
   B. 243 torr
   C. 232 torr
   D. 41 torr

3. How should the patient's $P(A-a)O_2$ results be interpreted?
   A. There is an error; check the blood gas analyzer.
   B. Normal oxygenation for 50% oxygen being inspired.
   C. Normal for a patient of this age.
   D. Larger than normal difference.

4. After performing a modified Allen's test on a patient's right wrist, it is found to take 25 seconds for the patient's hand to regain its color. What should be done now?
   A. Perform an Allen's test on the right wrist.
   B. Draw an arterial blood sample on the right wrist.
   C. Draw an arterial blood sample on the left wrist.
   D. Perform a modified Allen's test on the patient's left wrist.

5. A 45-year-old patient is brought by ambulance into the Emergency Department after being brought from a business where there is a carbon monoxide leak. The patient is obtunded and has an irregular pulse. Which of the following is the *least* important to evaluate at this time?
   A. Pulse oximeter value
   B. 12-lead electrocardiogram
   C. Arterial blood gases analyzed through a CO-oximeter
   D. Glasgow coma analysis

6. For which of the following conditions should an arterial line be inserted?
   I. Septic shock with vasopressor therapy.
   II. Suspected carbon monoxide poisoning.
   III. ARDS requiring mechanical ventilation with PEEP.
   IV. Anxiety induced hyperventilation.
   A. I and II only
   B. I and III only
   C. II, III, and IV only
   D. All of the above

7. A 45-year-old patient has been admitted to the emergency room after suffering smoke inhalation from a house fire. He is wearing a nonrebreather mask set at 10 L/min of oxygen. The most appropriate way to evaluate his oxygenation status is by:
   A. Pulse oximetry.
   B. Transcutaneous oxygen probe.
   C. Running an arterial blood gas sample through the blood gas analyzer.
   D. Running an arterial blood gas sample through the CO-oximeter.

8. You are working with a postanesthesia patient who has a transcutaneous carbon dioxide monitor. The correlation factor between the $PaCO_2$ and $PtcCO_2$ is 1.4. The patient's previous $PtcCO_2$ was 63 torr. The nurse has called you because it is now 76 torr. The patient's approximate $PaCO_2$ would be calculated as:
   A. 63 torr.
   B. 75 torr.
   C. 54 torr.
   D. 105 torr.

9. Interpret the following blood gas drawn when the patient was breathing in 45% oxygen: PaO_2, 64 torr; SaO_2, 91%; pH 7.38; $PaCO_2$ 59 torr; HCO_3^-, 39 mEq/L; and BE, +12 mEq/L.
   I. Corrected hypoxemia
   II. Uncorrected hypoxemia

III. Metabolic alkalosis
IV. Compensated respiratory acidosis
V. Metabolic acidosis
   A. I, IV
   B. I, III
   C. II, V
   D. II, IV

10. Interpret the following blood gas drawn when the patient was breathing in 30% oxygen: PaO_2, 82 torr; SaO_2, 94%; pH 7.32; $PaCO_2$, 39 torr; HCO_3^-, 16 mEq/L; and BE, −6 mEq/L.
   I. Corrected hypoxemia
   II. Uncorrected hypoxemia
   III. Compensated metabolic acidosis
   IV. Uncompensated metabolic acidosis
   V. Compensated respiratory acidosis
   A. II, IV
   B. I, IV
   C. II, V
   D. I, III

11. Interpret the following blood gas drawn when the patient was breathing in 24% oxygen: PaO_2, 125 torr; SaO_2, 99%; pH 7.52; $PaCO_2$, 25 torr; HCO_3^-, 25 mEq/L; and BE, +1 mEq/L.
   I. Normal oxygenation
   II. Excessively corrected hypoxemia
   III. Uncompensated respiratory alkalosis
   IV. Uncompensated metabolic acidosis
   V. Combined respiratory and metabolic alkalosis
   A. II, III
   B. II, V
   C. I, III
   D. I, IV

12. Interpret the following blood gas drawn when the patient was breathing in 40% oxygen: PaO_2, 75 torr; SaO_2, 93%; pH 7.15; $PaCO_2$, 55 torr; HCO_3^-, 20 mEq/L; and BE, −8 mEq/L.
   I. Uncorrected hypoxemia
   II. Corrected hypoxemia
   III. Uncorrected respiratory acidosis
   IV. Uncorrected metabolic acidosis
   V. Combined metabolic and respiratory acidosis
   A. I, V
   B. II, V
   C. II, III
   D. II, IV

13. Interpret the following blood gas drawn when the patient was breathing in 30% oxygen: PaO_2 65 mm Hg; SaO_2, 91%; pH 7.44; $PaCO_2$, 25 mm Hg; HCO_3^-, 17 mEq/L; and BE, −7 mEq/L.
   I. Corrected hypoxemia
   II. Uncorrected hypoxemia
   III. Compensated respiratory alkalosis
   IV. Uncompensated respiratory alkalosis
   V. Combined metabolic and respiratory acidosis
   A. I, III
   B. I, IV
   C. II, III
   D. II, V

14. Which of the following clinical values indicate that a patient's tissues are hypoxemic?
    A. PaO_2 55 torr
    B. $P\bar{v}O_2$ 25 torr
    C. $S\bar{v}O_2$ 80%
    D. SaO_2 88%

15. You are working with a neonate in an incubator who is being monitored with a transcutaneous oxygen electrode on her right upper chest. An hour ago the patient's oxygen value was 52 torr and now it is 115 torr. The nurse tells you that there has been no change in the neonate's condition. What is the most likely explanation of this difference?
    A. The patient has a patent ductus arteriosus.
    B. Air has leaked under the electrode.
    C. The temperature inside the incubator has been increased.
    D. The patient's cardiac output and lung condition have improved.

16. A 17-year-old patient is receiving mechanical ventilation because of apnea resulting from a drug overdose. While the patient is breathing 25% oxygen, the following arterial blood gas values are analyzed:

PaO_2	155 torr
SaO_2	100%
pH	7.42
$PaCO_2$	41 torr
HCO_3^-	26 mEq/L
BE	+2 mEq/L.

    What action should now be taken?
    A. Reduce the patient to 21% oxygen.
    B. Maintain the patient on present settings.
    C. Recheck the blood gas analyzer.
    D. Increase the tidal volume to hyperventilate the patient.

Answer Key

1. **B.** Rationale: The patient's PAO_2 (pressure of alveolar oxygen) can be calculated as follows:

$$PAO_2 = [(P_B - PH_2O)\ F_IO_2] - \frac{PaCO_2}{.8}$$
$$= [(750 - 54)\ .5] - \frac{36}{.8}$$
$$= [(696)\ .5] - 45$$
$$= [348] - 45$$
$$= 303\ torr$$

2. **B.** Rationale: The patient's $P(A - a)O_2$ (difference between alveolar and arterial pressure of oxygen) can be calculated as follows:
   The patient's PAO_2 = 303 torr
   The patient's PaO_2 = <u>–60 torr</u>
                                  243 torr

3. **D.** Rationale: The normal $P(A-a)O_2$ difference should be no more than 25 torr for a healthy person of this age. The patient's difference of 243 torr is far greater than normal. There is no indication that the blood gas analyzer needs recalibration. If a normal person were breathing 50% oxygen, the PaO_2 would be much higher (about 275 torr) than this patient's PaO_2. The difference is much larger than normal for a patient of this age. See Fig. 3-13.

4. **D.** Rationale: The modified Allen's test on the patient's right wrist is abnormal. It took 25 seconds for the return of adequate circulation through the ulnar artery. No arterial blood sample should be taken from the right radial artery because of poor collateral circulation through the ulnar artery. See Fig. 3-2. Check the circulation on the patient's left wrist by doing a modified Allen's test on it. Draw from the left radial artery if the test result is normal (less than 15 seconds for the return of circulation). The Allen's test is a test of circulation through the radial artery, whereas the modified Allen's test is a test of circulation through the ulnar artery.

5. **A.** Rationale: A pulse oximeter value is of no use in evaluating a patient with carbon monoxide poisoning. This is because pulse oximeter technology is unable to distinguish carboxyhemoglobin from oxyhemoglobin. Therefore the pulse oximeter value will show a higher oxygen saturation than is actually present in the patient. A 12-lead electrocardiogram is needed to help determine the cause of the patient's irregular pulse. The patient may have had a heart attack as the result of profound hypoxemia. To accurately evaluate the patient's oxygenation, an arterial blood sample should be drawn and analyzed with a CO-oximeter. A CO-oximeter can distinguish between carboxyhemoglobin and oxyhemoglobin so that the patient's actual SaO_2 can be determined. A Glasgow Coma Scale analysis should be done to evaluate the patient's neurologic status. The patient may have had a stroke as the result of profound hypoxemia.

6. **B.** Rationale: A patient with septic shock who is receiving vasopressor therapy needs an arterial line to continuously monitor blood pressure. This is because the disease condition and the drugs result in considerable variation in blood pressure. A patient with ARDS who requires mechanical ventilation with PEEP needs frequent arterial blood sampling for gas analysis. Rather than puncture the patient's arteries for each sample, it is more humane and efficient to place an arterial line. In addition, the patient's blood pressure can be continuously monitored for the effects of PEEP. A patient with suspected (or actual) carbon monoxide poisoning does not usually need more than one or two arterial blood samples taken for diagnosis and the evaluation of treatment effectiveness. An arterial line is not justified. A patient with anxiety induced hyperventilation is not hypoxic and does not need an arterial blood gas sample analyzed.

7. **D.** Rationale: The best way to assess the oxygenation status of a patient with carbon monoxide poisoning is to run an arterial blood gas sample through the CO-oximeter. The CO-oximeter is the only device that can accurately differentiate between carboxyhemoglobin and oxyhemoglobin (as well as other types of hemoglobin) and measure the amounts of each. Therefore it gives an accurate SaO_2 value. The pulse oximeter device is unable to distinguish between carboxyhemoglobin and oxyhemoglobin. This provides a false high value for SaO_2. The transcutaneous oxygen probe can be used to give an approximate tissue oxygen value. However, it is not the clinically accepted way to evaluate a patient with CO poisoning. Running an arterial blood gas sample through a standard blood gas analyzer results in measurements of oxygen, carbon dioxide, and pH. However, the SaO_2 value is calculated from the PaO_2. This can result in a falsely high value for the calculated SaO_2 if the patient is receiving

supplemental oxygen and has an elevated PaO_2 (measured from the blood plasma).

8. **C.** Rationale: Because the correlation factor between the $PaCO_2$ and $PtcCO_2$ is 1.4, the solution to the problem requires that the patient's current $PtcCO_2$ of 76 torr be divided by 1.4, as follows:

$$\text{approximate } PaCO_2 = \frac{PtcCO_2 \text{ of } 76 \text{ torr}}{1.4}$$
$$= 54 \text{ torr (actually 54.29 torr)}$$

9. **D.** Rationale: A PaO_2 of less than 80 torr is uncorrected hypoxemia. A compensated respiratory acidosis is indicated by the increased $PaCO_2$ coupled with an increased bicarbonate and increased base excess found with a normal pH. Review Table 3-2 and Table 3-9 if needed.

10. **B.** Rationale: A PaO_2 of greater than 80 torr with supplemental oxygen is corrected hypoxemia. An uncompensated metabolic acidosis is indicated by the normal $PaCO_2$ coupled with a decreased bicarbonate and decreased base excess found with an acidotic pH. Review Table 3-2 and Table 3-9 if needed.

11. **C.** Rationale: Normal oxygenation is indicated because the patient's PaO_2 is elevated secondary to hyperventilation ($PaCO_2$ of 25 torr). An uncompensated respiratory alkalosis is indicated by the low $PaCO_2$ coupled with a normal bicarbonate and normal base excess found with an alkalotic pH. Review Table 3-2 and Table 3-9 if needed.

12. **A.** Rationale: A PaO_2 of less than 80 mm Hg is uncorrected hypoxemia. A combined metabolic and respiratory acidosis is indicated by the increased $PaCO_2$ coupled with a decreased bicarbonate and decreased base excess found with an acidotic pH. Review Table 3-2 and Table 3-9 if needed.

13. **C.** Rationale: A PaO_2 of less than 80 mm Hg is uncorrected hypoxemia. A compensated respiratory alkalosis is indicated by the decreased $PaCO_2$ coupled with a decreased bicarbonate and decreased base excess found with a normal pH. Review Table 3-2 and Table 3-9 if needed.

14. **B.** Rationale: A $P\bar{v}O_2$ value of 25 torr is quite low. A $P\bar{v}O_2$ value of 40 torr is normal and a value below 30 torr usually indicates tissue hypoxemia. An $S\bar{v}O_2$ of 80% is above the normal value of 75% and indicates above normal tissue oxygenation. Review Table 3-11 if needed. Whereas a PaO_2 of 55 torr and SaO_2 of 88% are below normal, they do not necessarily indicate tissue hypoxemia. Many patients with chronic lung disease live acceptable lives with values in this range.

15. **B.** Rationale: Because the PO_2 of room air is 150 torr, the only possible explanation for the dramatic increase in the patient's transcutaneous oxygen value has to be a leak of room air under the electrode. When the electrode is sealed to the patient's skin the $PtcO_2$ value should drop to the actual value. If the patient had a patent ductus arteriosus, there would be a drop in the $PtcO_2$ value over the patient's left chest area and body. There is usually not a drop in the $PtcO_2$ value over the right chest because this area receives blood that is preductal. An increased temperature inside the incubator would have no effect on the $PtcO_2$ value. However, a drop in temperature inside the incubator could result in vasoconstriction and a resulting drop in $PtcO_2$ value. Even if the patient's cardiac output and lung condition have improved, the $PtcO_2$ value is too high for a neonate breathing room air. (It is important to also realize that if there is a leak of room air under the transcutaneous carbon dioxide electrode, there will be a drop in the $PtcCO_2$ value because room air contains virtually no carbon dioxide.)

16. **C.** Rationale: Recheck the blood gas analyzer for a problem with the PO_2 electrode. A calculation of the patient's PAO_2 shows that the maximum PaO_2 the patient can have is 127 torr. Until an accurate PaO_2 can be determined, there should be no change in the patient's inspired oxygen percentage. Although there is no reason to doubt the pH and $PaCO_2$ values, there can be no decision to maintain the patient on his or her present ventilator settings until a correct PaO_2 value is obtained. There is no indication to hyperventilate this drug overdose patient. Do not confuse this case with hyperventilation of a patient with a head injury and increased intracranial pressure.

4 | Pulmonary Function Testing

A review of the most recent Written Registry Examination has shown an average of five questions (5% of the exam) on pulmonary testing.

MODULE A | **Review the patient's record for data on the following tests**

1. Pulmonary function results (Code: IA1d) [Difficulty: An]

Be prepared to review the results of all types of pulmonary function test results.

2. Respiratory monitoring (Code: IA1f3) [Difficulty: An]

Patients at risk of respiratory failure, such as those with neurologic disease, should have their breathing monitored regularly.

3. Lung compliance (Code: IA1f4) [Difficulty: An]

Lung compliance is usually measured in patients with stiff lungs (as found with pulmonary fibrosis) or overly compliant lungs (as found with emphysema).

4. Airway resistance (Code: IA1f4) [Difficulty: An]

Patients with asthma or chronic bronchitis may need to have airway resistance measured as part of their bronchodilator therapy management. Airway resistance will decrease if the proper type and amount of medication is taken.

5. Pulmonary angiogram (Code: IA1i) [Difficulty: R, Ap, An]

This test is done to evaluate pulmonary blood flow if a pulmonary embolism is known or suspected.

MODULE B | **Ventilation to perfusion scan**

1. Recommend a ventilation to perfusion scan to get additional information (Code: IA2b) [Difficulty: An]

A ventilation scan (V scan) is performed to verify or refute the clinical suspicion that a patient has an area of the lung(s) that is underventilated. Abnormal ventilation is seen in the case of a bronchial obstruction from a tumor or foreign body or an alveolar problem such as atelectasis, consolidation, or emphysema. Radioactive xenon (^{133}Xe) is mixed with oxygen and inhaled to show the lung fields. A special scanner is used to "pick up" the radioactivity through the chest wall. Areas of normal ventilation can be compared with underventilated areas.

A perfusion scan (Q scan) is performed to verify or refute the clinical suspicion that a patient has an area of pulmonary circulation that is underperfused. Abnormal perfusion is seen in the case of a pulmonary embolism, tumor, or vascular problem such as pulmonary hypertension. Radioactive technetium (^{99m}Tc) is injected into the patient's venous system, where it is filtered out by the pulmonary circulation. As previously described, a special scanner is used to "pick up" the radioactivity through the chest wall. Areas of normal perfusion can be compared with underperfused areas. The ventilation scan and perfusion scan tests can be done singly or as a set.

2. Review the patient's record for data on ventilation to perfusion scan results (Code: IA1i) [Difficulty: R, Ap, An]

Comparing both results side by side enables the physician to look for areas of ventilation and/or perfusion mismatching. Normally, ventilation and perfusion match fairly closely and result in a 1:1 mix of air and blood at the alveolar capillary membrane. A pulmonary embolism results in a V:Q ratio of 2 (or greater):1 (or less) because normal ventilation is present and perfusion is reduced or absent. An obstructed airway with resulting atelectasis results in a V:Q ratio of 1 (or less):2 (or greater) because ventilation is reduced or absent and perfusion is normal.

MODULE C | **Bronchoprovocation**

1. Recommend the procedure to obtain additional information (Code: IA2d) [Difficulty: An]

Bronchoprovocation (also known as *bronchial provocation*) is indicated in patients suspected of having asthma, to determine the severity or changes in hyperresponsiveness in known asthma patients, and to assess a person before starting a job with occupational exposure to airborne irritants.

2. Interpret the results of the procedure (Code: IC2a) [Difficulty: An]

Current guidelines offer several ways to determine that the patient has had a positive response to the inhaled bronchospastic agonist (methacholine or histamine). In general, a drop in the patient's forced expiratory volume in one second (FEV_1) of greater than or equal to 10% to 20% indicates a bronchospastic condition. For example, after a methacholine challenge test, if a patient's FEV_1 dropped from 3000 mL to 2500 mL, the bronchoprovocation test would be abnormal.

| MODULE D | Perform the following types of bedside spirometry tests |

1. Lung mechanics tests

a. Review the patient's chart for data on the tests (Code: IA1f2) [Difficulty: An]

b. Recommend lung mechanics tests to obtain additional data (Code: IA2f) [Difficulty: An]

Different authors include various tests in the category of lung mechanics tests, including the following:

a. Lung volumes and capacities except for those requiring the residual volume (RV).

b. Spirometry for forced vital capacity (FVC) and flow values derived from the FVC. These values are needed to determine the degree of impairment in the obstructive diseases patient.

c. Spirometry for flow-volume loop. This test is used to determine obstructive problems in the lungs or upper airway.

d. Maximum inspiratory pressure (MIP) and maximum expiratory pressure (MEP). These values indicate the patient's overall respiratory muscle strength.

a. Perform any of the lung mechanics tests (Code: IB9d) [Difficulty: R, Ap]

b. Interpret the results (Code: IB10d) [Difficulty: R, Ap]

Discussion of the steps to perform and interpret the tests follow.

2. Tidal volume

a. Perform the procedure (Code: IIIA1h) [Difficulty: An]

The tidal volume (V_T) is the volume of gas breathed out in each respiratory cycle. Realize that individual tidal volumes are rarely identical. Fig. 4-1 shows several different tidal volumes before and after a nonforced (slow) vital capacity (VC). For that reason it is recommended that the tidal volumes be accumulated for 1 minute (thus providing a minute volume [V_E]) and the respiratory rate (f) counted. An average V_T is found by dividing the $\dot{V}_E$ by the respiratory f. If this cannot be done, find the average volume of at least six breaths. The average, predicted tidal volume for a resting, afebrile, alert adult should be about 3 to 4 mL/lb or 7 to 9 mL/kg of ideal body weight. For example, the predicted tidal volume range of a 154-lb (70-kg) patient is calculated as follows:

a. 3 to 4 mL/lb. × 154 lb. = 462 to 616 mL

b. 7 to 9 mL/kg × 70 kg = 420 to 630 mL

The patient should be allowed to relax before the test is performed so that the measured volume is accurate and not enlarged because of any undue stress or excitement. Keeping the instructions and demonstration simple and easy to follow help reduce the patient's anxiety. Some patients will not tolerate a full minute's tidal volume measurement. In that case, measure the accumulated tidal

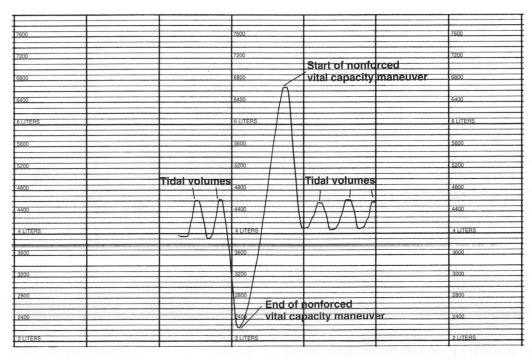

Fig. 4-1 Volume-time curve tracing of tidal volumes and nonforced vital capacity.

volumes for as long as possible, and divide by the number of respirations to obtain the average.

b. Interpret the results (Code: IB10b) [Difficulty: An]

A tidal volume that is larger or smaller than expected for the patient's size requires further evaluation. A small tidal volume may be seen in patients who have low metabolic rates, are asleep or in a coma, have neuromuscular diseases that make them unable to breathe deeply, or are alkalotic. A large tidal volume may be seen in patients with a high metabolic rate, fever, dead space producing diseases, increased intracranial pressure, or acidotic conditions.

3. Inspiratory/expiratory ratio

a. Perform the procedure (Code: IB9b and IIIA1h) [Difficulty: An]

The inspiratory/expiratory (I:E) ratio is the ratio of the patient's inspiratory time to the expiratory time. It can be simply measured at the bedside with a stopwatch. Again, make sure that the patient is relaxed and breathing in the normal pattern to get an accurate timing. Measure several of the patient's inspiratory times and expiratory times to figure an average for each. A spirometer that gives a printout is needed if a more complete analysis of the patient's breathing pattern is necessary.

📋 EXAM HINT

The National Board of Respiratory Care (NBRC) is known to test the examinee's ability to calculate: (1) the inspiratory time (T_I) and expiratory time (T_E) from a given I:E ratio and respiratory rate and (2) the I:E ratio from a given T_I and T_E. These examples should help.

---

1. Calculate the patient's inspiratory time and expiratory time when the I:E ratio is 1:2 and the respiratory rate is 12/min.
   a. $\dfrac{60 \text{ sec/min}}{12 \text{ breaths/min}} = 5$ seconds/respiratory cycle
   b. $\dfrac{5 \text{ sec/respiratory cycle}}{3 \text{ parts of I and E}} = 1.66$ seconds for one part
   c. Inspiratory time = 1 part = 1.66 seconds
   d. Expiratory time = 2 parts = 3.32 seconds
2. Calculate the neonatal patient's I:E ratio when the inspiratory time is 0.3 seconds and expiratory time is 0.9 seconds.
   a. $I:E = \dfrac{I}{E} = \dfrac{0.3 \text{ seconds}}{0.9 \text{ seconds}}$
   b. $\dfrac{I}{E} = \dfrac{1}{3}$ (The I:E ratio is 1:3.)

b. Interpret the results (Code: IB10b) [Difficulty: R, Ap]

A normal, spontaneously breathing patient has an I:E ratio of 1:2 to 1:4. A prolonged inspiratory time is often seen in patients with an upper airway obstruction. A prolonged expiratory time is often seen in patients with asthma or chronic obstructive pulmonary disease (COPD). Any abnormal I:E ratio should be investigated. For example, patients with Kussmaul's respiration, Cheyne-Stokes respiration, or Biot's respiration will have unusual I:E ratios.

4. Minute volume

a. Perform the procedure (Code: IB9b) [Difficulty: An]

The minute volume ($\dot{V}_E$) is the volume of gas exhaled in 1 minute. It is usually a more stable value than are individual tidal volumes. Minute volume is found by adding up the accumulated tidal volumes for 1 minute. A simple handheld spirometer is often used to accumulate the tidal volume breaths. If the patient cannot perform the test for 1 minute, do it for 30 seconds, and double the value.

b. Interpret the results (Code: IB10b) [Difficulty: An]

The predicted range for a minute volume in a resting, afebrile, alert adult should be 5 to 10 L/min. The wide range is found in part because it is a product of two factors: tidal volume and respiratory rate. It is possible for either one or both of these factors to be normal, abnormally high, or abnormally low. For these reasons, the minute volume must be evaluated along with the tidal volume and respiratory rate to reach any conclusion about the patient's condition. The same factors that have an impact on the tidal volume affects the patient's minute ventilation.

5. Alveolar ventilation

a. Perform the procedure (Code: IB9c) [Difficulty: An]

Alveolar ventilation (V_A) is the amount of tidal volume that reaches the alveoli. It is calculated by subtracting the physiologic dead space (anatomic plus alveolar dead space) from the measured exhaled tidal volume. For a bedside test, it is possible to subtract only the estimated anatomic dead space. It is estimated at 1 mL/lb or 2.2 mL/kg of ideal body weight. The alveolar dead space measurement requires sophisticated equipment, which is usually available only in the pulmonary function testing laboratory. Clinically normal people have very little alveolar dead space.

Example. A 154-lb/70-kg person has a measured tidal volume of 500 mL and an estimated anatomic dead space of about 154 mL. The calculated alveolar ventilation = 500 mL − 154 mL = 346 mL.

b. Interpret the results (Code: IB10c) [Difficulty: An]

The following examples show how the patient's alveolar ventilation can vary considerably because of changes in the respiratory rate and tidal volume even though the minute volume remains unchanged. These examples are included to show the importance of alveolar ventilation on the patient's $PaCO_2$ values.

Examples

1. Normal patient: f = 12, tidal volume = 500 mL, anatomic dead space = 154 mL

$$\text{minute alveolar ventilation } (\dot{V}_A) = 12 \times (500 \text{ mL} - 154 \text{ mL})$$
$$= 12 \times 346 \text{ mL}$$
$$= 4152 \text{ mL}$$

This patient should have a normal carbon dioxide level.

2. Tachypneic patient: f = 24, tidal volume = 250 mL, anatomic dead space = 154 mL minute volume = 24 × minute volume = 12 × 500 mL = 6000 mL

$$\text{minute alveolar ventilation } (\dot{V}_A) = 24 \times (250 \text{ mL} - 154 \text{ mL})$$
$$= 24 \times 96 \text{ mL}$$
$$= 2304 \text{ mL}$$

This patient should have a high carbon dioxide level.

3. Bradypneic patient: f = 6, tidal volume = 1000 mL, anatomic dead space = 154 mL

$$\text{minute volume} = 6 \times 1000 \text{ mL} = 6000 \text{ mL}$$
$$\text{minute alveolar ventilation } (\dot{V}_A) = 6 \times (1000 \text{ mL} - 154 \text{ mL})$$
$$= 6 \times 846 \text{ mL}$$
$$= 5076 \text{ mL}$$

This patient should have a low carbon dioxide level.

6. Measure and interpret the patient's maximum inspiratory pressure at the bedside

a. Recommend the procedure (Code: IA2d) [Difficulty: An]

The maximum inspiratory pressure (MIP) is the greatest amount of negative pressure that the patient can create when inspiring against an occluded airway. It is also known as negative inspiratory force (NIF). The following factors affect the test results: strength of the diaphragm and accessory muscles of inspiration, lung volume when the airway is occluded, ventilatory drive, and the length of time the airway is occluded. It is most commonly used to determine the weanability of mechanically ventilated patients. In addition, it is used to help monitor the strength of patients with a neuromuscular disease.

b. Perform the procedure (Code: IB9d) [Difficulty: An]

A study of the literature reveals that a number of measurement devices have been assembled and that different bedside techniques have been used to determine the effort of a patient breathing naturally, an intubated patient, and a patient breathing with assistance from a mechanical ventilator. Branson et al. and Kacmarek et al. make a strong case for the use of a double one-way valve to connect the intubated patient to the manometer (Fig. 4-2). Use of the one-way valve lets the patient exhale but prevents an inhalation when the practitioner occludes the opening. This forces the patient to inhale from closer to residual volume with each breathing effort. They also

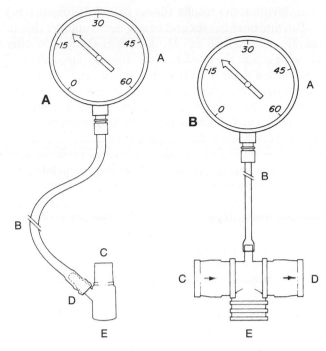

Fig. 4-2 Two systems for measuring maximum inspiratory pressure (MIP) on a patient with an artificial airway. System **A,** Simple occlusion. A, Pressure manometer; B, connecting tubing; C, port to be occluded during the MIP; D, connection of the adapter to the manometer; E, port to connect to the patient's airway. System **B,** One-way valve. A, Pressure manometer; B, connecting tubing; C, inspiratory port to be occluded during the MIP effort; D, expiratory port; E, port to be connected to the patient's artificial airway. (From Kacmarek RM, Cycyk-Chapman MC, Young-Palazzo PJ et al.: *Respiratory Care* 1989; 34:868–878.)

recommend that the patient make inspiratory efforts for 15 to 20 seconds.

Steps in the MIP procedure for a normally breathing patient include the following:

1. Obtain a pressure gauge capable of measuring at least −60 cm water pressure.
2. Have the patient sit upright. Place a note in the chart if the patient is lying down.
3. Describe the procedure to the patient.
4. Simulate a demonstration of the procedure.
5. Place nose clips over the patient's nose. Have the patient seal his or her lips and teeth around the mouthpiece and breathe through the open port.
6. Tell the patient to exhale completely. Seal the port when residual volume has been reached.
7. Tell the patient to breathe in as hard as possible and hold it for 1 to 3 seconds.
8. Reteach if necessary.
9. Repeat until at least three good efforts have been performed. Record the greatest stable value seen after the first second of effort. This eliminates any artifact created by the cheeks or by chest wall movement.

c. Interpret the results (Code: IB10d) [Difficulty: An]

Patients of either sex and of any age should be able to generate at least −60 cm H_2O. This is enough to offer assurance that the patient has enough strength and coordination to protect the airway, take a deep breath, and cough effectively. Patients with neuromuscular diseases, diseases of the respiratory muscles, thoracic injury or abnormality, and chronic obstructive lung diseases tend to have decreased strength. The patient who cannot generate at least −20 cm H_2O is at risk. This patient probably does not have the strength to cough effectively. Depending on the blood gas values and other physical parameters, the patient may need to be intubated and maintained on a mechanical ventilator.

Black and Hyatt have published the following MIP prediction formulas for spontaneous breathing in nonintubated adult subjects between 20 and 86 years old who are breathing from residual volume. The values are in centimeters of water pressure (cm H_2O). As can be seen, the older the patient, the lower the predicted negative inspiratory force.

	Lower limits of normal
Males: 143 − (0.55 × age)	−75 cm H_2O
Females: 104 − (0.51 × age)	−50 cm H_2O

d. Monitor the patient (Code: IIIA1h) [Difficulty: An]

A patient being weaned from mechanical ventilation or with a deteriorating neuromuscular condition should have the MIP measured on a regular, frequent basis. If the patient's pressure drops to −20 cm H_2O, the physician should be notified. Mechanical ventilation is probably needed.

It is important to monitor any patient for signs of undue stress and hypoxemia such as tachycardia, bradycardia, ventricular dysrhythmias, hypertension, hypotension, and decreasing saturation on pulse oximetry. If any of these are seen, the procedure should be stopped and the patient reoxygenated and ventilated. Some patients achieve their best effort on the first or second inspiration and have decreasing effort as they continue trying. This is probably because of fatigue. Stop the procedure and record the best effort.

7. Maximum expiratory pressure

a. Recommend the procedure (Code: IA2d) [Difficulty: An]

The maximum expiratory pressure (MEP) is the greatest amount of positive pressure that the patient can create when expiring from total lung capacity against an occluded airway. It is also known as a maximal expiratory force (MEF). The following factors affect the test results: patient cooperation and effort, strength of the expiratory muscles, lung volume when the airway is occluded, ventilatory drive, and the length of time the airway is occluded. It is used to determine the weanability of mechanically ventilated patients and to monitor the strength of patients with a neuromuscular disease.

b. Perform the procedure (Code: IB9d) [Difficulty: An]

As with the maximum inspiratory pressure test, a study of the literature reveals that a number of measurement devices have been assembled and that different bedside techniques have been used to determine the effort of a patient breathing naturally and the effort of one who is intubated and is breathing by way of a mechanical ventilator. A strong case can be made for the use of a double one-way valve to connect the intubated patient to the manometer (see Fig. 4-2). Use of the one-way valves lets the patient inhale but prevents an exhalation when the practitioner occludes the expiratory opening. This forces the patient to exhale from closer to total lung capacity with each breathing effort. However, the expiratory efforts should not be held for more than 3 seconds. This test is similar to Valsalva's maneuver and can cause a reduction in the cardiac output because of the high intrathoracic pressure.

Steps in the MEP procedure for a normally breathing patient include the following:
1. Obtain a pressure gauge capable of measuring at least + 60 cm water pressure.
2. Have the patient sit upright. Place a note in the chart if the patient is lying down.
3. Describe the procedure to the patient.
4. Simulate a demonstration of the procedure.
5. Place nose clips over the patient's nose. Have the patient seal his or her lips and teeth around the mouthpiece and breathe through the open port.
6. Tell the patient to inhale completely. Seal the port when total lung capacity has been reached.
7. Tell the patient to breathe out as hard as possible. Hold it for 1 to 3 seconds.
8. Reteach if necessary.
9. Repeat until at least three good efforts have been performed. Record the greatest stable value seen after the first second of effort. This eliminates any artifact created by the cheeks or chest wall movement.

It is important to monitor any patient for signs of undue stress and hypoxemia such as tachycardia, bradycardia, ventricular dysrhythmias, hypotension, and decreasing saturation on pulse oximetry. If any of these are seen, the procedure should be stopped and the patient reoxygenated and ventilated.

c. Interpret the results (Code: IB10d) [Difficulty: An]

Clinically normal people of either sex and of any age should be able to generate at least + 80 cm water pressure. Patients with neuromuscular diseases, thoracic injury or abnormality, and COPD tend to have decreased strength. A MEP value of + 40 cm water is probably enough to offer assurance that the patient has enough strength and coordination to cough effectively to clear secretions.

However, depending on the blood gas values and other physical parameters, the patient may need to be intubated and maintained on a mechanical ventilator.

Black and Hyatt have published the following MEP prediction formulas for spontaneously breathing non-intubated adult subjects between 20 and 86 years old who are breathing from total lung capacity. The values are in cm of water pressure. As can be seen, the older the patient, the lower the predicted maximal expiratory force.

	Lower limit of normal
Males: $268 - (1.03 \times$ age)	$+ 140$ cm H_2O
Females: $170 - (0.53 \times$ age)	$+ 95$ cm H_2O

8. Vital capacity

a. Perform the test (Code: IIIA1e) [Difficulty: An]

The nonforced (slow) vital capacity (VC or SVC) is the greatest volume of gas that the patient can exhale after the lungs have been completely filled. The therapist should demonstrate the procedure to the patient. He or she must understand that there is no need to blow out fast while emptying the lungs. The measurement device can be a simple, handheld spirometer if a printout of the result is not needed. A portable, computer-based spirometer can be used if needed to generate a printout of the results or a graphic tracing. Normally at least *three* efforts are made and the largest is recorded.

b. Interpret the results (Code: IB10d) [Difficulty: An]

See Fig 4-1 for a graphic tracing of a nonforced vital capacity. Compare it with the tracing on Fig. 4-3, which shows a forced vital capacity. In a patient without obstructive lung disease, the same volume should be found in a nonforced vital capacity and forced vital capacity. The following discussion on the forced vital capacity includes predicted values for male and female patients and guidelines on the interpretation of the patient's results.

MODULE E   **Advanced spirometry**

---

1. Forced vital capacity

a. Perform the test (Code: IB9d) [Difficulty: An]

The forced vital capacity (FVC) is the greatest volume of gas that the patient can exhale as rapidly as possible after the lungs have been completely filled. Normally, the FVC is the same volume as that found in a slow or nonforced vital capacity. Careful instructions, demonstrations, and coaching are needed to ensure that the patient's efforts are the best possible. At least *three* proper efforts must be obtained.

If the measurement instrument does not give a printout, simply record the patient's efforts in the chart. If the measurement instrument does give a printout, include copies of the efforts. See Fig. 4-3 for the tracing of a properly performed forced vital capacity. The tracing enables us to compare the volumes exhaled in a series of 1-second time intervals. Because of this, the tracing is often referred to as a *volume-time curve*. Notice that the start of the effort is smooth and without interruption. The initial fast flow of gas from the upper airway is seen as the nearly vertical part of the tracing. The rest of the tracing is smooth without any coughing or other interruptions in the patient's effort. The tracing becomes progressively more horizontal as the end of the effort is reached. Encourage

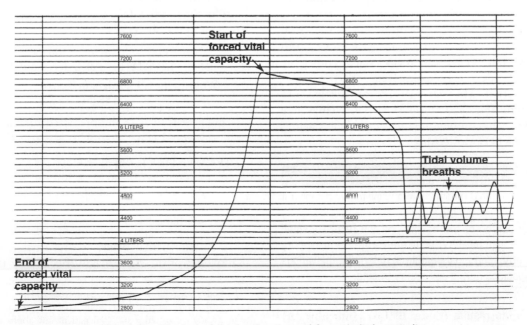

Fig. 4-3   Tracing of tidal volumes and forced vital capacity.

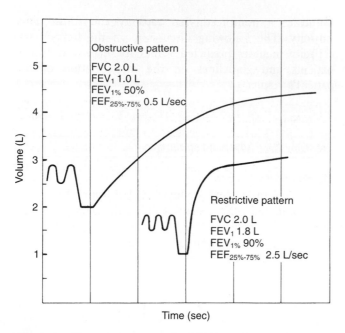

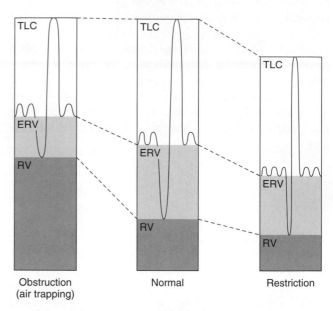

Fig. 4-4   Forced vital capacity (FVC) tracings showing an obstructed flow pattern and a restrictive flow pattern. Note how the patient with the obstructed pattern has a slower than normal exhalation whereas the patient with the restricted pattern has a faster-than-normal exhalation. (From Ruppel G: *Manual of Pulmonary Function Testing*, ed 6, St Louis, 1994, Mosby.)

Fig. 4-5   One method of determining the $FEF_{200-1200}$ value from a FVC tracing. First, mark the 200 mL and 1200 mL points from the start of the effort. Second, draw a line through these two points to intersect the dashed time lines at points A and B. Horizontal dashed lines are added from A and B to cross the volume scale. The $FEF_{200-1200}$ value is read as the distance between A and C or about 3 L/sec. BTPS correct this measurement. (From Ruppel G: *Manual of pulmonary function testing*, ed 5, St Louis, 1991, Mosby.)

the patient to try to push out as much air as possible as the end approaches. To be an acceptable FVC, the patient must show maximum effort without coughing or closing the glottis, and the expiratory effort must last at least 6 seconds. The patient's final two seconds of expiratory effort should show no appreciable airflow.

Fig. 4-3 was made on a chain-compensated, water-seal spirometry system. Notice how the tracing progresses from the right to the left. The Stead-Wells system shows the same tracing "upside down" compared with the chain-compensated system. The tracing starts on the left and moves to the right (Figs. 4-4 and 4-5). Other tracings may show either the chain-compensated or Stead-Wells tracings in a mirror image or opposite shape.

> **EXAM HINT**
>
> The NBRC can show a FVC tracing from any system and expect it to be interpreted. The start of the FVC effort can be determined by the near vertical portion of the tracing and the relatively small expiratory reserve volume (ERV) compared with the inspiratory reserve volume (IRV). You must be able to determine the various volumes and capacities from a spirometry tracing.

b. Interpret the results (Code: IB10d) [Difficulty: An]

Normal racial differences in the FVC must be taken into consideration. Most modern pulmonary function systems automatically adjust the measured values for racial differences when so programmed by the operator. If not, the predicted values should be mathematically adjusted by the therapist. The predicted white patient normal values in liters for the forced vital capacity* were reported by Morris, Koski, and Johnson (1971) as:

Men: $[(0.148 \times \text{height in inches}) - (0.025 \times \text{age})]$
      $- 4.24$ (SD [1 standard deviation] 0.58)

Women: $[(0.115 \times \text{height in inches}) - (0.024 \times \text{age})]$
      $- 2.85$ (SD 0.52)

Example. Calculate the predicted forced vital capacity of a 50-year-old white man who is 6 feet (72 inches) tall.

$$FVC = [(0.148 \times \text{height in inches}) - (0.025 \times \text{age})] - 4.24$$
$$= [(0.148 \times 72) - (0.025 \times 50)] - 4.24$$
$$= [10.656 - 1.25] - 4.24$$
$$= 9.406 - 4.24$$
$$= 5.166 \text{ L}$$

It is known that blacks have a smaller lung capacity than whites of the same height. Because of this, a 10% to

---

*The body, temperature, pressure, saturated (BTPS) correction has been calculated into these equations. Note: These and some other researchers have already calculated a standard patient and room temperature and barometric pressure into their formulas.

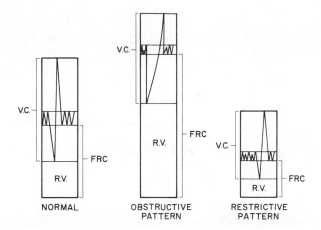

Fig. 4-6   Spirometry tracings of a normal, obstructed, and restricted patient. Note how the obstructed and restricted patients' volumes and capacities are out of proportion compared with the normal patient. *VC,* Vital capacity; *RV,* residual volume; *FRC,* functional residual capacity. (From Cherniak RM: *Pulmonary function testing,* Philadelphia, 1977, WB Saunders.)

15% adjustment should be made for the predicted FVC and total lung capacity (TLC) of a black patient. In other words, the predicted values for a black patient is 85% to 90% of those of a comparable white patient.

Adjustments for Hispanic and Asian populations are not as well documented. It has been reported that the predicted FVC values should be adjusted down by 20% to 25% for Asians.

It has been commonly accepted that a measured FVC that is at least 80% of the predicted FVC is considered to be within normal limits for adults of all races. In addition, the forced expiratory volume in 1 second (FEV_1) and total lung capacity (TLC) measurements have also been included in this 80% of predicted rule. More recent studies by Knudson, Kaltenborn, Knudson, and associates (1987) and Paoletti, Viegi, Pistelli, and associates (1985) suggest that normal values for most tests should be determined by finding the percent of predicted above which 95% of the population would be seen (the so-called "normal 95th percentile"). Even though this method finds 5% (1 in 20) of healthy nonsmokers to be abnormal, it offers more realistic predicted values. It is normal to see a decline in the FVC with age.

Restrictive problems such as advanced pregnancy, obesity, ascites, neuromuscular disease, sarcoidosis, and chest wall or spinal deformity can result in a small FVC. Patients with chronic obstructive lung diseases such as emphysema, bronchitis, asthma, cystic fibrosis, and bronchiectasis commonly have a small FVC. (Fig. 4-6 shows a comparison of the spirometry tracings of a normal, obstructed, and restricted patient.)

The limitations of this text prevent a discussion of back extrapolation to find the start of a less-than-perfect effort or

the calculations for converting volumes and flows from atmospheric temperature, pressure, saturated (ATPS) to BTPS. However, most pulmonary function textbooks discuss these topics.

📖 EXAM HINT

It is often necessary to calculate how close a patient's FVC or other breathing effort has come to his or her predicted value. This is known as the patient's percent of predicted. It is found by this equation:

$$\frac{\text{patient's actual test result}}{\text{patient's predicted test value}} \times 100 = \text{patient's \% of predicted}$$

For example, in the previous discussion on FVC, it was determined that a patient has a predicted FVC of 5.166 L. Calculate the percent of predicted if the actual FVC result is 4.65 L.

$$\frac{4.65\,\text{L}}{5.116} \times 100 = \text{patient's \% of predicted}$$
$$= .90 \times 100 = 90\%$$

Therefore the patient exhaled 90% of predicted FVC and is within the normal range for that test result.

---

2. **Peak flow**

   a. **Perform the procedure (Code: IB9d and IIIA1e) [Difficulty: An]**

   The peak flow (PF) is the greatest flow rate seen in a patient's forced expiratory effort. Some authors refer to the peak flow as the peak expiratory flow rate (PEFR). It is usually seen at the beginning of the FVC effort. The instructions for the test must emphasize that the patient must "blast" the air out as hard and fast as possible. It is not necessary to encourage the patient to completely empty the lungs to residual volume.

   The patient's effort is easily directly measured with a handheld peak flowmeter. Usually at least three efforts are required to find two that are acceptably close. Peak flow values that are consistent and low despite variable patient efforts probably indicate a malfunctioning unit that should not be used. It is reasonable to record the patient's effort in liters per second because the effort takes place in about that much time. However, do not be confused by some measurement instruments and other prediction equations giving the value in liters per minute. Simply multiply or divide by 60 to convert your patient's effort from one time frame to the other. For example, a young man's peak flow might be recorded as 10 L/sec or 600 L/min. Cherniack and Raber (1972) have published the following formula* for predicting peak flow in liters/second:

   Men: [(0.144 × height in inches) − (0.024 × age)] + 2.225
   Women: [(0.090 × height in inches) − (0.018 × age)] + 1.130

---

*The BTPS correction has been calculated into these equations.

b. Interpret the results (Code: IB10d) [Difficulty: An]

The peak flow is directly related to height and indirectly related to age. Therefore the taller the patient, the greater the peak flow. Peak flow decreases with age. The peak flow is a rather nonspecific measurement of airway obstruction. It measures flow through the upper airways and is reduced in patients with an upper airway problem like a tumor, vocal cord paralysis, or laryngeal edema.

The peak flow test is most often given to patients having an asthma attack as a quick and easy measurement of small-airways obstruction. Current asthma guidelines state that if an asthma patient's peak flow is 80% to 100% of predicted or personal best, he or she is in the "green zone." This means that the patient's medications are adequately controlling the asthma. If the peak flow is 50% to 79% of predicted or personal best, he or she is in the "yellow zone." This means that the patient's medications are not adequately controlling the asthma. Increased doses are indicated if ordered by the physician. If the peak flow is less than 50% of predicted or personal best he or she is in the "red zone." This means that the patient's medications are not adequately controlling the asthma. The patient should get medical help as soon as possible.

3. Timed, forced expiratory volumes

All of the timed, forced expiratory volume tests are derived from a properly performed forced vital capacity test. See Fig. 4-3. When the FVC is done correctly the following values can be properly calculated and evaluated to determine the patient's condition. As discussed earlier, a FVC that is within 80% of predicted is interpreted as within normal limits. Because of this, if the results of the following tests show patient values within 80% of predicted, the results are interpreted as being within normal limits.

a. Forced expiratory flow$_{200-1200}$ (FEF$_{200-1200}$)
1. Perform the procedure (Code: IB9d) [Difficulty: An]

The FEF$_{200-1200}$ is the mean forced expiratory flow between 200 mL and 1200 mL of an acceptable FVC (see Fig 4-5). The measurement is usually recorded in liters/second, but may be recorded in liters/minute. When performing the FEF$_{200-1200}$ test, the respiratory therapist must ensure that the patient gives his or her best effort. The results are effort-dependent and will not be valid if the patient does not give a full effort.

2. Interpret the results (Code: IB10d) [Difficulty: An]

The results of the test normally decline with age and are lower in women than men. A patient with a restrictive lung disease may have a normal or increased value. The patient with obstructive lung disease or with an upper airway, tracheal, or large bronchial obstruction will have a low value. A normal 150-lb/68-kg young man should have

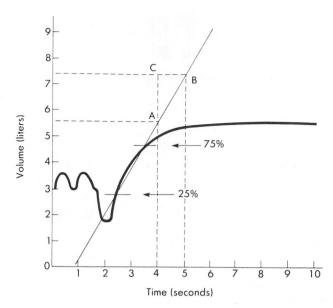

Fig. 4-7 One method of determining the FEF$_{25\%-75\%}$ value from a FVC tracing. First, mark the 25% and 75% points from the start of the effort. These are found by multiplying the FVC value by .25 and .75, respectively, and measuring from the start of the effort. Second, draw a line through these two points to intersect the dashed time lines at points A and B. Horizontal dashed lines are added from A and B to cross the volume scale. The FEF$_{25\%-75\%}$ value is read as the distance between A and C or about 2 L/sec. BTPS correct this measurement. (From Ruppel G: *Manual of pulmonary function testing,* ed 5, St Louis, 1991, Mosby.)

values of 6 to 7 L/sec or 360 to 420 L/min. The following formulas* have been developed by Morris, Koski, and Johnson (1971) to calculate predicted values in liters/second:

Men: [(0.109 × height in inches) − (0.047 × age in years)] + 2.010 (SD 1.66)

Women: [(0.145 × height in inches) − (0.036 × age in years)] + 2.532 (SD 1.19)

b. Forced expiratory flow$_{25\%-75\%}$ (FEF$_{25\%-75\%}$)
1. Perform the procedure (Code: IB9d) [Difficulty: An]

The FEF$_{25\%-75\%}$ is the mean forced expiratory flow during the middle half of an acceptable FVC (see Fig. 4-7). The FVC effort to use for this test is the one that has the greatest combination of FVC volume and FEV$_1$. As mentioned earlier, the patient must give his or her best effort. The measurement is usually recorded in liters/second but may be recorded in liters/minute.

2. Interpret the results (Code: IB10d) [Difficulty: An]

---

*The BTPS correction has been calculated into these equations.

The results are normally less than in the $FEF_{200-1200}$ and peak flow tests because the flow being measured comes from medium-size and small airways (less than 2 mm in diameter). The results should decline with age and be lower in women than men. A patient with a restrictive lung disease may have a normal or increased value whereas a low value is seen in a patient with obstructive lung disease. A small $FEF_{25\%-75\%}$ value when the FVC, FEV_1, and $FEF_{200-1200}$ values are normal is often taken to indicate early small airways disease. A normal 150-lb/68-kg young man should have values of 4 to 5 L/sec or 240 to 300 L/min. The following formulas* have been developed by Morris, Koski, and Johnson (1971) and can be used to calculate the predicted values in liters/second:

Men: [(0.047 × height in inches) − (0.045 × age in years)] + 2.513 (SD 1.12)

Women: [(0.060 × height in inches) − (0.030 × age in years)] + 0.551 (SD 0.80)

c. Forced expiratory volume, timed (FEV_T)
1. Perform the procedure (Code: IB9d) [Difficulty: An]

The FEV_T is the volume of air exhaled from an acceptable FVC in the specified time. The time increments are .5, 1, 2, and 3 seconds or more and are listed as $FEV_{.5}$, FEV_1, FEV_2, FEV_3, and so on. It is important that the FVC have a good start and a maximum effort to the end.

The FEV_1 is the most commonly used measurement along with the FVC value to judge the patient's response to inhaled bronchodilators, for bronchoprovocation testing to screen for asthmatic tendencies, to detect exercise-induced asthma, and for simple screening. BTPS correct all the measured values.

The timed forced expiratory volumes ($FEV_{.5}$, FEV_1, FEV_2, FEV_3) effectively "cut" the FVC into sections based on how much volume the patient forcibly exhales in .5, 1, 2, and 3 seconds. Some patients with severe obstructive lung disease require several more seconds to completely exhale. In these cases, simply keep measuring the volume exhaled in each additional second. See Fig. 4-8 for a FVC tracing that is subdivided at .5-, 1-, 2-, and 3-second intervals. Some bedside units give a numerical value for some or all of the timed intervals; however, it is best to have a spirometer that produces a printed copy of the patient's FVC effort. The individual volumes can be determined by marking the vertical distance on the volume scale from the baseline (total lung capacity) to the respective arrow tips.

2. Interpret the results (Code: IB10d) [Difficulty: An]

The FEV_T values are often reduced in both restrictive and obstructive lung diseases. Patients with a severe

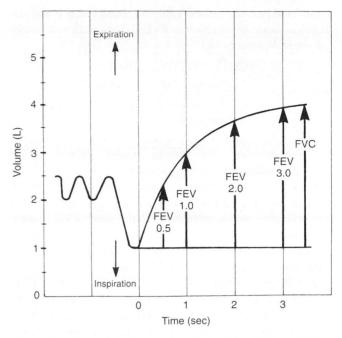

Fig. 4-8 Forced vital capacity divided into $FEV_{0.5}$, $FEV_{1.0}$, $FEV_{2.0}$, and $FEV_{3.0}$. (From Ruppel G: *Manual of Pulmonary Function Testing*, ed. 4, St. Louis, 1986, Mosby.)

restrictive lung disease exhale almost all of their small FVC within the first second. Patients with severe obstructive lung disease show low values at all time intervals with the volumes at $FEV_{2, 3, etc.}$ becoming progressively smaller. The most commonly evaluated values are the FEV_1 and the $FEV_{1\%}$. The following formulas* have been developed by Morris, Koski, and Johnson (1971) and can be used to calculate the predicted values for FEV_1 in liters:

Men: [(0.092 × height in inches) − (0.032 × age in years)] − 1.260 (SD .55)

Women: [(0.089 × height in inches) − (0.024 × age in years)] − 1.93 (SD 0.47)

d. Forced expiratory volume/forced vital capacity ratio (FEV_T / FVC or FEV_T%)
1. Perform the procedure (Code: IB9d) [Difficulty: An]

The FEV (timed) to FVC ratio compares by division the volume exhaled at .5, 1, 2, and 3 (or more) seconds (see Fig. 4-8) to the FVC. This results in a series of decimal fractions. These are multiplied by 100 to convert the answers to percentages.

It must be obvious that every person exhales different volumes for the FEV time intervals because each person's FVC is different. This procedure mathematically standardizes the results regardless of the patient's FVC. Therefore

---

*The BTPS correction has been calculated into these equations.

*The BTPS correction has been calculated into these equations.

these percentage values can be standardized for all individuals despite different FVCs. The predicted values for normal patients are:

$$FEV_{.5} = 50\% \text{ to } 60\% \text{ of the FVC}$$
$$FEV_1 = 75\% \text{ to } 85\% \text{ of the FVC}$$
$$FEV_2 = 94\% \text{ of the FVC}$$
$$FEV_3 = 97\% \text{ of the FVC}$$

2. Interpret the results (Code: IB10d) [Difficulty: An]

These values normally decrease slightly in the elderly patient. Most patients with normal lungs and airways are still able to completely exhale their FVC within 4 seconds.

Patients with restrictive lung diseases often exhale their FVC more quickly than expected. This abnormal finding is caused by these patients having a smaller-than-normal FVC and stiff lungs that recoil more quickly than expected to their resting volume. See Fig. 4-4 to compare the FVC curves of a patient with restrictive lung disease with the FVC curves of a patient with obstructive lung disease.

Patients with obstructive lung disease take longer than expected to exhale their FVC. As a result, the percentages of the FVC exhaled in the timed intervals listed are lower than normal. A FEV_1 of less than 65% to 70% of the FVC confirms obstructive lung disease. Obviously, the lower the percentage exhaled for any timed interval, the worse the obstruction to exhalation. A patient with restrictive lung disease exhales the FVC too quickly and all of the derived values are higher than expected.

 EXAM HINT

Of these tests, the FEV_1 is the most important to follow. A lower-than-normal value is widely used as an indicator of COPD.

MODULE F Special purpose pulmonary function tests

1. CO2 response curve
a. Recommend the procedure (Code: IA2d) [Difficulty: An]

The CO_2 response curve is also known as the *ventilatory response to CO_2 test*. The test is a measurement of the increase in minute volume caused by breathing different concentrations of carbon dioxide when the patient's oxygen level is normal. The test is performed on patients with obstructive lung disease to determine if their breathing will increase when their CO_2 level is increased. The change in breathing is recorded in L/min/mm Hg PCO_2.

b. Perform the procedure (Code: IC1a) [Difficulty: An]
Two methods of performing the test follow:
1. **Open-circuit technique.** While breathing 21%

oxygen, the patient is made to inhale increasing concentrations of CO_2 from 1% up to 7%. Breathing the set CO_2 percent continues until a steady state is reached. Measurements of end-tidal CO_2, $PaCO_2$, minute volume, and P_{100} are made at each increasing carbon dioxide level. (P_{100} is the symbol for occlusion pressure, or the pressure generated in the mouth during the first 100 milliseconds [1/10th second] of an inspiratory effort against an occluded airway.)
2. **Closed-circuit or rebreathing technique.** While breathing 21% oxygen, the patient is made to inhale 7% CO_2 from a reservoir. Rebreathing continues until the patient's end-tidal CO_2 value exceeds 9% or 4 minutes have passed. Measurements of end-tidal CO_2, $PaCO_2$, minute volume, and P_{100} are made periodically during the test. The patient's SpO_2 may also be monitored during the test.

With either method of testing, a curve is plotted by comparing the change in minute volume at each change in the patient's end-tidal CO_2 value.

c. Interpret the results (Code: IC2a) [Difficulty: An]

A normal person has a linear increase in minute volume of about 3 L/min/mm Hg PCO_2. The range is between 1 and 6 L/min/mm Hg PCO_2. Patients with COPD have a variable response to an increased carbon dioxide level. Some patients normally increase their breathing to try to maintain a steady PCO_2. Others have a less-than-normal increase in their breathing efforts as the PCO_2 increases. It is believed that this decreased reaction is because of the patient's increased airway resistance.

The curve plotted by comparing the change in minute volume at each change in the patient's end-tidal CO_2 value indicates a normal or decreased breathing effort. A normal curve shows an increased minute volume at each increased end-tidal CO_2 value. An abnormal curve shows a smaller than expected or no increase in minute volume at each increased end-tidal CO_2 value.

2. Spirometry before and after an aerosolized bronchodilator has been inhaled
a. Recommend the procedure (Code: IA2d) [Difficulty: An]

The following are common indications for the procedure:
1. Patient is known to have asthma or another type of chronic obstructive lung disease.
2. The patient has an $FEV_{1\%}$ of less than 70% (unless elderly).
3. The effectiveness of a new bronchodilator is being evaluated.

b. Perform the procedure (Code: IC1a) [Difficulty: An]

The most commonly administered tests are the peak flow and $FEV_{1\%}$ from a FVC. Before starting the test, make sure that the patient has not taken a bronchodilating drug in the previous 4 to 6 hours. If no bronchodilating drugs have been administered, the test can be performed. A peak flow or $FEV_{1\%}$ test should be performed and the value(s) should be measured. Then a fast onset sympathomimetic-type drug is given. The medication can be given by intermittent positive pressure breathing (IPPB), handheld nebulizer, or metered dose inhaler, as long as the method is done properly. Wait about 10 to 15 minutes for the medication to take effect and the patient's blood gas values to return to normal. Then repeat the peak flow or $FEV_{1\%}$ test. The percentage of improvement is calculated by using this formula:

percent of change
$$= \frac{\text{after drug airflow} - \text{before drug airflow}}{\text{before drug airflow}} \times 100$$

c. Interpret the results (Code: IC2a) [Difficulty: An]

To prove that the medication is effective, the current standard requires the patient to have at least a 12% improvement in peak flow and/or $FEV_{1\%}$ and a 200 mL increase in exhaled volume. (The old standard required a 15% to 20% improvement in flow.) It is not uncommon to see patients with asthma improve much more than this. Other patients may not have this much improvement but do show increases in airflow and FVC and say that they feel better. In these cases, the physician may decide to continue the medication.

3. Flow-volume loops

a. Recommend the procedure (Code: IA2d) [Difficulty: An]

The flow-volume loop is a graphic display of the flow and volume generated during a forced expiratory vital capacity (FEVC) that is immediately followed by a forced inspiratory vital capacity (FIVC). It is used to identify inspiratory or expiratory flow at any lung volume.

b. Perform the procedure (Code: IC1a) [Difficulty: An]

As with the FVC test, the patient should be coached to inhale completely and blast the air out until he or she is completely empty. When you are sure that the patient has exhaled to residual volume, coach him or her to inhale as quickly as possible until the lungs are completely full. There should not be any hesitation at the start, leaks, glottic closing, or coughing throughout the entire procedure.

The expiratory half of the curve is called the maximal expiratory flow-volume (MEFV) curve. It begins at total lung capacity and ends at residual volume. The inspiratory half of the curve is called the maximal inspiratory flow-volume (MIFV) curve. It begins at residual volume and ends at total lung capacity. Ideally, the two halves of the loop meet at the total lung capacity. Flow is recorded in L/sec and graphed on the vertical (ordinate or Y) axis.

Volume is recorded in liters and graphed on the horizontal (abscissa or X) axis. Both flow and volume should be BTPS adjusted.

c. Interpret the results (Code: IC2a) [Difficulty: An]

Flow-volume loops have gained great popularity because the shape of the curve is diagnostic of the patient's condition. In addition, peak inspiratory and peak expiratory flows can be determined. If the effort can be timed, all the parameters found on the previously discussed volume-time curves can be found on the flow-volume loop. The following examples show a normal flow-volume loop and representative abnormal loops.

Normal. A normal flow-volume loop is shown in Figs. 4-9 and 4-10. First look at Fig. 4-9, in which the various volumes are measured on the horizontal scale. The tidal volume (V_T) of 500 mL is the small loop within the larger vital capacity loop. The expiratory reserve volume (ERV) and inspiratory reserve volume (IRV) are shown on both sides of the tidal volume. The FVC is shown as the total of all three volumes. Finally, total lung capacity (TLC) and residual volume (RV) are marked.

Fig. 4-10 shows the same normal flow-volume loop in which the various flows are measured on the vertical scale. Starting from TLC with the FEVC, the peak expiratory flow rate (PEFR) is seen as the greatest flow that is generated; it is about 9 L/sec. Starting from RV with the forced inspiratory vital capacity, the peak inspiratory flow

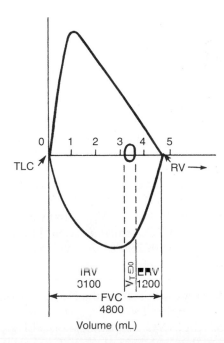

Fig. 4-9 Flow-volume loop tracing of a normal adult showing the positions and values of the lung volumes. *ERV,* Expiratory reserve volume; *FVC,* forced vital capacity; *IRV,* inspiratory reserve volume; *RV,* residual volume; *TLC,* total lung capacity.

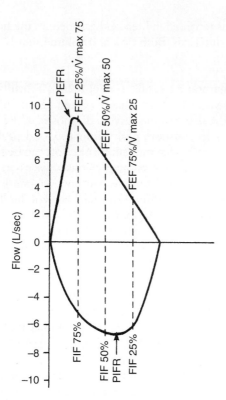

Fig. 4-10 Flow-volume loop tracing of a normal adult showing the positions and values of the various inspiratory and expiratory flows. *FEF,* Forced expiratory flow; *FIF,* forced inspiratory flow; *PEFR,* peak expiratory flow rate; *PIFR,* peak inspiratory flow rate.

rate (PIFR) is seen as the greatest flow that is generated; it is about 7 L/sec. It is normal for the PEFR to be greater than the PIFR.

To find the instantaneous flow at any FVC lung volume, the FVC must be divided by 4 to find the 25th, 50th, and 75th percentile points. In Fig. 4-10, the FVC is 4800 mL. Dividing by 4 gives 1200 mL per quarter of the FVC. These points are marked on the horizontal volume scale. If a vertical (dashed) line is drawn through these three points to the flow-volume tracing, the instantaneous flows at these volumes can be found. *Expiratory flows* are reported as:

1. Flow at 75% of the FEVC = $\dot{V}_{max75}$ (maximum flow with 75% of the FVC remaining) or $FEF_{25\%}$ (forced expiratory flow with 25% of the FVC exhaled)
2. Flow at 50% of the FEVC = $\dot{V}_{max50}$ (maximum flow with 50% of the FVC remaining) or $FEF_{50\%}$ (forced expiratory flow with 50% of the FVC exhaled)
3. Flow at 25% of the FEVC = $\dot{V}_{max25}$ (maximum flow with 25% of the FVC remaining) or $FEF_{75\%}$ (forced expiratory flow with 75% of the FVC exhaled)

Inspiratory flows are reported as:

1. Flow at 25% of the FIVC = $FIF_{25\%}$ (forced inspiratory flow with 25% of the FVC inhaled)

2. Flow at 50% of the FIVC = $FIF_{50\%}$ (forced inspiratory flow with 50% of the FVC inhaled)
3. Flow at 75% of the FIVC = $FIF_{75\%}$ (forced inspiratory flow with 75% of the FVC inhaled)

The PEFR and FEF_{25} or $\dot{V}_{max75\%}$ values should be about the same because they all measure flow through the large upper airways. Either test is a good gauge of the patient's effort because it will be low if the patient is not trying hard. The FEF_{50} or $\dot{V}_{max50\%}$ values should approximate the $FEF_{25\%-75\%}$ values because they both show flow through the medium to small airways in the middle half of the FVC effort. It is normal for the FIF_{50} to be greater than the FEF_{50}. The FEF_{75} or $\dot{V}_{max25\%}$ values are the best indicator of early small airways disease because both show flow through the small airways as the patient approaches the residual volume. Note that the tracing from the FEF_{25} or $\dot{V}_{max75\%}$ point to the residual volume is close to a straight line. In normal people, the flow decreases in proportion to the decreasing lung volume resulting in the straight-line tracing. Cherniack and Raber (1972) have published formulas for predicting adult MEFV flows in L/sec; see the bibliography.

Small airways disease. Examples of conditions resulting in small airways disease (less than 2 mm in diameter) include asthma, chronic bronchitis, bronchiectasis, cystic fibrosis, and emphysema. The obstruction can be from bronchospasm, mucus plugging, or damage to the alveoli and small airways leading to their collapse on expiration.

Fig. 4-11 shows representative flow-volume loops of asthma and emphysema superimposed over a normal flow-volume loop. Notice that both loops are shifted to the left toward the total lung capacity because the residual volumes are increased. Also notice that the flows are decreased more than normal as the patient exhales closer to the residual volume. This "scooped out" appearance is very characteristic of small airways disease. Having the patient inhale a bronchodilator and repeating the flow-volume loop shows the degree of reversibility. Some computer-based systems allow the before and after bronchodilator loops to be superimposed to further show the amount of improvement.

Restriction. A restriction can be caused by a pulmonary condition such as fibrosis; a thoracic condition such as pleural effusion, pneumothorax or hemothorax, or kyphoscoliosis; or obesity, advanced pregnancy, or ascites pushing up on the diaphragm. Only fibrosis and kyphoscoliosis are permanent. Fig. 4-11 shows a representative flow-volume loop for a patient with restrictive lung disease. Notice that the volume is small and shifted to the right toward the small residual volume.

Variable intrathoracic obstruction. A variable intrathoracic obstruction can be caused by a tumor or foreign body partially blocking a bronchus. Fig. 4-11 shows a representative flow-volume curve. Note that the forced vital capacity

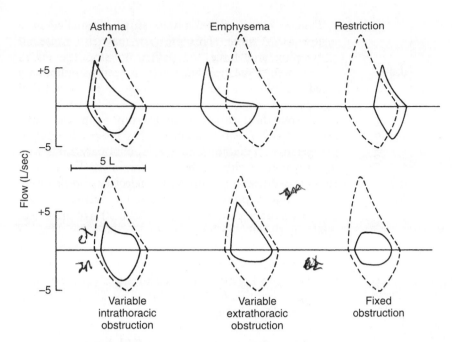

Fig. 4-11 A series of abnormal flow-volume loop tracings superimposed over a dashed line tracing of a normal loop. (From Ruppel G: *Manual of pulmonary function testing,* ed 6, St Louis, 1994, Mosby.)

volume is almost normal, and there is a greatly decreased peak expiratory flow rate.

Variable extrathoracic obstruction. A variable extrathoracic obstruction can be caused by vocal cord paralysis, laryngeal tumor, or a foreign body partially obstructing the upper airway. Fig. 4-11 shows a representative flow-volume curve. Note that the forced vital capacity volume is almost normal with a greatly reduced inspiratory flow. This same pattern is commonly seen in patients with obstructive sleep apnea. The $FEF_{50\%}$ will be greater than the $FIF_{50\%}$.

Fixed large airway obstruction. A fixed large airway obstruction is usually caused by a tumor in the trachea or a mainstem bronchus. Fig. 4-11 shows a representative flow-volume loop. Again, the forced vital capacity volume is close to normal. Note the abnormally reduced inspiratory and expiratory flow rates. The tracing looks almost "squared off" with the $FEF_{50\%}$ and $FIF_{50\%}$ values being about the same.

4. Maximum voluntary ventilation
a. Recommend the procedure (Code: IA2d) [Difficulty: An]

The maximum voluntary ventilation (MVV) is the volume of air exhaled in a specified period during a repetitive maximal respiratory effort. It is most commonly performed to evaluate a patient's ability to perform a stress test. It may also be used as a preoperative screening test to help determine the patient's chance of pulmonary complications.

b. Perform the procedure (Code: IC1a) [Difficulty: An]

The patient should breathe at a volume that is greater than the tidal volume but less than the vital capacity with a rate between 70 and 120 per minute. The minimal time for

the test is 5 seconds with a recommended time of 12 seconds. See Fig. 4-12 for two different tracings of the MVV effort. The total volume exhaled in the given time period is mathematically adjusted for 1 minute so that the derived value is in L/min. This is done by multiplying a 5-second effort by 12 or a 12-second effort by 5. The derived value is then BTPS corrected to give the final value.

c. Interpret the results (Code: IC2a) [Difficulty: An]

The results of the MVV test are among the most difficult to evaluate. This is because the patient's effort, the condition of the respiratory muscles, lung-thoracic compliance, neurologic control over the drive to breathe, and airway and tissue resistance all have an influence. Abnormalities in any of these can cause the MVV value to decrease. Also, because more than one problem can exist, a decreased MVV does not point out the exact difficulty. A healthy young man can have an MVV of 150 to 200 L/min. Women tend to have smaller values, and the values of both sexes decrease with age. Because of the many factors involved in the MVV, normal predicted values may vary by as much as ±30%. Therefore unless a patient has an MVV value that is less than 70% of predicted, he or she cannot really be considered abnormal.

Cherniack and Raber (1972) have published the following equations* for predicting the MVV in L/min:

Males: [(3.03 × height in inches) − (0.816 × age in years)] − 37.9

Females: [(2.14 × height in inches) − (0.685 × age in years)] − 4.87

When evaluating an abnormally low MVV result, the following considerations must be made:

*The BTPS correction has been calculated into these equations.

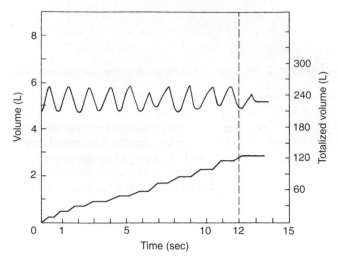

Fig. 4-12 Two tracings of the same maximum voluntary ventilation (MVV) effort. The saw-toothed tracing shows each individual volume effort and the respiratory rate. The stair-stepped tracing shows the cumulative volume during the effort. (From Ruppel G: *Manual of pulmonary function testing,* ed 6, St Louis, 1994, Mosby.)

1. Did the patient try his or her best? The respiratory therapist must make a professional judgment that the patient made his or her best effort. An objective way of judging this is to multiply the patient's $FEV_1 \times 35$ to estimate the MVV. They should be close to the same volume. For example, if the patient's FEV_1 is 3 L, the estimated MVV is 105 L/min (3 L × 35). An MVV value that is much less than this indicates that the patient did not try very hard. Conversely, an MVV value that is much greater than this indicates that the FEV_1 value is too low and should be repeated.
2. What is the condition of the patient's respiratory muscles? Patients with neuromuscular abnormalities probably will not be able to breathe much more deeply than the normal tidal volume or keep up the great effort required for the duration of the test. Because of this, their results will be low.
3. What is the patient's lung-thoracic compliance? Patients with low compliance probably will not be able to sustain the greater than normal workload required by the MVV test. However, some patients are able to compensate for a small tidal volume by increasing their respiratory rate enough to generate an MVV value within normal limits. A printout of the MVV test would show a smaller than expected volume moved at a higher than expected respiratory rate.
4. What is the patient's neurologic control over the drive to breathe? Patients who have had an injury to the brain may have an abnormal drive to breathe. Because of this, they produce a low MVV result.
5. What is the patient's airway and tissue resistance?

Patients with increased airway resistance usually have a low MVV result. This problem may also cause air trapping and force the patient to stop the effort. Increased tissue resistance such as seen in pulmonary edema, obesity, and ascites also results in a low MVV value.

Despite these difficulties in determining the cause of a decreased MVV value, doing so has proven helpful in preoperative evaluation and cardiopulmonary stress testing. Any patient with a lower-than-normal MVV value is at an increased risk of postoperative atelectasis and pneumonia. The risks of pulmonary complications related to MVV are low when the patient reaches 75% to 50% of predicted, moderate when the patient reaches 50% to 33% of predicted, and high when the patient reaches less than 33% of predicted. Patients with known moderate to severe COPD usually have to stop exercise testing because of their inability to breathe. An MVV value of less than 50 L/min is a good predictor of this.

5. **Single-breath nitrogen washout (SBN_2) test and closing volume**
   a. **Recommend the procedure (Code: IA2d) [Difficulty: An]**

   The single-breath nitrogen washout is used to measure two things: (1) the evenness of the distribution of ventilation into the lungs during inspiration, and (2) the emptying rates of the lungs during exhalation. It is a helpful diagnostic test in any adult patient who is known or suspected of having obstructive airways disease. The NBRC uses the phrase *nitrogen washout distribution test* for its examinations.

   The closing volume is one part of the SBN_2 test. It marks the lung volume when small airway closure begins and is used as an early indicator of small airways disease.

   b. **Perform the procedure (Code: IC1a) [Difficulty: An]**

   The SBN_2 test is done by analyzing the nitrogen (N_2) percentage that is exhaled after an inspiratory vital capacity of 100% oxygen. It is beyond the scope of this book to go into detail on all the steps of the procedure; however, the general steps include instructing the patient to perform an inspiratory vital capacity while inhaling oxygen. Without any breath holding, tell the patient to slowly and evenly exhale until his or her lungs are empty again. The exhaled gases are sent through a rapid N_2 analyzer to measure the percentage, a spirometer to measure the volume, and a graphing device.

   c. **Interpret the results (Code: IC2a) [Difficulty: An]**

   Refer to Fig. 4-13 for a normal tracing showing these phases:

   Phase I shows gas exhaled from the anatomic dead space of the upper airway. Because it is made up of 100% oxygen, the nitrogen percentage shows a zero reading.

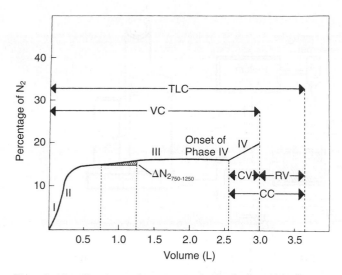

Fig. 4-13 Tracing of a normal single-breath nitrogen washout (SBN$_2$) test showing the four phases and other features. *CC*, Closing capacity; *CV*, closing volume; *ΔN_2 $_{750\text{-}1250}$*, nitrogen percentage found in the 500 mL of gas exhaled between 750 and 1250 mL of the vital capacity; *RV*, residual volume; *TLC*, total lung capacity; *VC*, vital capacity. (From Ruppel G: *Manual of pulmonary function testing,* ed 6, St Louis, 1994, Mosby.)

Phase II shows a mix of dead space gas and alveolar gas. The nitrogen percentage rises rapidly as the pure oxygen is exhaled and nitrogen rich gas from the alveoli is brought out. The first 750 mL of gas that includes these first two phases is not used in the evaluation of the distribution of ventilation.

Phase III shows a fairly level plateau as alveolar gas from the lower lobes with a stable mix of oxygen and nitrogen is exhaled. Phase III is further evaluated in the following two ways:

1. **ΔN_2 $_{750\text{-}1250}$** looks at the increase in the nitrogen percentage found in the 500 mL of gas exhaled between 750 mL and 1250 mL of the vital capacity. It is normally no more than 1.5% in healthy young adults. It increases to between 3% and 4.5% in healthy older adults. Patients with severe airways and lung disease, such as emphysema, may have a finding of 6% to 10% or more.

2. **Slope of Phase III** is found by drawing a straight line from the point where 30% of the vital capacity is exhaled to the point where phase IV begins. It is normally no more than .5% to 1% N$_2$ per liter of exhaled volume in healthy young adults, but may vary widely.

Phase IV is seen as a sharp increase in the nitrogen percentage and continues to residual volume. This is seen when the nitrogen-rich gas from the upper airways continues to be exhaled as the basilar airways became compressed and close off near the end of the vital capacity effort.

The start of phase IV is called the *closing volume* (CV). It marks the lung volume when small airway closure begins and is an early indicator of small airways disease. Closing volume does not occur in healthy young adults until after about 80% to 90% of the vital capacity has been exhaled. The closing capacity (CC) is found by adding the closing volume to the residual volume (found by another test). Healthy young adults have a closing capacity that is about 30% of their total lung capacity.

Problems can be indicated through the following: increases in the N$_2$ $_{750\text{-}1250}$, the slope of phase III, and especially early onset of phase IV; increased closing volume; and increased closing capacity. Included in the problems are small airways disease, congestive heart failure with pulmonary edema, or obesity.

6. Functional residual capacity (FRC) by the helium dilution method

a. Recommend the procedure (Code: IA2d) [Difficulty: An]

The functional residual capacity (FRC) is the volume of gas left in the lungs at the end of a normal expiration. It cannot be measured through spirometry. An FRC is needed to calculate a patient's residual volume (RV) and total lung capacity (TLC). It is necessary to know a patient's RV, FRC, and TLC to diagnose and determine the severity of obstructive lung disease and restrictive lung disease.

b. Perform the procedure (Code: IC1a) [Difficulty: An]

The helium (He) dilution method basically involves diluting the resident gases in the lungs (mainly nitrogen and oxygen) with helium to mathematically determine the FRC. This is also called the closed-circuit method because the patient and circuit are sealed off. Fig. 4-14 shows a schematic drawing of the components that make up the circuit. These include a two-way valve to switch the patient from breathing room air to the helium mix, soda lime to absorb the patient's exhaled carbon dioxide from the circuit, a combined CO$_2$ and water vapor absorber to prevent these gases from entering the helium analyzer, the helium analyzer, a variable speed blower to move the gases through the circuit, a spirometer for monitoring tidal volumes, attached kymograph to trace out the patient's breathing pattern, and an oxygen supply to meet the patient's needs. The helium supply is not shown.

It is beyond the scope of this text to cover all the steps in the helium dilution test; however, the following features of the procedure are important to know. Add enough helium to the room air in the circuit to create a 10% to 15% He mix. At the end of a normal elation, the patient is switched to breathing the mix so that the functional residual capacity can be determined. The patient breathes the gas mix until the helium is evenly distributed throughout the lungs and the helium percentage is stable. Typically, the test is performed for up to 7 minutes if

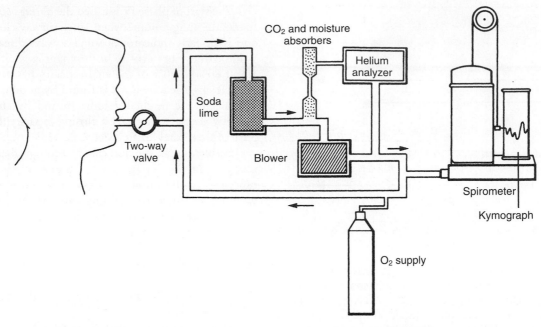

Fig. 4-14 Schematic drawing of the key components of a helium dilution system for measuring functional residual capacity. (From Beauchamp RK: Pulmonary function testing procedures. In Barnes TA, editor: *Respiratory care practice,* St Louis, 1988, Mosby.)

needed to reach an equilibrium point. Extending the test longer may help to reach a stable equilibrium point in abnormal patients. The calculation of residual volume is rather complex and is usually done through the computer built into the pulmonary function system. Spirometry must also be performed because the expiratory reserve volume is subtracted from the functional residual capacity to find the residual volume. Commonly the test is repeated. The patient should be allowed to breathe room air for 5 minutes between tests to clear the helium from the lungs. Patients with severe obstructive lung disease may need more time. Bates, Macklem, and Christie (1971) have published the following equations* for calculating the normal FRC in liters:

$$\text{Males} = (0.130 \times \text{height in inches}) - 5.16$$
$$\text{Females} = (0.119 \times \text{height in inches}) - 4.85$$

Goldman and Becklake (1959) have published the following equations† for calculating the normal RV in liters:

$$\text{Males} = [(0.069 \times \text{height in inches}) + (0.017 \times \text{age in years})] - 3.45$$
$$\text{Females} = [(0.081 \times \text{height in inches}) + (0.009 \times \text{age in years})] - 3.90$$

c. Interpret the results (Code: IC2a) [Difficulty: An]

A normal young man has an FRC volume of about 2400 mL. As shown in Fig. 4-15, it is composed of the expiratory reserve volume (ERV) and the residual volume (RV). The FRC and RV values are invaluable in diagnosing obstructive and restrictive lung diseases. See Fig. 4-6 for the relative volumes and capacities for a normal patient, a patient with an obstructive pattern, and a patient with a restrictive pattern. Note that the obstructive patient has a disproportionate increase in the residual volume with a resulting decrease in the FVC. The total lung capacity may be normal, as shown, or, more commonly, increased lung capacity. The patient with restrictive disease has a proportionate decrease in all the lung volumes and capacities. It is commonly accepted that the normal limits of total lung capacity are about ± 20% of the predicted value. This ± 20% of the normal limit applies to the FRC and RV values as well. In other words, obstructive lung disease can be diagnosed by an RV, FRC, or TLC that is more than 120% of the predicted value. Common examples of obstructive diseases include asthma, bronchitis, and emphysema. Restrictive lung disease can be diagnosed by an RV, FRC, or TLC that is less than 80% of the predicted value. Examples of restrictive diseases include fibrotic lung disease, air or fluid in the pleural space, obesity, kyphoscoliosis, pectus excavatum, and neuromuscular weakness or paralysis.

The following considerations should be accounted for to ensure that the measured values are accurate:
1. There should be no leaks in the system. A leak can result in an overestimation of the FRC because the lost helium results in a lower final helium percentage. Or, a

---

*The BTPS correction has been calculated into these equations.
†The BTPS correction has been calculated into these equations.

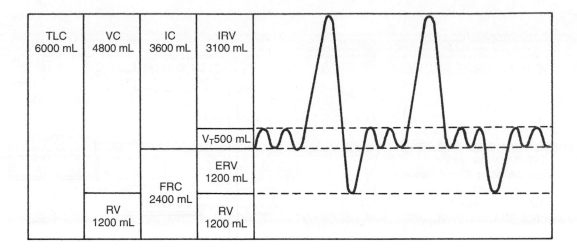

Volumes: Four primary

A. Tidal volume (V_T). The volume of gas inspired *or* expired during normal respiration.
B. Inspiratory reserve volume (IRV): The maximum volume of gas that can be inspired beyond a normal inspiration.
C. Expiratory reserve volume (ERV): The maximum volume of gas that can be exhaled after a normal expiration.
D. Residual volume (RV): The volume of gas remaining in the lungs after a maximum expiration.

Capacities: Four, which include two or more primary volumes

A. Total lung capacity (TLC): The total amount of gas contained in the lungs after maximum inspiration. Includes all four primary volumes (TLC = V_T + IRV + ERV + RV).
B. Vital capacity (VC): The maximum amount of gas that can be exhaled after a maximum inspiration. Includes three primary volumes (VC = V_T + IRV + ERV).
C. Inspiratory capacity (IC): The maximum amount of gas that can be inspired after a normal expiration. Includes two primary volumes (IC = V_T + IRV).
D. Functional residual capacity (FRC): The total amount of gas remaining in the lungs after normal expiration. Includes two primary volumes (FRC = ERV + RV).

Fig. 4-15 Lung volumes and capacities for a clinically normal young man.

leak can result in failure of the final helium percentage to stabilize as expected.

2. The patient must be breathing on the system long enough for the helium to reach all of the lung units and reach equilibrium. Usually this takes about 7 minutes; however, patients with severe obstructive lung disease will need more time and may never reach an equilibrium state. This results in an underestimation of the FRC.

7. Functional residual capacity (FRC) by the nitrogen washout method

a. Recommend the procedure (Code: IA2d) [Difficulty: An]

As discussed in the helium dilution method, the nitrogen (N_2) washout method is used to find the functional residual capacity so that the residual volume can be derived from it and total lung capacity calculated. It is necessary to know a patient's RV, FRC, and TLC to diagnose and determine the severity of obstructive lung disease and restrictive lung disease.

b. Perform the procedure (Code: IC1a) [Difficulty: An]

The nitrogen washout method basically involves having the patient breathe in 100% oxygen until all the resident nitrogen is removed from the lungs. It is also called the open-circuit method because the patient inspires as much oxygen as needed to displace the nitrogen to a reservoir for measurement.

Fig. 4-16 shows a schematic drawing of the components that make up the automated nitrogen washout system and circuit. These include a solenoid valve to switch the patient from breathing room air to pure oxygen, an oxygen source with demand valve, a nitrogen analyzer with recorder, a pneumotachometer, and a microprocessor that directs all the necessary activities for the test. It is beyond the scope of this text to go into the complete procedure for the test; however, the following features should be known. The circuit is filled with pure oxygen. The patient is switched from room air to oxygen at the end of a normal exhalation so that the nitrogen in the functional residual capacity can be determined. Typically, the test is performed for up to 7 minutes or until the nitrogen percentage

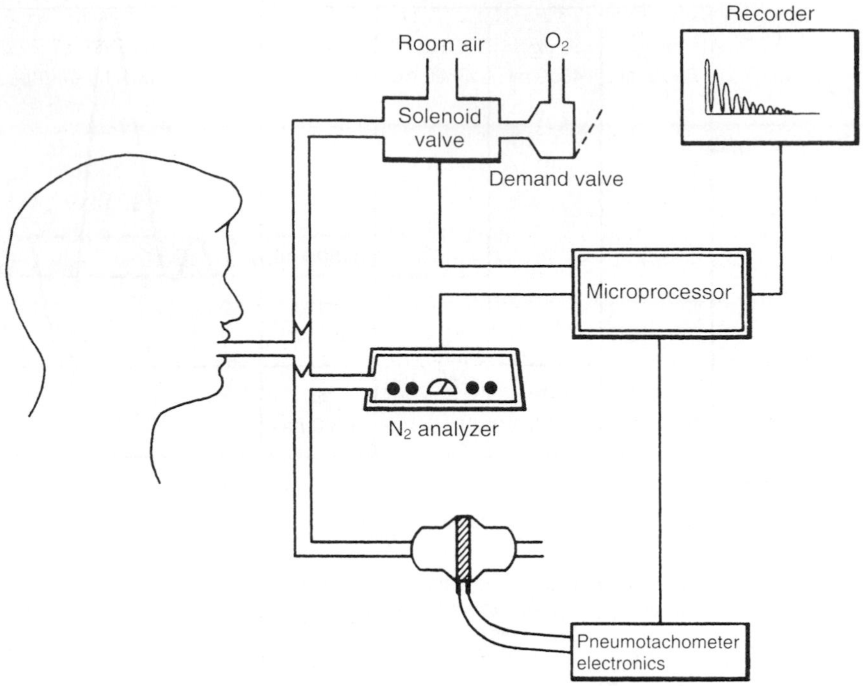

Fig. 4-16 Schematic drawing of the key components of the automated nitrogen washout system for measuring functional residual capacity. (From Beauchamp RK: Pulmonary function testing procedures. In Barnes TA, editor: *Respiratory care practice,* St Louis, 1988, Mosby.)

falls below a target level. This target percentage has been reported by various authors as 1% (best results) up to 3%. Extending the test longer may help to reach a target level in patients with increased airway resistance or an increased lung volume. As before, the calculation of residual volume is rather complex and is usually done through the computer built into the pulmonary function system. Spirometry must also be performed because the expiratory reserve volume is subtracted from the functional residual capacity to find the residual volume. Commonly the test is repeated. The patient should be allowed to breathe room air for at least 15 minutes between tests to clear the oxygen from the lungs. Patients with severe obstructive lung disease may need more time.

Predicted patient values for FRC and RV can be determined with the same equations listed in the previous discussion of the helium dilution method of determining FRC.

c. Interpret the results (Code: IC2a) [Difficulty: An]

As discussed earlier in the helium dilution test, the FRC and RV values are invaluable in diagnosing obstructive and restrictive lung diseases. When done properly, the helium dilution and nitrogen washout tests reveal similar patient values. If the nitrogen percentage is graphed over time, the shape of the washout curve can also be helpful in evaluating the degree of airway obstruction. Both the normal and abnormal tracings show rapid nitrogen washout from the upper airway dead space. However, as the test continues, the patient with obstructive lung disease shows a progressive slowing of the nitrogen washout rate.

The following considerations should be accounted for to ensure that the measured values are accurate:

1. There should be no leaks in the system. A leak would be noticed as a sudden increase in the nitrogen percentage after a steady decrease. This results in an overestimation in the FRC value.
2. The patient must be breathing on the system long enough for the nitrogen to be washed out of all the lung units. Usually this takes less than 7 minutes; however, patients with severe obstructive lung disease need more time and may never reach the targeted percentage. This results in an underestimation of the FRC.

8. Total lung capacity

a. Recommend the procedure (Code: IA2d) [Difficulty: An]

Total lung capacity is the volume of air in the lungs after inhaling a vital capacity. As discussed earlier, it is necessary to determine a patient's total lung capacity (TLC) to diagnose obstructive or restrictive lung disease.

b. Perform the procedure (Code: IC1a) [Difficulty: An]

Refer to Fig. 4-15 for the relationships of the lung volumes and capacities to each other. As can be seen, total lung capacity (TLC) can be found by adding several combinations of volumes and capacities. Most commonly it is calculated by adding the FRC to the inspiratory capacity (IC) found through spirometry. However, be prepared to add or subtract various combinations of volumes and capacities to find the TLC.

c. Interpret the results (Code: IC2a) [Difficulty: An]

The total lung capacity results cannot be interpreted without looking at the volumes and capacities that compose it. Fig. 4-6 shows representative TLC patterns for a normal patient and a patient with an obstructive pattern and a restrictive pattern. Note that with the abnormal patterns, the FRC and its components, the expiratory reserve volume and residual volume, are out of proportion. Patients with emphysema, bronchitis, or asthma often show the obstructive pattern with its large FRC of trapped gas. Patients with fibrotic lung disease, thoracic deformities, or obesity often show the restrictive pattern with its decreased FRC and other lung volumes.

Some practitioners use the general rule that a TLC that is more than 120% of predicted indicates an obstructive pattern, and a TLC that is less than 80% of predicted indicates a restrictive pattern. However, this may be an oversimplification. It is more reliable to calculate the residual volume:total lung capacity ratio (RV:TLC). This takes into account the interrelationship of the two. Normal healthy adults have a RV:TLC ratio that is .20 (20%) to .35 (35%). An increased RV:TLC ratio is commonly seen in patients with emphysema and an increased residual volume. However, if the patient's TLC is increased in proportion to the residual volume, the ratio may be within normal limits. A decreased RV:TLC ratio is commonly seen in patients with fibrotic lung disease. The ratio will be normal, however, if the patient's TLC is decreased in proportion to the residual volume. Table 4-1 shows the relationships of the lung volumes and capacities, TLC, and the RV:TLC ratio found in a number of conditions.

EXAM HINT

Most examinations have at least one table that must be interpreted to determine if the patient has obstructive lung disease, has restrictive lung disease, or has obstructive lung disease that is responsive to bronchodilator therapy. Expiratory flows that improve by at least 15% after inhaling a bronchodilating drug indicate a positive, clinical response.

9. Body plethysmography
a. Recommend the procedure (Code: IA2d) [Difficulty: An]

b. Perform the procedure (Code: IC1a) [Difficulty: An]

c. Interpret the results (Code: IC2a) [Difficulty: An]

The body plethysmography unit (sometimes called the *body bubble*) is a sealable chamber large enough for an adult to sit inside. Auxiliary equipment includes a differential pressure pneumotachometer, a monitor/storage oscilloscope, a computer, and a recording device (see Fig. 4-17). The plethysmograph can be used to measure: (1) the FRC and, from that, the RV and total lung capacity; (2) lung compliance; and (3) airway resistance. Each of these tests is discussed next.

10. Thoracic gas volume
a. Recommend the procedure (Code: IA2d) [Difficulty: An]

The volume of gas measured in the lungs at the end of exhalation by a plethysmograph is termed *thoracic gas volume* (TGV or VTG). When the unit is accurately calibrated and the test properly performed, the plethysmograph provides a more accurate FRC volume measurement than either the helium dilution or nitrogen washout methods. Once TGV is determined, the residual volume can be derived from it and total lung capacity calculated. It is necessary to know a patient's RV, FRC, and TLC to diagnose and determine the severity of obstructive lung disease and restrictive lung disease.

TABLE 4-1	Lung Volumes and Capacities Seen in Various Disorders						
Disorder	**VC**	**IC**	**ERV**	**FRC**	**RV**	**TLC**	**RV:TLC**
Asthma or airway disease	D	N	D	N,I	I	N,I*	I
Emphysema	N	N	N	I	I	I	N,I
Diffuse parenchymal disease							
Early	N	N	N	D	N	N	N
Advanced (all volumes and capacities are equally reduced)							
Space-occupying lesions	N	N	N	N	D	N	D
Obesity	N	N	D	N,I†	N	N	I
Thoracic/skeletal disease	D	D	D	D	N	D	I

D, Decreased; *ERV*, expiratory reserve volume; *FRC*, functional residual capacity; *I, increased*; *IC*, inspiratory capacity; *N*, normal; *RV*, residual volume; *TLC*, total lung capacity; *VC*, vital capacity.
*When airway resistance is greater than about 3.5 cm H_2O/L/sec.
†When the weight:height (pounds:inches) ratio is greater than 5:1.
Modified from Snow MG: Determination of functional residual capacity, *Respir Care* 34(7):586, 1989.

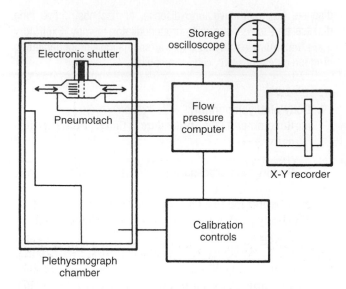

Storage oscilloscope

Electronic shutter

Pneumotach

Flow pressure computer

X-Y recorder

Calibration controls

Plethysmograph chamber

Fig. 4-17 Schematic drawing of the layout of a body plethysmograph with its components. The patient sits within the sealed plethysmograph chamber for the tests. (From Ruppel G: *Manual of pulmonary function testing*, ed 6, St Louis, 1994, Mosby.)

b. Perform the procedure (Code: IC1a) [Difficulty: An]

It is not possible to go into a complete discussion of the procedure; however, the following steps are important. The unit must be sealed so that it is airtight during the patient's breathing. The patient is instructed to breathe a normal tidal volume through the pneumotachometer. At the end of exhalation (FRC), a shutter is closed on the pneumotachometer so that no air leaks. The patient is instructed to continue to make tidal volume breathing efforts. The computer integrates the following two pressure changes: (1) a drop in mouth pressure as the patient attempts to inhale, and (2) an increase in plethysmograph chamber pressure as the patient's chest expands. The patient's TGV is then determined at functional residual capacity. Fig. 4-18, *A*, shows a normal TGV loop on the oscilloscope. Through spirometry the patient's expiratory reserve volume, residual volume, and total lung capacity can be calculated.

c. Interpret the results (Code: IC2a) [Difficulty: An]

The interpretation of the TGV and TLC results from a body plethysmograph are about the same as the interpretation of the FRC and TLC results from the helium dilution or nitrogen washout methods. (Review these earlier discussions if needed.) The only difference would be if the TGV were significantly larger than the FRC. This would indicate that the patient has trapped gas that was measured only in the plethysmograph. The TGV is commonly larger than the FRC measured by the preceding two methods when the patient has chronic obstructive pulmonary disease (COPD). This is because it includes *all* the gas

found in the thorax. That gas may be found in normal alveoli connected by a patent airway to the atmosphere, but it may also include gas trapped in emphysematous blebs and bullae, pneumothorax, pneumomediastinum, and so forth.

2. Lung compliance

a. Recommend the procedure (Code: IA2f) [Difficulty: An]

Lung compliance (C_L) is the volume change per unit of pressure change in the lungs. It is recorded in liters or milliliters per centimeter of water pressure (L[mL]/cm H_2O). A lung compliance test is indicated in a patient with a known or suspected condition that caused the lungs to be either overly compliant (such as emphysema) or noncompliant (such as pulmonary fibrosis).

b. Perform the procedure (Code: IIIA1e) [Difficulty: An]

The patient must swallow a 10-cm long balloon to the midthoracic level. A catheter connects the proximal end of the balloon to a pressure transducer outside of the patient. Air is injected into the balloon and the transducer is calibrated to accurately measure changes in intrathoracic pressure as the patient breathes. The patient is then placed into a body plethysmograph that is sealed. He or she is told to breathe through the differential pressure pneumotachometer to measure lung volumes. The patient is then instructed to slowly inhale from the resting level (FRC) to total lung capacity. As this is done, the pneumotachometer shutter is periodically closed to measure the intrathoracic pressure drop at the increasing volumes (see Fig. 4-19). As the patient slowly exhales from TLC, the shutter is again periodically closed to measure the increasing intrathoracic pressure as the patient returns to FRC volume. Lung compliance is usually calculated from the pressure and volume points of FRC and FRC + 500 mL (for a tidal volume).

c. Interpret the results (Code: IB10d, IC2i) [Difficulty: An]

Normal lung compliance (C_L) in an adult is 0.2 L/cm water. Through other methods, the normal adult's thoracic compliance (C_T) has been determined to also be .2 L/cm water. However, because the lungs tend to collapse smaller and the thorax cage tends to expand out, the two opposing forces offset each other somewhat. Because of this, the lung-thoracic compliance (C_{LT}) is calculated as 0.1 L (or 100 mL)/cm water.

A number of diseases and conditions can affect lung, thoracic, and lung-thoracic compliance. Patients with emphysema are known to have a higher-than-normal lung compliance. Their lungs are overly distended. Decreased lung compliance is seen in pulmonary fibrosis (from sarcoidosis, silicosis, or asbestosis), lung tumor, pulmonary edema, atelectasis, pneumonia, or decreased surfactant. Decreased thoracic compliance is seen in patients with

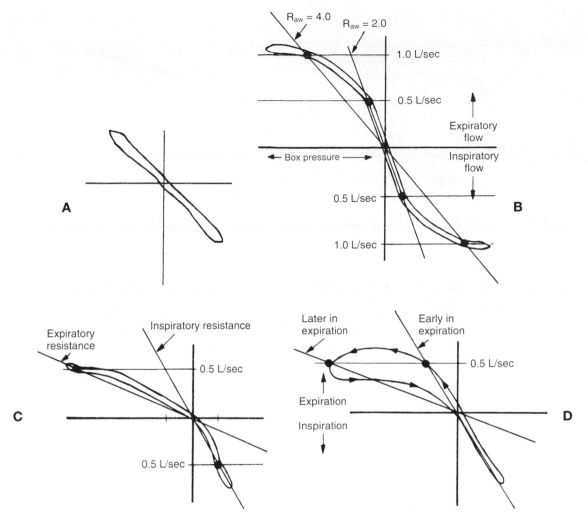

Fig. 4-18 Examples of body plethysmography tracings. Tracing **A** shows a normal thoracic gas volume loop. Tracing **B** shows a normal inspiratory and expiratory loop for airway resistance (Raw). Note that it is symmetrical. This patient has a Raw of 2 cm H_2O/L/sec at the standard flow of 0.5 L/sec. As the flow increases, the Raw increases as a result of the increased turbulence. So, the Raw of 4 cm H_2O/L/sec seen at the flow of 1 L/sec should not be recorded as the patient's value. Tracing **C** shows a patient who has an expiratory resistance that is greater than inspiratory resistance. In this case, either both resistances should be recorded in the chart or just the expiratory resistance if only one can be recorded. Tracing **D** shows a significant difference between early and late expiratory resistance. This is commonly seen in patients with obstructive airways disease such as emphysema. Record the late resistance because it better represents the patient's disease condition. (From Zarins LP, Clausen JL: Body plethysmography. In Clausen JL, editor: *Pulmonary function testing guidelines and controversies,* Orlando, 1984, Grune & Stratton.)

kyphoscoliosis, pectus excavatum, obesity, enlarged liver, or advanced pregnancy. All these conditions result in small, stiff lungs.

3. Airway resistance

a. Recommend the procedure (Code: IA2d and IA2f) [Difficulty: An]

Airway resistance (Raw) is the difference in pressure between the alveoli and the mouth that develops as air flows into and out of the lungs. It is recorded in centimeters of water pressure per liter of gas moved per second (cm water/L/sec). The test is performed on patients with a known or suspected condition of increased airway resistance. These include asthma, emphysema, and chronic bronchitis (COPD). The test confirms the patient's condition. Then it is used to help determine the proper dose of bronchodilator medications to help manage the problem.

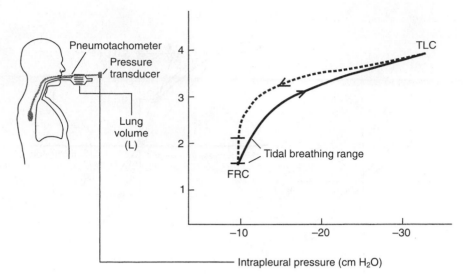

Fig. 4-19 Measurement of lung compliance (C_L) with the esophageal balloon technique. A balloon is swallowed to the midthoracic level, filled with air, and connected to a pressure transducer to measure intrapleural pressure. The patient sits within a body plethysmograph to measure inspiratory and expiratory volumes. (From Ruppel G: *Manual of pulmonary function testing,* ed 6, St Louis, 1994, Mosby.)

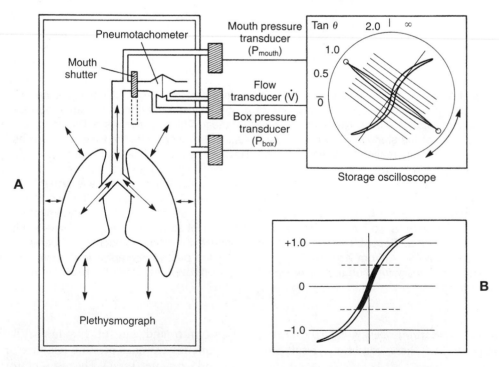

Fig. 4-20 Measurement of airway resistance (Raw). **A,** This represents the body plethysmograph that the patient sits within during the test. Tidal volume panting against an open and then closed pneumotachometer shutter is displayed on the storage oscilloscope. **B,** This represents a printout of the pressure changes as the patient pants a tidal volume of 500 mL/sec. (From Ruppel G: *Manual of pulmonary function testing,* ed 6, St Louis, 1994, Mosby.)

b. Perform the procedure (Code: IC1a and IIIA1e) [Difficulty: An]

The patient is placed into a plethysmograph that is sealed. He or she is instructed to breathe through a differential pressure pneumotachometer. With the pneumotachometer shutter open, the patient is told to pant several tidal volumes of about 500 mL at a rate of 1 breath per second. Data on flow rate, tidal volume, mouth pressure changes, and chamber pressure changes are recorded and graphed (see Fig. 4-20). Then the shutter is closed at the patient's resting FRC volume. The patient is told to continue panting at the same volume and rate. Again, flow rate, tidal volume, mouth pressure changes, and chamber pressures are recorded and graphed. The computer integrates the data to calculate the patient's airway resistance during tidal volume breathing.

c. Interpret the results (Code: IC2a) [Difficulty: An]

Airway resistance is the pressure difference developed per unit of flow. This pressure is required to overcome the friction of moving the tidal volume through the airways to the lungs. It can be thought of as the ratio of alveolar pressure to airflow. It is calculated by this formula:

$$Raw = \frac{\text{atmospheric pressure} - \text{alveolar pressure}}{\text{flow}}$$

Ruppel (1994) reports the normal adult's airway resistance to range from 0.6 to 2.4 cm H_2O/L/sec. The standard inspiratory and expiratory flow rate during the test is .5 L/sec (500 mL/sec). This is to standardize air turbulence during the test. The usual components of airway resistance found in an adult are as follows:

1. Upper airway including the nose and mouth = 50%
2. Trachea and bronchi larger than 2 mm in diameter = 30%
3. Airways less than 2 mm in diameter = 20%

Increased airway resistance is abnormal. It is most readily noticed if the problem is in the upper airway, trachea, or major bronchi because most resistance is normally found there. Patients with asthma, bronchitis, and emphysema have most of their resistance in the airways that are 2 mm or less in diameter. Because of this, significant disease must be present before a large enough airway resistance is noticed to alert the therapist or physician to the problem. Fig. 4-18, *B, C,* and *D,* show normal and increased expiratory resistance curves. Madama (1993) lists the following airway resistance values and their severity:

Raw (cm H_2O/L/sec)	Severity
2.8-4.5	mild
4.5-8	moderate
>8	severe

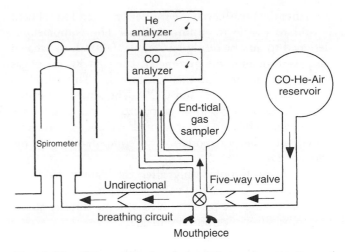

Fig. 4-21 Schematic drawing of the components and breathing circuit used when performing a single breath lung diffusion test ($D_{L\ CO}$SB). Analysis of the patient's exhaled helium (He) and carbon monoxide (CO) percentages is critical to the test. (From Ruppel G: *Manual of pulmonary function testing,* ed 6, St Louis, 1994, Mosby.)

4. Diffusing capacity

a. Recommend the procedure (Code: IA2d) [Difficulty: An]

The diffusing capacity (D_L or $D_{L\ CO}$) tests look at the capacity for carbon monoxide to diffuse through the lungs into the blood. Carbon monoxide is used because its high affinity for hemoglobin virtually eliminates blood as a barrier to diffusion. The measured value can then be correlated to the ability of oxygen to diffuse through the lungs. This test is indicated when it is important to know the extent of lung disability causing hypoxemia. This is most common with patients having emphysema, but it is also important in patients with fibrotic lung disease.

b. Perform the procedure (Code: IC1a) [Difficulty: An]

At the time of this writing, the single-breath carbon monoxide diffusing capacity test ($D_{L\ CO}$ SB) is the only version that has a widely adopted standard technique for administration. It is recorded in milliliters of carbon monoxide (CO) per minute per millimeter of mercury at 0 degrees C, 760 mm Hg, and dry standard temperature and pressure (STPD).

The following are key steps in the procedure. A reservoir or spirometer is filled with a mix of .3% CO, 10% He, 21% O_2, and the balance of N_2 (see Fig. 4-21). The patient is connected to the apparatus and breathes room air while being instructed in the test. After the patient is told to exhale completely (to residual volume), the practitioner switches the patient to the gas mix. The patient is instructed to inhale rapidly an inspiratory vital capacity. A shutter automatically closes so that the patient cannot exhale for 10 seconds. This allows time for some of the carbon monoxide to diffuse into the patient's bloodstream.

After the breath hold the shutter opens and the patient is told to exhale to resting volume. The equipment is designed to automatically let 750 to 1000 mL of exhaled gas pass through to the spirometer. The next 500 mL of gas is diverted into the end-tidal gas sampler. This sample is then analyzed for He% and CO%. The remainder of the patient's exhaled volume is passed through into the spirometer. The various measured parameters are integrated into the equations in the computer to give the patient's $D_{L\,CO}$ SB value.

This test is done only after the patient has been measured for both residual volume and total lung capacity. That is because the patient's lung volume directly affects the diffusibility of carbon monoxide.

c. Interpret the results (Code: IC2a) [Difficulty: An]

Interpretation is limited to the results of the $D_{L\,CO}$ SB test. Ruppel (1994) reports the average resting normal adult $D_{L\,CO}$ SB as 25 mL CO/min/mm Hg STPD. (All diffusing capacity values are reported in standard temperature, pressure, dry, conditions.) Gaensler and Wright (1966)

report the following $D_{L\,CO}$ SB prediction equations with values in mL CO/min/mm Hg STPD:

$$\text{Males: } [(0.250 \times \text{height in inches}) - (0.177 \times \text{age in years})] + 19.93$$

$$\text{Females: } [(0.284 \times \text{height in inches}) - (0.177 \times \text{age in years})] + 7.72$$

It should be noted that a number of other authors have developed their own prediction equations. In general, patients who show $D_{L\,CO}$ SB results within ± 20% of the predicted values (80% to 120% of predicted) are considered to be within normal limits. A patient who has actual results that are significantly below the predicted values has a problem with lung diffusion. Fig. 4-22 shows a number of common conditions that can lead to poor lung diffusion. The following factors should also be taken into consideration when interpreting the measured values:

1. Increased hematocrit and hemoglobin values result in an increased $D_{L\,CO}$ whereas decreased values result in a decreased $D_{L\,CO}$. An actual value should be used to calculate a patient's $D_{L\,CO}$.

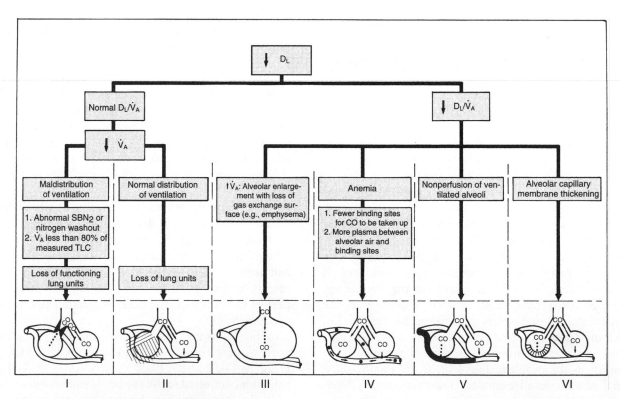

Fig. 4-22 Six factors that can cause decreased lung diffusion. Factors I and II result in a decrease in D_L that is in proportion to the decrease in alveolar volume. Factors III, IV, V, and VI result in a decrease in D_L that is greater than the decrease in alveolar volume. Therefore these later conditions are more harmful to the patient's pulmonary function and well-being. *SBN₂,* Single breath nitrogen washout; *TLC,* total lung capacity; V_A, alveolar ventilation. (From Ayers LN, Whipp BJ, Ziment I: *A guide to the interpretation of pulmonary function tests,* ed 2, New York, 1978, Roerig.)

2. An increased carboxyhemoglobin level results in a decreased $D_{L_{CO}}$ value. Patients who smoke should be instructed not to smoke the night before the test so that the COHb level will drop to normal.

3. An increased alveolar carbon dioxide level results in a lowered alveolar oxygen level. This, in turn, results in an increased $D_{L_{CO}}$ value. A decreased alveolar carbon dioxide level results in a decreased $D_{L_{CO}}$ value.

4. Increased altitude results in an increased $D_{L_{CO}}$. This is probably a concern only if the patient is tested in a mountainous area.

5. An increased pulmonary capillary blood volume results in an increased $D_{L_{CO}}$.

6. The patient should breathe room air for at least 4 minutes before the test is repeated.

It is well known that diffusibility is directly related to lung volume. This is the reason that blacks have lower diffusion rates than whites. To eliminate this as a factor in interpreting the D_L value, it is necessary to divide the diffusion value by the total lung capacity. Blacks have the same normal values as whites when this calculation is performed.

| MODULE G | Pulmonary Function Equipment |

EXAM HINT

Most examinations include one question that deals with either calibrating a piece of pulmonary function equipment or troubleshooting and fixing a problem with equipment.

1. **Water, mercury, and aneroid-type manometers (pressure gauges)**
   a. **Get the necessary equipment for the procedure (Code: IIA1n1) [Difficulty: An]**

   Mercury or water-type manometers have a vertical column of the liquid, as in a sphygmomanometer, for measuring blood pressure. An aneroid (spring-loaded) unit is most commonly used. This is because it does not have to be kept upright to measure accurately. Aneroid manometers can be calibrated in either mm of mercury (mm Hg) or cm of water (cm H_2O) pressure and look like a Bourdon gauge.

   b. **Put the equipment together, make sure that it works properly, and identify any problems with it (Code: IIB1n1) [Difficulty: An]**

   These pressure gauges come preassembled by the manufacturer. It is necessary to attach the pressure source only to the inlet port on the unit to measure a pressure change. This connection must be airtight or a leak will occur and the measured pressure will be less than actually exists. Accuracy of the unit can be checked by opening

the inlet port to room air and reading the pressure. A reading of zero should be seen (indicating no pressure change from atmospheric). Next, a known pressure is applied to the gauge. Often this is done by attaching it to a sphygmomanometer and pumping up the pressure to a known level such as 50 mm Hg. The pressure gauge should show the same.

   c. **Fix any problems with the equipment (Code: IIB2n1) [Difficulty: An]**

   If, during the calibration procedure, the set pressure does not match the pressure in the gauge, there may be a leak in the system or the pressure gauge is miscalibrated. Tighten all connections and attempt to calibrate again. Do not use a pressure gauge that cannot be calibrated.

2. **Inspiratory and/or expiratory force meters (pressure gauges)**
   a. **Get the necessary equipment for the procedure (Code: IIA1n1) [Difficulty: An]**

   The maximum inspiratory pressure and maximum expiratory pressure tests are usually recorded in centimeters of water pressure. However, millimeters of mercury can be used. If a centimeters of water pressure gauge is used, it should be able to record a negative and positive pressure of at least 100 cm H_2O. However, a unit that can record $\pm$ 60 cm H_2O is probably be adequate.

   b. **Put the equipment together, make sure that it works properly, and identify any problems with it (Code: IIB1n1)[Difficulty: An]**

   There is no standard setup for these devices. See Fig. 4-2 for a possible assembly. The system can be sealed and pressure checked with a known force to make sure that the pressure manometer is accurate and all the connections are airtight.

   c. **Fix any problems with the equipment (Code: IIA2n1) [Difficulty: An]**

   If, during the calibration procedure, the set pressure does not match the pressure in the gauge, there may be a leak in the system or the pressure gauge is miscalibrated. Tighten all connections and attempt to calibrate again. Do not use a pressure gauge that cannot be calibrated. The one-way valves must function so that the patient can exhale or inhale only as needed for the test.

3. **Pressure transducer**
   a. **Get the necessary equipment for the procedure (Code: IIA1n2) [Difficulty: An]**

   Pressure transducers are used in the body plethysmograph for measuring mouth pressure and chamber pressure. They come with the unit and are supplied by the manufacturer. Another type of transducer is used with an esophageal balloon when performing a lung compliance measurement. Follow the balloon manufacturer's recommendations for the proper transducer.

> **b. Put the equipment together, make sure that it works properly, and identify any problems (Code: IIB1n2) [Difficulty: R, Ap, An]**
>
> **c. Fix any problems with the equipment (NBRC Code: IIB2n2) [Difficulty: R, Ap, An]**

Each type of pressure transducer should be assembled as described by the manufacturer. As seen in Fig. 4-23, the differential pressure transducer has small-bore tubing connecting it before and after a resistive element. These small tubes transmit the pressures before and after the resistance element to the transducer as gas flows through the large, main tube. Make sure that the tubing is properly connected to the main tube and transducer. If a tube were to disconnect, the transducer would give a reading of zero.

> **4. Pneumotachometer respirometers**
> **a. Get the necessary equipment for the procedure (Code: IIA1o) [Difficulty: An]**
>
> **b. Put the equipment together, make sure that it works properly, and identify any problems (Code: IIB1o) [Difficulty: An]**
>
> **c. Fix any problems with the equipment (Code: IIB2o) [Difficulty: An]**

All pneumotachometers convert one type of physical information or signal to another, for example, converting an <u>airflow</u> or pressure signal to an electrical signal. Two common types are discussed next. Either type should be acceptable for performing bedside spirometry. Make sure that the unit you select is capable of performing the ordered test. Be sure that you select a unit capable of printing out a hard copy of the patient's test results and spirometry tracings if they are required for the chart.

Differential-pressure (flow sensing) pneumotachometer. Some articles refer to a differential pressure pneumotachometer as a *Fleisch-type* device. These units have a resistive element (tubes or mesh screen) in the flow tube. The faster the flow of gas through the flow tube the greater the pressure difference there is before and after the resistance. Hoses connect the flow tubes before and after the resistive element to the differential pressure transducer. The transducer converts this pressure difference into an electrical signal. A microprocessor calculates the various patient values from this information (see Fig. 4-23).

Assembly requires the addition of the patient's mouthpiece to the inspiratory port so that there is no air leak. The expiratory port should be kept completely open so that the only obstruction to the patient's airflow is from the resistive element. A volume calibration check is performed by forcing a known amount of air from a super-syringe (certified-volume standard syringe) through the pneumotachometer. Minimally, several repetitions of a known 3-L volume should reveal identical measured volumes. As long as the measured volumes are within ± 3% or 50 mL (whichever is less) the unit is acceptably accurate.

Common problems with accuracy include an air leak

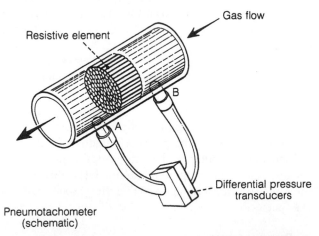

Fig. 4-23 Cutaway view of a differential pressure pneumotachometer. Flow is measured as the pressure drops between *A* and *B*, which are ports leading to a differential pressure transducer. The resistive element may consist of a mesh screen, a network of parallel capillary tubes, or other devices. (From Beauchamp RK: Pulmonary function testing procedures. In Barnes TA, editor: *Respiratory care practice*, St Louis, 1988, Mosby.)

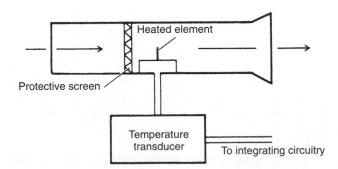

Fig. 4-24 Cutaway view of a heat-transfer pneumotachometer. (From Ruppel G: *Manual of pulmonary function testing*, ed 6, St Louis, 1994, Mosby.)

around the mouthpiece; cracked, disconnected, or obstructed pressure relaying hoses; water condensation or mucus on the resistive element; or obstructed upstream or downstream port. The resistive element is usually heated to minimize any condensation.

Heat-transfer pneumotachometer. Some articles refer to a heat-transfer pneumotachometer as a *thermistor-type device* or *hot wire anemometer.* These units have a heated thermistor that is cooled as the gas flows past it. The temperature transducer automatically increases and measures the flow of electricity to the thermistor to keep it at the required temperature. A microprocessor calculates the various patient values from this information. The earlier discussion on assembly, calibration, and troubleshooting applies to the heat-transfer-type pneumotachometers except that there are no pressure relaying hoses (see Fig. 4-24).

5. Volume displacement respirometers
a. Get the necessary equipment for the procedure (Code: IIA1o) [Difficulty: An]

b. Put the equipment together, make sure that it works properly, and identify any problems (Code: IIB1o) [Difficulty: An]

c. Fix any problems with the equipment (Code: IIB2o) [Difficulty: An]

Volume displacement (also called *positive displacement*) respirometers are mechanical devices. They are called *volume displacement respirometers* because the patient's exhaled gas fills and moves a sealed bell or accordian-like bellows. These systems are self-contained and sealed rather than being open to room air as the other devices. They can have residual volume and lung diffusion test hardware added on. There are three general categories that are discussed here: water-seal spirometers, dry rolling-seal spirometers, and wedge-type spirometers.

Water-seal spirometers. Water-seal spirometers are the commonly found chain-compensated and Stead-Wells units made by Collins Medical, Inc. (see Fig. 4-25 for the cutaway appearance of the chain-compensated type). The bell lowers and rises as the patient breathes in and out. A pulley system attached to the bell and the marking pens record the patient's efforts on the rotating kymograph paper. Note that the tracing is inverted from the patient's actual breathing effort. The Stead-Wells units have the marking pen attached directly to the bell; therefore the tracing directly shows the patient's breathing efforts (see Fig. 4-26). The newer chain-compensated and Stead-Wells units also have microprocessors for calculating patient information.

Gas analyzers for helium, nitrogen, carbon monoxide, and other extra equipment can be added for residual volume and lung diffusion measurements. The carbon dioxide absorber should be left out of the breathing circuit for forced vital capacity tests because it interferes with the fast flow of gas; however, it must be put in line for any testing that will last more than 15 seconds and involves

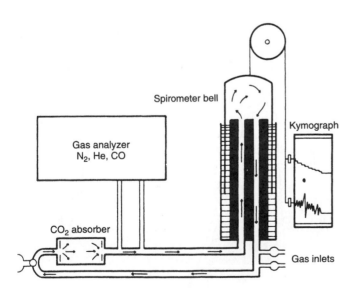

Fig. 4-25 Cutaway view of a chain-compensated water-seal spirometer. *CO,* Carbon monoxide; *CO₂,* carbon dioxide, *He,* helium; *N₂,* nitrogen. (From Ruppel G: *Manual of pulmonary function testing,* ed 6, St Louis, 1994, Mosby.)

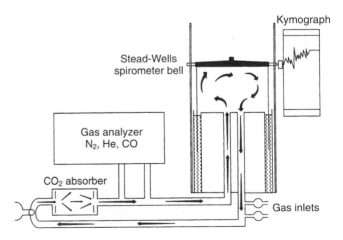

Fig. 4-26 Cutaway view of a Stead-Wells water-seal spirometer. *CO,* Carbon monoxide; *CO₂,* carbon dioxide, *He,* helium; *N₂,* nitrogen. (Courtesy Warren E. Collins, Inc, Braintree, Mass.)

breathing repeatedly into the closed system. Supplemental oxygen must be added to the circuit for any tests that require the patient to breathe repeatedly from the closed system. The following is a checklist for setup and where to look when problem solving:

1. Make sure the water level is correct (not too high or too low).
2. Use a 7-liter bell for children and a 14-liter bell for adults.
3. Make sure all circuit tubing and one-way valve connections are tight.
4. Check the following kymograph features: paper on correctly; pens contain ink; kymograph speeds are adjustable to 32, 160, and 1920 mm/sec.
5. The carbon dioxide absorber should be out of the circuit for FVC tests; it should be in the circuit for residual volume and lung diffusion tests.
6. Oxygen should be added to the system for residual volume and lung diffusion tests.
7. Make sure the various gas analyzers are calibrated properly.
8. As discussed earlier, do not be confused by the various ways the tracing is presented. Always find the start of the FVC by the near vertical slope of the tracing.

Dry rolling-seal spirometers. Dry rolling-seal spirometers are sometimes called *piston spirometers.* As can be seen in Fig. 4-27, these units use a flexible silastic or Teflon-coated rubber seal instead of water. The large-volume piston moves in and out as the patient breathes. The patient's efforts can be directly recorded by pen on paper. Newer units also have microprocessors for calculating the information.

They are still rather large and are best suited for the pulmonary function laboratory. These units can also be outfitted with a carbon dioxide absorber and various gas analyzers, So they too can be used for the full range of lung function tests. The previous checklist for setup and problem-solving ideas apply in this case except for those items that are specific to the chain-compensated and Stead-Wells systems.

Wedge-type spirometers. Wedge-type spirometers are sometimes called *bellows spirometers* (see Fig. 4-28). Note that these units have plastic or rubber bellows that are fixed on one side and are flexible like an accordion on other sides. The bellows move in and out as the patient breathes. The patient's efforts can be directly recorded by pen on paper. Newer units also have microprocessors for calculating the information.

All the earlier information on the dry rolling-seal spirometers applies here except what is specific to those units. The same setup and problem-solving ideas apply here also.

6. CO, He, O₂, and specialty gas analyzers

a. Get the necessary equipment for the procedure (Code: IIA1h5) [Difficulty: An]

These analyzers are needed for a variety of special-purpose tests as described earlier:

1. Carbon monoxide (CO) is analyzed in single-breath carbon monoxide diffusing capacity test.
2. Helium (He) is analyzed in the single-breath carbon monoxide diffusing capacity test and the helium dilution test to find FRC.
3. Oxygen (O₂) is analyzed in single-breath carbon monoxide diffusing capacity test and the helium dilution test to find FRC.
4. Nitrogen (N₂) is analyzed in the single-breath

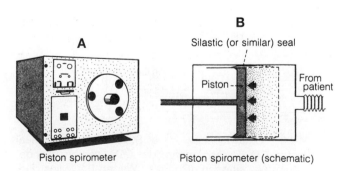

Piston spirometer   Piston spirometer (schematic)

Fig. 4-27 Outside **(A)** and cutaway **(B)** views of a dry rolling-seal or piston spirometer. (From Beauchamp RK: Pulmonary function testing procedures. In Barnes TA, editor: *Respiratory care practice,* St Louis, 1988, Mosby.)

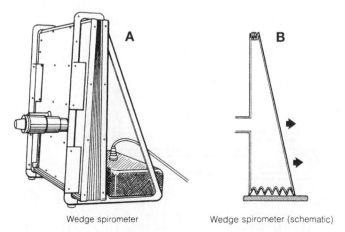

Wedge spirometer   Wedge spirometer (schematic)

Fig. 4-28 Outside **(A)** and cutaway **(B)** views of a wedge-type spirometer. (From Beauchamp RK: Pulmonary function testing procedures. In Barnes TA, editor: *Respiratory care practice,* St Louis, 1988, Mosby.)

nitrogen washout test and the nitrogen washout method of finding FRC.

b. Put the equipment together, make sure that it works properly, and identify any problems (Code: IIB1h5) [Difficulty: An]

Check the label on the tank to be sure it is the correct gas at the correct percentage. Review Table 6-1 for color codings for tanks, if needed. Each specialty gas has its own DISS reduction valve to connect to the tank. A high-pressure hose connects the reduction valve outlet to the pulmonary function testing machine inlet.

c. Fix any problems with the equipment (Code: IIB2h5) [Difficulty: An]

The problems that can occur with specialty gas cylinders, pressure reducing valves, and connecting high-pressure hoses are the same as can occur with oxygen cylinders. Review the discussion in Chapter 6 if needed.

7. Implement a quality improvement program (Code: IC3b) [Difficulty: An]

Every pulmonary function testing laboratory must have quality control/quality improvement program. Regular maintenance of equipment and calibration must be performed and documented.

a. Perform quality control procedures on pulmonary function equipment (Code: IIB3b) [Difficulty: An]

Spirometry equipment. The volume displacement respirometers should have the following quality control procedures performed on a regular basis:

a. A super-syringe with at least a 3-liter capacity should be pumped repeatedly into and out of the unit. A reading that is accurate to within ± 3% or ± 50 mL must be measured. The flow rates should be varied to ensure that they do not have any influence on the measured volumes. It is recommended that 1- and 2-liter volumes also be pumped into the unit to check for linearity.

b. To check for leaks in the circuit perform the following steps:
1. Pump a 3-L volume into the bellows.
2. Close the mouthpiece to atmosphere to seal the circuit.
3. Add a weight to the bell to speed up any small leaks.
4. Turn on the kymograph at a slow speed and put the pen on the paper to record any drop in volume.
5. If a leak is noted it must be discovered and sealed.

c. Turn on the kymograph to its various speeds and check its accuracy with a stopwatch. The manufacturer's literature should tell how far the kymograph will travel at its set speeds.

d. The thermometer reading should be compared with that of a laboratory quality unit.

Replace or repair any component that fails to meet the manufacturer's or established American Thoracic Society–American College of Chest Physicians (ATS–ACCP) standards.

Nitrogen washout equipment for measuring functional residual capacity. See Fig. 4-16 for the basic setup and breathing circuit of a nitrogen washout system. Review the troubleshooting of volume displacement and pneumotachometer spirometers; they are used with the nitrogen washout procedure to find the functional residual capacity. The nitrogen washout type residual volume test uses an emission spectroscopy ionization chamber analyzer for nitrogen. It is more commonly called a *Giesler tube ionizer.* It employs a vacuum pump to draw a gas sample into the ionization chamber. The intensity of the light spectrum given off by the ionized nitrogen directly relates to its percentage in the sample. A two-point calibration check should be performed at least every 6 months to check for linearity. It involves the following steps:

1. Draw a room air sample into the unit and check the nitrogen meter reading. It should read about 78% nitrogen.
2. Adjust the meter reading, if necessary, to the manufacturer's specified value.
3. Turn off the needle valve so that no air can be drawn into the unit.
4. Check to see that the nitrogen meter reading drops to 0% nitrogen as the vacuum pump removes all gas from the ionization chamber.

Linearity (three-point calibration) can be checked by introducing from 5% to 10% nitrogen into the unit to see if the nitrogen meter measures that value. Do not use an analyzer that is inaccurate.

Helium dilution equipment for measuring functional residual capacity. See Fig. 4-14 for the basic setup of the helium dilution equipment and breathing circuit. Again, review the troubleshooting of volume displacement and pneumotachometer spirometers; they are used with the helium dilution procedure to find the functional residual capacity. Both the helium dilution FRC test and the lung diffusion tests require the analysis of helium in the gas mixture. A thermal conductivity analyzer is typically used. It operates under the principal of a Wheatstone bridge, in which differences in gas density lead to different cooling rates of heated thermistor beads. The different rates of cooling change electrical resistances and cause different electrical currents to flow. In a helium analyzer, the greater the helium concentration, the faster the thermistor bead cools and the more electricity flows through the circuit. This is then read off a meter as the helium percentage.

The thermal conductivity helium analyzer should be linear over the clinically used range of helium to an accuracy of ± .2% He. Minimally, a two-point calibration should be performed. A room air sample can be drawn into the analyzer and should read 0% helium. A known helium concentration may then be added and analyzed, for example, heliox, which contains 80% helium and 20% oxygen. A third point can be checked if needed by analyzing another known helium percentage.

Body plethysmography. See Fig. 4-17 for the basic components of the system. The plethysmograph chamber must be airtight when the door and all vents are closed. This can be confirmed by attaching a pressure manometer to a chamber port and applying a known volume or pressure into the sealed chamber. The pressures should be identical between the chamber pressure gauges and outside pressure manometer. The differential-pressure pneumotachometer must also read accurately when a known volume is pumped through it. Most manufacturers have a series of calibration check procedures listed in the equipment literature.

MODULE H	Participate in the development of the patient's respiratory care plan [e.g., case management, development and application of protocols, disease management education] (Code: IC4) [Difficulty: An]

Even though a physician must legally determine the patient's diagnosis, a therapist must be able to understand the cause, pathophysiology, diagnosis, treatment, and prognosis for patients with cardiopulmonary disorders. Interpretation of patient data that is tested by the NBRC was discussed earlier. The following is a brief categorization of the conditions that may be diagnosed by pulmonary function testing.

Obstructive airways disease. The patient with severe obstructive lung disease shows low gas flow at all time intervals. However, a decreased FEV_3 and the $FEF_{25\%-75\%}$ are early markers of small airways disease. Quite commonly, the residual volume is increased as a result of air trapping. This increases the functional residual capacity and often the total lung capacity. Despite the increased lung volume, the patient's diffusing ability is decreased. Examples of conditions that cause obstructive lung disease include asthma, emphysema, bronchitis, and bronchiolitis. Excessive mucus, foreign bodies, and airway tumors also cause bronchospasm and air trapping.

EXAM HINT

Every past examination has had a least one question that deals with recommending tests for assessing a patient with airway obstruction or evaluating the results of pulmonary function tests on a patient with airway obstruction. This can include interpreting a table of data, a volume-time tracing, a flow-volume loop, or calculating the results of a before and after bronchodilator study.

Restrictive lung disease. In restrictive lung disease, all lung volumes and capacities are reduced and lung diffusion is reduced. Expiratory flows such as FEV_1 are increased. Examples of conditions that cause restrictive lung disease include fibrosis, pulmonary edema, hemothorax or pneumothorax, acute or infant respiratory distress syndrome, chest wall deformities, obesity, and various neuromuscular disorders.

EXAM HINT

Most examinations have tested the understanding and interpretation of data to determine whether a patient has obstructive or restrictive lung disease. This usually involves the assessment of patient data on a table.

Obviously the patient's care plan depends on the diagnosis and the degree of limitation of the patient. If the patient has reversible small airways disease, he or she should be counseled to stop smoking and avoid all airborne irritants. Inhaled and/or parenteral bronchodilators should be prescribed to relax the airways as much as possible. If the patient has restrictive lung disease, he or she should also be counseled to avoid any airborne irritants. Whether any medications or other procedures can be performed to offer some relief depends on the specific cause of the patient's disorder.

BIBLIOGRAPHY

AARC Clinical Practice Guideline: Spirometry, *Respir Care* 36(12):1414-1417, 1991.

AARC Clinical Practice Guideline: Single-breath carbon monoxide diffusing capacity, *Respir Care* 38(5):511-515, 1993.

AARC Clinical Practice Guideline: Single-breath carbon monoxide diffusing capacity, 1999 update, *Respir Care* 44(1):91-97, 1999.

AARC Clinical Practice Guideline: Static lung volumes, *Respir Care* 39(8):830-836, 1994.

AARC Clinical Practice Guideline: Infant/toddler pulmonary function tests, *Respir Care* 40(7):761-768, 1995.

AARC Clinical Practice Guideline: Bronchial provocation, *Respir Care* 37(8):902-906, 1992.

AARC Clinical Practice Guideline: Body plethysmography, *Respir Care* 39(12):1184-1190, 1994.

AARC Clinical Practice Guideline: Assessing response to bronchodilator therapy at point of care, *Respir Care* 40(12): 1300-1307, 1995.

American Thoracic Society: Standardization of spirometry: 1987 update, *Am Rev Respir Dis* 136:1285-1298, 1987.

Ayers LN, Whipp BJ, Ziment I: *A guide to the interpretation of pulmonary function tests,* ed 2, New York, 1978, Roerig.

Beauchamp RK: Pulmonary function testing procedures. In Barnes TA, editor: *Respiratory care practice,* St Louis, 1988, Mosby.

Black LF, Hyatt RE: Maximal respiratory pressures: normal values and relationship to age and sex, *Am Rev Respir Dis* 99:696-702, 1969.

Branson RD, Hurst JM, Davis K Jr et al.: Measurement of maximal inspiratory pressure: a comparison of three methods, *Respir Care* 34(9):789-794, 1989.

Buist SA, Ross BB: Predicted values for closing volumes using a modified single-breath nitrogen test, *Am Rev Respir Dis* 111:405, 1975.

Cherniack RM: *Pulmonary function testing,* ed 2, Philadelphia, 1992, WB Saunders.

Cherniack RM, Raber MD: Normal standards for ventilatory function using an automated wedge spirometer, *Am Rev Respir Dis* 106:38, 1972.

Clausen JL, editor: *Pulmonary function testing guidelines and controversies,* Orlando, 1984, Grune & Stratton.

Clausen JL: Clinical interpretation of pulmonary function test, *Respir Care* 34(7):638-650, 1989.

Crapo RO: Reference values for lung function tests, *Respir Care* 34(7):626-637, 1989.

Gaensler EA, Wright GW: Evaluation of respiratory impairment, *Arch Environ Health,* 12:146, 1966.

Gardner RM: Pulmonary function laboratory standards, *Respir Care* 34(7):651-660, July 1989.

Goldman HI, Becklake MR: Respiratory function tests: normal values at median altitudes and the prediction of normal results, *Am Rev Tuberculosis* 79:457, 1959.

Hess D: Measurement of maximal inspiratory pressure: a call for standardization, *Respir Care* 34:857-859, 1989.

Kacmarek RM, Cycyk-Chapman MC, Young-Palazzo PJ et al.: Determination of maximal inspiratory pressure: a clinical study and literature review, *Respir Care* 34:868-878, 1989.

Knudson RJ, Lebowitz MD, Holberg CJ et al.: Changes in the normal maximal expiratory flow- volume curve with growth and aging, *Am Rev Respir Dis* 127:725-734, 1983.

Knudson RJ, Kaltenborn WT, Knudson DE, et al: The single-breath carbon monoxide diffusing capacity, *Am Rev Respir Dis* 135:805-811, 1987.

Kory RC, Callahan R, Syner JC: The Veterans Administration-Army cooperative study of pulmonary function I. Clinical spirometry in normal men, *Am J Med* 30:243, 1961

MacIntyre NR: Diffusing capacity of the lung for carbon monoxide, *Respir Care* 34(6):489-499, 1989.

Madama VC: *Pulmonary function testing and cardiopulmonary stress testing,* ed 2, Albany, NY, 1998, Delmar.

Morris JF, Koski A, Johnson LC: Spirometric standards for healthy nonsmoking adults, *Am Rev Respir Dis* 103:57, 1971.

Paoletti P, Viegi G, Pistelli G et al.: Reference equations for the single-breath diffusing capacity, *Am Rev Respir Dis* 132: 806-813, 1985.

Practical guide for the diagnosis and management of asthma, National Institutes of Health, No. 97-4053, October, 1997.

Ruppel G: *Manual of pulmonary function testing,* ed 6, St Louis, 1994, Mosby.

Single breath carbon monoxide diffusing capacity (transfer factor): recommendations for a standard technique, *Am Rev Respir Dis* 136:1299-1307, 1987.

Snow MG: Determination of functional residual capacity, *Respir Care* 34(7):586-596, 1989.

Sue D: Exercise testing and the patient with cardiopulmonary disease. In Goldman AL, editor: *Problems in Pulmonary Disease* 2(1):1-7, Spring 1986.

Wanger J: *Pulmonary Function Testing,* ed 2, Baltimore, 1996, Williams & Wilkins.

Zamel N, Altose MD, Spcir WA: Statement on spirometry, *Chest* 3:547-550, 1983.

SELF-STUDY QUESTIONS

1. After performing complete spirometry on a 50-year-old patient, the following data are found:

	Predicted	Actual	% Predicted
TLC (St L)	5.9	8.1	137
RV (l)	1.1	1.8	164
FVC (l)	5.0	2.6	52
$FEF_{25\%-75\%}$ (L/sec)	4.2	1.5	36
FEV_1/FVC	75%	20%	27

How should the data be interpreted?
   A. Mild restrictive lung disease
   B. Severe restrictive lung disease
   C. Mild obstructive lung disease
   D. Severe obstructive lung disease

2. A nitrogen washout test for residual volume has been performed on a patient for 7 minutes and has not reached the desired nitrogen percentage. What could explain this situation?
   A. There is an oxygen leak into the system.
   B. The patient has an abnormally high respiratory exchange ratio.
   C. The patient has severe air trapping.
   D. Nitrogen has been absorbed into the patient's tissues.

3. An order is received to perform the following bedside spirometry tests on a patient: tidal volume, FVC, and peak flow. Which device would you take with you to perform the tests?
   A. Stead-Wells water-seal spirometer
   B. Maximum inspiratory pressure manometer
   C. Differential pressure pneumotachometer
   D. Body plethysmograph

4. Which section of the following spirometry tracing represents the inspiratory reserve volume?

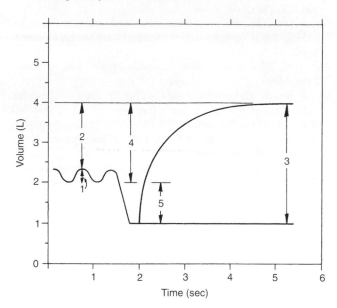

Time (sec)

A. 2
B. 3
C. 4
D. 5

5. Which section of the spirometry tracing in question 4 represents the functional residual capacity?
A. 1
B. 2
C. 3
D. 4

6. After performing spirometry, it is important that patient flow rates be reported at:
A. ATPS.
B. BTPS.
C. STPD.
D. ATPD.

7. Your patient is performing a residual volume test on a water-seal spirometer in the pulmonary function laboratory. After breathing on the system for 1 minute, he takes out the mouthpiece and complains of being short of breath. What is the most likely problem in the pulmonary function system?
A. The carbon dioxide absorber was accidentally left in the circuit.
B. There is too much water around the spirometer bell.
C. The carbon dioxide absorber has been left out of the circuit.
D. Nose clips were left off of the patient.

8. Which of the following studies produce the most accurate determination of the TLC in a patient with severe emphysema?
A. Single-breath nitrogen washout test
B. Seven-minute nitrogen washout test
C. Helium dilution test
D. Body plethysmography test

9. In which type of patient is a carbon dioxide response curve test indicated?
A. History of COPD

B. History of asthma attacks
C. History of ARDS
D. History of asbestos exposure

10. Before having a patient perform a forced vital capacity test, the water-sealed spirometer should have all the following done *except*:
A. Make sure that the circuit is airtight.
B. Place a carbon dioxide absorbing material in line with the circuit.
C. Pump a 3 L volume into and out of the circuit to check for leaks.
D. Check the kymograph speeds.

11. A properly performed FVC test will not have:
I. Any coughing or leaks
II. A weak patient effort
III. An unsatisfactory start to the test
IV. Excessive variability among test results
A. I, II
B. II, III
C. I, II, IV
D. I, II, III, IV

12. A patient has a suspected diagnosis of asthma. Which of the following tests would be the *least* helpful in assessing the patient for this condition?
A. Before and after bronchodilator study
B. Flow-volume loop
C. Diffusion study
D. Bronchoprovocation

13. A patient with a history of COPD has been admitted. To help clarify her diagnosis between emphysema and asthma, which of the following should the respiratory therapist recommend?
A. Flow-volume loop
B. Maximum voluntary ventilation
C. Spirometry before and after an inhaled bronchodilator
D. Peak flow test

14. Based on the flow-volume loops that are shown in the following figure, which one represents the most severe small airways obstruction?

A 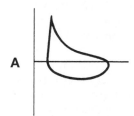   B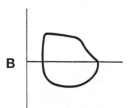

C 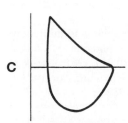   D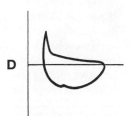

A. Tracing A
B. Tracing B
C. Tracing C
D. Tracing D

15. Based on the flow-volume loops that are shown in question 14, which one represents the fixed extrathoracic obstruction?
    A. Tracing A
    B. Tracing B
    C. Tracing C
    D. Tracing D

16. Based on the flow-volume loops that are shown in question 14, tracing **A** represents a patient with asthmatic bronchitis, and tracing **C** represents the same patient 1 hour after receiving an inhaled bronchodilator medication. What conclusion can be reached?
    A. The patient's condition is treatable.
    B. The patient is not giving his best effort.
    C. The patient's condition has worsened.
    D. The patient needs another bronchodilator treatment.

Answer Key

1. **D.** Rationale: All of the data on the table indicates severe obstructive lung disease. The TLC and RV are both greater than 120% of predicted indicating significant air trapping. All three flow measurements are far lower than predicted. If the patient had restrictive lung disease, the TLC and RV values would be smaller than predicted.

2. **C.** Rationale: Patients with severe air trapping, as found with emphysema, take much longer than normal to "wash" the nitrogen out of their lungs. Often the test needs to be prolonged for several minutes past the usual 7-minute duration to eliminate enough nitrogen to complete the test. The nitrogen washout test requires the patient breathe in 100% oxygen to displace the resident nitrogen found in the lungs. The respiratory exchange ratio has to do with oxygen consumption and carbon dioxide production; it has nothing to do with nitrogen elimination. Nitrogen is not active in metabolism. The normal amount of nitrogen found in the body is not significantly affected by the nitrogen washout test.

3. **C.** Rationale: A differential-pressure pneumotachometer is portable enough to be taken to a patient's bedside. It can be used to determine a patient's tidal volume, FVC, and peak flow. A Stead-Wells water-seal spirometer is not typically moved because it is large and the water will be splashed about while moving it. The device can be used for all three listed tests when done in the pulmonary function laboratory. A maximum inspiratory pressure manometer is used for the maximum inspiratory pressure (MIP) test. It may be reconfigured for a maximum expiratory test (MEP), but cannot measure any gas flows. A body plethysmograph is far too large to move to a patient's bedside. However, it can be used for all three listed tests when done in the pulmonary function laboratory.

4. **D.** Rationale: The inspiratory reserve volume (IRV) is found from the end of a tidal volume inspiration to the total lung capacity. It represents the additional volume that can be inhaled after a normal tidal volume. Review Fig. 4-15 if needed. Do not be confused by vital capacity efforts that look "upside down" compared with others. Review the various volume-time curve tracings in the chapter for extra practice determining volumes. Volume number 2 is the FRC. Volume number 3 is the vital capacity. Volume number 4 is the FRC and tidal volume combined. Volume number 1 is the tidal volume.

5. **B.** Rationale: The functional residual capacity (FRC) represents the volume of air found in the lungs after a normal tidal volume is exhaled. The FRC includes the expiratory reserve volume and residual volume. Review Fig. 4-15 if needed. Do not be confused by vital capacity efforts that look "upside down" compared with others. Review the various volume-time curve tracings in the chapter for extra practice determining volumes. Volume number 1 is the tidal volume. Volume number 3 is the vital capacity. Volume number 4 is the FRC and tidal volume combined.

6. **B.** Rationale: All patient flows, volumes, and capacities must be mathematically converted from ATPS (atmospheric temperature, pressure, saturated) to BTPS (body temperature, pressure, saturated) conditions. This results in the exhaled flows or volumes measured at room temperature being adjusted for the expansion of gas found at the patient's body temperature. STPD (standard temperature, pressure, dry) conditions are used only with diffusing capacity tests. ATPS (atmospheric temperature, pressure, dry) is not used for reporting any pulmonary function results.

7. **C.** Rationale: It is necessary to place a carbon dioxide absorber in the PFT system when the patient has to breathe on a closed system for an extended period. Without one, the patient will rebreathe his or her own exhaled carbon dioxide. If there is too much water around the spirometer bell there may be some splashing. However, too much water will not cause the patient to feel short of breath. If nose clips were left off the patient he or she may breathe through the nose instead of the mouth. This will not cause a feeling of shortness of breath.

8. **D.** Rationale: A body plethysmography test for total lung capacity (TLC) will be the most accurate for a patient with severe emphysema because it can measure the volume of *all* gas within the chest. This includes gas in damaged parts of the lungs that do not ultimately connect to larger airways and the outside atmosphere. The 7-minute nitrogen washout test and helium dilution test measure only the gas in areas of the lungs that connect to the larger airways and outside atmosphere. This may result in an undermeasurement of the patient's true lung volumes. The single-breath nitrogen washout test is not used to measure the TLC. It is used to assess the evenness of inspiratory and expiratory gas flow.

9. **A.** Rationale: A patient with a history of COPD can have a carbon dioxide response curve test performed to determine if his or her central chemoreceptors are responding normally to the stimulation of carbon dioxide. Some COPD patients do not increase their breathing as much as expected when exposed to higher than normal levels of carbon dioxide. Patients with a history of asthma, acute respiratory distress syndrome (ARDS), and asbestos exposure do not have their central chemoreceptors affected adversely.

10. **B.** Rationale: Because the FVC test lasts for only a few seconds the patient will not rebreathe significant amounts of carbon dioxide. Therefore a carbon dioxide absorber is not needed. In addition, in some pulmonary function systems, a carbon dioxide absorber slows down the flow of exhaled gas and results in lower reported FVC values than are actually present. The PFT circuit

must be airtight to prevent any leakage and resulting lower volumes and flows. Volume calibration is done by pumping a known volume (3 liters) into and out of the spirometer. Any leak will result in a lower-than-expected volume being found. The kymograph should have its speed settings checked to make sure that the timing of the test is accurate.

11. **D.** Rationale: All listed items must be avoided to ensure an accurate FVC test. Coughing causes variable flows and cuts off the full FVC volume. A leak results in a loss of volume. A weak patient effort results in a slower expiratory flow than the patient can optimally provide. When tests are done properly, they show consistent results. Excessive variability shows inconsistent patient effort.

12. **C.** Rationale: A diffusion study measures carbon monoxide diffusion to evaluate oxygen diffusion across the alveolar-capillary membrane. It is not helpful in the diagnosis of asthma. The other three listed tests can be very useful in diagnosing asthma. With a before and after bronchodilator study, an asthmatic who is responsive to inhaled bronchodilator medications shows improved flows after inhaling the medication. A patient with an asthma problem often reveals a distinctive flow-volume loop tracing. See Fig.4-11. A bronchoprovocation test often produces decreased expiratory flows in a patient with asthma.

13. **C.** Rationale: Spirometry before and after an inhaled bronchodilator is the best test to differentiate between asthma and emphysema. Most asthmatic patients have some reversibility to their bronchospasm. Their spirometry should show improved expiratory flows after inhaling a bronchodilating medication. Patients with emphysema have very little if any improvement in expiratory flows after inhaling a bronchodilating medication. This is because it is the alveoli and not the airways that are damaged. The other three listed tests may not show significant differences between patients with asthma or emphysema.

14. **D.** Rationale: Tracing **D** shows a severe "scoop" during the expiratory part of the patient effort after the peak flow. This dramatic drop in expiratory flow is characteristic of severe small airways obstruction. Tracing **A** shows a less-severe drop in expiratory flow after the peak flow. Tracing **B** shows a severely reduced peak flow that is characteristic of a fixed extrathoracic obstruction. Tracing **C** shows a normal flow-volume loop. Review Fig. 4-11 if needed for a comparison of different flow-volume loops.

15. **B.** Rationale: Tracing B shows a severely reduced peak flow that is characteristic of a fixed extrathoracic obstruction. This might be caused by a laryngeal tumor, paralyzed vocal cord, or other upper airway problem. Tracing **D** shows a severe "scoop" during the expiratory part of the patient effort after the peak flow. This dramatic drop in expiratory flow is characteristic of severe small airways obstruction. Tracing **A** shows a less severe drop in expiratory flow after the peak flow. Tracing **C** shows a normal flow-volume loop. Review Fig. 4-11 if needed for a comparison of different flow-volume loops.

16. **A.** Rationale: Tracing **C** shows an increased peak flow compared with tracing **A** and correction of the expiratory "scoop" seen in tracing **A**. In addition, the inspiratory flow on tracing **C** is greater than that on tracing **A**. All of these changes show significant improvement indicating that the patient's condition is treatable. The patient's effort or lack of effort cannot be determined by looking at the two tracings. Tracing **C** is normal and does not justify the patient receiving another bronchodilator treatment.

5 Advanced Cardiopulmonary Monitoring

A review of the most recent Written Registry Examinations has shown an average of 13 questions (13% of the exam) on advanced cardiopulmonary monitoring.

MODULE A   Cardiopulmonary monitoring procedures

1. Capnography (exhaled CO_2 monitoring)

a. Review capnography data in the patient's chart (Code: IA1f5) [Difficulty: An]

Capnography is the analysis of graphic and numerical data showing the pattern and amount of exhaled carbon dioxide (CO_2). It is wise to look for previous capnography data before measuring the patient's exhaled CO_2 level again. Look for numerical values as well as a printout of the tracing of exhaled CO_2. Be prepared to compare the previous information with the new data to help evaluate the patient's condition. It is also useful to compare the patient's pressure of CO_2 in arterial blood ($PaCO_2$) with the capnography information, even though they should not be expected to be the same.

b. Perform the bedside procedure (Code: IB9a and IIIA1b) [Difficulty: An]

The capnometer is a device that measures the concentration of CO_2 in a gas sample from a patient. The principle of operation of most bedside units is based on carbon dioxide's absorption of infrared light in a narrow wavelength band (4.3 μ). Infrared light at this wavelength is passed through the gas sample to a receiving unit. The difference between what is sent out and what is received is directly related to how much carbon dioxide is in the gas sample. In other words, the greater the difference between the sent and the received infrared light, the greater the concentration of carbon dioxide in the gas sample.

The capnometer is calibrated by comparing a gas sample without carbon dioxide (possibly room air) with a second gas sample containing a known amount of carbon dioxide. The first gas sample without CO_2 should give a "zero" reading. Adjust the calibration control to zero if needed. The second sample usually contains 5% to 10% carbon dioxide. The capnometer should read out a CO_2 level that matches the amount in the known gas sample. Adjust the calibration control as necessary. The carbon dioxide level can be read as a percent or fraction (F_ACO_2) or as partial pressure (P_ACO_2).

The capnograph is a strip chart recorder that provides a copy of the patient's exhaled carbon dioxide curve. There are at least two paper speeds that are useful for different purposes. The fast speed is most useful for evaluating sudden changes in the patient's condition. Each individual breath is easily seen (Fig. 5-1). The slow speed is most useful for trend monitoring (Fig. 5-2).

Two different gas sampling methods exist: mainstream and sidestream. The mainstream method involves having the infrared sensing unit at the airway; usually it is attached directly to the endotracheal/tracheostomy tube. If the patient is on a ventilator, the sampling adapter must be placed between the endotracheal tube and the ventilator circuit (with or without mechanical dead space). All inspired and expired gas passes through the sensor (Fig. 5-3).

The sidestream method employs a capillary tube placed so that a small sampling of the patient's exhaled gas can be drawn into the capnometer for analysis. It is not necessary for the patient's entire breath to pass through the sampling adapter; therefore it can be used in an unintubated patient by taping the sampling catheter a short distance into a nostril. If the patient is on a ventilator, the sampling adapter must be placed between the endotracheal tube and the ventilator circuit (with or without mechanical dead space). Remember that the patient's exhaled tidal volume (V_T) and minute volume ($\dot{V}_E$) is reduced by the amount that is drawn into the capnometer (Fig. 5-4).

c. Note and interpret the results from the procedure (Code: IB10a, IIIA1b, IIIA1m, and IIIA2a4,) [Difficulty: An]

Box 5-1 lists normal values and Fig. 5-5 shows the normal physiology behind capnography. Three factors influence capnography's use and the interpretation of the results. First is the patient's metabolism. The average resting adult produces about 200 mL of CO_2 per minute, and fever and exercise increase this value. Hypothermia, sleep, and sedation decrease CO_2 production. Lastly, exhaled CO_2 is monitored during a cardiopulmonary resuscitation attempt to determine the effectiveness of circulation and ventilation attempts and to determine if the efforts should be continued or stopped. If no carbon dioxide is being exhaled, a patient's metabolism has stopped altogether and death has occurred. There is nothing to be gained by continuing cardiopulmonary resuscitation (CPR) efforts.

Second, although not a major factor, is the patient's cardiac output. Sepsis, which might double a patient's cardiac output, reduces the PCO_2 only a few torr

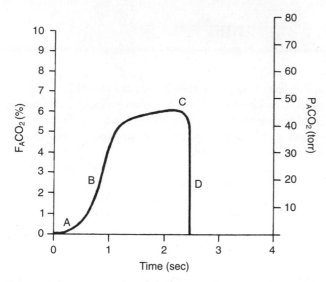

Fig. 5-1 Normal capnograph tracing taken at a fast speed. The percentage of exhaled alveolar CO_2 is shown on the left vertical scale as F_ACO_2. The partial pressure of exhaled alveolar CO_2 is shown on the right vertical scale as P_ACO_2. The tracing of exhaled gas can be divided into these four components: *A*, the beginning of exhalation, which shows no carbon dioxide in the upper airway anatomic dead space; *B,* the addition of alveolar gas, rich in carbon dioxide, to the anatomic dead space gas causes a rapid rise in measured CO_2; *C,* pure alveolar gas with a stable amount of CO_2 causes a plateau—the end-tidal CO_2 point is shown at C just before inspiration; and *D,* inspiration with a rapid drop in carbon dioxide to zero. A fast-speed tracing is more useful for determining the cause of a patient's changing condition than a slow-speed tracing.

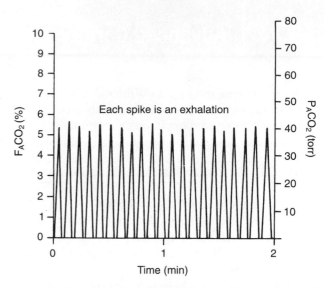

Fig. 5-2 Normal capnograph tracing taken at a slow speed. The percentage of exhaled alveolar CO_2 is shown on the left vertical scale as F_ACO_2. The partial pressure of exhaled alveolar CO_2 is shown on the right vertical scale as P_ACO_2. The slow speed results in a blending of parts *A, B,* and *C* of the fast-speed tracing (Fig. 5-1). Each spike is part *C* of the curve and marks an exhalation. A slow-speed tracing is more useful in trend monitoring of a patient than a fast-speed tracing.

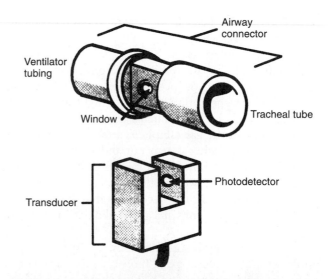

Fig. 5-3 Schematic drawing of a mainstream exhaled carbon dioxide analyzer sensor. The infrared sensor is attached to the patient's airway so that all of the exhaled and inhaled gas passes through it. (From Szaflarski NL, Cohen NH: *Heart Lung* 20:363–374, 1991.)

(millimeters of mercury [mm Hg]). Cardiogenic shock, which reduces the cardiac output, raises the partial pressure of CO_2 (PCO_2) only a few torr.

Third, and most important, is alveolar ventilation. A doubling of alveolar ventilation, under steady-state conditions for carbon dioxide production, results in a halving of the PCO_2 in arterial blood and alveolar gas. However, a reduction of alveolar ventilation to half of its previous level will result in the $PaCO_2$ and P_ACO_2 being doubled (Fig. 5-6).

V_T and respiratory rate are directly related to alveolar ventilation. Of the two, tidal volume is more important because it relates to the patient's dead space (V_D) to V_T ratio (V_D/V_T). A decrease in the patient's V_T results in less alveolar ventilation and a rise in PCO_2. Conversely, an increase in the V_T results in more alveolar ventilation and a drop in the PCO_2.

Capnography is most accurate and correlates best with the $PaCO_2$ if the patient's ventilation and perfusion match. The more ventilation and perfusion mismatching there is, or the more unstable the pulmonary perfusion is, the wider

or less reliable the gradient between the patient's arterial carbon dioxide and alveolar carbon dioxide levels. The following procedures should be performed to help understand the patient's condition and interpret the capnography results.

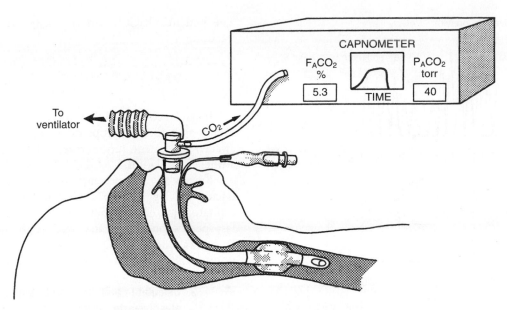

Fig. 5-4 Representation of a sidestream capnometry system. A capillary tube is placed into the ventilator circuit to sample the exhaled and inhaled gases.

BOX 5-1	Normal Blood Gas and Capnography Values (Based on a Sea Level Barometric Pressure of 760 torr)

$PaCO_2$ is approximately 40 torr.
$P\bar{v}CO_2$ is approximately 46 torr.
P_ACO_2 ranges from approximately 40 to 46 torr with the breathing cycle. This shows the carbon dioxide level varying between the arterial and mixed venous blood levels.
(end-tidal) P_ACO_2 ranges from 40 to 46 torr and correlates with the $PaCO_2$.
(end-tidal) F_ACO_2 is approximately 5.3% to 6.1% and correlates with the $PaCO_2$.

Both P_ACO_2 and F_ACO_2 may be seen listed in the literature as end-tidal CO_2. Note: The NBRC uses the abbreviation $P_{ET}CO_2$ for end-tidal CO_2.

🖹 EXAM HINT

Remember that mm Hg (millimeters of mercury) and torr (Torricelli) are equivalent units of pressure. The National Board of Respiratory Care (NBRC) uses these two units for different items in its questions. It uses mm Hg for blood pressure measurements and torr for blood gas values (such as $PaCO_2$ and $P\bar{v}O_2$). However, in questions dealing with capnography, the NBRC has used both mm Hg and torr in its questions that relate to exhaled CO_2 (such as P_ACO_2 and $P_{ET}CO_2$).

1. Calculate and interpret the end-tidal alveolar-arterial carbon dioxide gradient

The end-tidal alveolar-arterial carbon dioxide gradient [ET (A – a) CO_2] is useful, because once it is reliably

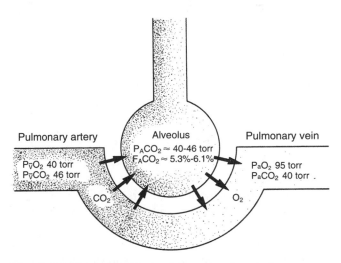

Fig. 5-5 Representation of the alveolar-capillary membrane showing the diffusion of oxygen and carbon dioxide and the arterialization of venous blood. Also shown are alveolar CO_2 values measured by capnography.

determined, the patient's ventilatory condition can be monitored by capnography alone. Drawing an arterial blood sample to measure the $PaCO_2$ level is less necessary if the patient is stable.

The normal gradient is 6 torr or less. However, most patients using capnography are not normal. The possible gradient ranges from −6 to + 20 torr in unstable patients with cardiopulmonary abnormalities. For example, the patient who is breathing shallowly may have an end-tidal CO_2 that is less than the arterial CO_2. This is because the patient is not exhaling completely to empty alveolar gas.

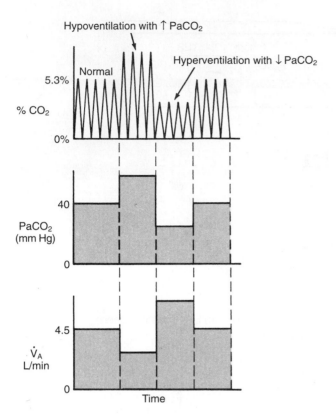

Fig. 5-6 Relationship between alveolar ventilation, $PaCO_2$, and exhaled CO_2 percent. (From Pilbeam SP: *Mechanical ventilation: physiological and clinical applications,* ed 3, St Louis, 1998, Mosby.)

Therefore determining each patient's own gradient is important.

Follow these steps:

a. Simultaneously draw an arterial blood gas (ABG) sample for $PaCO_2$ measurement and take an end-tidal gas sample for P_ACO_2 measurement.

b. The difference is the ET $(A - a)$ CO_2 gradient. The alveolar sample commonly shows a higher CO_2 level than the arterial sample.

Example 1. A patient is seen in the recovery room after surgery and has the following PCO_2 levels:

$$P_ACO_2 = 46 \text{ torr}$$
$$PaCO_2 = \underline{-40 \text{ torr}}$$
$$\text{ET } (A - a) \text{ } CO_2 = 6 \text{ torr}$$

The usefulness of this gradient is demonstrated when monitoring a patient's spontaneous breathing during weaning or making ventilator changes in the tidal volume or minute volume. It may be possible to avoid drawing as many ABG samples.

Example 2. The patient in Example 1 is seen later and has the following capnography reading: $P_ACO_2 = 56$ torr.

The patient's $PaCO_2$ can be easily calculated by subtraction:

$$P_ACO_2 = 56 \text{ torr}$$
$$\text{ET } (A - a) \text{ } CO_2 \text{ gradient} = \underline{- 6 \text{ torr}}$$
$$\text{estimated } PaCO_2 = 50 \text{ torr}$$

It can be concluded that the patient is not breathing as deeply as before. Appropriate action should be taken to awaken the patient, further reverse the anesthesia, or begin artificial ventilation.

Review the components of a fast-speed capnography tracing in Fig. 5-1 to understand a normal person's expiratory pattern. Fig. 5-7 shows eight different abnormal fast-speed capnography tracings. See the figure legend for an explanation of each problem. As the patient returns to normal, the tracing should approach that shown in Fig. 5-1.

2. Calculate and interpret the residual volume alveolar-arterial carbon dioxide gradient

If the patient is cooperative and will exhale maximally to residual volume (RV), this measurement provides more clinically useful information. The usual RV $(A - a)$ CO_2 gradient in a normal person is less than 7 torr. The wider the gradient, the more ventilation to perfusion (V/Q) mismatching there is. A gradient of more than 13 torr is considered to be markedly abnormal. This may be the case in patients with chronic obstructive pulmonary disease (COPD), pulmonary emboli, left heart failure (LHF), or hypotension.

When comparing the normal (solid line) tracing in Fig. 5-8 with the V/Q mismatching (dashed line) tracing, note the increased gradient at end-tidal CO_2. With continued exhalation to residual volume, the left heart failure and COPD patients have a narrowing of the gradient. This can be used clinically to follow these patients' progress and response to treatment. The patient with large pulmonary emboli will not have such a narrowing of the gradient as he or she exhales to residual volume. This patient's gradient will narrow to normal as the emboli are resolved and the physiologic dead space returns to normal.

EXAM HINT

Expect to see at least one question on the examination that requires the interpretation of capnography results, especially the end-tidal CO_2 value ($P_{ET}CO_2$). Examples include a change in alveolar ventilation, shallow breathing, and CPR attempt.

---

2. Dead space to tidal volume ratio

a. Recommend the measurement of dead space to tidal volume (Code: IA2h) [Difficulty: R, Ap, An]

The dead space to tidal volume test (V_D/V_T) is most commonly performed to document the amount of dead

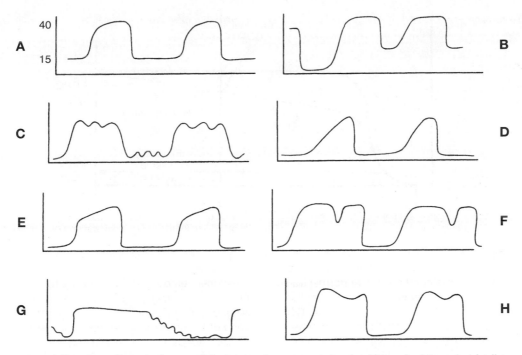

Fig. 5-7   A series of abnormal fast-speed capnography tracings. *A,* A mechanically ventilated patient with a malfunctioning exhalation valve. Note that the baseline CO_2 level is elevated because the patient's exhaled breath is measured during an inspiration. Correction of the exhalation valve should result in normal inhalation and exhalation. *B,* This rapidly rising baseline gas pressure and failure to return to baseline is usually seen when moisture or secretions block the capillary tube. Clearing the obstruction enables the patient's gas to again reach the analyzer. *C,* Distortions in the tracing from incomplete exhalation. These may be caused by hiccups, chest compressions during CPR, or inconsistent tidal volume efforts during an asthma attack. *D,* An obstructive lung disease patient with ventilation and perfusion mismatching. There is no alveolar plateau with a stable CO_2 level. Inhaling a bronchodilator should result in the tracing returning closer to normal. *E,* A patient with restrictive lung disease showing no plateau of alveolar gas emptying. This is because the alveoli do not empty evenly. *F,* A sudden drop in carbon dioxide level in the middle of an exhalation indicates that the patient attempted inspiration. This "cleft" is usually seen when a patient who has been pharmacologically paralyzed begins to regain movement. *G,* uneven carbon dioxide levels seen at the end of exhalation can be caused by: (1) The patient's heartbeat pumping fresh blood and CO_2 to the emptying lungs. The cardiogenic oscillations should match the heart rate. (2) The ventilator's exhalation valve is fluttering open and closed. *H,* The alveolar plateau is biphasic. This has been seen in patients with lungs that are different in compliance and ventilation/perfusion matching (e.g., single lung transplantation). (From Shapiro BA, Peruzzi WT, Templin R: *Clinical application of blood gases,* ed 5, St Louis, 1994, Mosby.)

space (wasted ventilation) in a patient with a pulmonary embolism. There are a number of other clinical situations, discussed later, that can justify the procedure. Review previous data before repeating the test to understand if the patient's condition has changed or is abnormal. Be prepared to compare the previous information with the new data to help evaluate the patient's current condition.

b. Perform the bedside procedure (Code: IB9c and IC1c) [Difficulty: An]

The procedure is the mathematical comparison of a person's dead space volume with tidal volume. Steps in the procedure follow (Fig. 5-9):

1. Determine the *average* exhaled CO_2 ($P_{\bar{E}} CO_2$) value by either of these methods:
   a. Collect the patient's entire exhaled gas sample over several minutes in a large airtight bag. Count the number of breaths that occurred. Calculate the average tidal volume breath by dividing the total exhaled volume by the total rate. Put all or part of this gas sample through the blood gas analyzer for the PCO_2 value.

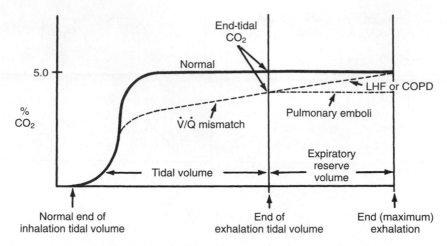

Fig. 5-8 Comparison of several fast-speed capnograph tracings showing how the exhaled carbon dioxide level changes as the patient exhales to residual volume. A normal tracing is matched against abnormal tracings of pulmonary emboli, left heart failure (LHF), and chronic obstructive pulmonary disease (COPD). The normal patient has the same end-tidal CO_2 as residual volume CO_2, showing good matching of ventilation and perfusion. LHF and COPD patients have a narrowing of the gradient as residual volume is approached. The patient with a pulmonary embolism keeps the same gradient at the residual volume as that found at the end of the tidal volume. (From Pilbeam SP: *Mechanical ventilation: physiological and clinical applications, ed 3, St Louis,* 1998, Mosby.)

Fig. 5-9 A schematic presentation of the procedure for gathering patient samples for calculating the dead space to tidal volume ratio (V_D/V_T). An anesthesia or other airtight bag is used to gather all exhaled gas to determine the average exhaled carbon dioxide pressure. An arterial sample is collected for $PaCO_2$. (From Pilbeam SP: *Mechanical ventilation: physiological and clinical applications, ed 2, St Louis,* 1992, Mosby.)

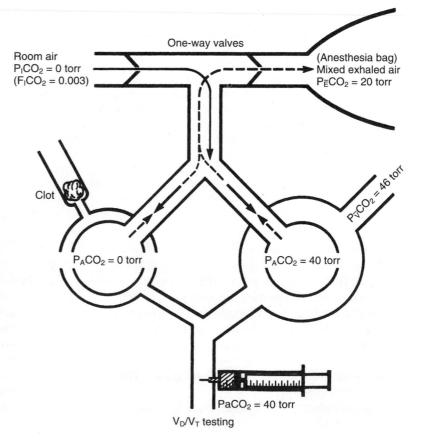

b. Have the patient's exhaled gas pass through a capnometer that can give you an average value (not end-tidal CO_2). A number of breaths should be averaged for greater PCO_2 accuracy. Measure or calculate the patient's average tidal volume over the time of the test.

2. Draw an arterial sample at the same time that you are performing either step 1a or 1b. Have the blood sample analyzed for $PaCO_2$.

3. Calculate the results using either of two methods.

Determine the decimal fraction or percentage of dead space.

Place both carbon dioxide values into this formula, which is derived from the original Bohr formula:

$$V_D/V_T \text{ (or } V_D) = \frac{(PaCO_2 - P_{\bar{E}}CO_2)}{PaCO_2}$$

In which:

V_D/V_T or V_D = The patient's physiologic dead space
$PaCO_2$ = The patient's arterial carbon dioxide pressure
$P_{\bar{E}}CO_2$ = The patient's average exhaled carbon dioxide pressure

The following example is based on an abnormal adult:
$PaCO_2$ = 45 torr
$P_{\bar{E}}CO_2$ = 18 torr

$$V_D = \frac{(45 - 18)}{45}$$
$$= \frac{27}{45} = .6$$

The patient's V_D fraction can be recorded as .6 or 60%. (Note that this equation must be used when the patient's tidal volume is not known.)

Determine the dead space volume.

Place both carbon dioxide values into this formula, which is derived from the original Bohr formula:

$$V_D/V_T \text{ (or } V_D) = \frac{(PaCO_2 - P_{\bar{E}}CO_2)}{PaCO_2} \times \dot{V}_E$$

In which:

V_D/V_T or V_D = The patient's physiologic dead space
$\dot{V}_E$ = Average exhaled tidal volume
$PaCO_2$ = The patient's arterial carbon dioxide pressure
$P_{\bar{E}}CO_2$ = The patient's average exhaled carbon dioxide pressure

The following example is based on a normal adult:
$\dot{V}_E$ = 500 mL
$PaCO_2$ = 40 torr
$P_{\bar{E}}CO_2$ = 28 torr

$$V_D = \frac{(40 - 28)}{40}$$
$$= \frac{12}{40} \times 500 = .3 \times 500 \text{ mL} = 150 \text{ mL}$$

The patient's physiologic V_D volume = 150 mL (Note that this equation must be used when the patient's tidal volume is known.)

In addition, the preceding equation allows for calculation of the patient's V_D/V_T ratio. In this example it is 150/500, .3, or 30%, depending on how it is written.

📑 EXAM HINT

Every recent examination has had at least one V_D/V_T calculation. Be able to calculate the value by either method. In addition, know the information needed to make the calculation, for example, average exhaled carbon dioxide value ($P_E CO_2$) rather than end-tidal carbon dioxide value ($P_{ET}CO_2$).

---

c. **Interpret the results (Code: IC2c and IIIA1m2) [Difficulty: An]**

The normal adult's V_D/V_T ratio ranges from .2 (20%) to .4 (40%). Anatomic dead space is normally greater in men than in women. The normal 3 kg neonate's dead space to tidal volume ratio is .3 (30%). Physiologic dead space (also known as respiratory dead space) is gas that is ventilated into the lungs but does not take part in gas exchange. This is because the alveoli are not perfused or are underperfused for the amount of gas that they receive.

Physiologic dead space is made up of the following:

1. Anatomic dead space, or the gas in the connecting airways from the nose and mouth to the terminal bronchioles. Generally it is assumed to be about 1 mL/lb of ideal body weight, or 2.2 mL/kg of ideal body weight.

2. Alveolar dead space that is made up of nonfunctioning alveoli that are ventilated but not perfused is minimal in a normal person. The previous "normal" adult example has the expected amount of dead space for his or her weight.

The following conditions or pulmonary disorders can cause the ratio to vary from the normal range:

1. Decreased V_D/V_T ratio
   a. Lung resection or pneumonectomy because the airways are removed; the patient will maintain his or her tidal volume in the other lung segments.
   b. Asthma attack because the airways are narrowed.
   c. Insertion of an endotracheal or tracheostomy tube because the upper airway is bypassed.
   d. Exercise in the normal person because the increased blood pressure increases perfusion of the apices (Zone 1).

2. Increased V_D/V_T ratio
   a. Vascular tumor because of decreased perfusion to ventilated alveoli.
   b. Pulmonary embolism because of lack of blood flow to ventilated alveoli. Consider this if the patient is a candidate for a pulmonary embolism and suddenly deteriorates.
3. Increased dead space effect with ventilation greater than perfusion (V > Q)
   a. Rapid, shallow ventilations because the upper airway dead space is overventilated compared with the alveoli.
   b. Mechanical dead space added to the ventilator circuit. This is an intentional effort to have the patient retain some of his or her exhaled carbon dioxide to correct for a respiratory alkalosis.
   c. COPD (bronchitis, bronchiectasis, cystic fibrosis, emphysema) because varying degrees of bronchospasm, mucous plugging, and tissue destruction lead to increased ventilation and perfusion mismatching.

Many clinicians believe that a dead space/tidal volume ratio of .6 (60%) or more is an indication for mechanically ventilating the patient. A person who is wasting 60% or more of his or her ventilation will soon tire from the work of breathing and go into ventilatory failure.

EXAM HINT

Remember that a pulmonary embolism is the most likely cause of a sudden increase in dead space. This concept is usually tested. In addition, there is usually a question that relates to identifying that a COPD patient will have an increased V_D/V_T value.

---

3. **Central venous pressure (CVP) monitoring**
   a. **Review the patient's chart for data on previous central venous pressure measurements (Code: IA1g2) [Difficulty: An]**

Review previous patient data to understand whether there is an abnormality. Compare the current data with the earlier information to determine if there has been a change in the patient's condition. See Box 5-2 for normal values.

   b. **Recommend the insertion of a central venous pressure catheter to obtain additional data (Code: IA2e) [Difficulty: An]**

A central venous catheter (also called a CVP line) is inserted into many patients for one or more reasons: (1) to monitor the patient's right sided heart pressure, (2) to rapidly administer a large volume of intravenous fluids, and (3) for giving cardiac medications during a CPR attempt (preferred route).

   c. **Measure central venous pressure at the bedside and note the results (Code: IB9e) [Difficulty: R, Ap, An]**

The catheter is usually inserted into the right jugular

BOX 5-2 Normal Cardiopulmonary Values

CENTRAL VENOUS PRESSURE (CVP)
Range for a normal adult is 2-8 cm water or 1-6 mm Hg
Range for a normal infant is 1-5 mm Hg
Range for a normal neonate is 0-3 mm Hg

PULMONARY ARTERY PRESSURE (PAP)
Range for a normal adult is 15-28/5-16 mm Hg (about 25/10 mm Hg)
Range for a normal adult mean PAP is 10-22 mm Hg
Range for a normal child is 15-30/5-10 mm Hg
Range for a normal neonate is 30-60/2-10 mm Hg

PULMONARY CAPILLARY WEDGE PRESSURE (PCWP)
Range for a normal PCWP (mean) is 6-15 mm Hg (about 8 mm Hg)

CARDIAC OUTPUT
Range for a normal adult is 4-8 L/min
Range for a normal neonate is 0.6-0.8 L/min

STROKE VOLUME
Adults: 50-120 mL/beat
School-age children: 35 mL/beat
Preschoolers: 15 mL/beat
Neonates: 5 mL/beat

CARDIAC INDEX
2.5-4.0 L/min/square meter of body surface area.

ARTERIAL-VENOUS OXYGEN CONTENT DIFFERENCE
$[C(a - v)O_2]$
Range of normal is 3.0-5.5 vol % of O_2

SHUNT
5% or less of cardiac output

PULMONARY VASCULAR RESISTANCE
80-240 dynes/seconds/cm^{-5}

SYSTEMIC VASCULAR RESISTANCE
900-1400 dynes/seconds/cm^{-5}

---

vein or right subclavian vein and advanced to just above the superior vena cava. When set up for monitoring pressure, it measures the right atrial pressure (see Fig. 5-10 for how to perform the procedure). Note that the stopcock must be kept at the midchest level. Usually a mark is placed there for consistency. Raising the stopcock above the mark results in an incorrectly low reading. Lowering the stopcock below the mark results in an incorrectly high reading. Clinical practice is very important in learning how to perform this procedure. It is important that the patient breathes spontaneously if at all possible. Peak pressures during inspiration on a mechanical ventilator may artificially raise the CVP reading. Positive end-expiratory pressure (PEEP) may also raise the CVP reading. If the patient cannot be removed from the ventilator, take the reading during exhalation. Make a note of the settings and that the reading was taken with the patient on the

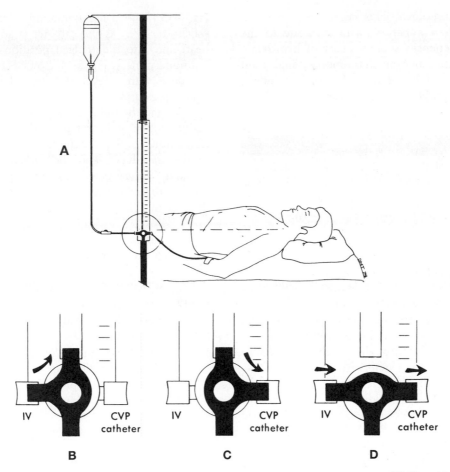

Fig. 5-10 Procedure for determining the central venous pressure (CVP) with a manometer. **A,** Water-column manometer marked in centimeters, IV tubing, and patient in place. **B,** Turn the stopcock so that the manometer fills with fluid above the expected pressure. **C,** Turn the stopcock off to the IV so that the fluid flows from the manometer into the patient. Look at the stable fluid level for the CVP reading. **D,** Turn the stopcock so that the fluid flows from the IV into the patient. (From Daily EK, Schroeder JS: *Techniques in bedside hemodynamic monitoring,* ed 5, St Louis, 1994, Mosby.)

ventilator. Record the data in the patient's chart or flow sheet.

d. Interpret the results of the central venous pressure measurement (Code: IB10e and IIIA1f) [Difficulty: R, Ap, An]

As noted earlier, the CVP is a measure of the pressure in the right atrium. The two main factors that influence the right atrial pressure are the blood volume returning to it and the functioning of the right ventricle (see Box 5-2 for the normal CVP readings).

A decreased CVP reading usually means that the patient is hypovolemic. Hypotension confirms this. An increased CVP may suggest one of the following possibilities:

a. Fluid overload. Check for an elevated blood pressure and crackles in the bases of the lungs. Unfortunately, an elevated CVP is a late finding with this problem.

b. Tricuspid valve or pulmonic valve insufficiency or stenosis. Abnormal electrocardiogram or echocardiogram findings or abnormal heart sounds (heart murmur) help to specify the problem.

c. Right ventricular failure. A right ventricular heart attack can be identified on an electrocardiogram. If a COPD patient with pulmonary hypertension has right ventricular failure, the condition is called *cor pulmonale.*

d. Cardiac tamponade (blood filling the pericardium). Watch for a fall in the blood pressure, tachycardia, and distended jugular veins. This problem can be rapidly fatal if not quickly corrected.

e. Atrial septal defect or ventricular septal defect with a left to right intracardiac shunt. These congenital conditions are usually detected in a young child by an abnormal electrocardiogram or echocardiogram finding or an abnormal heart sound (heart murmur).

f. Pulmonary embolism. This condition should be suspected when a patient who is prone to the problem experiences sudden onset of hypoxemia and clinical deterioration. A pulmonary angiogram showing blocked blood flow through the lung(s) confirms the problem.

📋 EXAM HINT

Memorize the values listed in Box 5-2. Expect to see several questions in which these values are used as patient data or as options to answer a question. The normal values must be understood to identify abnormal values and know why they are abnormal.

---

4. Pulmonary artery pressure (PAP) monitoring

a. Review the patient's chart for data on the pulmonary artery pressure (Code: IA1g2) [Difficulty: An]

The pulmonary artery pressure (PAP) is the systolic and diastolic pressure found in either pulmonary artery. It can be measured only through a pulmonary artery catheter. (The NBRC often refers to this as a flow-directed pulmonary artery catheter.) Review the patient's previous values before taking another to make a comparison. Box 5-2 shows normal cardiopulmonary values.

b. Recommend the insertion of a pulmonary artery catheter for additional data (Code: IA2e) [Difficulty: An]

PAP is important to measure in patients with severe pulmonary or cardiovascular problems, pulmonary hypertension, myocardial infarction, congestive heart failure, hypertension, and hypotension.

To read the PAP, a pulmonary artery catheter (PAC) must be inserted through a vein and passed through the right atrium and right ventricle into the pulmonary artery. The common insertion sites, in descending order of preference, are the basilic vein in either the right or left arm, the right internal jugular or subclavian vein, or the right or left femoral vein. The pulmonary artery catheter is also commonly called a Swan-Ganz catheter after the inventors who lent their names to a particular brand. The catheters come in different lengths and diameters for pediatric and adult patients. See Fig. 5-11 for a typical adult catheter.

c. Perform pulmonary artery pressure monitoring at the bedside (Code: IB9e) [Difficulty: R, Ap, An]

Fig. 5-11 is an illustration of a 7-French quadruple lumen thermodilution pulmonary artery catheter. Beside PAP, it is capable of being used to measure cardiac output. Fig. 5-12 shows how a pulmonary artery catheter could be arranged with a pressure transducer and pressure monitor.

Fig. 5-13 shows a representation of the series of pressure waveforms seen as the catheter is advanced through the heart and into the wedged position in a branch of the pulmonary artery. Fig. 5-14 shows a larger cutaway view of the heart with a PAC and normal heart chambers and related pressures.

To read the pulmonary artery pressure accurately, the equipment must be set up and calibrated properly, the distal lumen of the catheter must be patent and connected to the transducer, and the catheter's balloon must be deflated. Clinical practice is very important in understanding how to perform this procedure. Record the PAP data in the patient's chart or flow sheet.

d. Interpret the results of pulmonary artery pressure monitoring (Code: IB10e and IIIA1f) [Difficulty: R, Ap, An]

Again, the PAP is the systolic and diastolic pressure found in the pulmonary artery (see Box 5-2 for normal values). Elevated PAP values are usually seen with the following conditions:

1. Left ventricular failure/congestive heart failure, acute myocardial infarction, or fluid overload. To better determine the pathophysiologic problem, it is necessary to evaluate the following kinds of clinical information:
   a. Known history of heart disease or of sudden illness suggesting a heart attack
   b. Crackles heard in the bases of the lungs
   c. Decreased static lung compliance
   d. Elevated pulmonary capillary wedge pressure
   e. Decreased cardiac output and/or low blood pressure
   f. The normal gradient (difference) between the pulmonary artery diastolic pressure (PAd) and the pulmonary capillary wedge pressure (PCWP) is 5 mm Hg or less.

   Example. An adult patient has the following pulmonary artery catheter values: PAP is 35/24 mm Hg and PCWP is 22 mm Hg. Calculate the patient's pulmonary artery diastolic pressure minus pulmonary capillary wedge pressure (PAd – PCWP) gradient as follows:

Pulmonary artery diastolic is:	25 mm Hg
Pulmonary capillary wedge pressure is:	−22 mm Hg
The PAd – PCWP gradient is:	3 mm Hg

   It can be concluded that this person's PAd – PCWP gradient is normal.

2. Pulmonary hypertension from COPD (usually emphysema). To better determine the pathophysiologic problem, it is necessary to evaluate the following kinds of clinical information:
   a. The patient usually has a known history of COPD.
   b. Systolic PAP may exceed 40 mm Hg if the problem is long standing.
   c. The gradient (difference) between the pulmonary artery diastolic pressure and the pulmonary capil-

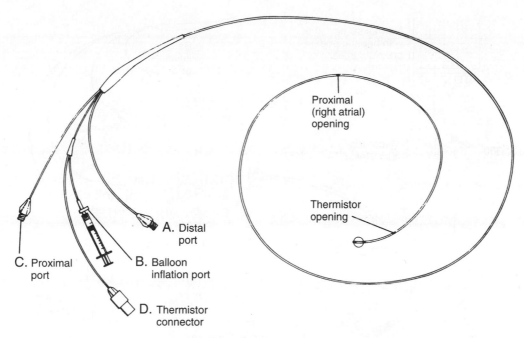

Fig. 5-11 A 7-French quadruple lumen thermodilution pulmonary artery catheter. *A,* Distal port goes to the tip of the catheter. It is used for measuring PAP, PCWP, and sampling blood for $P\bar{v}O_2$. *B,* Balloon inflation port is used to inflate the balloon for inserting the catheter and for obtaining a PCWP reading. *C,* Proximal port is used for measuring central venous pressure and for injecting iced saline for a thermodilution cardiac output study. The iced saline exits from the right atrial opening. *D,* Thermistor connector attaches to the cardiac output computer. A bimetalic wire runs through the catheter to the thermistor opening, where it is exposed to temperature changes of the blood and cold injectate. (Note: Not all catheters are capable of measuring cardiac output. Some catheters have other special features such as continuously measuring venous saturation or cardiac pacemaker leads.) (From Oblouk Darovic G: *Hemodynamic monitoring,* Philadelphia, 1987, WB Saunders.)

lary wedge pressure (Pad − PCWP) is greater than 5 mm Hg.

Example. An adult patient has the following pulmonary artery catheter values: PAP is 35/25 mm Hg and PCWP is 8 mm Hg. Calculate the patient's pulmonary artery diastolic pressure minus pulmonary capillary wedge pressure (Pad − PCWP) gradient as follows:

Pulmonary artery diastolic is:	25 mm Hg
Pulmonary capillary wedge pressure is:	− 8 mm Hg
The Pad − PCWP gradient is:	17 mm Hg

It can be concluded that this person's Pad − PCWP gradient is elevated.

3. Pulmonary hypertension from a pulmonary embolism. To better determine the pathophysiologic problem, it is necessary to evaluate the following kinds of clinical information:
   a. The patient's history matches that of a sudden onset of shortness of breath and other pulmonary problems.
   b. The systolic PAP is less than 40 mm Hg. This is because the relatively thin-walled right ventricle cannot rapidly increase its muscle mass to increase the driving pressure.
   c. The gradient (difference) between the pulmonary artery diastolic pressure and the pulmonary capillary wedge pressure (Pad − PCWP) is greater than 5 mm Hg if the embolism is large.

4. Pulmonary hypertension in the neonate with persistent pulmonary hypertension of the newborn (PPHN). This condition is often seen in the premature neonate with the infant respiratory distress syndrome (RDS). When these neonates become hypoxic, the pulmonary vascular bed constricts. This causes the infant to revert back to fetal circulation. Giving 100% oxygen and hyperventilating the infant usually reverses the processes. The PAP then returns to normal.

Decreased pulmonary artery pressure values are not frequently seen. Patients with hypovolemic shock, anaphylaxis (allergic shock), or excessive use of vasodilating drugs may have a decreased pulmonary artery pressure. The most obvious clinical sign in these patients is a low systemic blood pressure.

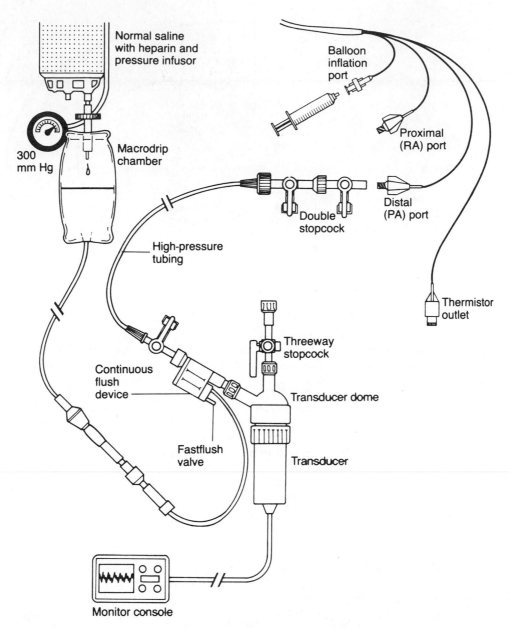

Normal saline with heparin and pressure infusor

300 mm Hg

Macrodrip chamber

High-pressure tubing

Double stopcock

Balloon inflation port

Proximal (RA) port

Distal (PA) port

Thermistor outlet

Threeway stopcock

Continuous flush device

Transducer dome

Fastflush valve

Transducer

Monitor console

Fig. 5-12 The various components of the pulmonary artery monitoring system. It includes a fluid source such as normal saline that is pressurized to 300 mm Hg to maintain a flow of fluid through the tubing system. The continuous flush device (made by Sorenson) is designed to allow three drips of fluid per minute through the tubing system; pulling on the fast-flush valve gives a continuous flow of fluid to clear air or blood from the system. The transducer converts a pressure signal to an electrical signal that is sent to the monitor for display as numerical data and a pressure waveform. The high-pressure tubing transfers the patient's pressure accurately to the transducer. The double stopcocks are used to close off the tubing system or sample blood from the patient. This then connects to the distal port of the pulmonary artery catheter. This same monitoring system can be used with an arterial catheter for continuous pressure monitoring and blood sampling. (From Oblouk Darovic G: *Hemodynamic monitoring,* Philadelphia, 1987, WB Saunders.)

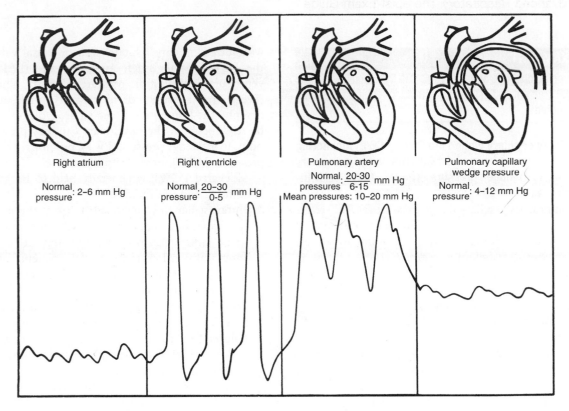

Fig. 5-13 Sequence of pressures and pressure waveforms seen as the pulmonary artery catheter advances through the *right atrium, right ventricle,* and *pulmonary artery* until it wedges. Be observant of premature ventricular contractions (PVC) as the catheter is advanced through the right ventricle. (From Wilkins RL, Sheldon RL, Krider SJ: *Clinical assessment in respiratory care,* ed 4, St Louis, 2000, Mosby.)

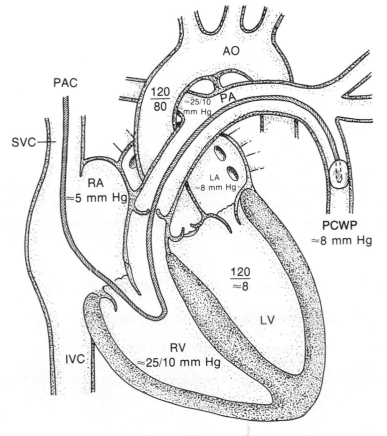

Fig. 5-14 Pulmonary artery catheter (PAC) through a heart with normal chamber pressures. *SVC,* superior vena cava; *IVC,* inferior vena cava; *RA,* right atrium; *RV,* right ventricle; *PA,* pulmonary artery; *PCWP,* pulmonary capillary wedge pressure; *LA,* left atrium; *LV,* left ventricle; and *Ao,* aorta.

5. Pulmonary capillary wedge pressure (PCWP) monitoring

a. Review the patient's chart for data on the pulmonary capillary wedge pressure (Code: IA1g2) [Difficulty: An]

The pulmonary capillary wedge pressure (PCWP) refers to the pressure measured in the pulmonary capillary bed under no-flow conditions. It is important to review previous patient data before measuring another pressure. Normal values are listed in Box 5-2.

b. Recommend the insertion of a pulmonary artery catheter for additional data (Code: IA2e) [Difficulty: An]

A pulmonary artery catheter must be placed into a patient's pulmonary artery for the PCWP to be measured. Measuring the PCWP is important in patients with severe pulmonary or cardiovascular problems, including pulmonary hypertension, myocardial infarction, congestive heart failure, hypertension, and hypotension.

c. Measure pulmonary capillary wedge pressure at the bedside (Code: IB9e) [Difficulty: R, Ap, An]

The PCWP is obtained by inflating the balloon at the tip of the catheter. This blocks off that branch of the pulmonary artery so that the downstream pressure from the left ventricle is seen on the monitor (see Fig. 5-13 and Fig. 5-14). The balloon volume varies with the diameter of the catheter. The needed volume is printed on the catheter near where the air is injected into the balloon. For example, the 5-French catheter balloon holds .8 mL of air and the 7-French catheter balloon holds 1.5 mL of air. It is important to put in only the required amount. Overinflating may burst the balloon or rupture the pulmonary artery. If the balloon wedges at less than the required volume, the catheter is probably too far down in the artery and may need to be withdrawn a short distance. The balloon is only inflated long enough to obtain the PCWP and then the balloon is deflated. Pulmonary infarction will occur if the balloon is left inflated and the blood in the pulmonary artery is stagnant and allowed to clot. Record the PCWP value in the patient's chart or flow sheet.

d. Interpret the pulmonary capillary wedge pressure results (Code: IB10e and IIIA1f) [Difficulty: R, Ap, An]

As noted earlier, the PCWP refers to the pressure measured in the pulmonary capillary bed under no-flow conditions. This pressure reflects downstream pressure from the left side of the heart. At diastole, in the patient without pulmonary hypertension or mitral valve disease, the PCWP parallels left atrial pressure (LAP) and left ventricular end diastolic pressure (LVEDP). The literature reveals that a variety of terms and initials are used to describe the same physiologic value. Do not be confused by reading about the pulmonary capillary pressure (PCP), pulmonary wedge pressure (PWP), pulmonary artery wedge pressure (PAWP), or wedge pressure.

Elevated PCWP is generally held to be greater than 10 mm Hg and can indicate:

1. Intravascular fluid overload: Look at the patient's history to see if the patient is in renal failure or has recently had a large amount of oral or intravenous fluids. Perform a physical exam to see if the patient has edema in the ankles or back if he or she has been lying down. Look for jugular vein distension when the patient lies down. Listen for crackles in the bases of the lungs.
2. Left ventricular dysfunction with congestive heart failure: Perform the same steps listed in point 1. In addition, look for a history of chronic heart failure or acute myocardial infarction.
3. Mitral valve insufficiency: Blood regurgitating back into the left atrium is shown as an elevated PCWP.

These conditions result in serious problems for the patient's lung function. When the PCWP reaches 20 to 25 mm Hg, fluid begins to leak into the pulmonary interstitium. This makes the lungs less compliant and increases the patient's work of breathing. A PCWP of 25 to 30 mm Hg results in frank pulmonary edema and dramatically decreases the patient's PaO_2.

Decreased PCWP is commonly held to be less than 4 mm Hg and can indicate:

1. Low intravascular volume: Look in the patient's history for an illness resulting in dehydration (vomiting and diarrhea). A physical examination will show tachycardia, low blood pressure, low urine output with a high specific gravity, tenting of the skin when pinched showing poor turgor, and flat jugular veins when the patient is lying down.
2. Sepsis: The patient's history will reveal infection, usually a septicemia. The physical examination will reveal tachycardia, hypotension, and oliguria, as noted in point 1. A major difference is that the patient will appear to be fluid overloaded because of the peripheral edema. This finding is produced when an infectious organism (often *Staphylococcus aureus*) causes a dilation of the peripheral vascular bed and leakage of fluids out of the vascular bed into the tissues. The patient will have weak peripheral pulses and feel warm.

6. Cardiac output

a. Review the patient's chart for data on cardiac output (Code: IA1g2) [Difficulty: An]

Cardiac output (CO) is defined as the product of heart rate for 1 minute and stroke volume (CO = HR × SV). It is

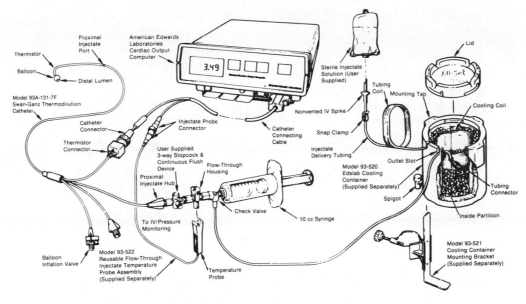

Fig. 5-15 Complete system for performing thermodilution cardiac output studies. (From Edwards Lifesciences LLC, Santa Ana, CA. 1985.)

a measurement of the heart's pumping ability to meet the body's needs. As always, review previous data before repeating the test. Box 5-2 lists normal values.

b. Recommend a cardiac output procedure for additional patient data (Code: IA2h) [Difficulty: R, Ap, An]

A cardiac output measurement is performed on patients with serious cardiovascular disease to assess the patient's condition. A major change in vital signs or new treatment justifies a measurement. The patient must have a pulmonary artery catheter in place that is capable of measuring cardiac output.

c. Perform a cardiac output procedure at the bedside (Code: IIIA1f) [Difficulty: R, Ap, An]

The bedside procedure involves the use of a special four-lumen pulmonary artery catheter designed for thermodilution cardiac output studies. Both catheter types require additional hardware and supplies, including a computer designed to calculate the CO. The first type of thermodilution catheter that was developed is used to inject a cool solution into the heart. This cool solution is diluted with the patient's blood. As the blood and cool solution mix passes a thermistor at the catheter tip, the computer calculates the patient's cardiac output based on the time required to pump the cooler blood past the thermistor (Fig. 5-11).

This procedure requires an injectable saline solution or 5% dextrose, ice water bath to cool the injectate, necessary tubing and connections, thermometer, 10 cc

syringes, and injector system (see Fig. 5-15). It is beyond the scope of this text to describe all of the steps in the different types of adult and neonatal thermodilution cardiac output procedures. Hands-on experience is necessary. Only the most important and common features are presented here:

a. The usual injectate volume is 10 cc. The neonatal injectate volume may be reduced to 3 cc in an attempt to prevent fluid overloading the patient. The right atrial lumen is used for the injection.

b. The usual injectate temperature is 0° to 4° C. Some clinicians use room air temperature injectate because it is easier to work with. The cold injectate cardiac output result may be more accurate because of the greater difference between it and the patient's body temperature. If the patient is hypothermic, the cold injectate must be used for greater accuracy.

c. Three injections are usually performed. The results are then averaged for the final CO value. Individual CO measurements that vary by more than 10% from each other probably indicate an error in the procedure. A compressed CO_2 "gun" is preferred to hand injection because the injector gun provides a smoother and more reliable injection. The injection must be completed within 4 seconds.

The "cool solution" thermodilution cardiac output procedure has been available for more than 20 years and is widely used clinically. Its main disadvantages are that the CO value is available only intermittently, it is a time-

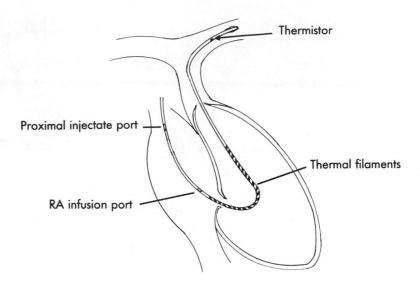

Fig. 5-16 View of the right side of the heart showing a continuous cardiac output thermodilution pulmonary artery catheter in proper position. Note the thermal filaments that heat the passing blood. The resulting temperature change is detected by the thermistor in the pulmonary artery. (From Daily EK, Schroeder JS: *Techniques in bedside hemodynamic monitoring,* ed 5, St Louis, 1994, Mosby.)

consuming procedure, and patients with heart failure are given significant amounts of additional fluid for each cardiac output calculation.

A newer thermodilution cardiac output catheter has been developed that makes use of a thermal filament (a heated wire) that wraps around the catheter (Fig. 5-16). With this catheter, the computer periodically directs electricity to the filament. This results in periodic warming of the blood from the heated wire. The computer calculates the patient's cardiac output by determining the time needed to pump the heated blood past the thermistor at the tip of the catheter. The advantages of the "heated wire" cardiac output catheter are that it gives an updated cardiac output value every 30 seconds, requires no additional time from the nurse or respiratory therapist after the initial set up, and does not add any additional fluid to the patient's intake.

d. Calculate the patient's cardiac output value (Code: IIIA1l) [Difficulty: R, Ap, An]

The following formula can be used to calculate a predicted cardiac output for the adult patient. This value can then be compared with the actual patient cardiac output.

$$CO = \frac{BSA \times 125}{.045}$$

BSA stands for body surface area and can be calculated mathematically or determined from a data table (see Fig. 5-17). See the following discussion on cardiac index for information on calculating BSA.

The following two methods can be used to calculate the patient's cardiac output:
1. A computer calculates the cardiac output (CO) when either thermodilution method is used. As long as the procedural steps are done properly and the patient and

catheter variables are programmed into the computer, the results should be reliable. This method is widely used at the bedside.
2. The Fick method of measuring cardiac output is the "gold standard" by which all others are measured. Unfortunately, it is difficult to perform at the bedside. The patient's inhaled and exhaled gases must be analyzed for PO_2 to calculate his or her oxygen consumption. In addition, arterial and mixed venous blood samples must be taken and analyzed for oxygen to calculate the arterial-venous oxygen content difference $[C(a - v)O_2]$. The following example shows fairly standard values for an adult:

$$CO \; (mL/min) = \frac{oxygen \; consumption \; (mL/min)}{arterial \; O_2 \; content \; (vol\,\%) - venous \; O_2 \; content \; (vol\,\%)}$$

In which:
Vol % = volumes % or mL of oxygen/100 mL of blood
Oxygen consumption = 250 mL/min
Arterial oxygen content = 20 vol %
Mixed venous oxygen content = 15 vol %
$C(a - v)O_2 = 5$ vol %
Therefore:

$$CO = \frac{250 \; mL/min}{20 \; vol\,\% - 15 \; vol\,\%} = \frac{250 \; mL/min}{5 \; vol\,\%} = \frac{250}{.05} =$$
$$5000 \; mL/min = 5 \; L/min$$

e. Interpret the patient's cardiac output measurement results (Code: IIIA1m3) [Difficulty: R, Ap, An]

As listed in Box 5-2, the normal, resting adult has a cardiac output in the range of 4 to 8 L/min and a normal, resting neonate has a cardiac output in the range of .6 to .8 L/min.

Cardiac output can increase markedly in a person with

a normal heart who is stressed, exercising, has a fever, or has any other reason for an increased metabolism. All these conditions increase the person's demand for oxygen, which is primarily met by increasing cardiac output. (To a lesser extent, the tissues extract more oxygen from the blood.) Sepsis is the one serious condition that results in a high cardiac output.

There are many possible causes of a decreased cardiac output. The most common are hypovolemia, increased peripheral resistance, and heart failure. A patient with low cardiac output often has a low blood pressure. If the cardiac output and blood pressure are too low, the patient will develop metabolic acidosis from peripheral hypoxemia. Death can result if this is not corrected.

7. Stroke volume

a. Calculate a patient's stroke volume (Code: IIIA1l) [Difficulty: R, Ap, An]

Stroke volume (SV) is defined as the volume of blood ejected with each heartbeat. It is the difference between the volume of blood in each ventricle at the end of diastole and the volume left in the ventricles at the end of systole (after ejection). The normal stroke volume is based on a person's age. See Box 5-2 for normal values. Stroke volume can be determined through a cardiac ultrasound procedure or calculated from the patient's heart rate and cardiac output.

For example, calculate an adult patient's stroke volume when the heart rate is 100/min and cardiac output is 8 liters:

$$SV = \frac{CO}{HR} = \frac{8000 \text{ mL}}{100} = 80 \text{ mL}$$

b. Interpret the patient's stroke volume calculation (Code: IIIA1m3) [Difficulty: R, Ap, An]

The stroke volume is the same for both ventricles except under pathologic conditions. Usually, however, only the left ventricle is of concern. The Frank-Starling curve shows us that as the heart muscle is stretched with greater volume, it contracts and pumps more completely resulting in a larger stroke volume. A left ventricle that has been damaged by a myocardial infarction does not pump as effectively and the stroke volume decreases. A drop in stroke volume results in a drop in cardiac output unless the heart rate can increase to make up the difference. This is seen in many patients with heart disease. In addition, when a normal right ventricle continues to pump more blood than the damaged left ventricle, the unpumped blood backs up into the pulmonary circulation and results in pulmonary edema (congestive heart failure).

8. Cardiac index

a. Calculate the patient's cardiac index value (Code: IIIA1l) [Difficulty: R, Ap, An]

The cardiac index (CI) is the cardiac output per square meter of body surface area. Cardiac output is usually measured by the thermodilution cardiac output method via a special pulmonary artery catheter. The body surface area (BSA) can be determined from the DuBois Body Surface Chart as shown in Fig. 5-17. The body surface area can also be determined with this equation:

$$BSA = \frac{1 + \text{weight in kilograms} + (\text{height in centimeters} - 160)}{100}$$

Example. A 166-lb/75-kg, 5'10"/152-cm man has a cardiac output of 6 L/min. According to the DuBois Body Surface Chart, he has a BSA of 1.92 m². His cardiac index is calculated as:

$$CI = \frac{CO}{BSA} = \frac{6 \text{ L/min}}{1.92 \text{ m}^2} = 3.125 \text{ L/min/m}^2$$

b. Interpret the patient's cardiac index results (Code: IIIA1m3 [Difficulty: R, Ap, An]

A normal, resting cardiac index is 2.5 to 4 L/min/m² of BSA. The cardiac index is a much more accurate way of determining if the patient's oxygen demands are being met than by simply looking at the cardiac output. For example, a resting cardiac output of 4 L/min is considered normal. This cardiac output might be fine for a small adult but not for a large one. The CI takes into account the difference in body sizes. A normal cardiac index indicates that the patient is receiving enough oxygen to meet the body's needs. A low cardiac index should be a cause for concern; it usually indicates that the patient is not getting enough blood and oxygen to his or her tissues. Check to see if the patient's cardiac output and blood pressure are also low and if he or she has hypoxemia or acidemia. If these exist, they must be corrected as quickly as possible to prevent dire consequences. A high cardiac index indicates that the patient is pumping more blood than appears necessary. Investigate why this is so. See the earlier discussion on cardiac output and the factors that affect it to understand the factors that affect cardiac index as well.

9. Mixed venous blood sampling

a. Review the patient's chart for data on mixed venous oxygen values (Code: IA1g2) [Difficulty: An]

A patient with a functioning pulmonary artery catheter can have a sample of blood withdrawn through it and analyzed for the mixed venous oxygen ($P\bar{v}O_2$) value (and the other blood gas values as well). As always, the $P\bar{v}O_2$ value(s) should be reviewed before measuring it again. (See Chapter 3 for information on mixed venous blood gas values.)

b. Perform mixed venous oxygen sampling at the bedside (Code: IA1b and IIID3) [Difficulty: An]

There are currently three methods of performing the bedside procedure.

Perform the procedure through the distal lumen of a PAC as it is being inserted. This method is employed when trying to

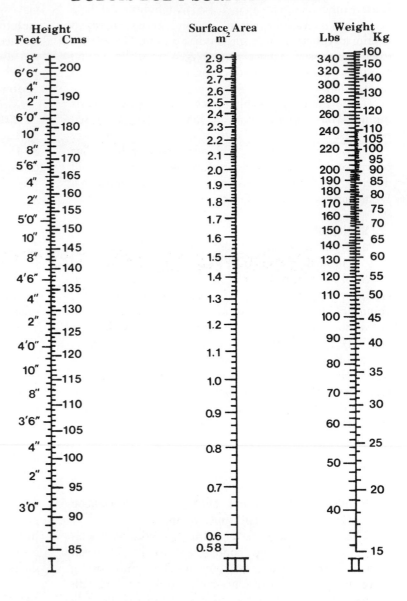

DUBOIS BODY SURFACE CHART

Fig. 5-17 DuBois Body Surface Chart (as prepared by Boothby and Sandiford of the Mayo Clinic). Directions: To find the body surface of a patient, locate the height in inches (or centimeters) on scale I and weight in pounds (or kilograms) on scale II. Place a straightedge (ruler) between these two points, which will intersect scale III at the patient's surface area. (From Boothby WM, Sandiford RB: *Boston Med Surg J* 185: 337, 1921.)

determine whether there is a ventricular septal defect. The procedure is commonly done on neonates with suspected congenital heart defects, but may be used in adults as well. Using sterile technique, blood samples are withdrawn serially from the right atrium, right ventricle, and sometimes from the pulmonary artery.

Normally, the $P\bar{v}O_2$ and $S\bar{v}O_2$ values are the same in all blood samples. The patient with a ventricular septal defect shows an increase in $P\bar{v}O_2$ and $S\bar{v}O_2$ values going from the right atrium to the right ventricle and pulmonary artery. This is because the oxygenated blood from the left ventricle is forced though the ventricular septal defect to raise the oxygen value of the right ventricular blood.

Use a pulmonary artery catheter with reflectance oximetry capability. These catheters have fiber optic bundles built into them and use technology similar to that used in pulse

oximeters. See Fig. 5-18. The processing unit sends a narrow waveband of light down the transmitting fiber optic bundle to be shined on the passing blood in the pulmonary artery. Oxyhemoglobin in the red blood cells absorbs some of the light. The rest is reflected off. The receiving fiber optic bundle picks up some of this light and transmits it back to the monitoring unit.

$S\bar{v}O_2$ is determined by the monitoring unit based on the light waves that were transmitted and what was received. Care must be taken when using this catheter in patients with elevated carboxyhemoglobin or methemoglobin levels. As with pulse oximetry, COHb and MetHb will be interpreted as oxyhemoglobin. Thus inaccurately high readings will be seen.

An actual mixed venous blood sample can be taken with this catheter through the distal lumen as described

PRINCIPLES OF REFLECTION
SPECTROPHOTOMETRY

Fiber optic catheter oximetry (*in vivo*)

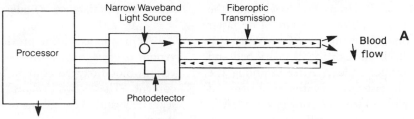

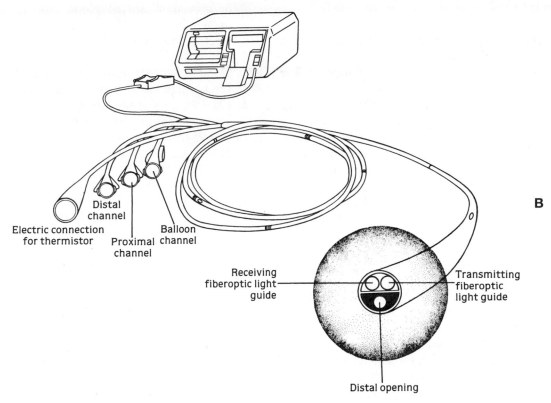

Fig. 5-18   Continuous monitoring of $S\bar{v}O_2$ by reflection spectrophotometry. **A,** Specific wavelengths of light are directed at passing blood. Some of the light is absorbed by the red blood cells and some is reflected back to the photodetector. **B,** Details of the fiber optic pulmonary artery catheter used for continuous $S\bar{v}O_2$ monitoring. The catheter tip detail shows a channel for the withdrawal of a mixed venous blood sample or the measurement of pulmonary artery pressure, a fiber optic channel for transmitting light to the blood, and a fiber optic channel for receiving the reflected light. The proximal ends of the fiber optic channels connect to a processor that determines the $S\bar{v}O_2$ value. (From Oximetric, Inc., Mountain View, CA.)

next. The advantage of the reflectance oximetry system is that it gives continuous monitoring of the patient's venous oxygen level. In addition, high and low saturation alarms can be set. If the tip should become lodged in the wall of the artery or if a clot should form at the tip, the $S\bar{v}O_2$ will drop or fluctuate dramatically. The alarms should warn the clinician of a problem with the equipment.

Use the distal lumen of a "standard" pulmonary artery catheter. A true mixed venous blood sample is obtained by withdrawing blood from the distal lumen of the catheter. This is the same lumen that is used for the PAP and PCWP readings. Using sterile technique, a 5- to 10-mL syringe is used to pull out the heparinized solution in the lumen until about 1 to 2 mL of blood are removed. A second preheparinized syringe is then used to withdraw about 2 mL of mixed venous blood. It is important to withdraw the intravenous (IV) solution and blood at a rate of no faster than .5 mL per second. Drawing any faster can pull preoxygenated blood back through the capillary bed and give falsely elevated oxygen values. After sampling the blood, the lumen must be fast-flushed with the heparinized solution to prevent the blood from clotting (see Fig. 5-12). Flush for several seconds until the solution flows freely. This blood sample may be reliably analyzed for $S\bar{v}O_2$, $P\bar{v}O_2$, and $P\bar{v}CO_2$.

c. Interpret the mixed venous blood sample results (Code: IB10c) [Difficulty: An]

This topic is discussed in some detail in Chapter 3. The normal values follow:

$P\bar{v}O_2$ of 40 torr (range of 37 to 43 torr)

$S\bar{v}O_2$ of 75% (range of 70% to 76%)

Mixed venous blood oxygen values are useful for following the patient's oxygen consumption. The most accurate methods of calculating percent shunt and cardiac output (Fick method) use mixed venous blood oxygen values with arterial blood oxygen values. A $P\bar{v}O_2$ value of less than 30 torr or $S\bar{v}O_2$ of less than 56% is considered to show tissue hypoxemia. Quick steps must be taken to reverse this. Increase the inspired oxygen percentage as needed. Low stroke volume and cardiac output can be increased by giving digoxin (Lanoxin) or other inotropic agents. Low blood pressure can be increased by giving vasopressors such as dopamine HCl (Intropin).

10. Arterial-venous oxygen content difference

a. Review the patient's chart for data on any previous arterial-venous oxygen content difference measurements. (Code: IA1g2) [Difficulty: An]

The arterial-venous oxygen content difference $[C(a - v)O_2]$ is a calculation of oxygen consumption by the body. It is the difference between the oxygen content of arterial blood and the oxygen content of mixed venous blood. Box 5-2 lists the normal value. As always, check for previous values to compare with present values to understand if the patient's condition has changed.

b. Perform the measurement of arterial-venous oxygen content difference (Code: IC1c) [Difficulty: R, Ap, An]

The following must be performed to make the arterial-venous oxygen content calculation:

1. Draw and analyze an arterial blood gas sample.
2. Simultaneously draw and analyze a mixed venous blood gas sample.
3. Determine the patient's hemoglobin value.

4. Place the data into the calculations shown in the next discussion.

c. Calculate the patient's arterial-venous oxygen content difference (Code: IIIA1m1) [Difficulty: R, Ap, An]

As mentioned in the previous discussion, the arterial-venous oxygen content difference is found by subtracting venous blood oxygen content from arterial blood oxygen content. These two values must first be calculated separately and then subtracted as shown in these three steps:

1. CaO_2 = The content of oxygen in arterial blood = vol % of oxygen in arterial blood (vol % means mL of oxygen/100 mL of blood.)
$CaO_2 = (Hb \times 1.34 \times SaO_2) + (PaO_2 \times 0.003)$
2. $C\bar{v}O_2$ = The content of oxygen in mixed venous blood = vol % of oxygen in mixed venous blood
$C\bar{v}O_2 = (Hb \times 1.34 \times S\bar{v}O_2) + (P\bar{v}O_2 \times 0.003)$
3. $C(a - \bar{v})O_2 = CaO_2 - C\bar{v}O_2$

Example. Your patient has the following clinical data:

PaO_2 = 95 torr

SaO_2 = 97% or .97

$P\bar{v}O_2$ = 40 torr

$S\bar{v}O_2$ = 75% or .75

15 g/dl = The patient's hemoglobin concentration

1.34 = mL of oxygen/g Hb in the patient (The value of 1.39 mL of oxygen/g Hb is occasionally used.)

0.003 = The oxygen carrying capacity of blood plasma per torr PO_2

Therefore:

1. $CaO_2 = (Hb \times 1.34 \times SaO_2) + (PaO_2 \times 0.003)$
$= (15 \times 1.34 \times .97) + (95 \times 0.003)$
$= (19.5) + (0.3)$
$= 19.8$ vol %

2. $C\bar{v}O_2 = (Hb \times 1.34 \times S\bar{v}O_2) + (P\bar{v}O_2 \times 0.003)$
$= (15 \times 1.34 \times .75) + (40 \times 0.003)$
$= (15.1) + (.1)$
$= 15.2$ vol %

3. $C(a - \bar{v})O_2$ difference = (CaO_2 of 19.8 vol %) −
(C$\bar{v}O_2$ of 15.2 vol %)
$= 4.6$ vol %

d. Interpret the patient's arterial-venous oxygen content difference (Code: IIIA1m1) [Difficulty: R, Ap, An]

The normal range for the $C(a - \bar{v})O_2$ difference is 3 to 5.5 vol %. Figures in this range show normal oxygen consumption by the tissues, cardiac output, and cardiopulmonary function. (See Fig. 5-19 for a graphic presentation of $C(a - \bar{v})O_2$ on the oxyhemoglobin dissociation curve.) A $C(a - \bar{v})O_2$ difference of greater than 5.5 to 6 vol % is seen in patients with a low cardiac output. As the blood flows more slowly than normal through the tissues, more oxygen is consumed per mL of blood. The $S\bar{v}O_2$ and $P\bar{v}O_2$ values drop and the $C(a - \bar{v})O_2$ difference widens.

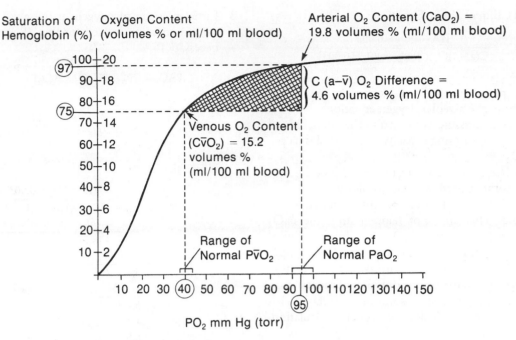

Fig. 5-19 Oxyhemoglobin dissociation curve showing normal oxygen saturations and pressures in arterial and venous blood. From these, the normal $C(a - v)O_2$ difference of 4.6 vol % can be calculated.

A $C(a - \bar{v})O_2$ difference of less than 4 vol % in the healthy patient commonly indicates good cardiovascular reserve with an increased cardiac output. As the blood flows more quickly than normal through the tissues, less oxygen is consumed per mL of blood. The $S\bar{v}O_2$ and $P\bar{v}O_2$ values increase and the $C(a - \bar{v})O_2$ difference narrows. The septic patient may have a narrowed $C(a - \bar{v})O_2$ difference because of peripheral shunting and decreased oxygen consumption by the tissues caused by the infection. The $C(a - \bar{v})O_2$ difference is necessary to accurately calculate the percent of pulmonary shunting as discussed next.

11. Shunt study

a. Review the patient's chart for data on previous shunt studies (Code: IA1g2) [Difficulty: An]

Shunt ($\dot{Q}s/\dot{Q}t$) is the amount of blood pumped by the heart that passes through the lungs but does not participate in gas exchange. A pulmonary artery catheter must be inserted into the patient for a shunt study to be performed. Review previous $\dot{Q}s/\dot{Q}t$ study results and compare with current information to see if there has been a change in the patient's status. See Box 5-2 for normal values.

b. Recommend a shunt study for added data (Code: IA2h) [Difficulty: R, Ap, An]

A shunt study is very useful to find out how much ventilation to perfusion mismatch a patient has. Most patients with refractory hypoxemia and requiring mechanical ventilation have an increased amount of pulmonary shunting. When an optimal PEEP study is performed a shunt study should be performed with each change in the PEEP level.

c. Perform the bedside shunt study procedure (Code: IB9C and IIIA1l) [Difficulty: R, Ap, An]

Steps in the bedside shunt procedure include:

1. Measure the patient's fractional concentration of inspired oxygen (F_IO_2).
2. Simultaneously draw arterial and mixed venous blood samples.
3. Have both blood samples analyzed for SO_2 and PO_2.
4. Calculate the percent of shunt as shown next.

d. Calculate the patient's shunt percentage (Code: IIIA1l) [Difficulty: R, Ap, An]

📝 EXAM HINT

To date the NBRC has not had an examination question that requires all of the calculations needed to determine a patient's shunt percentage. However, examinations have had questions that relate to calculating components of the shunt equations. These have included calculating CaO_2, $C\bar{v}O_2$, and $C(a - \bar{v})O_2$.

There are a number of possible variations on the methods and equations for calculating shunt percentage. Only the two most commonly used equations are presented here.

Modified Clinical Shunt Equation

$$\dot{Q}_s/\dot{Q}_t = \frac{P(A-a)O_2 \times 0.003}{C(a-\bar{v})O_2 + [P(A-a)O_2 \times 0.003]}$$

In which:

PAO_2 = The partial pressure of oxygen in the alveoli calculated from the alveolar oxygen equation

PaO_2 = The partial pressure of oxygen in the arterial blood

0.003 = The oxygen carrying capacity of blood plasma per mm Hg PO_2

$C(a-\bar{v})O_2$ = The oxygen content of arterial blood minus the oxygen content of mixed venous blood

This formula requires that the patient's hemoglobin be 100% saturated. This does not happen until the PaO_2 reaches 150 torr at any given F_IO_2. An obvious clinical limitation is that very ill patients never reach 100% saturation even on 100% oxygen. Also, putting patients on more than 80% oxygen, even for just the duration of the test, may lead to some denitrogenation absorption atelectasis. This results in an incorrectly high shunt percentage calculation.

Modified Clinical Shunt Equation Example

The following example shows the modified clinical shunt calculation with the following environmental and patient information:

P_B = Local barometric pressure; 760 torr for sea level in this example

PH_2O = 47 torr; water vapor pressure in the lungs at normal body temperature

F_IO_2 = inhaled oxygen percent of 100% or 1.0

PaO_2 = 155 torr

$PaCO_2$ = 40 torr

SaO_2 = 100% or 1.0

$P\bar{v}O_2$ = 40 torr

$S\bar{v}O_2$ = 75% or .75

.8 = The normal respiratory quotient (An exact value can be determined by a metabolic study.)

15 g/dl = The patient's hemoglobin concentration

0.003 = The oxygen carrying capacity of blood plasma per torr PO_2

1.34 = mL of oxygen/g Hb in the patient (The value of 1.39 mL of oxygen/g Hb is occasionally used.)

Preliminary calculations:

1. Oxygen content of arterial blood

$$\begin{aligned} CaO_2 &= (Hb \times 1.34 \times SaO_2) + (PaO_2 \times 0.003) \\ &= (15 \times 1.34 \times 1.0) + (155 \times 0.003) \\ &= (20.1) + (0.5) \\ &= 20.6 \text{ vol \%.} \end{aligned}$$

2. Oxygen content of mixed venous blood

$$\begin{aligned} C\bar{v}O_2 &= (Hb \times 1.34 \times S\bar{v}O_2) + (P\bar{v}O_2 \times 0.003) \\ &= (15 \times 1.34 \times .75) + (40 \times 0.003) \\ &= (15.1) + (.1) \\ &= 15.2 \text{ vol \%.} \end{aligned}$$

3. Partial pressure of oxygen in the alveoli. The alveolar oxygen equation is used for this. (Review Chapter 3 if necessary.)

$$\begin{aligned} PAO_2 &= [(P_B - PH_2O) \times F_IO_2] - \frac{PaCO_2}{.8} \\ &= [(760 - 47) \times 1.0] - \frac{40}{.8} \\ &= [713] - 50 \\ &= 663 \text{ torr} \end{aligned}$$

Final calculation:

$$\begin{aligned} \dot{Q}_s/\dot{Q}_t &= \frac{P(A-a)O_2 \times 0.003}{C(a-\bar{v})O_2 + [P(A-a)O_2 \times 0.003]} \\ &= \frac{(663 - 155) \times 0.003}{(20.6 - 15.2) + [(663 - 155) \times 0.003]} \\ &= \frac{(508) \times 0.003}{5.4 + [(508) \times 0.003]} \\ &= \frac{1.5}{5.4 + 1.5} \\ &= \frac{1.5}{6.9} \\ &= .217 \text{ or } 21.7\% \text{ shunt} \end{aligned}$$

Classic Shunt Equation

This equation is widely used because of the clinical limitations of the clinical shunt equation.

$$\dot{Q}_s/\dot{Q}_t = \frac{CcO_2 - CaO_2}{CcO_2 - C\bar{v}O_2}$$

In which:

CcO_2 = The content of oxygen in the end pulmonary capillary blood

CaO_2 = The content of oxygen in the arterial blood

$C\bar{v}O_2$ = The content of oxygen in the mixed venous blood

The patient should be inspiring 30% oxygen or more to calculate the oxygen content of end pulmonary capillary blood. This much oxygen should cause the PAO_2 of the ventilated alveoli to reach 150 torr or more. That results in 100% saturation of the hemoglobin of the end pulmonary capillary blood (ScO_2). Most patients who are sick enough to warrant a shunt determination will be on at least 30% oxygen. If not, the ScO_2 must be found using the oxyhemoglobin dissociation curve.

A pulmonary artery catheter is needed to sample mixed venous blood for $P\bar{v}O_2$ and $S\bar{v}O_2$ in both of these equations. An arterial blood gas sample is also needed. There are clinical situations in which either of these equations will work and will result in the same answer.

Classic shunt equation example. The following example shows the classic shunt calculation with the following environmental and patient information:

P_B = Local barometric pressure; 760 torr for sea level in this example.

PH_2O = 47 torr; water vapor pressure in the lungs at normal body temperature.

F_IO_2 = Inhaled oxygen percent of 30% or .3
PaO_2 = 95 torr
$PaCO_2$ = 40 torr
SaO_2 = 97% or .97
$P\bar{v}O_2$ = 40 torr
$S\bar{v}O_2$ = 75% or .75
.8 = The normal respiratory quotient (An exact value can be determined by a metabolic study.)
15 g/dl = The patient's hemoglobin concentration
0.003 = The oxygen carrying capacity of blood plasma per torr PO_2
1.34 = mL of oxygen/g Hb in the patient. (The value of 1.39 mL of oxygen/g Hb is occasionally used.)

Preliminary calculations:
1. Oxygen content of arterial blood

$$CaO_2 = (Hb \times 1.34 \times SaO_2) + (PaO_2 \times 0.003)$$
$$= (15 \times 1.34 \times .97) + (95 \times 0.003)$$
$$= (19.5) + (0.3)$$
$$= 19.8 \text{ vol \%}$$

2. Oxygen content of mixed venous blood

$$C\bar{v}O_2 = (Hb \times 1.34 \times S\bar{v}O_2) + (P\bar{v}O_2 \times 0.003)$$
$$= (15 \times 1.34 \times .75) + (40 \times 0.003)$$
$$= (15.1) + (.1)$$
$$= 15.2 \text{ vol \%}$$

3. Partial pressure of oxygen in the alveoli the alveolar oxygen equation is used for this.

$$PAO_2 = [(P_B - PH_2O) \times F_IO_2] - \frac{PaCO_2}{.8}$$
$$= [(760 - 47) \times .3] - \frac{40}{.8}$$
$$= [214] - 50$$
$$= 164 \text{ torr}$$

4. Oxygen content of pulmonary capillary blood

$$CcO_2 = (Hb \times 1.34 \times ScO_2) + (PAO_2 \times 0.003)$$
$$= (15 \times 1.34 \times 1.0) + (164 \times 0.003)$$
$$= 20.1 + .492$$
$$= 20.1 + .5 \text{ (Rounded off to one decimal place)}$$
$$= 20.6 \text{ vol \%}$$

Final calculation:

$$\dot{Q}_s/\dot{Q}_t = \frac{CcO_2 - CaO_2}{CcO_2 - C\bar{v}O_2}$$
$$= \frac{20.6 - 19.8}{20.6 - 15.2}$$
$$= \frac{.8}{5.4}$$
$$= .15 \text{ or } 15\% \text{ shunt}$$

e. Interpret the results of the shunt study (Code: IIIA1m1) [Difficulty: An]

As noted earlier, shunt is the amount of blood pumped by the heart that does not participate in gas exchange through the lungs. It is wasted cardiac output and wasted effort by the heart. The normal person has a shunt of 5% of cardiac output or less. This shunted blood has a low oxygen content and dilutes down the oxygen content of all the blood. The larger the percentage of shunted blood, the more the heart and body are stressed. Many clinicians believe that an indication for mechanical ventilation is a shunt of 15% to 20%. Most agree that 30% or more shunt can be life threatening. The ventilator is used to reduce the patient's work of breathing and oxygen consumption. Also, supplemental oxygen can be more carefully controlled, and PEEP may be added to increase the patient's functional residual capacity (FRC) as needed.

12. Pulmonary vascular resistance

a. Perform the pulmonary vascular resistance procedure. (Code: IB9f) [Difficulty: R, Ap, An]

Pulmonary vascular resistance (PVR) is the total resistance of the pulmonary vascular bed to the blood being pumped through it by the right ventricle. Cardiac output and pulmonary blood pressure determine the PVR. To gather the necessary hemodynamic information, the patient must have a thermodilution-type cardiac output pulmonary artery catheter.

b. Calculate the patient's pulmonary vascular resistance value. (Code: IB10f and IIIA1) [Difficulty: R, Ap, An]

The patient must have mean pulmonary artery pressure (PAm), pulmonary capillary wedge pressure (PCWP), and cardiac output (CO) measured and placed into this formula:

$$PVR = \frac{\begin{array}{c}\text{mean pulmonary artery pressure (PAm)} - \\ \text{pulmonary capillary wedge pressure (PCWP)}\end{array}}{\text{cardiac output (CO)}} \times 80$$

The answer will be in units of dynes/sec/cm^{-5}.

c. Interpret the results of the pulmonary vascular resistance calculation (Code: IIIA1m3) [Difficulty: R, Ap, An]

The normal range for PVR in the adult is 1 to 3 mm Hg/L/min. Multiplying this value by 80 gives the units of dynes/sec/cm^{-5}. PVR is listed this way in some cardiology studies. The normal range of PVR in an adult is between 20 to 30 and 120 to 240 dynes/sec/cm^{-5}.

With a normal PVR, the difference between the pulmonary artery diastolic pressure and the pulmonary capillary wedge pressure is 5 mm Hg or less. Any of the following can cause an elevated pulmonary vascular resistance:
1. Decreased oxygen in the lungs
2. Chronic obstructive lung disease (COPD)
3. Acute respiratory distress syndrome (ARDS)
4. Persistent pulmonary hypertension of the newborn/persistent fetal circulation

5. Primary pulmonary hypertension
6. Pulmonary embolism
7. Excessive positive end-expiratory pressure (PEEP)
8. Increased pulmonary blood flow from a left to right intracardiac shunt such as an atrial septal defect or ventricular septal defect

Additional clinical data must be gathered to confirm the diagnosis. An increased PVR is a serious problem because it can lead to right ventricular hypertrophy. The COPD patient is at risk for developing cor pulmonale. This is right ventricular failure secondary to lung disease and increased pulmonary vascular resistance.

13. Systemic vascular resistance
a. Perform the systemic vascular resistance procedure. (Code: IB9f) [Difficulty: R, Ap, An]

Systemic vascular resistance (SVR) is the total resistance of the systemic vascular bed to the blood being pumped through it by the left ventricle. Cardiac output and systemic blood pressure determine the SVR. To gather the necessary hemodynamic information, the patient must have a thermodilution-type cardiac output pulmonary artery catheter, arterial line, and central venous pressure line (if this cannot be measured from the pulmonary artery catheter).

b. Calculate the patient's systemic vascular resistance value. (Code: IB10f and IIIA1) [Difficulty: R, Ap, An]

The patient must have mean arterial pressure (MAP), central venous pressure (CVP), and cardiac output (CO) measured and placed into this formula:

$$SVR = \frac{\text{mean arterial pressure (MAP)} - \text{central venous pressure (CVP)}}{\text{cardiac output (CO)}} \times 80$$

The answer will be in units of dynes/sec/cm^{-5}.

c. Interpret the results of the systemic vascular resistance calculation (Code: IIIA1) [Difficulty: R, Ap, An]

The normal range of SVR in the adult is 15 to 20 mm Hg/L/min. Multiplying this value by 80 gives us the units of dynes/sec/cm^{-5}. SVR is listed this way in some cardiology studies. When multiplied by 80, an adult's SVR has a range between 770 to 900 and 1400 to 1500 dynes/sec/cm^{-5}.

A patient with hypertension will have an elevated SVR. It will also increase if the patient is given a vasoconstricting drug and decrease if the patient is given a vasodilating drug. Some allergic reactions result in anaphylaxis with a dramatic drop in the SVR and blood pressure despite an increase in the cardiac output.

EXAM HINT

Know both sets of normal values for pulmonary and systemic vascular resistance. To date, the NBRC has not expected the examinee to perform all of the calculations to determine a patient's PVR or SVR. Know that a COPD patient has a chronically increased PVR and a patient with a large pulmonary embolism will have a sudden increase in the PVR. There are several ways that the cardiology version of the PVR or SVR values can be found. The preferred versions have units listed in "dynes/sec/cm^{-5}" or "dyne sec/cm^{-5}". However, the NBRC has also listed these values in units of "dynes seconds cm^{-5}", "dynes·seconds·cm^{-5}", and "mm Hg/L/min."

MODULE B Cardiopulmonary monitoring equipment

1. Capnography equipment
a. Get the necessary equipment for the procedure (Code: IIA1h4) [Difficulty: An]

As discussed earlier, a capnograph is used to measure a patient's exhaled carbon dioxide level and expiratory pattern. There are two different types of capnography systems. Their main difference is in how the gas is sampled from the patient. Fig. 5-3 shows the patient connection for a mainstream capnograph. Fig. 5-4 shows a sidestream capnograph. Both work equally well if the patient is intubated. The capnography connector is attached between the endotracheal tube and the ventilator circuit or T-piece (Brigg's adapter). The sidestream unit may also be used with a spontaneously breathing patient because the capillary tube may be taped into a patient's nostril for gas sampling.

b. Put the capnography equipment together, make sure that it works properly, and identify any problems (Code: IIB1h4) [Difficulty: An]

The following are components of a capnography system:
1. Airway attachment: The mainstream and sidestream units must have both inhaled and exhaled gas pass through the sensor or connector, respectively. Connections must be airtight and free of obstructions.
2. The gas sampling capillary tube of the sidestream unit must be kept clear of water or secretions.
3. Capnometer: Periodically calibrate the unit with two gases of different CO_2 content. Room air is used for the "zero" value, and either 5% or 10% CO_2 in a preanalyzed cylinder is used for the "high" value. Both values should calibrate within the manufacturer's specifications.
4. Capnograph: Check that the paper speeds and marker work properly.

c. Fix any problems with the capnography equipment (Code: IIB2h4) [Difficulty: An]

Relatively few things can go wrong with capnography systems. The sidestream capnometer units must be kept dry. An external water trap is located between the capillary tube and the capnometer itself. Make sure that the water is drained periodically. Either capnography system can be disconnected from the patient. This is seen as a drop in exhaled carbon dioxide to zero. The alarm should activate if it has been set.

d. Perform quality control procedures on capnography equipment (Code: IIB3d) [Difficulty: R, Ap, An]

As presented earlier, both capnography units are calibrated using two points. Room air is used to set the zero point, and either 5% or 10% carbon dioxide from a cylinder is used to set the high point. Follow the manufacturer's guidelines regarding how much adjustment for low or high point can be tolerated. Do not use a machine that cannot be properly calibrated.

3. Pressure transducer

a. Get the necessary equipment for the procedure (Code: IIB1n2) [Difficulty: An]

Hemodynamic monitoring requires a transducer that converts a blood pressure signal into an electrical signal. Select a strain gauge type transducer to do this. The strain gauge transducer uses a fine wire screen that bends proportionately to the pressure put against it.

b. Put the strain gauge transducer equipment together, make sure that it works properly, and identify any problems (Code: IIB2n2) [Difficulty: R, Ap, An]

Check to see that the wire screen of the transducer is not bent, damaged, or fouled with old blood or other debris. The transducer's wire cable and monitor connecting prongs should not be bent or damaged. Carefully insert the prongs into the receiving jack on the monitor.

A disposable, sterile, clear plastic dome should be firmly screwed onto the transducer. Noncompliant pressure tubing should connect the transducer with the patient's arterial or pulmonary artery catheter. The automatic fluid drip system (Sorenson) should be pressurized to 300 mm Hg. Heparin must be added to the fluid (usually normal saline) to prevent clotting in the patient's catheter. Because this is a continuous fluid "plumbing" system, all connections must be tightly screwed together to be watertight. (See Figs. 5-12 and 5-20.)

The transducer must be kept at the patient's midchest (midheart) level during calibration and measurement. Calibrate the electronics in the monitor by putting known pressures against the fluid system. The electronics should first be adjusted to "zero" pressure by opening the transducer to room air (atmospheric pressure). Adjust the

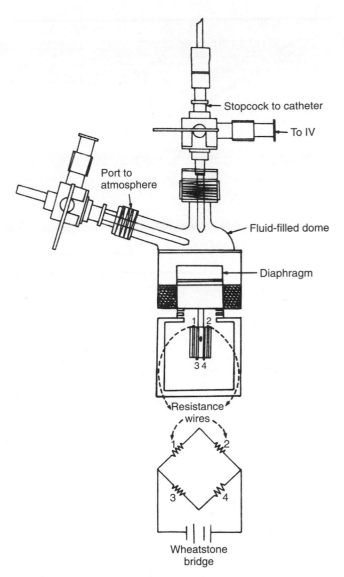

Fig. 5-20 Schematic diagram of a strain gauge pressure transducer. The wire mesh resistance wires are arranged like a Wheatstone bridge so that a pressure change results in a proportional change in the electrical resistance. (From Armstrong PW, Baigrie RS: *Hemodynamic monitoring in the critically ill,* Philadelphia, 1980, Harper & Row.)

electronic controls as needed. A sphygmomanometer is then used to pressurize the fluid system. A pulmonary artery catheter system is pressurized to relatively low pressures such as 30 and 50 mm Hg. An arterial system is adjusted to higher pressures such as 100 and 150 mm Hg. The monitored pressure should match the sphygmomanometer pressure. If not, adjust the electronic controls on the monitor to match.

c. Fix any problems with the equipment (Code: IIB2n2) [Difficulty: R, Ap, An]

As mentioned earlier, all connections must be water-

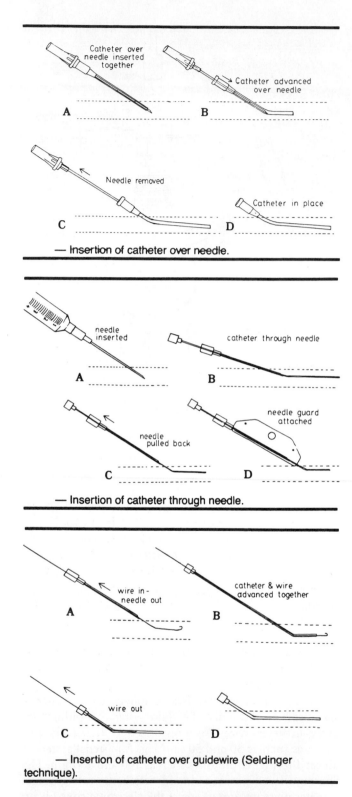

— Insertion of catheter over needle.

— Insertion of catheter through needle.

— Insertion of catheter over guidewire (Seldinger technique).

Fig. 5-21 Steps in the procedure for the percutaneous insertion of an arterial catheter for the continuous measurement of arterial pressure. Once inserted into the artery, the proximal end of the catheter is connected to a tubing circuit and pressure transducer as shown in Figs. 5-22 and 5-23. (From Oblouk Darovic G: *Hemodynamic monitoring*, Philadelphia, 1987, WB Saunders.)

tight. If not, the IV solution will drip out when it is pressurized. This can also result in the patient's measured pressures being less than true. Stopcocks must be opened or closed properly to allow the patient's pressure to be measured by the transducer. Electronics that will not calibrate to match the known pressures should not be used.

4. Central venous catheters
a. Get the necessary equipment for central venous catheterization (Code: IIA1q1) [Difficulty: R, Ap, An]

Get the catheter type and gauge that is requested by the physician. Additional equipment includes a water-column manometer, stopcock, intravenous tubing, and IV solution system.

b. Put the equipment together, make sure that it works properly, and identify any problems (Code: IIB1q) [Difficulty: R, Ap, An]

See Fig. 5-10 for the assembly of the equipment and the procedure for measuring the central venous pressure (CVP). The equipment must be properly calibrated to ensure that the data are accurate. Calibrating a central venous pressure water-column manometer usually involves only making sure that it reads zero at atmospheric pressure.

c. Correct any problems with the equipment (Code: IIB2q) [Difficulty: R, Ap, An]

Make sure that all connections are watertight. Check the position of the stopcock if the CVP cannot be measured.

5. In-dwelling arterial catheters
a. Get the necessary equipment for arterial catheterization (Code: IIA1q2) [Difficulty: R, Ap, An]

As discussed earlier, a neonate can have its umbilical artery catheterized. An adult usually has the radial artery catheterized. Following are the general supplies necessary for catheterizing either of these arteries for drawing blood gases and continuously monitoring blood pressure:

1. Sterile 20-gauge or 21-gauge needle with a flexible plastic sheath. After placement into the artery, the needle is withdrawn and the sheath is left in place. See Fig. 5-21. A neonate needs a long catheter of the correct gauge based on its body weight.
2. Sterile surgical drape for covering the area surrounding the insertion site.
3. Disinfectant such as 70% isopropyl alcohol or Betadine solution.
4. Local anesthetic such as 4% lidocaine in a syringe and needle for injection into the insertion site.
5. One or two sterile 3 mL or 5 mL syringes for blood sampling.
6. Equipment for setting up a pressurized intravenous drip system so that the catheter does not clot.

b. Put the equipment together, make sure that it works properly, and identify any problems (Code: IIB1q2) [Difficulty: R, Ap, An]

See Figs. 5-12 and 5-22 for illustrations of how the pressure transducer, connecting tubing, stopcocks, infusion system, and monitoring electronics are assembled. See Fig. 5-23 for a completed radial artery system. Clinical experience is needed with these types of systems.

The process of calibrating the monitor for systemic artery pressures was briefly discussed earlier. Regardless of whether the catheter is placed into a systemic artery, pulmonary artery, umbilical artery, or superior vena cava, the equipment must be properly calibrated to ensure accurate data. When performing two-point calibration, all pressures should read "zero" when exposed to atmospheric pressure. This is the low point. The high point pressure for arterial pressure monitoring is commonly 100 mm Hg.

c. Correct any problems with the equipment (Code: IIB2q2) [Difficulty: R, Ap, An]

Table 5-1 lists problems, causes, prevention, and treatment for inaccurate pressure measurements with arterial or pulmonary artery catheters. Table 5-2 specifically lists problems with arterial lines. Fig. 5-24 shows common problem areas with arterial lines. Pulmonary artery catheters can have problems in the same areas.

d. Interpret the results of the insertion of arterial and umbilical monitoring lines (Code: IC2h) [Difficulty: R, Ap, An]

As discussed previously, if the equipment is properly assembled, the pressure readings will be accurate.

6. Pulmonary artery catheters
   a. Get the necessary equipment for the procedure (Code: IIA1q1) [Difficulty: R, Ap, An]

Pulmonary artery catheters come in several diameter sizes. The smallest can be advanced into a pediatric patient's vein. Most adults will have either a 5-French or 7-French catheter inserted. Once the appropriate size is determined, select a catheter that provides the information that is needed. A standard 5-French catheter can be used to measure pulmonary artery pressure and pulmonary capillary wedge pressure, and a mixed venous blood sample can be withdrawn from it for analysis. A 7-French thermodilution cardiac output catheter can do all these things and can give a central venous pressure and measure cardiac output through the computer (see Figs. 5-11 and 5-15). A 7-French fiber optic catheter can measure continuous $S\bar{v}O_2$ as well as PAP, PCWP, CVP, and cardiac output by the thermodilution method. Mixed venous blood can also be sampled for analysis.

b. Put the equipment together, make sure that it works properly, and identify any problems (Code: IIB1q1) [Difficulty: R, Ap, An]

The 5-French and 7-French catheters come self-contained as a single unit. The general assembly of the related tubing circuit and pressure transducer was discussed earlier and illustrated in Figs. 5-12 and 5-22. Clinical experience is needed. Make sure that all connections are watertight, the transducer calibrates accurately, and the balloon inflates and deflates properly.

The process of calibrating the monitor for pulmonary artery pressures or systemic artery pressures was briefly discussed earlier. Regardless of whether the catheter is placed into a systemic artery, pulmonary artery, umbilical artery, or superior vena cava, the equipment must be properly calibrated to ensure accurate data. When performing two-point calibration, all pressures should read "zero" when exposed to atmospheric pressure. This is the low point. The high point pressure for pulmonary artery pressure monitoring is commonly 30 mm Hg.

c. Correct any problems with the pulmonary artery catheter equipment (Code: IIB2q1) [Difficulty: R, Ap, An]

See Table 5-3 for a listing of the problems seen with pulmonary artery catheters and their causes, prevention, and treatment. Fig. 5-24 shows common problem areas with the related pressure tubing and equipment.

7. Cardiac output computer
   a. Get the correct cardiac output computer for the procedure (Code: IIA1q1) [Difficulty: R, Ap, An]

The makers of cardiac output pulmonary artery catheters (e.g., American Edwards Laboratories) also make thermodilution cardiac output computers. However, the computer is usually designed only for use with their brand of catheter. Make sure that you have a compatible catheter and computer.

b. Put the equipment together, make sure that it works properly, and identify any problems (Code: IIB1q1) [Difficulty: R, Ap, An]

Fig. 5-11 shows a thermodilution cardiac output pulmonary artery catheter. Note the thermistor connection to the cardiac output computer and the proximal port where the cooled solution is injected. See Fig. 5-15 for the assembly of the cardiac output computer to the catheter.

In addition, the computer must be programmed with the size of catheter, injectate volume, and injectate temperature.

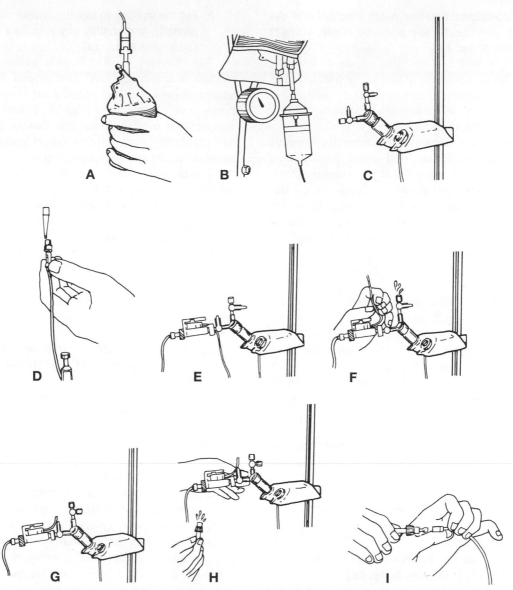

Fig. 5-22 Common steps in the assembly of the tubing circuit and pressure transducer to attach to an arterial or pulmonary artery catheter. Sterile technique must be maintained at all times. (Note: Individual institutions will vary these steps. Clinical practice is very important in this assembly.) **A,** Obtain a 250 to 500 mL bag of sterile, normal saline. Add 1 to 2 units of heparin per mL of solution. Attach an IV line with a macrodrip chamber. **B,** Insert the solution bag into a pressure bag. Inflate the pressure to about 100 mm Hg to force the fluid through the IV tubing. The pressure bag will be pumped up to 300 mm Hg at the end of this procedure to ensure that 3 drops of fluid flow through the tubing per minute to keep it patent. **C,** Attach the strain gauge pressure transducer to an IV pole. Let it and the monitor warm up. **D,** Attach the IV tubing to the continuous flush device (Sorenson Intraflow). **E,** Screw the continuous flush device into the transducer stopcock. **F,** Backflush the continuous flush device and transducer, with open stopcocks, so that all air is removed and replaced with the saline solution. **G,** Zero and calibrate the pressure transducer and monitor. **H,** Attach high-pressure tubing to the continuous flush device. Flush the air out of it. **I,** Attach the high-pressure tubing to the patient's arterial line or pulmonary artery catheter. Ensure that no air bubbles are present and that there is a continuous saline to blood connection. Accurate patient pressures should now be seen on the monitor. (From Oblouk Darovic G: *Hemodynamic monitoring,* Philadelphia, 1987, WB Saunders.)

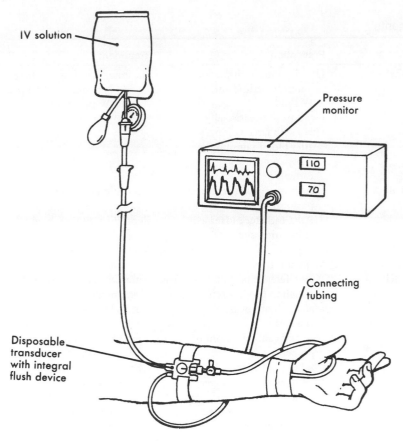

Fig. 5-23   Example of a complete setup for monitoring the arterial pressure. (From Daily EK, Schroeder JS: *Techniques in bedside hemodynamic monitoring,* ed 5, St Louis, 1994, Mosby.)

c. Correct any problems with the pulmonary artery catheter equipment and cardiac output computer (Code: IIB2q1) [Difficulty: R, Ap, An]

An error in the cardiac output value can be caused by an error in programming the computer or by not injecting the cooled solution through the proximal port in the required four seconds.

8. Continuous mixed venous oxygen saturation monitor
a. Get the correct monitor for the procedure (Code: IIA1q1) [Difficulty: R, Ap, An]

The makers of continuous mixed venous oxygen saturation pulmonary artery catheters (e.g., American Edwards Laboratories) also make the required monitor. However, the monitor is usually designed only for use with their brand of catheter. Make sure that you have a compatible catheter and monitor.

b. Put the equipment together, make sure that it works properly, and identify any problems (Code: IIB1q1) [Difficulty: R, Ap, An]

See Fig. 5-18 for a drawing of the continuous mixed venous oxygen saturation pulmonary artery catheter and its connection to the required monitor. Make sure the monitor is properly connected to the catheter. Calibrate the processor as directed by the manufacturer so that the monitor will give accurate patient values.

c. Correct any problems with the pulmonary artery catheter equipment (Code: IIB2q1) [Difficulty: R, Ap, An]

Errors can result from the catheter and monitor not being properly connected or the processor not being properly calibrated.

MODULE C   Patient assessment

---

1. Participate in the development of the patient's respiratory care plan (e.g., case management, developing and applying protocols, disease management education) (Code: IC4) [Difficulty: An]

Each clinical problem presented in this section requires its own individualized treatment. Be prepared to make recommendations to change the inspired oxygen percentage, give fluids if the patient is dehydrated, give diuretic medications to increase urine output if the patient is fluid overloaded, give vasodilator medications if the patient is hypertensive, or give vasoconstrictor medications if the patient is hypotensive.

See Fig. 5-25 for examples of diagnostic pathways. These can be used to help the clinician evaluate all the patient data. The diagnosis or pathophysiologic state can be determined by following the data down a given pathway. Normal values and common conditions associ-

Text continued on p. 156

| TABLE 5-1 | Inaccurate Pressure Measurements |

Problem	Cause	Prevention	Treatment
Damped waveforms and inaccurate pressures	Partial clotting at catheter tip	Use continuous drip with 1 unit heparin/1 mL IV fluid. Hand flush occasionally. Flush with large volume after blood sampling. Use heparin-coated catheters.	Aspirate, then flush catheter with heparinized fluid (*not* in PAW position).
	Tip moving against wall	Obtain more stable catheter position.	Reposition catheter.
	Kinking of catheter	Restrict catheter movement at insertion site.	Reposition to straighten catheter. Replace catheter.
Abnormally low or negative pressures	Incorrect air-reference level (above midchest level)	Maintain transducer air-reference port at midchest level; rezero after patient position changes.	Remeasure level of transducer air-reference and reposition at midchest level; rezero.
	Incorrect zeroing and calibration of monitor	Zero and calibrate monitor properly.	Recheck zero and calibration of monitor.
	Loose connection	Use Luer-Lok stopcocks.	Check all connections.
Abnormally high pressure reading	Pressure trapped by improper sequence of stopcock operation	Turn stopcocks in proper sequence when two pressures are measured on one transducer.	Thoroughly flush transducers with IV solution; rezero and turn stopcocks in proper sequence.
	Incorrect air-reference level (below midchest level)	Maintain transducer air-reference port at midchest level; recheck and rezero after patient position changes.	Check air-reference level; reset at midchest and rezero.
Inappropriate pressure waveform	Migration of catheter tip (e.g., in RV or PAW instead of in PA)	Establish optimal position carefully when introducing catheter initially. Suture catheter at insertion site and tape catheter to patient's skin.	Review waveform; if RV, inflate balloon; if PAW, deflate balloon and withdraw catheter slightly. Check position under fluoroscope and/or radiograph after reposition.
No pressure available	Transducer not open to catheter	Follow routine, systematic steps for pressure measurement.	Check system, stopcocks.
	Amplifiers still on *cal*, *zero*, or *off*		
Noise or fling in pressure waveform	Excessive catheter movement, particularly in PA	Avoid excessive catheter length in ventricle.	Try different catheter tip position.
	Excessive tubing length	Use shortest tubing possible (<3 to 4 feet).	Eliminate excess tubing.
	Excessive stopcocks	Minimize number of stopcocks.	Eliminate excess stopcocks.

From Daily and Schroeder: *Techniques in bedside hemodynamic monitoring,* ed 5, Mosby 1995.
PAW, Pulmonary artery wedge; *RV,* right ventricle; *PA,* pulmonary artery.

| TABLE 5-2 | Problems Encountered with Arterial Catheters | | |

Problem	Cause	Prevention	Treatment
Hematoma after withdrawal of needle	Bleeding or oozing at puncture site	Maintain firm pressure on site during withdrawal of catheter and for 5-15 min (as necessary) after withdrawal. Apply elastic tape (Elastoplast) firmly over puncture site.	Continue to hold pressure to puncture site until oozing stops.
		For femoral arterial puncture sites, leave a sandbag on site for 1-2 hr to prevent oozing.	Apply sandbag to femoral puncture site for 1-2 hr after removal of catheter.
		If patient is receiving heparin, discontinue 2 hr before catheter removal.	
Decreased or absent pulse distal to puncture site	Spasm of artery	Introduce arterial needle cleanly, nontraumatically.	Inject lidocaine locally at insertion site and 10 mg into arterial catheter.
	Thrombosis of artery	Use 1 unit heparin/1 mL IV fluid	Arteriotomy and Fogarty catheterization both distally and proximally from the puncture site result in return of pulse in more than 90% of cases if brachial or femoral artery is used.
Bleedback into tubing, dome, or transducer	Insufficient pressure on IV bag	Maintain 300 mm Hg pressure on IV bag. Use Luer-Lok stopcocks; tighten periodically.	Replace transducer. "Fast flush" through system.
	Loose connections		Tighten all connections.
Hemorrhage	Loose connections	Keep all connecting sites visible. Observe connecting sites frequently. Use built-in alarm system. Use Luer-Lok stopcocks.	Tighten all connections.
Emboli	Clot from catheter tip into bloodstream	Always aspirate and discard before flushing. Use continuous flush device. Use 1 unit heparin/1 mL IV fluid. Gently flush <2-4 mL.	Remove catheter.
Local infection	Forward movement of contaminated catheter	Carefully suture catheter at insertion site. Always use aseptic technique. Remove catheter after 72-96 hr.	Remove catheter. Prescribe antibiotic.
	Break in sterile technique Prolonged catheter use	Inspect and care for insertion site daily, including dressing change and antibiotic or iodophor ointment.	
Sepsis	Break in sterile technique Prolonged catheter use	Use percutaneous insertion. Always use aseptic technique. Remove catheter after 72-96 hr.	Remove catheter. Prescribe antibiotic.
	Bacterial growth in IV fluid	Change IV fluid bag, stopcocks, dome, and tubing every 24-48 hr. Do not use IV fluid containing glucose. Use sterile dead-ender caps on all ports of stopcocks. Carefully flush remaining blood from stopcocks after bloodsampling.	

From Daily and Schroeder: *Techniques in bedside hemodynamic monitoring,* ed 5, Mosby, 1995.

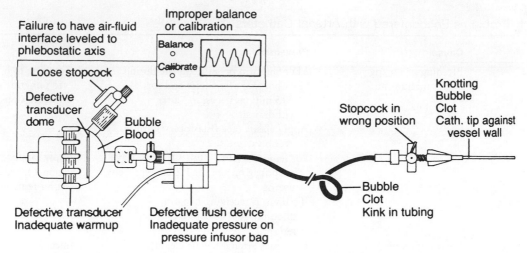

Fig. 5-24   Common problem areas with arterial and pulmonary artery catheters. (From Oblouk Darovic G: *Hemodynamic monitoring,* Philadelphia, 1987, WB Saunders.)

TABLE 5-3   Problems Encountered With PA Catheters

Problem	Cause	Prevention	Treatment
Phlebitis or local infection at insertion site	Mechanical irritation or contamination	Prepare skin properly before insertion. Use sterile technique during insertion and dressing change. Insert smoothly and rapidly. Use Teflon-coated introducer. Attach silver-impregnated cuff to introducer. Change dressings, stopcocks, and connecting tubing every 24 to 48 hr. Remove catheter or change insertion site every 4 days.	Remove catheter. Apply warm compresses. Give pain medication as necessary.
Ventricular irritability	Looping of excess catheter in right ventricle Migration of catheter from PA to RV Irritation of the endocardium during catheter passage	Suture catheter at insertion site; check chest film. Position catheter tip in main right or left PA. Keep balloon inflated during advancement; advance gently.	Reposition catheter; remove loop. Inflate balloon to encourage catheter flotation out to PA. Advance rapidly out to PA.
Apparent wedging of catheter with balloon *deflated*	Forward migration of catheter tip caused by blood flow, excessive loop in RV, or inadequate suturing of catheter at insertion site	Check catheter tip by fluoroscopy; position in main right or left PA. Check catheter position on radiography film if fluoroscopy is not used. Suture catheter in place at insertion site.	Aspirate blood from catheter; if catheter is wedged, sample will be arterialized and obtained with difficulty. If wedged, slowly pull back catheter until PA waveform appears. If not wedged, gently aspirate and flush catheter with saline; catheter tip can partially clot, causing damping that resembles damped PAW waveform.

From Daily and Schroeder: *Techniques in bedside hemodynamic monitoring,* ed 5, Mosby, 1995.
PA, Pulmonary artery; *RV,* Right ventricle; *PAW,* pulmonary artery wedge

TABLE 5-3 Problems Encountered With PA Catheters—cont'd

Problem	Cause	Prevention	Treatment
Pulmonary hemorrhage or infarction, or both	Distal migration of catheter tip Continuous or prolonged wedging of catheter Overinflation of balloon while catheter is wedged Failure of balloon to deflate	Check chest film immediately after insertion and 12-24 hr later; remove any catheter loop in RA or RV. Leave balloon deflated. Suture catheter at skin to prevent inadvertent advancement. Position catheter in main right or left PA. Pull catheter back to pulmonary artery if it spontaneously wedges. Do not flush catheter when in wedge position. Inflate balloon slowly with only enough air to obtain a PAW waveform. Do not inflate 7-Fr catheter with more than 1-1.5 cc air. Do not inflate if resistance is met.	Deflate balloon. Place patient on side (catheter tip down). Stop anticoagulation. Consider "wedge" angiogram. Intubate with double-lumen ET. Surgery, if severe hemorrhage.
"Overwedging" or damped PAW	Overinflation of balloon Eccentric inflation of balloon	Watch waveform during inflation; inject only enough air to obtain PAW pressure. Do not inflate 7-Fr catheter with more than 1-1.5 cc air. Check inflated balloon shape before insertion.	Deflate balloon; reinflate slowly with only enough air to obtain PAW pressure. Deflate balloon; reposition and slowly reinflate.
PA balloon rupture	Overinflation of balloon Frequent inflations of balloon Syringe deflation damaging wall of balloon	Inflate slowly with only enough air to obtain a PAW pressure. Monitor PAd pressure as reflection of PAW and LVEDP. Allow passive deflation of balloon. Remove syringe after inflation.	Remove syringe to prevent further air injection. Monitor PAd pressure.
Infection	Nonsterile insertion techniques Contamination via skin	Use sterile techniques. Use sterile catheter sleeve. Prepare skin with effective antiseptic (chlorhexidine). Apply iodophor ointment and sterile gauze dressing daily. Do not use clear semipermeable dressing. Inspect site daily. Reassess need for catheter after 3 days. Avoid internal jugular approach.	Remove catheter. Use antibiotics.
	Contamination through stopcock ports or catheter hub	Use sterile dead-ender caps on all stopcock ports. Change IV solution, stopcock, and tubing every 24-48 hr. Do not use IV solution that contains glucose.	
	Fluid contamination from transducer through cracked membrane of disposable dome	Check transducer domes for cracks. Change transducers every 48 hr. Change disposable dome after countershock. Do not use IV solution that contains glucose.	
	Prolonged catheter placement	Change catheter insertion site every 4 days.	
Heart block during insertion of catheter	Mechanical irritation of His bundle in patients with preexisting left bundle branch block	Insert catheter expeditiously with balloon inflated. Insert transvenous pacing catheter before PA catheter insertion.	Use temporary pacemaker or flotation catheter with pacing wire.

PAd, Pulmonary artery diastolic; *LVEDP,* left ventricular end-diastolic pressure; *ET,* endotracheal tube.

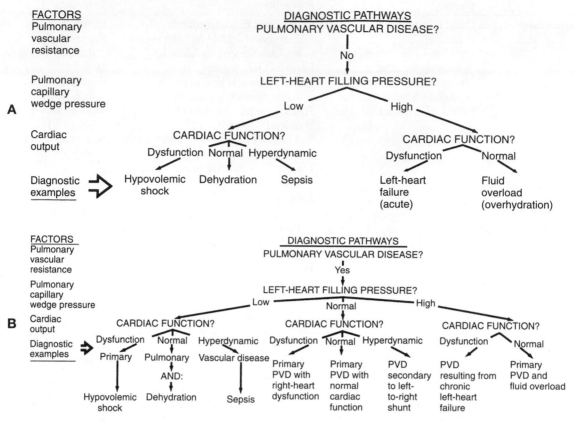

Fig. 5-25 Possible diagnostic pathways for patients with (A) and without (B) pulmonary vascular disease (PVD). In both cases, the pulmonary vascular resistance, pulmonary capillary wedge pressure, and cardiac output are measured. High, normal, or low values lead down different pathways. Previous discussions and clinical experience are needed to determine the final diagnosis. Sepsis may be associated with normal left-heart filling pressures. Primary PVD may be caused by pulmonary emboli, pulmonary artery disease (vasculitis, "primary" pulmonary hypertension), respiratory distress syndromes, hypoxic vasoconstriction, or drugs. (From Osgood CF, Watson MH, Slaughter MS et al: *Respir Care* 29(1):25–34, 1984.)

ated with abnormal values were discussed earlier in this chapter. Interpret the information given by the intravascular monitor.

EXAM HINT

Closely review the following concepts because they have been tested on previous examinations.
1. Interpretation of pulmonary artery pressure (PAP)
   An increased PAP is usually associated with one of the following: fluid overload, heart failure or pulmonary hypertension (increased pulmonary vascular resistance) from COPD (emphysema), pulmonary embolism, or persistent pulmonary hypertension of the newborn (PPHN).
2. Interpretation of pulmonary capillary wedge pressure (PCWP)
   An increased PCWP is usually associated with one of the following: fluid overload, heart failure, mitral valve insufficiency, cardiac tamponade, or constrictive pericarditis.

Treatment for fluid overload and/or heart failure usually includes fluid restriction and diuretics (Lasix) and digitalis-type drugs (Lanoxin). A decreased PCWP is usually associated with dehydration, treated with increased fluids, or vasodilation, treated with vasoconstricting drugs. When interpreting the PAP and PCWP together, it is very important to calculate the difference between the PAP diastolic pressure and the PCWP. Normally, the difference, or gradient, is 5 mm Hg or less. In other words, if the PAP diastolic pressure minus the PCWP is 5 mm Hg or less, the patient does not have pulmonary hypertension. A gradient of more than 5 mm Hg indicates pulmonary hypertension.
3. Interpretation of cardiac output
   A decreased cardiac output is usually caused by hypovolemia, treated with increased fluids, or heart failure, treated with digitalis-type drugs (Lanoxin). Cardiac output may also be decreased on a ventilator dependent patient with high peak

pressures or PEEP level because of the increased intrathoracic pressure. When this is presented in an NBRC question and a request for care is called for, the best response is to decrease the PEEP level.

BIBLIOGRAPHY

AARC Clinical Practice Guideline: Capnography/capnometry during mechanical ventilation. *Respir Care,* 40(12):1321-1324, 1995.

Anton WR, Raghu G: Measuring end-tidal carbon dioxide tension at maximal exhalation to improve its utility during T-piece weaning trials, *Respir Care* 35(11):1082-1083, 1990.

Bakow ED: A limitation of capnography, *Respir Care* 27(2):167-168, 1982.

Branson RD, Campbell RS: Cardiovascular monitoring. In Branson RD, Hess DR, Chatburn RL, editors: *Respiratory care equipment,* ed 2, Philadelphia, 1999, Lippincott Williams & Wilkins.

Cairo JM: Assessment of physiologic function. In Cairo JM, Pilbeam SP: *Mosby's respiratory care equipment,* ed 6, St Louis, 1999, Mosby.

Carlon GC, Ray C, Miodownik S et al: Capography in mechanically ventilated patients, *Crit Care Med* 16(5):550-556, 1988.

Clark DB, Marshall SG: Mixed venous oxygen saturation measurement. II. General and specific clinical applications, *Respir Ther* 81-86, Nov/Dec 1986.

Daily EK, Schroeder JS: *Techniques in bedside hemodynamic monitoring,* ed 5, St Louis, 1994, Mosby.

Deshpande VM, Pilbeam SP, Dixon RJ: *A comprehensive review in respiratory care,* Norwalk, Conn, 1988, Appleton & Lange.

Divertie MB, McMichan JC: Continuous monitoring of mixed venous oxygen saturation, *Chest* 85(3):423-428, 1984.

Fahey PJ, Harris K, Vanderwarf C: Clinical experience with continuous monitoring of mixed venous oxygen saturation in respiratory failure, *Chest* 86(5):748-752, 1984.

Harris K: Noninvasive monitoring of gas exchange, *Respir Care* 32(7):544-557, 1987.

Hess D: Capnometry and capnography: technical aspects, physiologic aspects, and clinical applications, *Respir Care* 35(6):557-576, 1990.

Hess DR, Branson RD: Noninvasive respiratory monitoring equipment. In Branson RD, Hess DR, Chatburn RL, editors: *Respiratory care equipment,* ed 2, Philadelphia, 1999, Lippincott Williams & Wilkins.

Hess D: Respiratory care monitoring. In Burton GC, Hodgkin JE, Ward JJ, editors: *Respiratory care: a guide to clinical practice,* ed 4, Philadelphia, 1997, Lippincott-Raven.

Hunt GE: Diagnostic procedures at the bedside. In Fink JB, Hunt GE, editors: *Clinical practice in respiratory care.* Philadelphia, 1999, Lippincott-Raven.

Jaquith SM: The oximetric opticath: what is it and how can it facilitate nursing management of the critically ill patient? *Crit Care Nurse,* 55-58, May/June 1984.

Kandel G, Aberman A: Mixed venous oxygen saturation: its role in the assessment of the critically ill patient, *Arch Intern Med* 143:1400-1402, 1983.

Kinasewitz GT: Use of end-tidal capnography during mechanical ventilation, *Respir Care* 25(2):169-171, 1982.

Krider SJ: Cardiac output assessment. In Wilkins RL, Sheldon RL, Krider SJ, editors: *Clinical assessment in respiratory care,* ed 4, St Louis, 2000, Mosby.

Krider SJ: Invasively monitored hemodynamic pressures. In Wilkins RL, Sheldon RL, Krider SJ, editors: *Clinical assessment in respiratory care,* ed 4, St Louis, 2000, Mosby.

Malinowski T: Respiratory monitoring in the intensive care unit. In Wilkins RL, Krider SJ, Sheldon RL, editors: *Clinical assessment in respiratory care,* ed 3, St Louis, 1990, Mosby.

Marini JJ: Obtaining meaningful data from the Swan-Ganz catheter, *Respir Care* 30(7):572-585, 1985.

Mathews PJ, Gregg BL: Monitoring and management of the patient in the ICU. In Scanlan CL, Wilkins RL, Stoller JK, editors: *Egan's fundamentals of respiratory care,* ed 7, St Louis, 1999, Mosby.

McMichan JC: Continuous monitoring of mixed venous oxygen saturation in clinical practice, *Mount Sinai J Med* 51(5):569-572, 1984.

Nuzzo PF, Anton WR: Practical applications of capnography, *Respir Ther,* 12-17, Nov/Dec 1986.

Oblouk Darovic G: *Hemodynamic monitoring,* Philadelphia, 1987, WB Saunders.

Osgood CF, Watson MH, Slaughter MS et al: Hemodynamic monitoring in respiratory care, *Respir Care* 29(1):25-34, 1984.

Paulus DA: Invasive monitoring of respiratory gas exchange: continuous measurement of mixed venous oxygen saturation, *Respir Care* 32(7):535-543, 1987.

Pilbeam SP: *Mechanical ventilation: physiological and clinical applications,* ed 3, St Louis, 1998, Mosby.

Ruppel G: *Manual of pulmonary function testing,* ed 6, St Louis., 1994, Mosby.

Shapiro BA, Harrison RA, Cane RD et al: *Clinical application of blood gases,* ed 4, St Louis, 1989, Mosby.

Shapiro BA, Kacmarek RM, Cane RD, et al., editors: *Clinical application of respiratory care,* ed 4. St Louis, 1991, Mosby.

Whitaker K: *Comprehensive Perinatal & pediatric respiratory care,* ed 2, Albany, NY, Delmar, 1997.

White GC: *Equipment theory for respiratory care,* ed 3, Albany, NY, Delmar, 1999.

Wiedemann HP: Invasive monitoring techniques in the ventilated patient. In Kacmarek RM, Stoller JK, editors: *Current respiratory care,* Toronto, 1988, BC Decker.

SELF-STUDY QUESTIONS

1. The wave form sequence seen during the insertion of a pulmonary artery catheter is:
   A. RA, RV, PAP, PCWP
   B. RV, RA, PAP, PCWP
   C. RA, RV, PCWP, PAP
   D. Ao, RA, RV, PAP

2. A patient with advanced emphysema is admitted to the respiratory intensive care unit. He is placed on a 24% Venturi-type mask and has a pulmonary artery catheter inserted. His initial pulmonary vascular resistance (PVR) is 9 mm/Hg/L/min and PaO_2 is 57 torr. The physician orders him increased to 28% oxygen. The resulting PVR is

5 mm Hg/L/min and PaO_2 is 63 torr. Based on this information, what would you recommend?
A. Decrease the oxygen to 24%.
B. Place the patient on a ventilator.
C. Administer a bronchodilating agent such as albuterol.
D. Keep the patient on 28% oxygen.

3. Stroke volume:
A. Is an indicator of the adequacy of perfusion of the body tissues.
B. Is the output of blood for a minute.
C. Has a range of 60 to 120 mL in the adult.
D. Is the resistance to flow.

4. Your patient is in the intensive care unit and is being monitored with a pulmonary artery catheter. She has the following parameters: PAP of 35/20 mm Hg, PCWP of 9 mm Hg, central venous pressure of 9 cm water. You would interpret the data to indicate that she:
A. Has right ventricular failure/cor pulmonale.
B. Has left ventricular failure.
C. Has increased pulmonary vascular resistance.
D. Is hypovolemic.

5. A 40-year-old patient receiving mechanical ventilation has an arterial line in place. It is noticed that there is a significant difference between the blood pressure taken by cuff on the left arm and blood pressure taken by arterial line on the right arm. What could explain this difference?
I. A clot is at the tip of the catheter.
II. There is an air bubble in the arterial line.
III. The ventilator's peak pressure is too high.
IV. The patient has a ventricular septal defect.
A. I and II only
B. II and III only
C. I, III, and IV only
D. I, II, III, and IV

6. An adult patient is receiving mechanical ventilation when the following data are gathered:

	9:00 A.M.	11:00 A.M.
PaO_2	75 torr	53 torr
pulmonary vascular resistance	120 dynes/sec/cm^{-5}	340 dynes/sec/cm^{-5}
pulmonary capillary wedge pressure	8 mm Hg	10 mm Hg
pulmonary artery pressure	25/10 mm Hg	42/21 mm Hg

How should the results be interpreted?
A. Pulmonary edema
B. Pulmonary embolism
C. Pneumonia
D. Cardiac tamponade

7. A patient is receiving mechanical ventilation with the SIMV mode and a mandatory rate of 10/minute. End-tidal carbon dioxide monitoring is being done and the following data are recorded:

	4:00 P.M.	6:00 P.M.
Set tidal volume	700 mL	700 mL
Set rate	10	10
$P_{ET}CO_2$	33 torr	41 torr
$PaCO_2$	42 torr	43 torr

How can this data be explained?
A. Alveolar ventilation has decreased.
B. Pulmonary edema has developed.
C. The patient is hyperventilating.
D. The patient's cardiac output has increased.

8. A patient with chronic bronchitis is being monitored with regular measurements of arterial blood gas values and capnometry. The following data are available:

$PaCO_2$	53 torr
PaO_2	67 torr
$P_{ET}CO_2$	33 torr
$P_{\bar{E}}CO_2$	20 torr

Calculate the patient's V_D/V_T.
A. .30
B. .38
C. .62
D. .71

9. A patient has had an arterial line inserted. What should be done to ensure that accurate blood pressure readings are obtained?
I. Open the stopcock to room air to "zero" the transducer.
II. Make sure that air fills the transducer dome.
III. Have the patient lie flat to measure the blood pressure.
IV. Fill the pressure tubing with saline solution.
A. I and II only
B. II and IV only
C. I, II, and III only
D. I, III, and IV only

10. A 40-year-old patient recovering from ARDS is receiving mechanical ventilation with a tidal volume of 650 mL. The patient has an arterial line, a pulmonary artery catheter, and capnometry for monitoring. The following information is gathered after a change in PEEP level:

$PaCO_2$	43 torr
PaO_2	79 torr
$P\bar{v}O_2$	32 torr
$P_{ET}CO_2$	38 torr
$P_{\bar{E}}CO_2$	22 torr

Calculate the patient's V_D.
A. 273 mL
B. 319 mL
C. 338 mL
D. 384 mL

11. A 35-year-old patient in the intensive care unit has the following hemodynamic data. Which of them indicates a problem with the patient?
A. SVR of 600 dynes/sec/cm^{-5}
B. CI of 3 L/min/m^2 of body surface area
C. $P\bar{v}O_2$ of 38 torr
D. Shunt of 4%

12. A patient with a history of congestive heart failure is inadvertently given intravenous fluids of 2000 mL instead of the ordered amount of 200 mL. Which of the following is most likely to be seen?
A. Decreased lung markings on chest radiograph
B. Increased pulmonary capillary wedge pressure
C. Increased PaO_2
D. Decreased pulmonary artery pressure

13. A patient hospitalized with leg vein thrombosis experiences sudden shortness of breath. Which of the following should be recommended to evaluate the patient's situation?
    A. Lung compliance
    B. Electrocardiogram
    C. Chest radiograph
    D. V_D/V_T

14. An unconscious 25-year-old patient is admitted with viral pneumonia, vomiting, and diarrhea. Mechanical ventilation is initiated and a flow-directed pulmonary artery (Swan-Ganz) catheter is inserted. The following data are gathered:

Pulmonary artery pressure	22/8 mm Hg
Pulmonary capillary wedge pressure	3 mm Hg
Central venous pressure	0 mm Hg
Blood pressure	90/60 mm Hg
Pulse	142/min

    What is the most likely cause of these findings?
    A. Hypovolemia
    B. High ventilating pressures
    C. Bronchospasm
    D. Rupture of the balloon on the catheter

Answer Key

1. **C.** Rationale: The pulmonary artery catheter first enters the right atrium (RA) of the heart. It then follows the flow of blood through the heart by entering the right ventricle (RV). Next the catheter enters the pulmonary artery and the pulmonary artery pressure (PAP) is seen. When the balloon at the tip of the catheter advances as far into the pulmonary artery as it can, it "wedges" in place. The resulting pressure is the called the pulmonary capillary wedge pressure (PCWP). See Fig. 5-13 to see the sequence.

2. **D.** Rationale: The patient should be kept on 28% oxygen because the pulmonary vascular resistance decreased from 9 to 5 mm Hg/L/min and PaO_2 increased from 57 to 63 torr when the patient was increased from 24% oxygen. The patient is not hypoxemic; there is no indication to begin mechanical ventilation. A bronchodilating agent such as albuterol may help the patient's breathing somewhat, but it is not effective at reducing pulmonary vascular resistance.

3. **C.** Rationale: Stroke volume is the volume pumped by each ventricle with each heartbeat and has a range of 60 to 120 mL in the adult. Cardiac index (CI) is an indicator of the adequacy of perfusion of the body tissues. Cardiac output (CO) is the output of blood for 1 minute. Afterload is the resistance to flow. It is caused by the level of tone in the blood vessels and the viscosity of the blood.

4. **C.** Rationale: The patient's pulmonary vascular resistance can be found by calculating the pulmonary artery diastolic pressure minus the pulmonary capillary wedge pressure (PAd – PCWP) as follows:

PAd	20 mm Hg
PCWP	– 9 mm Hg
	11 mm Hg

    Because a normal PAd – PCWP gradient is no more than 5 mm Hg, this patient's value of 11 mm Hg indicates increased pulmonary vascular resistance. Even though the patient's PAP is elevated at 35/20 mm Hg, that pressure alone does not give enough information to determine that the patient has right ventricular failure/cor pulmonale. An increased right ventricular pressure in a patient with COPD indicates right ventricular failure/cor pulmonale. Because the patient has a normal PCWP of 9 mm Hg she does not have left ventricular failure. This problem is identified by an increased PCWP. This same normal PCWP of 9 mm Hg indicates normal blood volume. Hypovolemia is identified by a PCWP that is less than 4 mm Hg.

5. **A.** Rationale: If a clot is at the tip of the catheter it will prevent the patient's blood pressure from being transmitted back to the transducer to be measured. By withdrawing the clot, the lumen of the catheter will be open and the blood pressure can be measured. If an air bubble is in the arterial line, the measured blood pressure will be less than actual. This is because the patient's blood pressure will partially collapse the gas bubble (Boyle's law) and transmit a lower pressure to the transducer. Withdrawing the air bubble allows the patient's blood pressure to be accurately sent to the transducer. If the ventilator's peak pressure is too high, the patient's cardiac output will be reduced. This will result in a drop in blood pressure that will be measured equally on both arms. There is no evidence that the patient has a ventricular septal defect. Even if a septal defect were present, the blood pressure would be the same in both arms.

6. **B.** Rationale: There are two significant changes in the patient's parameters that indicate that the patient has a pulmonary embolism. First, the patient's pulmonary vascular resistance has almost tripled in 2 hours. Second, the patient's pulmonary artery diastolic pressure minus the pulmonary capillary wedge pressure (PAd – PCWP) difference has increased significantly.

	9:00 A.M.	11:00 A.M.
PAd	10 mm Hg	21 mm Hg
PCWP	– 8 mm Hg	–10 mm Hg
	2 mm Hg	11 mm Hg
	(Normal)	(Increased)

    The fact that both of these parameters have quickly increased significantly, combined with the sudden drop in the patient's oxygen level, indicates a cause that can be only a pulmonary embolism. Because the patient's pulmonary capillary wedge pressure (PCWP) remains normal at 8 mm Hg and 10 mm Hg, pulmonary edema is not supported as a diagnosis. Pulmonary edema results in an increased PCWP. Pneumonia will result in hypoxemia. However, the other parameters do not match this diagnosis. Cardiac tamponade will decrease the patient's cardiac output but will not increase pulmonary vascular resistance or PCWP.

7. **A.** Rationale: The increase in the patient's $P_{ET}CO_2$ from 35 torr to 45 torr indicates that alveolar ventilation has decreased. There is no data that correlates with pulmonary edema (such as an increased pulmonary capillary wedge pressure). If the patient were hyperventilating, the $P_{ET}CO_2$ would have decreased instead of increased. Also the $PaCO_2$ would have decreased. There is no data that correlates with an increased cardiac output (such as a decreased difference between the oxygen content of arterial blood and the oxygen content of venous blood).

8. **C.** Rationale: This problem requires the calculation of the decimal fraction or percentage of dead space. To do so, place

both the patient's arterial and end-tidal carbon dioxide values into this formula:

$$V_D/V_T = \frac{(PaCO_2 - P_{\bar{E}}CO_2)}{PaCO_2}$$

In which:

V_D/V_T (or V_D) = The patient's physiologic dead space
$PaCO_2$ = The patient's arterial carbon dioxide pressure
$P_{\bar{E}}CO_2$ = The patient's average exhaled carbon dioxide pressure

Calculate the V_D/V_T as follows:

$$V_D/V_T = \frac{(53 - 20)}{53}$$
$$= \frac{33}{53} = .62$$

The patient's V_D/V_T or V_D fraction can be recorded as .62 or 62%. (Note that this equation must be used when the patient's tidal volume is not known.)

9. **D.** Rationale: It is necessary to "zero" the transducer by exposing it to local barometric pressure. Adjust the transducer so that it reads zero when exposed to room barometric pressure. The patient must lie flat in bed with the transducer at midchest level to give accurate blood pressure readings. If the patient sits up, the blood pressure will read low. If the patient's head is lower than his or her body, the blood pressure will read too high. Saline must fill the pressure tubing, transducer dome, and arterial catheter so that the patient's blood pressure is measured accurately. If air fills the transducer dome, it will be variably compressed based on the patient's systolic and diastolic blood pressure changes. This is the result of Boyle's law and results in a lower-than-actual blood pressure being measured.

10. **B.** Rationale: This problem requires the calculation of the patient's dead space volume. To do so, place both the patient's arterial and end-tidal carbon dioxide values into this formula:

$$V_D = \frac{(PaCO_2 - P_{\bar{E}}CO_2)}{PaCO_2} \times \dot{V}_E$$

In which:

V_D = The patient's physiologic dead space
$\dot{V}_E$ = Average exhaled tidal volume
$PaCO_2$ = The patient's arterial carbon dioxide pressure
$P_{\bar{E}}CO_2$ = The patient's average exhaled carbon dioxide pressure

Calculate the V_D as follows:

$$V_D = \frac{(43 - 22)}{43}$$
$$= \frac{21}{43} \times 650 = .49 \times 650 \text{ mL} = 319 \text{ mL}$$

The patient's physiologic V_D volume equals 319 mL. (Note that this equation must be used when the patient's tidal volume is known.)

11. **A.** Rationale: A normal adult's systemic vascular resistance (SVR) has a range of 900 to 1400 dynes/sec/cm^{-5}. This patient's SVR value of 600 dynes/sec/cm^{-5} is well below normal. This may result from vasodilation or hypovolemia. All of the other values are within the normal range. See Box 5-2, Table 3-11, and discussion earlier in the chapter.

12. **B.** Rationale: If excessive fluid is given to a patient with congestive heart failure, the fluid is likely to back up into the pulmonary vessels because the left ventricle cannot pump effectively. This backup of fluid into the lungs will increase the pulmonary capillary wedge pressure. The patient should be watched for pulmonary edema. If the patient develops pulmonary edema, a chest radiograph will show increased rather than decreased lung markings and fluid in the lungs. The patient's PaO_2 can be expected to decrease rather than increase if pulmonary edema develops. If fluid backs up from the left ventricle into the pulmonary vessels the pulmonary artery pressure will increase along with the pulmonary capillary wedge pressure.

13. **D.** Rationale: The patient's history and current situation suggest that a pulmonary embolism has occurred. The V_D/V_T test should be performed to determine whether the patient's dead space has increased. If it has, this will match the clinical suspicion of a pulmonary embolism. It is doubtful that the patient's lung compliance will change if a pulmonary embolism occurred. There is no specific change in the electrocardiogram that corresponds with a pulmonary embolism or other sudden cause of shortness of breath. Chest radiograph changes are unlikely soon after a pulmonary embolism has occurred.

14. **A.** Rationale: The patient's history of vomiting and diarrhea would lead to a loss of body fluids. Hypovolemia correlates with tachycardia and all of the patient's low blood pressure values. High ventilating pressures can result in a drop in the cardiac output. This can cause the systemic blood pressure to drop, but is unlikely to result in all of the hemodynamic values being low. In addition, there is no information given that relates to the patient's ventilating pressures. There is no mention of the patient's breath sounds revealing bronchospasm. Even if bronchospasm were present, it would not cause all of the low hemodynamic values. If the balloon on the catheter were to rupture there would be a small volume of gas released into the pulmonary circulation. This would act as a small gas embolism. Although not good for the patient, this small gas embolism is unlikely to cause a drop in all of the hemodynamic pressures.

6 Oxygen and Medical Gas Therapy

A review of the most recent Written Registry Exams has shown an average of six questions (6% of the exam) on oxygen and medical gas therapy.

<hr/>

MODULE A	**Ensure that the patient is adequately oxygenated**

1. Oxygen administration

a. Minimize hypoxemia by positioning the patient properly (Code: IIB4c) [Difficulty: An]

Usually a patient who is short of breath when lying supine should be repositioned to sit more upright in a Fowler's or semi-Fowler's position. This seems to work best in patients with bilateral pulmonary problems such as congestive heart failure or pneumonia. If the patient cannot sit up and the lung problem is one sided, roll the patient so that the more-functional lung is down. The good lung should be positioned up in the following exceptions:

1. Undrained pulmonary abscess that should not be drained into the good lung.
2. Neonatal congenital diaphragmatic hernia in which the good lung should not be compressed by the bowel in the chest cavity.
3. Pulmonary interstitial emphysema in which, by lying on the bad lung, the air leak and functional residual capacity can be reduced.

In either case, always ask the patient whether the new position helps to make breathing easier. If not, reposition the patient until breathing is more comfortable with less shortness of breath.

b. Administer oxygen as needed and make a recommendation to change the fractional inspired oxygen concentration or oxygen flow to spontaneously breathing patients. (Code: IIIB4c and IIIC3a) [Difficulty: An]

Oxygen (O_2) must be administered in doses (up to 100%) that are adequate to treat hypoxemia, decrease the patient's work of breathing, or decrease the work of the heart. Because the Food and Drug Administration has declared supplemental oxygen to be a drug, there must be a physician's order to give it to a patient or to make a change in the percentage. The only exceptions are when there are recognized protocols in your institution to give oxygen under certain limited conditions. For example, all patients with a diagnosed heart attack are given a nasal cannula at 2 L/min, or all patients undergoing cardiopulmonary resuscitation (CPR) receive 100% oxygen.

See Chapter 3 (Module A) for a listing of indications for drawing blood for an arterial blood gas (ABG) measurement. This list should be fairly complete for conditions that justify the need for supplemental oxygen. In general, the goal of giving supplemental oxygen is to keep the patient's PaO_2 level between 60 and 100 torr. Exceptions include carbon monoxide poisoning, severe anemia, and CPR, when the hope is to fully saturate the hemoglobin and increase the plasma oxygen content as much as possible. Oxygen should not be given without proof of hypoxemia or another clinical justification. When those conditions have been corrected, the oxygen percentage should be adjusted accordingly.

Giving supplemental oxygen is not without risk. The following is a list of oxygen-related problems that may be clinically seen:

O_2-induced hypoventilation. This is something to watch for in patients who have an elevated carbon dioxide level because of severe emphysema, chronic bronchitis, or both (known as chronic obstructive pulmonary disease [COPD]). A common clinical goal is to keep the PaO_2 level between 50 and 60 torr. Check the blood gases frequently for the oxygen and carbon dioxide level.

Retinopathy of prematurity (ROP) (formerly called retrolental fibroplasia or RLF). This type of blindness is found in some premature neonates who were given high levels of supplemental oxygen. The exact cause is not completely understood, but is related primarily to the degree of prematurity. Keeping the PaO_2 in the range of 50 to 60 torr for the first week and 50 to 70 torr after that should help to prevent the problem.

Denitrogenation absorption atelectasis. Giving more than 80% oxygen can result in atelectasis of underventilated alveoli after the oxygen has been taken up by the blood.

Central nervous system abnormalities. A patient who is breathing 100% oxygen in a hyperbaric chamber can have muscle tremors and seizures.

Pulmonary O_2 toxicity. In general, it appears that patients can breathe up to 50% oxygen for prolonged periods without significant damage. If clinically possible, many practitioners try to limit their patients to no more than 48 to 72 hours of breathing more than 50% oxygen.

<hr/>

📖 EXAM HINT

The National Board of Respiratory Care (NBRC) is known to ask questions that relate to the proper use of oxygen and the hazards associated with its use. Expect to see at least one question that deals with the need to decrease the oxygen percentage for a

COPD patient who has shown an increased $PaCO_2$ when given too much supplemental oxygen.

---

c. Measure the patient's oxygen percentage, oxygen liter flow, or both (Code: IIIA1I) [Difficulty: An]

Always measure the patient's inspired O_2 percentage (F_IO_2) if possible. The gas sample should be taken as close as possible to the patient to minimize the chance of dilution from room air. Record the oxygen percentage on the arterial blood gas order slip, in the department records, and in the patient's chart if needed. As discussed in Chapter 3, the oxygen percentage must be known to interpret the patient's PaO_2 level.

The oxygen liter flow is all that can be recorded with the following devices: nasal cannula, nasal catheter, simple mask, partial rebreather mask, nonrebreather mask, and transtracheal oxygen catheter. There is a direct relationship between the liter flow and the oxygen percentage, but it is not predictably accurate.

d. Prevent the patient from becoming hypoxemic by using proper technique (Code: IIIB4c) [Difficulty: An]

Use caution and plan ahead to minimize any time that the oxygen supply to the patient is cut off or reduced. When changing equipment of any kind, have the replacement set up and tested for proper function before replacing the current setup.

It is well known that suctioning the airway reduces the patient's oxygen level. This can result in dangerous dysrhythmias. Remember to increase the patient's inspired oxygen percentage about 1 minute before, during, and for at least 1 minute after suctioning. It is acceptable and safe to give 100% oxygen for short periods like this. Remember to reduce the oxygen percentage or liter flow to the previous level once the patient is stable after the procedure. Reanalyze the percentage if possible.

2. Oxygen and specialty gas analyzers

a. Get the necessary equipment for the procedure (Code: IIA1h5) [Difficulty: An]

b. Put the equipment together, make sure that it works properly, and identify any problems with it (Code: IIB1h5) [Difficulty: An]

c. Fix any problems with the equipment (Code: IIB2h5)[Difficulty: R, Ap, An]

Because there are so many different models available, consult an equipment book or the manufacturer's literature for details of the various analyzers. All portable, handheld analyzers fall into one of the following categories: electric, physical/paramagnetic, and electrochemical.

Calibration is done on all oxygen analyzers by sampling room air, adjusting a calibration control if necessary to have the unit show 21% oxygen, sampling 100% oxygen, and adjusting a calibration control if necessary to have the unit show 100% oxygen. In general, always follow the manufacturer's guidelines for setup and calibration.

Electric analyzers. These analyzers basically operate by comparing the cooling effects of an oxygen-enriched gas sample on a heated wire with the cooling effects of a room air gas sample on a heated wire. The oxygen-enriched gas cools faster than the room air gas. This is known as the principle of thermal conductivity. Each sample must be drawn into the analyzer through a capillary line. These analyzers are designed to work only in oxygen and nitrogen gas mixes. Do *not* use them around flammable gases such as those found in anesthesia. Failure to calibrate can be caused by a weak battery, a plugged capillary line, or a defect in an electrical component.

Physical/paramagnetic analyzers. These analyzers make use of the fact that oxygen is attracted toward a magnetic field (paramagnetic property). The more oxygen there is in a sample gas, the more the magnetic field is altered. These units can be used with all types of gases and are safe in the operating room with flammable and explosive anesthetics. A silica gel-filled container is in line with the capillary tube to dry out the sample gas before it gets to the analyzing chamber. Failure to calibrate can be caused by water or a defect in the analyzing chamber, a weak battery, or a plugged capillary line.

Electrochemical analyzers: polarographic and galvanic fuel cell. Both the polarographic an galvanic fuel cells make use of the fact that each oxygen molecule accepts up to two electrons and becomes chemically reduced. The more oxygen in the gas sample, the more electrons are released from an oxidizing electrolyte solution. This is measured as an electrical current that is proportional to the oxygen percentage. These analyzers can continuously monitor and display the oxygen percentage. Both types are safe by themselves in the presence of flammable gases, but the added alarm systems are electrically powered and may make the units unsafe. Polarographic analyzers use a battery to polarize the gas sampling probe. Because of this, they have a faster response time than do the galvanic fuel cell types. Galvanic fuel cell analyzers do not need a battery for power. However, they usually include alarms that are battery powered.

Failure to calibrate either type can be caused by a weak battery, an exhausted supply of chemical reactant in the gas sampling probe, or an electronic failure. The galvanic units must have their probes kept dry to read accurately. Both types are pressure sensitive. High altitude causes them to display a lower-than-true oxygen percentage, and high pressure as seen in a ventilator circuit with positive end-expiratory pressure (PEEP) causes the units to display a higher-than-true oxygen percentage.

Specialty gas analyzers. The specialty gas analyzers (helium, nitrogen, and carbon monoxide) are mainly used with pulmonary function testing procedures and are discussed in Chapter 4. It may be necessary to use a helium analyzer if a helium and oxygen mix is given to a patient.

Nitric oxide (NO) is delivered through the INOvent delivery system. It is able to deliver set amounts of therapeutic NO and continuously monitor the amount of NO given to the patient along with nitrogen dioxide (NO_2) and oxygen.

MODULE B	Storage, hardware, and distribution of medical gases

1. **Oxygen and other gas cylinders, bulk storage systems, and manifolds**
   a. **Get the necessary equipment for the procedure (Code: IIA1h3)[Difficulty: An]**

   b. **Put the equipment together, make sure that it works properly, and identify any problems (Code: IIB1h3) [Difficulty: An]**

   c. **Fix any problems with the equipment (Code: IIB2h3) [Difficulty: An]**

   Oxygen and other gas cylinders. The different types of gases in cylinders are identified by the color code of the cylinder and the cylinder's label. Note that only E cylinders have mandatory color coding. The color codings on the other cylinders are voluntary but are usually followed by the manufacturers. However, always read the label to be sure of the contents of the cylinder. The most important cylinder colors to remember are those of oxygen and air, but all are included in Table 6-1 for the sake of completeness.

TABLE 6-1	Color Codes for Gas Cylinders

Gas	Color
Oxygen	Green (white for international)
Air	Yellow
Helium	Brown
Helium and oxygen	Brown and green (check the label for the percentage of each gas)
Carbon dioxide	Gray
Carbon dioxide and oxygen	Gray and green (check the label for the percentage of each gas)
Nitrous oxide	Light blue
Cyclopropane	Orange
Ethylene	Red

EXAM HINT

The NBRC is known to ask the examinee to calculate how long a certain cylinder lasts at a given gas flow. To date, only the durations of E-, H-, and K-sized oxygen cylinders have had to be calculated.

To review how to calculate the duration of flow of a type of cylinder, see Table 6-2, the following equation, and the following examples.

Minutes of flow (divide by 60 to calculate hours) =
$$\frac{\text{gauge pressure in psig} \times \text{cylinder factor}}{\text{liter flow}}$$

1. Calculate the duration of flow of an E cylinder with 1500 pounds per square inch gauge (psig) that is running at 6 L/min.

$$\text{Minutes of flow (divide by 60 to calculate hours)} = \frac{1500 \text{ psig} \times 0.28}{6 \text{ L}}$$

$$= \frac{420}{6}$$

$$\text{Minutes of flow} = 70 \left(\begin{array}{c} 1.16 \text{ hr, or 1 hr} \\ \text{and 10 min} \end{array} \right)$$

2. Calculate the duration of flow of an H cylinder with 1950 psig that is running at 9 L/min.

$$\text{Minutes of flow (divide by 60 to calculate hours)} = \frac{1950 \text{ psig} \times 3.14}{9 \text{ L}}$$

$$= \frac{6123}{9}$$

$$\text{Minutes of flow} = 680.33 \left(\begin{array}{c} 11.34 \text{ hr, or 11 hr} \\ \text{and 20 min} \end{array} \right)$$

Bulk storage systems. The bulk liquid oxygen (LOX)-storage system is the main source of a hospital's oxygen. A reducing valve is used to decrease the gas pressure to 50 psig before it is piped throughout the hospital for easy

TABLE 6-2	Oxygen Cylinder Duration of Flow Factors

Cylinder size	Factor (L/psig)
E	0.28
H	3.14
K	3.14
D	0.16
M	1.36
G	2.41

psig, Pounds per square inch gauge.

access. Alarms will sound if the pressure falls low or goes too high. Pressure relief valves will open if the pressure is greater than 75 psig. Zone valves are located throughout the hospital to turn off the gas if a leak develops or there is a fire.

Manifolds. A manifold is a piping system that connects the bulk storage system and hospital gas piping system with a bank of H- or K-sized cylinders. These free-standing cylinders are a backup source of oxygen in case the bulk system fails. A 24-hour supply of gas must be available.

The manifold system includes a reducing valve to decrease the gas pressure to 50 psig. Check valves are built into the manifold so that a leak in one cylinder connection cannot result in all of the gas cylinders leaking out.

2. **Adjunct hardware: reducing valves, flowmeters, regulators, pulse-dose systems, and high-pressure hose connectors**
   a. **Get the necessary equipment for the procedure (Code: IIA1h1) [Difficulty: An]**

   b. **Put the equipment together, make sure that it works properly, and identify any problems with it (Code: IIB1h1) [Difficulty: An]**

   c. **Fix any problems with the equipment (Code: IIB2h1) [Difficulty: An]**

Reducing valves. Reducing valves are used to reduce the high pressure seen in a bulk oxygen storage system, manifold, or gas cylinder. One or more stages (pressure-reducing steps) can be used to reach the working pressure of 50 psig. Single-stage reducing valves reach the pressure in a single step. Multiple-stage reducing valves give finer control over pressure and flow by dropping pressure in the first stage to about 200 psig and to 50 psig in the second stage. Occasionally, three stages are seen. All reducing valves (and regulators [combined reducing valve and flowmeter]) have the following built-in safety features:
a. A frangible disk that breaks to release gas pressure in the event of a mechanical failure or breakage.
b. A fusible plug that melts to release gas pressure in the event of a fire.
c. American Standard Compressed Gas Cylinder Valve Outlet and Index Connections (usually called the American Standard system), which prevent the accidental connection of the wrong reducing valve (or regulator) to a large gas cylinder.
d. The Pin Index Safety System (PISS) is a special section of the American Standard system that applies to gas cylinders that are E-sized and smaller. It is designed to prevent an accidental connection of the wrong gas to a reducing valve or regulator. These reducing valves and regulators are designed with a specifically pinned yoke to wrap around the valve stem of a gas cylinder. A soft plastic O-ring washer is included to help ensure a tight

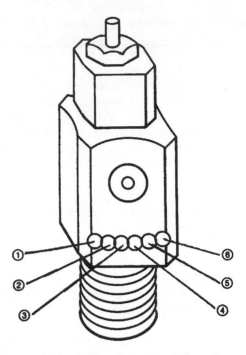

Fig. 6-1 Locations of the Pin Index Safety System holes in the cylinder valve face. (From Branson RD, Hess DR, Chatburn RL: *Respiratory care equipment,* ed 2, Philadelphia, 1999, Lippincott Williams & Wilkins.)

TABLE 6-3	Pin-Index Safety System Gases and Pinhole Locations
Gas	**Pinhole locations**
Oxygen	2-5
Air	1-5
Oxygen/carbon dioxide (≤7%)	2-6
Oxygen/carbon dioxide (>7%)	1-6
Oxygen/helium (not >80% helium)	2-4
Oxygen/helium (helium >80%)	4-6
Nitrous oxide	3-5
Ethylene	1-3
Cyclopropane	3-6

seal. Fig. 6-1 shows the location of the pinholes in the cylinder valve face. Table 6-3 shows the gases and pinhole positions. It is important to know the positions for oxygen and air; the others are included for the sake of completeness.

It is necessary to "crack" or blow some gas out of a cylinder before putting any reducing valve or regulator onto it to prevent any dust or debris from being forced into the reducing valve or regulator, which might cause a fire.

Flowmeters. Flowmeters are designed to regulate and indicate flow. They also come with the following safety

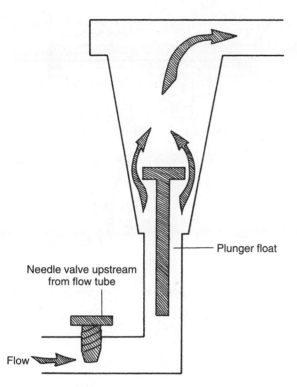

Fig. 6-2 Kinetic-type non–backpressure-compensated (pressure-uncompensated) flowmeter. (Modified from McPherson SP: *Respiratory care equipment,* ed 4, St Louis, 1990, Mosby.)

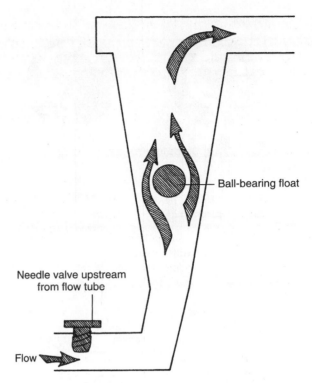

Fig. 6-3 Thorpe-type non–backpressure-compensated (pressure-uncompensated) flowmeter. (Modified from McPherson SP: *Respiratory care equipment,* ed 4, St Louis, 1990, Mosby.)

features so that they cannot be attached to the wrong reducing valve, regulator, high-pressure hose, or appliance:

   a. Diameter-Index Safety System (DISS) inlets and outlets that are specific to the various gases so that a mix-up cannot be made with the wrong appliance or connector. The DISS system applies to flowmeters that attach to all American Standard and DISS reduction valves.

   b. Flowmeters with quick-connect inlet adapters instead of DISS inlets. These quick-connects are designed specifically for the hospital's piped-in oxygen and air outlets. They are not interchangeable between gases or between manufacturers. Occasionally a piped oxygen outlet will jam open and let gas rapidly escape. Insert the proper flowmeter into the outlet and turn the flowmeter off. This stops the leak until the defective wall outlet can be repaired.

Flowmeters are usually categorized by how they react to backpressure. To complicate matters further, we must remember that there are three different manufactured types of flowmeters that may or may not be backpressure compensated.

   A. Non–backpressure-compensated (pressure-uncompensated) flowmeters will *inaccurately* indicate the flow through them in the face of backpressure. Figs. 6-2 and 6-3 show non–backpressure-compensated kinetic and Thorpe types of flowmeters, respectively. Note that the Thorpe and kinetic flowmeters have the flow control valve upstream from the meter. They read accurately if they are kept upright and do not have to "push" against any backpressure. If laid on their sides, the plunger and ball bearing do not indicate the set flow. They both read a *lower* flow than what is actually delivered when faced with a backpressure.

   B. The Bourdon flowmeter is designed like the Bourdon gauge in the reducing valve. See Fig. 6-4. The face piece is marked in liters of flow rather than pressure. It is the flowmeter of choice in a transport situation because it may be laid flat without affecting its flow if there is no backpressure. These flowmeters will display a *higher* flow than what is actually delivered when faced with a backpressure.

   C. Backpressure-compensated (pressure-compensated) flowmeters *accurately* indicate the flow through them in the face of backpressure. For this reason they should be used whenever possible. Figs. 6-5 and 6-6 show backpressure-compensated kinetic and Thorpe types of flowmeters, respec-

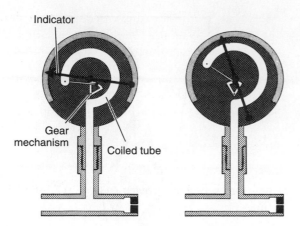

Fig. 6-4 Bourdon-type non–backpressure-compensated (pressure-uncompensated) flowmeter. (From McPherson SP: *Respiratory care equipment,* ed 4, St Louis, 1990, Mosby.)

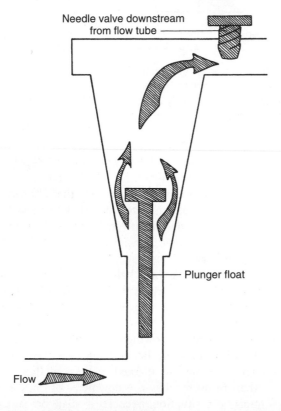

Fig. 6-5 Kinetic-type backpressure-compensated (pressure-compensated) flowmeter. (Modified from McPherson SP: *Respiratory care equipment,* ed 4, St Louis, 1990, Mosby.)

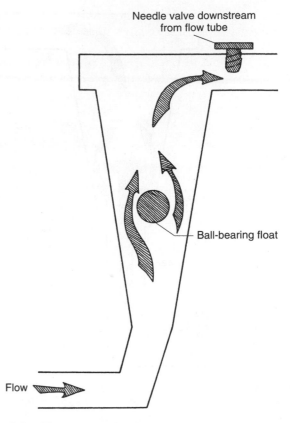

Fig. 6-6 Thorpe-type backpressure-compensated (pressure-compensated) flowmeter. (Modified from McPherson SP: *Respiratory care equipment,* ed 4, St Louis, 1990, Mosby.)

tively. Note that both of these flowmeters have the flow-control valve downstream from the meter. Because of this, they read accurately in the face of backpressure as long as they are kept upright. Besides reading the label, this simple test enables the practitioner to tell whether a flowmeter is backpressure compensated:

1. Make sure the flowmeter is turned off.
2. Plug the flowmeter into a gas outlet.
3. If the float or ball bearing bounces, the flowmeter is backpressure compensated.

EXAM HINT

Choose a backpressure-compensated flowmeter in all situations except during patient transport when the oxygen tank and flowmeter might be laid flat.

Regulators. Regulators combine a reducing valve and a flowmeter. Everything that has been discussed so far relates to regulators. Bourdon gauge reducing valves are usually seen and can have either a second Bourdon gauge added as a flowmeter or a Thorpe or kinetic flowmeter. As mentioned earlier, use a backpressure-compensated flowmeter in all situations except for patient transport.

Pulse-dose systems. A pulse-dose oxygen delivery system is used in the home-care setting to reduce the patient's oxygen use and to save money. The unit takes the place of a regulator and flowmeter on the oxygen source. Some units are designed for a low-pressure liquid oxygen system. Others are designed for a high-pressure E tank of oxygen. Be careful to not place a low-pressure unit on a high-pressure gas source, because it will be damaged. In all units, the distal end of a regular nasal cannula is attached to a pressure sensor on the pulse-dose system. It senses a drop in pressure as the patient inspires. The sensor then triggers a solenoid valve that delivers a burst of oxygen to the cannula. A pulse-dose unit can be adjusted to change several factors such as how long the oxygen is delivered, how much is delivered, and if the patient receives oxygen every breath or every second or third breath.

Make sure that the patient can feel a flow of gas from the cannula after he or she starts to inhale. The gas should stop during exhalation. Check the patient's pulse oximetry value at rest and during exercise to ensure that desaturation does not occur. Adjust the pressure sensor or solenoid if needed to meet the patient's oxygen needs.

If the patient cannot feel any oxygen flowing, the following should be considered: (1) the source of oxygen might be empty, (2) the tubing might be disconnected or kinked, or (3) the sensor is not detecting the patient's effort. The patient or therapist can switch to a second oxygen source and look for disconnections or kinks in the tubing. The therapist must adjust the nasal cannula or pulse-dose unit to correct for a sensitivity problem. Do not use a system that is malfunctioning and cannot be adjusted.

High-pressure hose connectors. These connectors and other adapters connect high-pressure hoses, flowmeters, and oxygen appliances. They have DISS inlets and outlets so that the gases cannot be cross-fitted to the wrong equipment.

3. Perform quality control procedures for gas metering devices: flowmeters and regulators (Code: IIB3c) [Difficulty: An]

When performing a quality control procedure on a flowmeter, it is critical that an accurately known flow be sent through it so that the flowmeter can be checked for accuracy. This should be done without any backpressure. When a backpressure is placed against a flowmeter the following is seen:

a. Non–backpressure-compensated (pressure-uncompensated) Thorpe and kinetic flowmeters show an inaccurately *low* flow in the face of backpressure. In other words, they show less flow than is actually being delivered.

b. Bourdon regulators (Bourdon reducing valve and flowmeter) show an inaccurately *high* flow in the face of backpressure. In other words, they show more flow than is actually being delivered.

c. Backpressure-compensated (pressure-compensated) Thorpe and kinetic flowmeters show an accurate flow in the face of backpressure. If the gas flow is

restricted, the ball bearing or plunger float drops to mark the reduced flow. If the flow is completely blocked off, the float drops to zero showing no flow.

Reducing valves and regulators must have a known pressure directed against them to check for accuracy. The known pressure should be seen on the regulator gauge. Any flowmeter or regulator that is not reading accurately should not be used until after it has been repaired.

4. Air compressors
a. **Get the necessary equipment for the procedure (Code: IIA1h2) [Difficulty: An]**

b. **Put the equipment together, make sure that it works properly, and identify any problems (Code: IIB1h2) [Difficulty: An]**

c. **Fix any problems with the equipment (Code: IIB2h2) [Difficulty: An]**

Air compressors are used whenever a high-pressure gas source other than oxygen is needed. All three systems are alike in that they employ an electrically powered motor, filter the room air as it enters and exits the compressor, and have a condenser to remove water vapor as it leaves the compressor.

Rotary-type compressors. Rotary-type compressors generate pressure with a rotating fan. They are commonly used in volume ventilators and in the home to power handheld medication nebulizers and intermittent positive-pressure breathing (IPPB) units.

Diaphragm-type compressors. Diaphragm-type compressors generate pressure with a diaphragm that moves up and down within a cylinderlike piston. They also are commonly used in the home to power handheld medication nebulizers and IPPB units.

Piston-type compressors. Piston-type compressors generate pressure by piston action within a cylinder. They are much more powerful than the previous two types of compressors. Because they are designed to generate pressures of 50 psig or greater, they are used in the hospital with its piped air system. They are also used in the home setting in oxygen concentrators.

Make sure that all of these units are operational by checking that the inlet and outlet filters are cleaned. Dirty filters prevent proper airflow. Check the unit's pressure gauge to make sure that it is able to meet its manufacturer's specified pressure. Empty the water trap on the condensing unit as needed.

5. Air/oxygen proportioners (blenders)
a. **Get the necessary equipment for the procedure (Code: IIA1h1) [Difficulty: An]**

b. **Put the equipment together, make sure that it works**

properly, and identify any problems (Code: IIB1h1) [Difficulty: An]

c. Fix any problems with the equipment (Code: IIB2h1) [Difficulty: An]

These units are designed to change the ratio of oxygen and air to blend the specific percentage of oxygen from 21% to 100%. To do that, both source gases must be pressurized to 50 psig. The oxygen percentage will remain close to that desired even if there is a small drop in either one or both line pressures. Always analyze the oxygen percentage to confirm that it is correct. The blended gas can be sent directly to a ventilator or other device that uses 50 psig or through an added flowmeter.

Keep the gas inlets and outlets clear of any debris. All current units give an audible whistle if either one or both of the line pressures drop to an unsafe level (often about 30 psig). If the unit has a water trap at the compressed air inlet, keep it emptied of any condensate.

6. Oxygen concentrators (enrichers)
a. Get the necessary equipment for the procedure (Code: IIA1h2) [Difficulty: An]

There are two different types of oxygen concentrators available for the delivery of continuous low-flow oxygen in the home: molecular sieve and permeable plastic membrane.

Molecular sieve. Molecular sieve-type oxygen concentrators use an air compressor to push room air through two canisters of zeolite pellets (inorganic sodium-aluminum

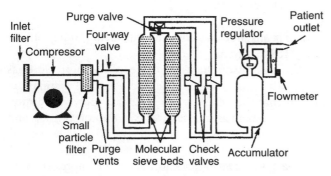

Fig. 6-7 Drawing of the components of a molecular sieve oxygen concentrator. The molecular sieve beds remove nitrogen and pass oxygen through to the patient. (Courtesy Sunrise Medical, Inc., Somerset, PA.)

TABLE 6-4	Comparison of Flow Rates and Oxygen Percentages in Oxygen Concentrators

MOLECULAR SIEVE CONCENTRATOR

Flow (L/min)	*Oxygen percentage*
1-2	>90%
3-5	80%-90%
6	about 74%
8	about 60%
10	50%

(PERMEABLE MEMBRANE CONCENTRATOR)

1-10	40%

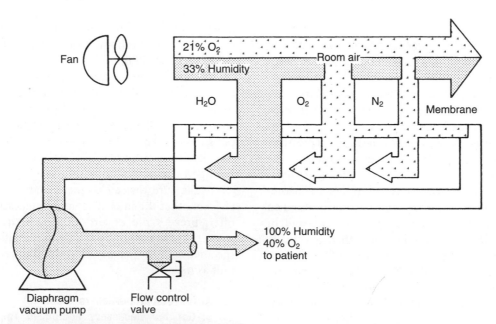

Fig. 6-8 Functional schematic of a semipermeable membrane oxygen concentrator. The membrane permits more oxygen and water vapor to pass through than nitrogen. (Courtesy of the Oxygen Enrichment Company, Schenectady, NY.)

silicate) to remove nitrogen and water vapor. The remaining oxygen is delivered to the patient through a flowmeter (see Fig. 6-7). Be aware that with this unit the oxygen percentage varies inversely with the flow that is delivered (see Table 6-4).

Permeable plastic membrane. Permeable plastic membrane oxygen concentrators make use of a 1-μm-thick plastic membrane as a filter. Room air is pulled through it by a vacuum pump. Molecular oxygen and water vapor can pass through the membrane faster than nitrogen. Any excess water vapor is removed by a simple condenser system. There is no need to add an external humidification system to the flowmeter (see Fig. 6-8). The oxygen percentage is fixed at 40% in these units; however, the flow can be varied from 1 to 10 L/min as shown in Table 6-4.

When deciding which type of concentrator to use, it is important to know the patient's required oxygen percentage and flow. As can be seen from Table 6-4, the molecular sieve types can deliver a higher oxygen percentage at any liter flow as compared with the permeable plastic membrane units.

b. Put the equipment together, make sure that it works properly, and identify any problems with it (Code: IIB1h2 and IIIC3b) [Difficulty: An]

c. Fix any problems with the equipment (Code: IIB2h2) [Difficulty: An]

The molecular sieve-type units deliver dry gas; therefore, a humidification system is frequently added to the flowmeter. With the permeable plastic membrane type units, the condensed water vapor must be emptied from the collection jar. In both types of oxygen concentrators it is important to check the air inlet filter on a monthly basis to keep it clean of dust and debris. Follow the manufacturer's requirements for when filters should be replaced. The delivered oxygen concentration should also be checked each month. Follow the manufacturer's guidelines for its preventative maintenance needs. The molecular sieve-type units must have the zeolite pellet canisters replaced on a scheduled basis.

Some units have a visual or audio alarm that warns when there is a problem such as decreased flow. Because this is not a low-oxygen percentage alarm, some home-care practitioners have recommended the addition of an external analyzer with an alarm system. This alerts the patient to call the home-care company to repair the equipment. If a patient says that he or she cannot feel any gas coming out of the cannula, have the patient place the prongs into a glass of water. If no bubbling is seen, have the patient check the tubing for any disconnections. If the concentrator is malfunctioning, have the patient turn it off and switch to oxygen from the backup oxygen cylinder until repairs can be made.

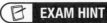

EXAM HINT

Most past examinations have included a question related to a malfunctioning oxygen concentrator used in the home. A patient may be expected to check for oxygen flowing through a cannula by placing the prongs under water to look for bubbling or switching from the concentrator to a backup source of oxygen such as an oxygen cylinder (tank). The patient should not be expected to troubleshoot problems with the concentrator or perform maintenance work on it. That is the home-care respiratory therapist's job.

7. Portable liquid oxygen systems
a. Get the necessary equipment for the procedure (Code: IIA1h2) [Difficulty: An]

A liquid oxygen (LOX) system is used in the home when it is found to be more cost effective than an oxygen concentrator or battery of oxygen cylinders. An additional advantage is that the patient can carry a smaller portable unit in a shoulder bag for added mobility. It is also less conspicuous than wheeling an E cylinder about. The best-known unit is the Linde (Union Carbide) Walker System. Fig. 6-9 shows the large reservoir that is kept in the patient's home. Fig. 6-10 shows its smaller companion, the portable Linde Walker.

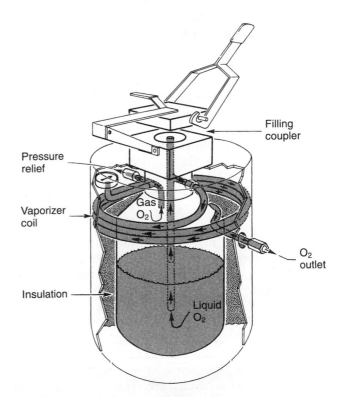

Fig. 6-9 Drawing of the components of a home liquid oxygen supply unit. (From Lampton LM: Home and outpatient oxygen therapy. In Brashear RE, Rhodes ML, editors: *Chronic obstructive lung disease,* St Louis, 1978, Mosby.)

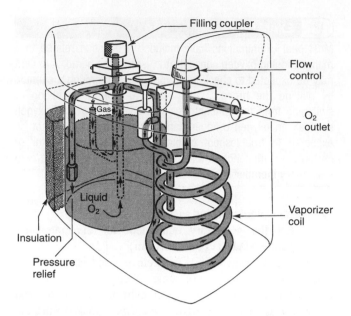

Fig. 6-10 Drawing of the components of a portable liquid oxygen unit. (From Lampton LM: Home and outpatient oxygen therapy. In Brashear RE, Rhodes ML, editors: *Chronic obstructive lung disease,* St Louis, 1978, Mosby.)

b. Put the equipment together, make sure that it works properly, and identify any problems (Code: IIB1h2 and IIIC3b) [Difficulty: An]

The Linde Walker reservoir tank weighs about 11 pounds and can be carried over the shoulder by a strap. It can be refilled from the larger reservoir tank kept in the home. The flow rate can be adjusted to meet most patients' needs. Humidification is provided by the patient's own airway. As with any pressurized system, all fittings must be kept tight to prevent leakage.

The National Fire Protection Agency (NFPA) has established a number of regulations to ensure that home liquid oxygen systems are safely installed. The key safety regulations include:

1. Stabilize the unit to prevent it from being tipped over.
2. The reservoir unit should not be set up near any radiators, steam pipes, or heat ducts to reduce the rate of oxygen loss.
3. There can be no open flames or sources of ignition within 5 feet of the unit.
4. "No smoking" signs must be posted.
5. The patient and family must be instructed in how to use the equipment. This includes how to fill the Walker from the large reservoir tank. The person filling the Walker should wear safety goggles with side shields, loose-fitting insulated gloves, and high-top boots.
6. If liquid oxygen spills and contacts skin it can cause frostbite. Medical attention should be sought immediately.

7. Avoid contact for at least 15 minutes with any equipment or the floor where liquid oxygen has spilled.

c. Fix any problems with the equipment (Code: IIB2h2) [Difficulty: An]

Check that all connections are airtight to avoid spills and minimize the loss of oxygen. Make sure that the unit is functioning at its designed working pressure. The Linde unit operates at 90 psig. Make sure that the pressure relief valve operates properly and that the proper flow is delivered.

📖 EXAM HINT

Most past examinations have questioned either the need to set up a liquid oxygen supply unit and portable unit for a home-care patient or troubleshooting problems with the system. A patient may be expected to check for oxygen flowing through a cannula by placing the prongs under water to look for bubbling or switching from the liquid oxygen system to a backup source of oxygen such as an oxygen cylinder (tank). The patient should not be expected to troubleshoot problems with the liquid oxygen system or perform maintenance work on it. That is the home-care respiratory therapist's job.

---

8. Other therapeutic gases

a. Get the necessary equipment for the procedure (Code: IIA1m) [Difficulty: R, Ap, An]

The NBRC lists O_2/CO_2 (carbogen) and He/O_2 (heliox) as therapeutic gases besides oxygen that may be administered to patients. However, inhaled NO (nitric oxide) is now being used and may be tested. The discussion of patient indications for each of these is presented in Module D.

All of these gases come in high-pressure cylinders and require the use of an American Standard system reducing valve (or regulator) designed specifically for the gas or gas mix. As shown in Table 6-3 and Fig. 6-1, a reducing valve or regulator for an E-cylinder must match the appropriate pinholes on the cylinder valve face. Corresponding high-pressure hoses may also be needed. Table 6-1 shows the color codes for the various gas cylinders. Note that pure carbon dioxide comes in a gray colored cylinder whereas a carbon dioxide and oxygen mix (carbogen) has a gray and green colored cylinder. Pure helium comes in a brown cylinder whereas helium and oxygen mixes come in brown and green cylinders. Always check the cylinder label for the exact percentage of the gases within it. For example, heliox comes in mixes of 80% He/20% O_2, 70% He/30% O_2, and 60% He/40% O_2.

If carbogen is needed for a carbon dioxide response curve test (see Chapter 4), the gas mix can be delivered from the cylinder flowmeter to the pulmonary function testing breathing circuit through small-bore tubing and a silicate) to remove nitrogen and water vapor. The remaining oxygen is delivered to the patient through a flowmeter (see Fig. 6-7). Be aware that with this unit the oxygen percentage varies inversely with the flow that is delivered (see Table 6-4).

Permeable plastic membrane. Permeable plastic membrane oxygen concentrators make use of a 1-μm-thick plastic membrane as a filter. Room air is pulled through it by a vacuum pump. Molecular oxygen and water vapor can pass through the membrane faster than nitrogen. Any excess water vapor is removed by a simple condenser system. There is no need to add an external humidification system to the flowmeter (see Fig. 6-8). The oxygen percentage is fixed at 40% in these units; however, the flow can be varied from 1 to 10 L/min as shown in Table 6-4.

When deciding which type of concentrator to use, it is important to know the patient's required oxygen percentage and flow. As can be seen from Table 6-4, the molecular sieve types can deliver a higher oxygen percentage at any liter flow as compared with the permeable plastic membrane units.

b. Put the equipment together, make sure that it works properly, and identify any problems with it (Code: IIB1h2 and IIIC3b) [Difficulty: An]

c. Fix any problems with the equipment (Code: IIB2h2) [Difficulty: An]

The molecular sieve-type units deliver dry gas; therefore, a humidification system is frequently added to the flowmeter. With the permeable plastic membrane type units, the condensed water vapor must be emptied from the collection jar. In both types of oxygen concentrators it is important to check the air inlet filter on a monthly basis to keep it clean of dust and debris. Follow the manufacturer's requirements for when filters should be replaced. The delivered oxygen concentration should also be checked each month. Follow the manufacturer's guidelines for its preventative maintenance needs. The molecular sieve-type units must have the zeolite pellet canisters replaced on a scheduled basis.

Some units have a visual or audio alarm that warns when there is a problem such as decreased flow. Because this is not a low-oxygen percentage alarm, some home-care practitioners have recommended the addition of an external analyzer with an alarm system. This alerts the patient to call the home-care company to repair the equipment. If a patient says that he or she cannot feel any gas coming out of the cannula, have the patient place the prongs into a glass of water. If no bubbling is seen, have the patient check the tubing for any disconnections. If the concentrator is malfunctioning, have the patient turn it off and switch to oxygen from the backup oxygen cylinder until repairs can be made.

EXAM HINT

Most past examinations have included a question related to a malfunctioning oxygen concentrator used in the home. A patient may be expected to check for oxygen flowing through a cannula by placing the prongs under water to look for bubbling or switching from the concentrator to a backup source of oxygen such as an oxygen cylinder (tank). The patient should not be expected to troubleshoot problems with the concentrator or perform maintenance work on it. That is the home-care respiratory therapist's job.

7. Portable liquid oxygen systems

a. Get the necessary equipment for the procedure (Code: IIA1h2) [Difficulty: An]

A liquid oxygen (LOX) system is used in the home when it is found to be more cost effective than an oxygen concentrator or battery of oxygen cylinders. An additional advantage is that the patient can carry a smaller portable unit in a shoulder bag for added mobility. It is also less conspicuous than wheeling an E cylinder about. The best-known unit is the Linde (Union Carbide) Walker System. Fig. 6-9 shows the large reservoir that is kept in the patient's home. Fig. 6-10 shows its smaller companion, the portable Linde Walker.

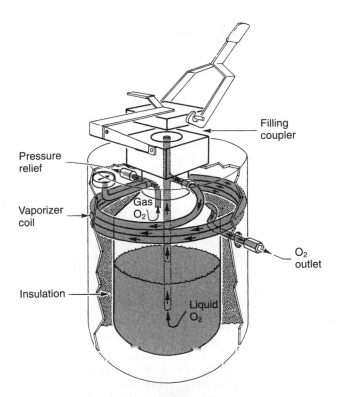

Fig. 6-9 Drawing of the components of a home liquid oxygen supply unit. (From Lampton LM: Home and outpatient oxygen therapy. In Brashear RE, Rhodes ML, editors: *Chronic obstructive lung disease,* St Louis, 1978, Mosby.)

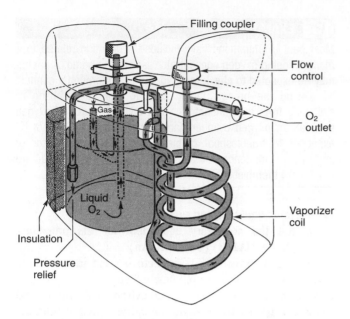

Fig. 6-10 Drawing of the components of a portable liquid oxygen unit. (From Lampton LM: Home and outpatient oxygen therapy. In Brashear RE, Rhodes ML, editors: *Chronic obstructive lung disease,* St Louis, 1978, Mosby.)

b. Put the equipment together, make sure that it works properly, and identify any problems (Code: IIB1h2 and IIIC3b) [Difficulty: An]

The Linde Walker reservoir tank weighs about 11 pounds and can be carried over the shoulder by a strap. It can be refilled from the larger reservoir tank kept in the home. The flow rate can be adjusted to meet most patients' needs. Humidification is provided by the patient's own airway. As with any pressurized system, all fittings must be kept tight to prevent leakage.

The National Fire Protection Agency (NFPA) has established a number of regulations to ensure that home liquid oxygen systems are safely installed. The key safety regulations include:

1. Stabilize the unit to prevent it from being tipped over.
2. The reservoir unit should not be set up near any radiators, steam pipes, or heat ducts to reduce the rate of oxygen loss.
3. There can be no open flames or sources of ignition within 5 feet of the unit.
4. "No smoking" signs must be posted.
5. The patient and family must be instructed in how to use the equipment. This includes how to fill the Walker from the large reservoir tank. The person filling the Walker should wear safety goggles with side shields, loose-fitting insulated gloves, and high-top boots.
6. If liquid oxygen spills and contacts skin it can cause frostbite. Medical attention should be sought immediately.

7. Avoid contact for at least 15 minutes with any equipment or the floor where liquid oxygen has spilled.

c. Fix any problems with the equipment (Code: IIB2h2) [Difficulty: An]

Check that all connections are airtight to avoid spills and minimize the loss of oxygen. Make sure that the unit is functioning at its designed working pressure. The Linde unit operates at 90 psig. Make sure that the pressure relief valve operates properly and that the proper flow is delivered.

EXAM HINT

Most past examinations have questioned either the need to set up a liquid oxygen supply unit and portable unit for a home-care patient or troubleshooting problems with the system. A patient may be expected to check for oxygen flowing through a cannula by placing the prongs under water to look for bubbling or switching from the liquid oxygen system to a backup source of oxygen such as an oxygen cylinder (tank). The patient should not be expected to troubleshoot problems with the liquid oxygen system or perform maintenance work on it. That is the home-care respiratory therapist's job.

---

8. Other therapeutic gases

a. Get the necessary equipment for the procedure (Code: IIA1m) [Difficulty: R, Ap, An]

The NBRC lists O_2/CO_2 (carbogen) and He/O_2 (heliox) as therapeutic gases besides oxygen that may be administered to patients. However, inhaled NO (nitric oxide) is now being used and may be tested. The discussion of patient indications for each of these is presented in Module D.

All of these gases come in high-pressure cylinders and require the use of an American Standard system reducing valve (or regulator) designed specifically for the gas or gas mix. As shown in Table 6-3 and Fig. 6-1, a reducing valve or regulator for an E-cylinder must match the appropriate pinholes on the cylinder valve face. Corresponding high-pressure hoses may also be needed. Table 6-1 shows the color codes for the various gas cylinders. Note that pure carbon dioxide comes in a gray colored cylinder whereas a carbon dioxide and oxygen mix (carbogen) has a gray and green colored cylinder. Pure helium comes in a brown cylinder whereas helium and oxygen mixes come in brown and green cylinders. Always check the cylinder label for the exact percentage of the gases within it. For example, heliox comes in mixes of 80% He/20% O_2, 70% He/30% O_2, and 60% He/40% O_2.

If carbogen is needed for a carbon dioxide response curve test (see Chapter 4), the gas mix can be delivered from the cylinder flowmeter to the pulmonary function testing breathing circuit through small-bore tubing and a

Some patients may complain that the gas coming through the mask is dry. To resolve this problem, some manufacturers have designed an aerosol adapter to add at the jet. A separate bland aerosol is then added to the room air that enters the jet stream. Make sure that the adapter fits properly and does not interfere with or block the jet or room air-entrainment ports. Do *not* add a bubble-type humidifier to the jet on the mask because the high backpressure through the jet will cause the pressure relief (pop-off) valve to open, and the oxygen will leak out.

There are two different types of air-entrainment devices based on the physical principles seen in the Bernoulli effect. It is important to know about the two different types to understand what can go wrong with them and how they can be fixed. Make sure that the correct liter flow of oxygen, jet size, and air-entrainment port setting are selected to get the desired total flow and oxygen percentage.

Variable jet diameter. Notice that the jets have different diameters, but the room air-entrainment ports are the same size. You will see that the *smaller* the jet diameter is, the *lower* the oxygen percentage is. This is because as the jet becomes smaller, the lateral pressure is lower. This results in more room air being brought into the entrainment ports to dilute the oxygen and raise the total flow.

Make sure that the jets are not obstructed by mucus or anything else, or the oxygen percentage will be decreased. An obstruction downstream from the jet prevents the appropriate amount of room air from being brought into the mask. This results in the oxygen percentage increasing and the total flow decreasing.

Variable air-entrainment ports. Notice that the jet size is fixed, but the room air-entrainment ports have different sizes. The smaller the entrainment ports, the *higher* the oxygen percentage. This is because less room air can be entrained to dilute the oxygen. The total flow is also reduced when the entrainment ports are smaller.

Make sure that the entrainment ports are not obstructed by the patient's sheet or anything else, or the oxygen percentage will increase. An obstruction downstream from the jet prevents the appropriate amount of air from being brought into the mask. This results in the oxygen percentage increasing and the total flow decreasing.

Nasal cannula
a. Get the necessary equipment for the procedure (Code: IIA1a1) [Difficulty: An]

b. Put the equipment together, make sure that it works properly, and identify any problems (Code: IIB1a1) [Difficulty: An]

c. Fix any problems with the equipment (Code: IIB2a1) [Difficulty: An]

A nasal cannula is an oxygen delivery tube that has two short prongs to deliver oxygen to

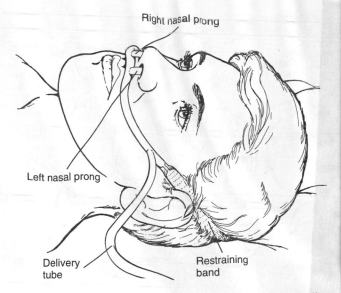

Fig. 6-14 Adult wearing a nasal cannula. (From Thalken FR: Medical gas therapy. In Scanlan CL, Spearman CB, Sheldon RL, editors: *Egan's fundamentals of respiratory care,* ed 5, St Louis, 1990, Mosby.)

the nostrils (Fig. 6-14). They come in neonatal, pediatric, and adult sizes based on the diameter of the prongs. Care must be taken to make sure that the nares are patent and not plugged by a common cold, deviated septum, or other unseen problem. This low-flow oxygen delivery device is very widely used because it is more comfortable for many patients than an air entrainment or other types of face masks.

If a humidifier is used, make sure that it is properly filled with sterile water and that the oxygen bubbles through it. Check the high-pressure pop-off valve for pressure release and a whistling sound. Before placing the cannula on the patient, check to see that the oxygen is flowing through the tubing. If available, use a cannula with curved prongs. They direct the gas flow toward the back of the nasal passages for better natural humidification, as well as better patient comfort. Take care not to pull the elastic restraining band too tightly around the head. Some brands loop the oxygen tubing over the ears to be drawn up snugly under the chin. Often this is more comfortable than the types that have an elastic band.

The problem with a nasal cannula is that the delivered oxygen percentage is unreliable. Variations in the patient's respiratory rate, I:E ratio, tidal volume, and minute volume result in different inhaled oxygen percentages. This is clearly unacceptable in an unstable patient in whom the PaO_2 values are being used to help judge the changing cardiopulmonary status. Because of this clinical limitation, this device and the other low-flow oxygen delivery systems in the discussions that follow should be used only with stable patients. In the adult, the delivered oxygen percentage can be *estimated* at approximately 4% for each

T-piece. The same simple assembly can deliver the carbogen to a patient's face mask or ventilator circuit. In both cases, the carbon dioxide level should be monitored by a capnometer added into the system (see Chapter 5).

A helium flowmeter can be used to set a flow of one of the heliox mixes to a patient's face mask. However, if a helium flowmeter is not available, an oxygen flowmeter can be added to the reducing valve on a heliox mix cylinder to set the flow of gas to the patient. (The calculation for determining the flow of a heliox mix through an oxygen flowmeter is shown in the following discussion.) If a patient requires helium through a mechanical ventilator, an air/oxygen proportioner (blender) is needed. Substitute 100% helium for the air side; oxygen will go through on its side of the unit, as usual. Simply dial the oxygen percentage as needed to adjust the mix of the two gases. For example, giving the patient 35% oxygen results in the patient also receiving 65% helium. Be aware that some ventilators do not accurately read the tidal volume when a helium/oxygen mix is delivered rather than the standard nitrogen/oxygen mix. The ventilator volume-measuring device (usually a flow-type pneumotachometer) may need to be recalibrated. Or, use a bellows-type spirometer to measure the exhaled tidal volume. Use a polarographic or galvanic fuel cell oxygen analyzer to monitor the patient's oxygen percentage.

The Food and Drug Administration (FDA) has granted approval of therapeutic inhaled nitric oxide (NO) and its delivery system to INO Therapeutics, Inc. The gaseous mixture is called INOmax and contains 0.8% nitric oxide and 99.2% nitrogen. The INOvent delivery system is needed to deliver inhaled nitric oxide to a mechanical ventilator or anesthesia machine. It is designed to deliver a precise dose of nitric oxide to either unit as well as to monitor the NO level, nitrogen dioxide (NO_2) level, and oxygen level.

b. Put the equipment together, make sure that it works properly, and identify any problems (Code: IIB1m) [Difficulty: R, Ap, An]

c. Fix any problems with the equipment (Code: IIB2m) [Difficulty: R, Ap, An]

Each of the therapeutic gases discussed earlier needs its own particular hardware accessories as described. In addition, other types of respiratory care equipment such as face masks, pulmonary function testing equipment, or a mechanical ventilator are needed based on the patient's situation.

A helium-oxygen mix is the most widely used of the therapeutic gases besides oxygen. With heliox therapy, the type of mask, delivery tubing, and humidifier chosen depends on whether the patient needs an aerosol delivered or not. If an aerosol is not needed, a nonrebreather mask with all of its one-way valves and small-bore oxygen tubing

is used. Attach a bubble humidifier with sterile water to the flowmeter. Connect the small-bore tubing to the humidifier nipple and to the nonrebreather mask nipple. If aerosol is required, an aerosol mask with one-way exhalation valves and reservoir is needed. Screw the nebulizer filled with sterile water to the flowmeter. Make sure that the air entrainment control is set to deliver 100% source gas of heliox (no room air should be entrained). Connect the large-bore, aerosol tubing to the nebulizer and the mask. Make sure the mask is adjusted to give as tight a fit to the face as is practical and comfortable. In either system it is extremely important that all connections be tight because helium easily leaks out of any openings.

If an oxygen flowmeter is used with a helium/oxygen regulator, the following adjustments must be made to the flow seen on the flowmeter. This is done because helium is less dense than oxygen.

1. When using an 80% helium and 20% oxygen mix, multiply the observed flow by 1.8. For example, an observed flow of 10 L/min × 1.8 = 18 L/min actual flow.
2. When using a 70% helium and 30% oxygen mix, multiply the observed flow by 1.6. For example, an observed flow of 10 L/min × 1.6 = 16 L/min actual flow.
3. When using a 60% helium and 40% oxygen mix, multiply the observed flow by 1.4. For example, an observed flow of 10 L/min × 1.4 = 14 L/min actual flow.

MODULE C **Administration of oxygen therapy**

1. Oxygen hoods and oxygen tents
a. Get the necessary equipment for the procedure. (Code: IIA1a2) [Difficulty: An]

b. Put the equipment together, make sure that it works properly, and identify any problems with it. (Code: IIB1a2) [Difficulty: An]

c. Fix any problems with the equipment. (Code: IIB2a2) [Difficulty: An]

Oxygen hoods. Oxygen hoods are used to provide a warmed aerosol, humidity, and a controlled oxygen percentage to pediatric patients who weigh no more than 18 lb. (8.2 kg) (Fig. 6-11). When using an oxygen hood, the following procedures should be observed:
a. Use an air/oxygen proportioner with a flowmeter to control the oxygen percentage and flow to the hood. The flow should be at least 7 L/min to prevent the buildup of exhaled carbon dioxide. A flow of 10 to 15 L/min is needed to keep a stable oxygen percentage. Keeping the hood sealed as much as possible and minimizing the gap between the infant's neck and the opening to the hood also helps to stabilize the oxygen percentage.
b. A warmed humidifier is needed to provide a high

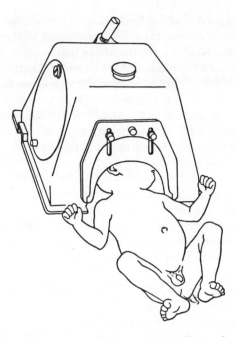

Fig. 6-11 Infant in an oxygen hood. (From Gaebler G, Blodgett D: Gas administration. In Blodgett D, editor: *Manual of pediatric respiratory care procedures,* Philadelphia, 1982, Lippincott.)

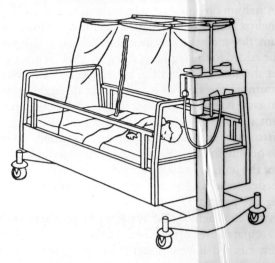

Fig. 6-12 Child in an oxygen tent. (From Gaebler G, Blodgett D: Gas administration. In Blodgett D, editor: *Manual of pediatric respiratory care procedures,* Philadelphia, 1982, Lippincott.)

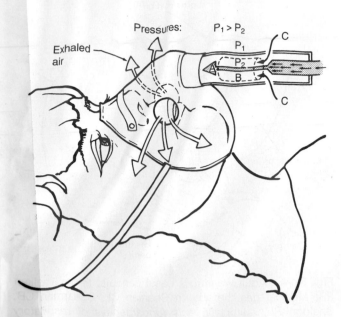

Fig. 6-13 Adult wearing an air-entrainment mask. *A,* High velocity jet; *B,* an area of reduced lateral pressure (Bernoulli's principle); *C,* room air entrainment. (From White GC: *Basic clinical lab competencies for respiratory care, an integrated approach,* Albany, NY, 1988, Delmar.)

humidity level and to warm the oxygen to the infant's body temperature. Care must be taken with infants to ensure that they are neither heated nor cooled by the gas blowing over their heads. A thermometer should be kept in the hood to note the temperature.

c. An oxygen analyzer should continuously monitor how much oxygen is inside the hood. The analyzer probe should be placed at the same level as the infant's nose. This is because oxygen is heavier than air and tends to settle toward the bottom of the hood.

The advantages of the hood over the tent are that the patient's body is accessible, and the head can be reached by lifting the top off of the hood. Be aware of the noise level inside the hood to minimize damage to the infant's hearing. The sound level should be monitored and kept well below 65 dB.

Oxygen tents. Oxygen tents were formerly used for adults, but are now used only for children who are too large and active for a hood. The tent is used to control the environment by providing a cooled aerosol, humidity, and controlled oxygen percentage (Fig. 6-12). In addition, the following procedures should be observed:

a. Set an oxygen flowmeter to deliver 8 to 10 L/min to small tents and 12 to 15 L/min to large tents. Flows of 30 L/min or greater are needed to keep the oxygen percentage close to the 50% maximum that can be reliably maintained. (Commonly, between 35% and 50% oxygen can be kept in a tent.)

b. The oxygen should flow through a nebulizer or

ultrasonic unit to provide the needed humidity. Try to keep the relative humidity at 60% or greater to minimize any risk of a spark causing a fire inside the tent.

c. The tent must be cooled to prevent the patient from overheating the enclosed space. Also, if the infant put into a tent has croup, the cooled air is therapeutic. Be careful not to chill the infant.

d. As with hoods, an oxygen analyzer should continuously monitor how much oxygen is inside the tent. The analyzer probe should be placed at the same level as the infant's nose. Keep the tent sealed and the bottom edges tucked under the mattress to try to keep the oxygen percentage as high and stable as possible. The child should not be allowed to have any electrically powered toys inside the tent to minimize the risk of a spark and fire.

2. Air-entrainment devices and masks

a. Get the necessary equipment for the procedure (Code: IIA1a2) [Difficulty: An]

b. Put the equipment together, make sure that it works properly, and identify any problems with it (Code: IIB1a2) [Difficulty: An]

c. Fix any problems with the equipment (Code: IIB2a2) [Difficulty: An]

Air-entrainment masks are designed to provide the patient with a controlled oxygen percentage at a flow rate high enough to ensure that all of the patient's needs are met

expiratory (I:E) ratio, tidal volume, or minute volume. Common situations include a COPD patient and a patient in respiratory failure who needs increasing oxygen percentages. Because it is difficult to ensure that the patient's peak inspiratory flow is matched by the gas flow through the mask, the following guidelines are recommended:

a. Make sure that the total flow through the mask is at least 40 L/min in a resting patient. More may be needed if the patient is breathing rapidly.

b. Provide the patient with a total flow that is four to six times his or her measured minute volume.

The total flow through the mask can be raised by increasing the oxygen flow. This should not significantly change the oxygen percentage because more room air is entrained to keep the same ratio. However, to be certain, analyze the oxygen percentage inside the mask to ensure that it is as prescribed. The total flow through the mask can be calculated by adding the total of the ratio parts and multiplying by the oxygen flow rate.

Math review of air-entrainment mask calculations:

Example 1. Your patient has on a 28% air-entrainment mask with an oxygen flow of 4 L/min. His condition worsens, and he increases his minute volume to 15 L/min. To ensure that he still receives his prescribed oxygen percentage, someone makes a recommendation to you to increase the oxygen liter flow to 6 L/min. The new total flow through the mask can be calculated as follows:

A 28% air-entrainment mask has an air/oxygen ratio of 10:1.

a. The sum of the ratio parts is 10 + 1 = 11.

b. Total flow = 11 × 6 L/min oxygen flow = 66 L/min.

c. This flow is more than four times the patient's current minute volume. He should have all of flow needs met.

d. Reanalyze the delivered oxygen percentage certain that it is as prescribed.

Example 2. Your patient is wearing entrainment mask that has the manufac 8 L/min of oxygen running into it. H flow is about 48 L/min (0.75 L/sec oxygen flow be changed to ensure greater than her peak inspirat flow to the mask can be calc

a. 40% air-entrainme of 3:1.

b. The sum of t

c. Divide the inspirat

d. Increa

TABLE 6-5 Specifications for Air-Entrainment Devices and Masks

Oxygen (%)	Approximate air/oxygen ratio	Total ratio parts	Oxygen flow rate (L/min)*	Total flow (L/min)
24	25:1	26	4	104
28	10:1	11	4	44
30	8:1	9	6	54
35	5:1	6	8	48
40	3:1	4	10	40
45	2:1	3	15	45
50	1.7:1	2.7	15	40.5

*These flow rates were selected to ensure that the minimum total flow through the system would be at least 40 L/min. The manufacturers may recommend other minimal O₂ flow rates.

(Fig. 6-13). To be sure that this happens, the total flow through the mask must be equal or greater than the patient's peak inspiratory flow. (The interested learner is encouraged to read about the Bernoulli principle, which regulates the mixing of fluids as a result of a drop in pressure caused by a jet.) These masks are sometimes called Venturi masks, Venti masks, jet-mixing, and high airflow with oxygen enrichment (HAFOE) systems. See Table 6-5 for specific information on available air-entrainment masks.

These masks are recommended in any clinical situation where a known, certain oxygen percentage must be given to the patient who has a variable respiratory rate, inspiratory/

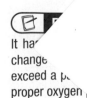

It ha change exceed a p proper oxygen ,

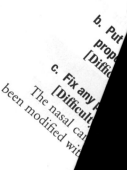

3. Na

a.

b. Put prop [Diffi

c. Fix any The nasal ca been modified wi

TABLE 6-6	Estimated Delivered Oxygen Percentage in Adults Based on the Oxygen Liter Flow Through a Nasal Cannula

Oxygen (L/min)	Estimated delivered oxygen (%)
1	24
2	28
3	32
4	36
5	40
6	44

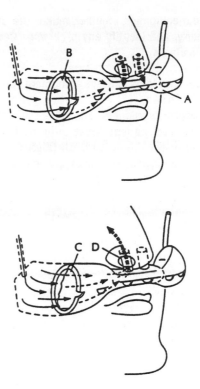

Fig. 6-15 Drawing of the Oximizer reservoir nasal cannula and its functions. (Courtesy of CHAD Therapeutics, Chatsworth, Calif.)

liter of oxygen per minute (Table 6-6). Flows are usually limited to 6 L/min to avoid excessive irritation to the nasal passages.

Flows are usually limited to no more than 1 to 2 L/min in infants and 4 L/min in older children. The pulse oximetry value or PaO_2 level should be checked in patients of any age whenever a flow change is made or the patient's condition changes significantly.

The traditional cannulas just described are commonly used in hospitals for short-term patient use. However, in the home setting for long-term use, it is more economical to use one of the newer cannulas with a built-in oxygen reservoir because less oxygen is used.

Oxygen-conserving nasal cannula. Oxygen-conserving nasal cannulas are employed for patients who need long-term oxygen therapy and wish to reduce their costs. When such a cannula is combined with a pulse-dose oxygen delivery system, the patient's oxygen delivery costs can be significantly cut. There are at least two different types of oxygen-conserving cannulas. Fig. 6-15 shows a reservoir nasal cannula and how it operates. It has an 18-mL reservoir that fills when the patient exhales and gives up its oxygen bolus during the next inspiration. Fig. 6-16 shows a pendant nasal cannula with its reservoir that hangs on the chest. Both types can have problems with tubing disconnections or kinks that can happen with any type of cannula. The only problem that is unique to both of these units is failure of the diaphragm that moves back and forth as the reservoir fills and empties. This membrane may wear out after about a week and prevent the reservoir from filling or emptying properly. Watch as the patient breathes to make sure that the diaphragm is moving properly. If not, replace the cannula.

4. Oxygen masks: simple oxygen mask, partial rebreathing mask, nonrebreathing mask, and face tent
    a. Get the necessary equipment for the procedure (Code: IIA1a1) [Difficulty: An]

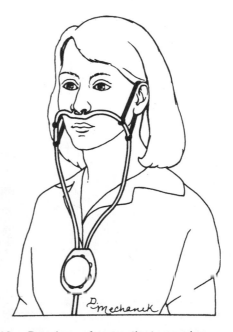

Fig. 6-16 Drawing of a patient wearing a pendant reservoir nasal cannula made by CHAD Therapeutics. (From Wyka KA: Respiratory home care. In Scanlon CL, Spearman CB, Sheldon RL: *Egan's fundamentals of respiratory care,* ed 5, St Louis, 1990, Mosby.)

b. Put the equipment together, make sure that it works properly, and identify any problems (Code: IIB1a1) [Difficulty: An]

c. Fix any problems with the equipment (Code: IIB2a1) [Difficulty: An]

Simple oxygen mask. This mask, like all others, is designed to fit over the patient's nose and mouth and act as an oxygen reservoir for the next breath (Figs. 6-17 and 6-18). Various adult and pediatric sizes are available, and the patient should wear one that best fits the facial contours and size of the face. This is for comfort, as well as to try to increase the inspired oxygen percentage by decreasing the amount of room air that is inspired. Exhaled breath escapes through the exhalation ports. The patient's breathing pattern affects the amount of room air that is breathed in through the same exhalation ports. These ports are also important in case the oxygen flow to the mask is cut off.

Because the oxygen reservoir in the mask is not large enough to meet the patient's tidal volume, the inspired

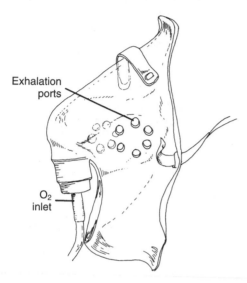

Fig. 6-17 Close up view of a simple oxygen mask. (From McPherson SP: *Respiratory care equipment,* ed 4, St Louis, 1990, Mosby.)

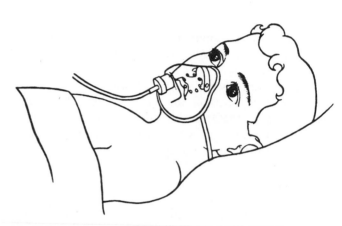

Fig. 6-18 Child wearing a simple oxygen mask. (From Gaebler G, Blodgett D: Gas administration. In Blodgett D, editor: *Manual of pediatric respiratory care procedures,* Philadelphia, 1982, Lippincott.)

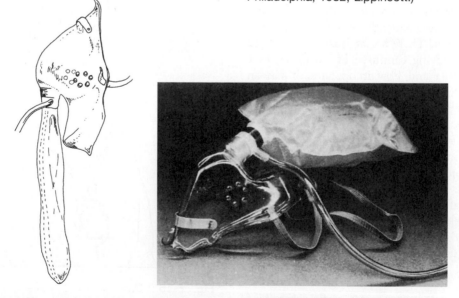

Fig. 6-19 Outside view of a partial rebreathing mask. (From McPherson SP: *Respiratory care equipment,* ed 4, St Louis, 1990, Mosby.)

oxygen percentage is unpredictable. Oxygen flows between 5 and 10 L/min should provide *approximately* 35% to 60% inspired oxygen. The pulse oximetry value or PaO_2 level should be checked whenever a flow change is made or the patient's condition changes significantly.

A bubble humidifier is often added so that the gas is not dry. Make sure that it works properly and that oxygen is flowing through the tubing before putting it on the patient. This and all other masks use an adjustable elastic strap that goes behind the head to hold it in place. Make sure that the mask fits snugly but not so tight as to cut off circulation.

Partial-rebreathing mask. The partial-rebreathing mask has a 500- to 1000-mL plastic bag added to the mask to act as an oxygen reservoir for the next breath (Figs. 6-19 to 6-21). Child and adult size masks are commonly available. When properly applied, the first third of the patient's exhaled gas from the anatomic dead space is exhaled back into this bag. This gas is close to pure oxygen and has no carbon dioxide. Exhaled breath escapes through the exhalation ports. The patient's breathing pattern affects the amount of room air that is breathed in through the same exhalation ports. These ports are also important in case the oxygen flow to the mask is cut off. The added reservoir of oxygen results in a higher percentage being given to the patient than a simple oxygen mask. An oxygen flow of between 6 and 10 L/min should provide *approximately* 35% to 80% inspired oxygen.

A bubble humidifier is often added so that the gas is not dry. Make sure that it works properly, that the oxygen is flowing through the tubing, and that the reservoir bag has been filled before putting it on the patient. Adjust the flow as needed to ensure that the reservoir does not collapse by more than one-third on inspiration. This ensures that the mask and reservoir are filled with as much oxygen as possible. A pulse oximetry value or PaO_2 level should be checked whenever a flow change is made or the patient's condition changes significantly.

Nonrebreathing mask. The nonrebreathing mask looks initially like the partial-rebreathing mask with its plastic bag added as an oxygen reservoir for the next breath (Figs. 6-22 and 6-23). However, notice that a one-way valve has been added between the mask and the reservoir bag. This allows the bag to be filled with pure oxygen that is available for the next breath. No exhaled gas can enter the reservoir. Two (sometimes one) one-way valves are added to the exhalation ports on the mask. These ensure that the patient breathes in only oxygen and not room air. Exhaled breath escapes through the exhalation ports as with the partial-rebreathing mask. Not shown is an emergency pop-in valve that allows room air to be drawn into the mask if the oxygen supply is cut off. Adult and pediatric sizes are available. The mask should be conformed to fit the patient's facial contours and size as much as possible. As mentioned earlier, this is for comfort and to try to increase the inspired oxygen percentage by decreasing the amount of room air that is inspired. It is, in theory, possible to deliver 100% oxygen with this mask if the oxygen flow is high enough and the mask is airtight over the face. However, experience has shown that the disposable masks that are usually available in the hospital do not prevent room air from being drawn in. Oxygen flows between 8

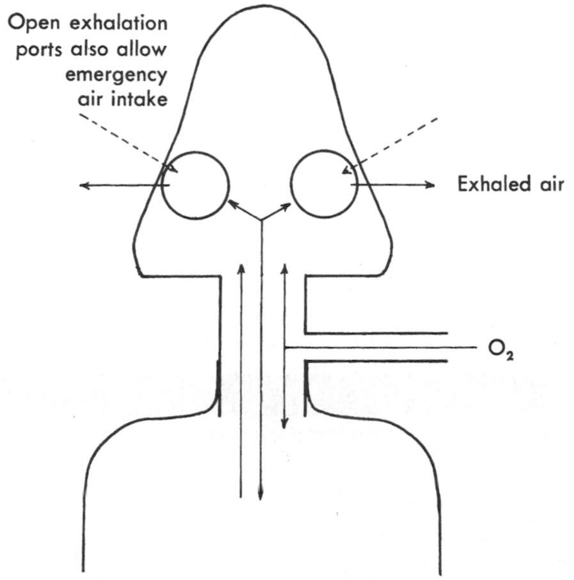

Open exhalation ports also allow emergency air intake

Exhaled air

O_2

Fig. 6-20 Cutaway view of a partial rebreathing mask showing gas flow. (From Thalken FR: Medical gas therapy, in Scanlan CL, Spearman CB, and Sheldon RL, editors: *Egan's fundamentals of respiratory care*, ed 5, St Louis, 1990, Mosby.)

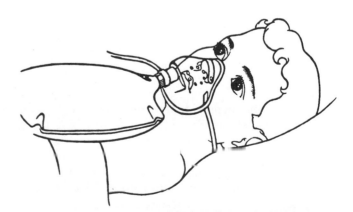

Fig. 6-21 Child wearing a partial rebreathing mask. (From Gaebler G, Blodgett D: Gas administration. In Blodgett D, editor: *Manual of pediatric respiratory care procedures*, Philadelphia, 1982, Lippincott.)

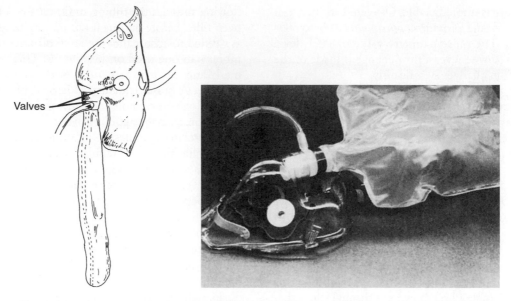

Valves

Fig. 6-22 Outside view of a nonrebreathing mask. (From McPherson SP: *Respiratory care equipment,* ed 4, St Louis, 1990, Mosby.)

Fig. 6-23 Cutaway view of a nonrebreathing mask showing gas flow. (From Thalken FR: Medical gas therapy. In Scanlan CL, Spearman CB, Sheldon RL, editors: *Egan's fundamentals of respiratory care,* ed 5, St Louis, 1990, Mosby.)

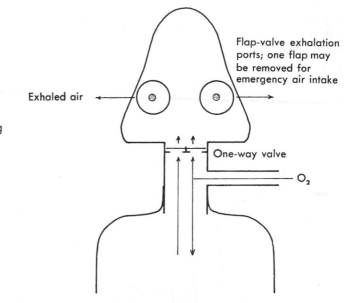

Flap-valve exhalation ports; one flap may be removed for emergency air intake

Exhaled air

One-way valve

O_2

and 10 L/min should provide *approximately* 60% to 80% (or more) inspired oxygen.

A bubble humidifier is often added so that the gas is not dry. Make sure that it works properly, that the oxygen is flowing through the tubing, and that the reservoir bag has been filled before putting it on the patient. Adjust the flow as needed to ensure that the reservoir does not collapse by more than one-third on inspiration. This ensures that the mask and reservoir are filled with oxygen and that the patient's tidal volume comes completely from the reservoir bag. The patient's pulse oximetry value or PaO_2 level should be checked whenever a flow change is made or the patient's condition changes significantly.

EXAM HINT

Expect to see one question that deals with the need to switch from a low oxygen percentage mask to a nonrebreather mask to give the seriously hypoxemic patient as much oxygen as possible. Also expect to see one question dealing with the reservoir bag collapsing on inspiration. Usually this involves the patient receiving a helium and oxygen (heliox) mix. Solve the problem by increasing the flow of therapeutic gas to the mask and bag.

Face tent. These masks are designed to fit around the patient's neck, under the jaw, and around the cheeks in front of the ears. The front edge should be higher than the

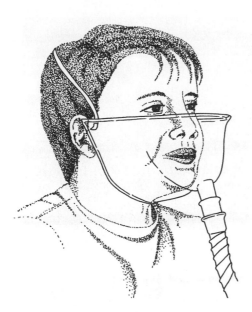

Fig. 6-24 Young adult wearing a face tent.

level of the patient's nostrils (Fig. 6-24). These are sometimes used to provide oxygen to a patient who cannot wear a mask or cannula because of oral and nasal trauma, burns, or surgery. The patient using a face tent should be sitting as upright as possible. This is because oxygen is heavier than air and tends to settle in the mask around the patient's nose and mouth if the fit is tight. If the patient is lying flat or if the mask fits loosely, the oxygen will simply "pour" down out of it. This makes it difficult to know with any certainty what inspired oxygen percentage is available to the patient. Flows of 5 to 10 of oxygen L/min are commonly used with adults.

A face tent is usually ordered with the oxygen run through a humidifier or nebulizer so that the gas is not dry. Make sure that the humidifier or nebulizer is filled with sterile water, that the high-pressure pop-off works, and that gas is flowing through the tubing before it is put on the patient. Try to analyze the oxygen percentage close to the patient's nose and mouth with as much accuracy as possible. A pulse oximetry value or PaO_2 level should be checked whenever a change in the oxygen percentage is made or the patient's condition changes significantly.

5. Transtracheal oxygen catheter
   a. Get the necessary equipment for the procedure (Code: IIA1a1) [Difficulty: An]

   b. Put the equipment together, make sure that it works properly, and identify any problems with it (Code: IIB1a1) [Difficulty: An]

The transtracheal oxygen (TTO_2) catheter is a 20-cm long flexible, hollow plastic tube (see Fig. 6-25, **A**). It is inserted into the trachea via a puncture procedure at the suprasternal notch. To date, only adults with COPD have

had the procedure performed. Oxygen is delivered directly into the trachea. The patient's oxygenation can be maintained at lower oxygen flows than needed by a regular face mask or nasal cannula. The following equipment is needed:

1. Proper size transtracheal catheter (9 French is the usual adult size)
2. Guide wire/stylet
3. Chain-link necklace to hold the catheter in place
4. Regular small-bore oxygen tubing to connect to the distal end of the catheter
5. Flowmeter and oxygen source
6. Optional bubble humidifier with sterile water for patient comfort

Under normal working conditions, regular oxygen tubing is used to connect the oxygen source to the catheter. The oxygen flow to the catheter is set high enough to keep a satisfactory PaO_2 or SpO_2 level. Usually this is less than previously needed by nasal cannula. When combined with a portable liquid oxygen system or a pulse-dose oxygen delivery system, the patient has a real opportunity for increased mobility and decreased cost.

   c. Fix any problems with the equipment (Code: IIB2a1) [Difficulty: An]

The patient needs to be instructed to disconnect the oxygen tubing and flush the catheter with 3 mL of sterile saline twice a day. A cleaning rod can also be pushed through the catheter to make sure that no mucus accumulates. As with any tubing system, the components can become disconnected. Make sure that all connections are tight. If the saline or cleaning rod cannot be pushed through the catheter, an obstruction is likely. The patient should come into the hospital to have the catheter removed and replaced if necessary. It is possible that the proximal catheter tip has twisted into the tracheal mucosa. This can lead to subcutaneous emphysema. The patient should be instructed on how to identify the signs of this and to turn off the oxygen to the catheter. He or she should go back to using a nasal cannula for oxygen and call the physician for guidance.

6. Tracheostomy appliances: mask/collar and Brigg's adapter/ T-piece
   a. Get the necessary equipment for the procedure (Code: IIA1a2) [Difficulty: An]

   b. Put the equipment together, make sure that it works properly, and identify any problems (Code: IIB1a2) [Difficulty: An]

   c. Fix any problems with the equipment (Code: IIB2a2) [Difficulty: An]
   Tracheostomy mask/collar. The adult or pediatric tracheostomy mask or collar is shaped to fit over a tracheostomy tube or stoma to provide oxygen and aerosol (Fig. 6-26).

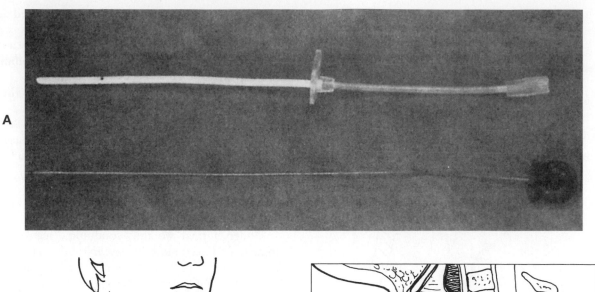

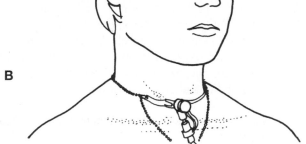
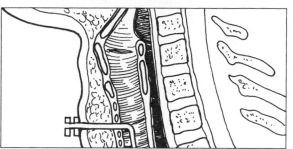

Fig. 6-25 Transtracheal oxygen catheter. **A (top),** Photograph of a flexible, plastic transtracheal oxygen catheter. The part to the left of the flange is inserted into the patient's trachea. The part to the right of the flange is attached to standard oxygen tubing. **A (bottom),** The metal stylet may be used to help keep the catheter stiff during insertion and to clear the catheter of an obstruction. **B,** Drawing of a chain-link necklace keeping the external part of the catheter and flange secure. **C,** Cutaway drawing showing the catheter inserted into the trachea. (From White GC: *Equipment theory for respiratory care,* Albany, NY, 1992, Delmar.)

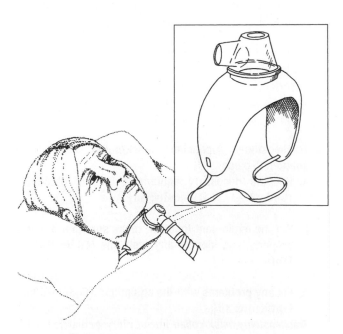

Fig. 6-26 Adult wearing a tracheostomy mask/collar.

Because the patient's upper airway is bypassed, a nebulizer is used for humidity. It is usually an air-entrainment type, so the oxygen percentage can be adjusted. Make sure that the nebulizer is filled with sterile water, that the high-pressure pop-off valve is working, and that adequate mist is flowing through to the mask before putting it on the patient.

Because the tracheostomy mask is an open system without reservoir, it is difficult to guarantee the patient's inspired oxygen percentage. Set the gas flow high enough to make a "cloud" of aerosol around the tracheostomy. If an excess of aerosol can be seen around the tracheostomy during inspiration, there is a good likelihood that the desired oxygen percentage is being delivered. Analyze the oxygen percentage from inside the mask to try for as much accuracy as possible. A pulse oximetry value or PaO_2 level should be checked whenever a flow change or oxygen percentage change is made or the patient's condition changes significantly.

Brigg's adapter/T-piece. The Brigg's adapter or T-piece is designed to provide air or supplemental oxygen and aerosol to an endotracheal or tracheostomy tube. It has one 15-mm inner-diameter (ID) opening that fits over any endotracheal or tracheostomy tube adapter. The other two openings are 22 mm outer diameter (OD) so that aerosol tubing can be added (Fig. 6-27). A nebulizer is commonly used for humidity because the patient's upper airway is bypassed. Make sure that the nebulizer is filled with sterile water, that the high-pressure pop-off valve is working, and that adequate mist is flowing through to the adapter before putting it on the patient. The nebulizer is usually an air-entrainment type, so the oxygen percentage can be adjusted.

The addition of a length of aerosol tubing downstream from the adapter acts as a reservoir so that the inspired oxygen percentage is ensured. A reservoir of 50 to 100 mL of aerosol tubing is commonly needed for the adult. Care must be taken to adjust the gas flow so that it is high enough to meet the patient's peak inspiratory flow rate. This can be determined by watching the aerosol flow past the adapter and reservoir. Make sure that during inspiration the aerosol is still flowing past the tracheostomy/endotracheal tube and into the reservoir. Inadequate flow could result in the patient rebreathing gas from the reservoir. This gas has just been exhaled and is high in carbon dioxide and low in oxygen.

🖺 EXAM HINT

Know to increase the aerosol flow to either a tracheostomy mask or Brigg's adapter/T-piece if the aerosol cannot be seen during a patient's inspiration. The NBRC usually calls this a T-piece rather than a Brigg's adapter in its questions.

MODULE D	Modify specialty gas therapy by changing the mode of administration, adjusting the flow, and adjusting the gas concentration (Code: IIIC4) [Difficulty: Ap, An]

The indications for all of the specialty gases are listed in Box 6-1. Although none of these gases are widely used in respiratory care, they can be very beneficial when indicated.

O₂/CO₂ (carbogen) therapy. A child with hypoplastic left-heart syndrome (HLHS) is usually being mechanically ventilated. The infant with this congenital heart defect must maintain an open foramen ovale and patent ductus arteriosus (PDA) for adequate systemic circulation. Carbogen is added by small-bore tubing connecting the gas cylinder with a T-piece connected into the ventilator circuit. Usually enough carbogen flow is added to result in 1% to 4% carbon dioxide being measured on a capnometer. Because increased carbon dioxide is a pulmonary vasoconstrictor, the PDA can be maintained. The infant's

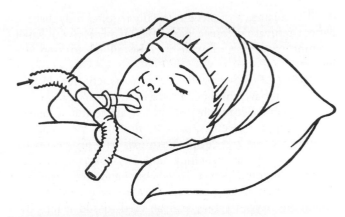

Fig. 6-27 Child with intubated airway with a Brigg's adapter/T-piece and aerosol tubing added to the endotracheal tube. (From Gaebler G, Blodgett D: Gas administration. In Blodgett D, editor: *Manual of pediatric respiratory care procedures,* Philadelphia, 1982, Lippincott.)

BOX 6-1	Indications for the Special Therapeutic Gases: O_2/CO_2 (Carbogen), He/O_2 (Heliox), and NO (Nitric Oxide)

CARBOGEN USES
  Hypoplastic left-heart syndrome (HLHS)
  Carbon dioxide response curve test
  Singultus (hiccup)

HELIOX USES
Upper-airway obstruction:
  Tracheal tumor
  Laryngotracheobronchitis (croup)
  Postextubation stridor
Lower-airway obstruction:
  Status asthmaticus
  May reduce work of breathing in other conditions such as COPD, bronchiolitis, or small endotracheal tube

NITRIC OXIDE USES
  Treatment of term and near-term (>34 weeks) neonates with hypoxic respiratory failure associated with clinical or echocardiographic evidence of pulmonary hypertension
  Possible use in acute respiratory distress syndrome (ARDS)

vital signs and arterial blood gas values must be closely monitored to guide the adjustment in carbogen.

The carbon dioxide response curve test is discussed in Chapter 4. Depending on the method of test performed, the patient inhales between 1% and 7% carbon dioxide. The flow and concentration must be adjusted to maintain the desired carbon dioxide level as measured on a capnometer. An oxygen analyzer should also be included in the system to make sure that the patient does not inhale less than 21% oxygen.

The treatment of hiccups usually requires only that the patient rebreathe from a paper bag. If necessary, a small amount of carbon dioxide can be added to stop the hiccups.

He/O$_2$ (heliox) therapy. Patients who benefit from He/O$_2$ therapy can have an upper-airway or lower-airway obstruction problem. Because helium atoms are so much smaller than nitrogen molecules, patients find that their work of breathing is greatly reduced. Normoxic patients are usually given a mix of 80% helium and 20% oxygen, whereas hypoxic patients are given 70% helium and 30% oxygen or 60% helium and 40% oxygen. If more oxygen is needed, small-bore oxygen tubing can be used to add it into the mask or reservoir bag, or a special closed system will have to be assembled from components.

Ideally any helium/oxygen delivery system should have a reservoir bag. Usually the nonrebreathing mask and reservoir are used. The reservoir should be filled with the He/O$_2$ mix before the mask is placed on the patient's face. Again, the fit should be as tight as possible to minimize leaks. Adjust the flow so that the reservoir bag does not collapse by more than one-third during an inspiration. If it does, increase the flow. The flow should be increased if the patient complains of shortness of breath. Signs of increased work of breathing include agitation, increased use of accessory muscles of respiration, sweating, and increased respiratory rate, heart rate, and blood pressure.

Nitric oxide (NO) therapy. Because nitric oxide is a pulmonary vasodilator, it has been shown to be effective in the treatment of newborns with pulmonary hypertension (persistent pulmonary hypertension of the newborn [PPHN]). The Food and Drug Administration has approved the use of INOmax (0.8% nitric oxide and 99.2% nitrogen) to deliver inhaled nitric oxide to these patients. The currently recommended dose of INOmax is 20 parts per million (ppm). To deliver this concentration of nitric oxide and supplemental oxygen the INOvent delivery system is also needed. It is used to set the desired mix of INOmax to the newborn's ventilator and monitor the level of NO, nitrogen dioxide (NO$_2$), and oxygen delivered.

INOmax has not been approved for adult patients. However, there are reports of nitric oxide being administered to patients with acute respiratory distress syndrome (ARDS) with promising results.

MODULE E	Participate in the development of the respiratory care plan [e.g., case management, develop and apply protocols, disease management education] (Code: IC4) [Difficulty: An]

Look for signs of hypoxemia and be prepared to recommend a change in the patient's oxygen delivery system or oxygen percentage to correct the problem. Tachycardia and tachypnea are common findings in hypoxemic patients. Proper oxygen therapy should relieve the problem so that the patient's vital signs return toward normal. An abnormal heart rhythm as a result of hypoxemia should return to normal with the relief of the problem. Check the patient's pulse oximetry or PaO$_2$ value whenever there is a change in the inspired oxygen percentage or a significant change in the patient's clinical condition.

a. Change the oxygen percentage (Code: IIIC3a) [Difficulty: An]

b. Change the flow of oxygen (Code: IIIC3a) [Difficulty: An]

c. Change the method of administering the oxygen (Code: IIIC3a) [Difficulty: An]

Every patient's oxygen percentage or flow must be tailored to meet the patient's clinical goals. Usually this means keeping the patients who are acutely hypoxemic with a PaO$_2$ level between 60 and 100 torr and a SpO$_2$ value between 90% and 97%. Exceptions, when the blood oxygen level is kept as high as possible, include cardiopulmonary resuscitation and the treatment of carbon monoxide poisoning. Another exception is the chronic obstructive lung disease (COPD) patient who is hypoxemic and hypercarbic. Usually these patients' conditions are maintained with a moderate hypoxemia. The PaO$_2$ level should be between 50 and 60 torr and the SpO$_2$ value between 85% and 90%. It is imperative to keep the oxygen in this relatively narrow range. Further hypoxemia will result in pulmonary hypertension and cor pulmonale. Cardiac dysrhythmias or arrest and death can occur if the hypoxemia is severe (<40 torr). Oxygen levels in the normal range (>60 torr) may result in blunting of the hypoxic drive. This can result in bradypnea and even greater carbon dioxide retention with corresponding acidemia. When the carbon dioxide pressure (PaCO$_2$) level exceeds 80 to 90 torr, many patients become drowsy or somnolent. The treatment is to decrease the FIO$_2$ to lower the PaO$_2$ level to 50 to 60 torr. This, in turn, stimulates the hypoxic drive so that the patient increases his or her ventilation.

☞ EXAM HINT

Know the advantages, disadvantages, and possible oxygen ranges for the various oxygen appliances discussed earlier. Be prepared to make recommendations to change from one appliance to another or to change the oxygen percentage or flow. Expect to see one question that deals with the need to reduce the inspired oxygen percentage to a COPD patient with hypercarbia. In addition, there is usually one question that deals with needing to raise the inspired oxygen percentage to a COPD patient who is too hypoxemic.

BIBLIOGRAPHY

AARC clinical practice guideline: Oxygen therapy in the acute care hospital. *Respir Care* 36:1410-1413, 1991.

AARC Clinical Practice Guideline: Oxygen therapy in the home or extended care facility. *Respir Care* 37(8):918-922, 1992.

Bageant RA: Oxygen analyzers. *Respir Care* 21:410-416, 1976.

Burton GG, Hodgkin JE, Ward JJ, editors: *Respiratory care, a guide to clinical practice*, ed 4, Philadelphia, 1997, Lippincott-Raven.

Dantzker DR, MacIntyre NR, Bakow ED, editors: *Comprehensive respiratory care*, Philadelphia, 1995, WB Saunders.

Datex-Ohmeda. INOvent delivery system. Available at: http://www.datex-ohmeda.com. Accessed January 1, 2001.

Eubanks DH, Bone RC: *Comprehensive respiratory care*, ed 2, St Louis, 1990, Mosby.

Fink JB, Hunt GE, editors: *Clinical practice in respiratory care.* Philadelphia, 1999, Lippincott-Raven.

Gaebler G, Blodgett D: Gas administration. In Blodgett D, editor: *Manual of pediatric respiratory care procedures.* Philadelphia, 1982, Lippincott.

Gluck EH et al: Helium-oxygen mixture in intubated patients with status asthmaticus and respiratory acidosis, *Chest* 98(3): 693-698, 1990.

Hill KV: Oxygen Therapy. In Aloan CA, Hill TV, editors: *Respiratory care of the newborn and child*, ed 2, Philadelphia, 1997, Lippincott-Raven.

Holman GA et al: Helium-oxygen improves clinical asthma scores in children with acute bronchiolitis, *Crit Care Med* 26(10):1731-1736, 1998.

INOTherapeutics, Inc. Homepage. Available at: http://www.inotherapeutics.com. Accessed January 1, 2001.

Kass JE, Castriotta RJ: Heliox therapy in acute severe asthma, *Chest* 107(3): 757-760, 1995.

Kemper KJ et al: Helium-oxygen mixture in the treatment of postextubaton stridor in pediatric trauma patients, *Crit Care Med* 19(3): 356-359, 1991.

Kudukis TM et al: Inhaled helium-oxygen revisited: effect of inhaled helium-oxygen during the treatment of status asthmaticus in children, *J Pediatri* 131(2): 333-334, 1997.

McPherson SP: *Respiratory care equipment*, ed 5, St Louis, 1995, Mosby.

Scanlan CL, Heuer A: Medical gas therapy. In Scanlan CL, Wilkins RL, Stoller JK, editors: *Egan's fundamentals of respiratory care*, ed 7, St, Louis, 1999, Mosby.

Schaffer EM et al: Oxygenation in status asthmaticus improves during ventilation with helium-oxygen, *Crit Care Med* 27(12): 2666-2670.

Shapiro BA, Kacmarek RM, Cane RD et al, editors: *Clinical application of respiratory care*, ed 4, St Louis, 1991, Mosby.

Shapiro BA, Harrison RA, Cane RD et al: *Clinical application of blood gases*, ed 4, St Louis, 1989, Mosby.

Tassaux D et al: Calibration of seven ICU ventilators for mechanical ventilation with helium- oxygen mixtures, *Am J Respir Crit Care Med* 160:22-32, 1999.

Ward JJ: Equipment for mixed gas and oxygen therapy, In Branson RD, Hess DR, Chatburn RL, editors: *Respiratory care equipment*, ed 2, Philadelphia, 1999, Lippincott Williams & Wilkins.

Ward JJ: Medical gas therapy. In Burton GC, Hodgkin JE, Ward JJ, editors: *Respiratory care: a guide to clinical practice*, ed 4, Philadelphia, 1997, Lippincott-Raven.

Whitaker K: *Comprehensive perinatal & pediatric respiratory care*, ed 2, Albany, NY, 1997, Delmar.

White GC: *Equipment theory for respiratory care*, ed 3, Albany, NY, 1999, Delmar

Wojciechowski WV: *Respiratory care sciences: an integrated approach*, ed 3, Albany, NY, 2000, Delmar.

Youtsey JW: Oxygen and mixed gas therapy. In Barnes TA, editor: *Core textbook of respiratory care practice*, ed 2, St Louis, 1994, Mosby.

SELF-STUDY QUESTIONS

1. A COPD patient is going home. After doing a hospital exercise test, it has been determined that she will require 1 L/min of supplemental oxygen when exercising on her stationary bicycle or when she feels short of breath. Which of the following oxygen delivery systems should the respiratory therapist recommend?
   A. Molecular sieve oxygen concentrator
   B. Linde Walker portable liquid oxygen system
   C. Semipermeable membrane oxygen concentrator
   D. Piston compressor

2. You are attempting to calibrate a polarographic oxygen analyzer but find that it cannot be done. Possible reasons for this include:
   I. The membrane is torn on the probe.
   II. The gas sampling capillary tube is plugged with debris.
   III. The electrode solution has evaporated.
   IV. The battery needs to be replaced.
   V. Water has condensed on the membrane.
   A. I and III only
   B. II and III only
   C. III, IV, and V only
   D. I, III, IV, and V only

3. A 3-year-old child with bronchitis is being kept in an oxygen tent. He is supposed to be in a 40% oxygen environment. When analyzing the percentage you find the tent to contain 35% oxygen. To increase the oxygen percentage you would do all the following *except*:
   A. Make sure that the bottom edge of the tent canopy is tucked under the mattress.
   B. Increase the flow of oxygen.
   C. Adjust the air entrainment nebulizer to give a more dense mist
   D. Make sure that all patient access ports are closed.

4. An adult patient who was rescued from a house fire is being received in the emergency department. He is wearing a simple oxygen mask at 5 L/min. The SpO_2 value by pulse oximeter is 100%, and his SaO_2 value from an arterial blood gas sample analyzed on a CO-oximeter is 73%. What would you recommend be done at this time?
   A. Maintain the simple oxygen mask at the present flow.
   B. Change the patient to a nonrebreather mask.

C. Decrease the oxygen flow to the simple oxygen mask to 4 L/min.

D. Maintain present therapy and recalibrate the CO-oximeter.

5. Which of the following is the best device for giving 35% oxygen to an alert 2-year-old?
   A. Oxygen tent
   B. Nasal cannula at 3 L/min
   C. Simple mask at 3 L/min
   D. Incubator

6. You are called to evaluate a patient known to have advanced emphysema. She is wearing a nasal cannula at 6 L/min. The nurse says that she has become drowsy and less responsive since the oxygen was given to her an hour ago. Her arterial blood gas (ABG) results on the oxygen show:

   PaO_2 84 torr
   $PaCO_2$ 65 torr
   pH 7.32.

   Which of the following would you would recommend?
   I. Leave her on the cannula.
   II. Change her to 24% O_2 on an air-entrainment mask and repeat the ABGs in 20 minutes.
   III. Change her to a simple oxygen mask and repeat the ABGs in 20 minutes.
   IV. Let her rest undisturbed.
   V. Monitor her closely for becoming more alert.
   A. I and IV only
   B. III and IV only
   C. II and V only
   D. III and V only

7. You are assisting with a bronchoscopy to biopsy a suspicious laryngeal node on your patient. Afterward, the patient complains of shortness of breath and a "tight" throat. Which of the following recommendations could you give to the physician?
   A. Give the patient a 20% oxygen/80% helium mix to breathe.
   B. Put the head of the bed down 30 degrees.
   C. Give the patient a carbogen mix to breathe.
   D. Do a 7-minute helium dilution test.

8. You receive a call at the office from one of your home-care patients. She reports that the high-pressure pop-off valve on the bubble humidifier to her transtracheal oxygen catheter is venting. In addition, she cannot flush out the catheter with saline or push the cleaning rod through it. What should you tell her to do?
   A. Remove the humidifier and double the oxygen flow rate to the catheter.
   B. Force the saline through the catheter until the obstruction is cleared.
   C. Force the cleaning rod through the catheter until the obstruction is cleared.
   D. Come in to the outpatient area of the hospital to have the catheter replaced.

9. You are working with a patient who has a tracheal tumor. He is wearing a nonrebreather mask with 20% oxygen and 80% helium. The patient says that it is harder to breathe and has increased his respiratory rate. You notice that the reservoir bag has collapsed. The most appropriate action is to:

A. Decrease the flow of gas.
B. Switch to an air entrainment mask and deliver 24% oxygen.
C. Increase the flow of gas.
D. Switch to a 30% oxygen/70% helium mix.

10. A 58-year-old patient with advanced emphysema is admitted with an acute exacerbation of his condition. While breathing 2 L/min of oxygen through a transtracheal oxygen catheter, he has the following arterial blood gas results:

pH	7.38
$PaCO_2$	57 torr
HCO_3^-	31 mEq/liter
PaO_2	47 torr
SaO_2	80%

    Based on these findings, what do you think should be done?
    A. Change the patient to 24% oxygen by an air-entrainment mask.
    B. Initiate bilevel mask ventilation.
    C. Change the patient to a nonrebreathing mask with 10 L/min of oxygen.
    D. Increase the oxygen flow to the current system to 3 L/min.

11. A 36-week gestational age neonate is hypoxic despite mechanical ventilation and has clinical evidence of persistent pulmonary hypertension of the newborn. What can be done to correct the hypoxemia?
    A. Instill intratracheal surfactant.
    B. Begin nitric oxide (NO) therapy.
    C. Begin 10 cm water PEEP.
    D. Begin carbogen therapy.

12. While working as the respiratory therapist assigned to the emergency department, a 24-year-old patient with status asthmaticus is transferred by ambulance from a small, rural hospital. The patient has been given continuous bronchodilator therapy and intravenous corticosteroids and aminophylline. She is becoming exhausted but refuses to allow intubation and mechanical ventilation. What should be recommended?
    A. Begin heliox therapy.
    B. Begin nitric oxide therapy.
    C. Intubate and ventilate the patient despite her protests.
    D. Allow the patient to expire.

Answer Key

1. **A.** Rationale: At a flow of 1 L/min a molecular sieve oxygen concentrator delivers at least 90% oxygen to the patient. A Linde Walker portable liquid oxygen system is not needed if the patient is not actively and frequently mobile. A semipermiable membrane oxygen concentrator delivers only about 40% oxygen to the patient. A piston compressor is useful to deliver pressurized air to power a small volume nebulizer. It does not deliver more than 21% oxygen (room air) to the patient.

2. **D.** Rationale: A polarographic oxygen analyzer does not have a gas sampling capillary tube; the paramagnetic type does. The other four listed problems can cause a polarographic analyzer to fail. The probe has a membrane through which oxygen diffuses. It must not be torn or have water, blood, or mucus covering it. There must an adequate amount of electrolyte solution within the probe for the oxygen-

related chemical reaction to take place. A functional battery is needed to drive the chemical reaction within the electrolyte solution.

3. **C.** Rationale: Because an air entrainment nebulizer is powered by air and entrains air, it cannot affect the oxygen percentage. The three other items can affect the patient's oxygen percentage inside the tent. Because oxygen is more dense than air, it will leak out the bottom of the tent unless the plastic canopy is tightly tucked under the mattress. Increasing the flow of oxygen into the tent directly increases the oxygen percentage. All patient access ports must be closed to prevent oxygen from leaking out and lowering the oxygen percentage.

4. **B.** Rationale: The significant discrepancy between the pulse oximeter reading and the CO-oximeter can only be explained by the patient having carbon monoxide poisoning. In this situation only the CO-oximeter reading will be accurate. A CO-oximeter reading of 73% indicates severe hypoxemia. Therefore the patient should be changed to a nonrebreather mask with enough flow to keep the reservoir bag inflated. This maximizes the inspired oxygen percentage to the patient. Maintaining the simple oxygen mask at the present flow or decreasing the oxygen flow to the simple oxygen mask to 4 L/min will worsen rather than improve the patient's condition. There is no indication that the CO-oximeter is malfunctioning and needs to be recalibrated.

5. **A.** Rationale: An oxygen tent will provide 35% oxygen to an alert 2-year-old patient without restricting normal movement. It is doubtful that an alert, active 2-year-old will keep either a nasal cannula or simple mask in place as needed. In addition, the actual oxygen percentage cannot be measured through these devices. This child is too large for an incubator.

6. **C.** Rationale: The patient's arterial blood gas results show her PaO_2 to be 84 torr. This is too high for many COPD patients. It is likely that her hypoxic drive to breathe has become blunted. This has resulted in her hypoventilating, with a rising carbon dioxide level and secondary drowsyness. Although it is not possible to know the patient's inspired oxygen percentage with a 6 L/min nasal cannula, this flow has resulted in the PaO_2 being too high. It is best to switch her to an air entrainment mask so that a known low oxygen percentage (24%) can be administered. She should then be closely monitored for returning alertness and another arterial blood gas sample should be obtained. This should be evaluated for a lower, but safe, PaO_2 and a lower $PaCO_2$. The patient should not be left on her present oxygen flow though the nasal cannula because of her unnecessarily high oxygen level, hypoventilation, rising carbon dioxide level, and secondary drowsyness. Changing her from a cannula to a simple face mask at the same oxygen flow will not correct these problems. She needs to be awakened because her drowsiness is not the result of simple fatigue.

7. **A.** Rationale: It is likely that the biopsy site has developed some edema which is causing the shortness of breath and "tight" throat feeling. Giving the patient 20% oxygen and 80% helium should help to ease the patient's shortness of breath because helium is less dense than nitrogen. Putting the patient's head down 30 degrees is commonly used when a patient's blood pressure is low; it is unlikely to ease a feeling of shortness of breathing. Carbogen (carbon dioxide and oxygen mix) stimulates the breathing center of the brain but will not relieve the patient's shortness of breath caused by laryngeal edema. The 7-minute helium dilution test is performed in the pulmonary function laboratory to measure the patient's residual volume. It is not intended to relieve the patient's feeling of shortness of breath from laryngeal edema.

8. **D.** Rationale: Because there is a major obstruction in the transtracheal oxygen catheter it should be replaced and the patient evaluated. This should be done by a practitioner, not the patient. Attempts to force out the obstruction by doubling the oxygen flow or forcing the saline or cleaning rod through the catheter can result in injury to the airway if the catheter ruptures or the obstruction is blown down the airway.

9. **C.** Rationale: Because the reservoir bag has collapsed, the flow of helium and oxygen must be increased. Ideally, the reservoir bag should not collapse by more than one-third on inspiration. Decreasing the flow of gas to the patient will worsen the problem of shortness of breath, not improve it. When the flow of gas to the mask is inadequate it does not matter if the patient is given 24% oxygen or changed to a 30% oxygen and 70% helium mix. In addition, there is no indication that the patient is hypoxemic.

10. **D.** Rationale: The patient's current blood gases show unacceptable hypoxemia with a PaO_2 of 47 torr and SaO_2 of 80%. Increasing the patient from 2 to 3 L/min through the transtracheal oxygen catheter should help to correct the situation. The patient should be monitored for a possible rising carbon dioxide level as well as an improving oxygen level. Changing the patient to 24% oxygen by an air entrainment mask will probably not change his actual inspired oxygen percentage. In addition, there is no indication that the transtracheal oxygen catheter has failed. The patient's ventilation is stable and there is no indication that bilevel mask ventilation is needed. Changing the patient to a nonrebreathing mask with 10 L/min of oxygen is potentially dangerous. This much oxygen may blunt his hypoxic drive to breathe.

11. **B.** Rationale: Inhaled nitric oxide (INOmax) is indicated to dilate the pulmonary vascular bed of a newborn with persistent pulmonary hypertension of the newborn (PPHN). When the pulmonary vascular bed dilates, more blood flows through the lungs and oxygenation should improve. The instillation of intratracheal surfactant is indicated only in a newborn with infant respiratory distress syndrome (RDS). Surfactant therapy is not indicated in PPHN. Although PEEP increases the functional residual capacity of an infant with RDS and improves oxygenation, PEEP must be used with great care, if at all, in a newborn with PPHN. Too much water PEEP may over expand the alveoli of a newborn with PPHN and prevent blood from flowing through the capillary bed. Oxygenation will worsen rather than improve. Carbogen (carbon dioxide and oxygen mix) may be harmful to a newborn with PPHN. This is because an increased carbon dioxide level further constricts the newborn's pulmonary vascular bed. Carbogen is indicated in a newborn with hypoplastic left-heart syndrome.

12. **A.** Rationale: Heliox therapy should be helpful in reducing

the patient's work of breathing. This should allow more time for the corticosteroid and aminophylline medications to begin working. Nitric oxide therapy is a pulmonary vasodilator and not indicated for status asthmaticus. Review Box 6-1 if needed. It is not necessary at this time to go against a patient's wishes and begin mechanical ventilation without first trying heliox therapy. There is absolutely no reason to allow this patient to die from status asthmaticus! It should not be fatal if managed appropriately and aggressively.

7 Humidity and Aerosol Therapy

A review of the most recent Written Registry Exams has shown an average of two questions (2% of the exam) on humidity and aerosol therapy.

MODULE A	Humidity and aerosol generators and administrative devices

1. Humidity delivered through small-bore tubing

a. Bubble-type humidifiers

1. Get the necessary equipment for the procedure (Code: IIA1b) [Difficulty: An]

The bubble-type humidifiers are used on patients with a normal upper airway who need some supplemental humidity because of the dryness of medical oxygen. These devices are not usually heated and, in fact, deliver gas cooled to less than room temperature. They provide around 40% relative humidity (RH) at the delivered gas temperature. The rest of the humidity has to be made up by the patient (Figs. 7-1 and 7-2). It is possible to add a wraparound type of heater if it is clinically indicated to raise the temperature of the delivered gas and reduce the patient's humidity deficit.

There are three different types of these humidifiers designed to add some humidity to dry oxygen delivered through small-bore tubing: tradition bubble humidifiers, jet humidifiers, and underwater jet humidifiers.

Bubble humidifiers. Bubble humidifiers use a perforated capillary tube or porous diffusion head to break the oxygen into small bubbles (Fig. 7-2). This allows for more surface area contact of the oxygen with the water and raises the RH by evaporation. It is important to keep the water level in the reservoir within the manufacturers' specifications and, if possible, as full as possible. The lower the water level, the lower the RH because there is less time for evaporation. The faster the oxygen flow, the lower the RH.

Jet humidifiers. Jet humidifiers create an aerosol that is baffled out of the delivered gas flow. The RH is increased by evaporation of some of the aerosol droplets. These units deliver a higher RH than the bubble humidifiers. They have the additional advantage of delivering the same RH at higher flow levels and as the water level drops.

Underwater jet humidifiers. Underwater jet humidifiers create water vapor and an aerosol. The aerosol is not baffled out as it is in the jet humidifiers. Because of this, these units deliver the highest RH. They can deliver the same humidity level at high gas flows and as the water level drops. The aerosol particles can carry pathogens, so stricter infection control standards must be met to protect the patient. The water and humidifier must be changed at least every 24 hours. If the patient needs the highest possible delivered RH, a jet humidifier or underwater jet humidifier is a better choice than a bubble type.

2. Put the equipment together, make sure that it works properly, and identify any problems (Code: IIB1b) [Difficulty: An]

3. Fix any problems with the equipment (Code: IIB2b) [Difficulty: An]

Many of the simple bubble humidifiers come prepackaged with sterile water. They can be used for many short-term patients (e.g., those in the recovery room) or for a single long-term patient. When the water runs low, they are discarded. The bubble and other types of humidifiers consist of a reservoir jar for the water and a Diameter-Index Safety System (DISS) oxygen connector lid that screws on. Turn on the flowmeter, and make sure that oxygen flows through the delivery tube and bubbles into the water. Failure to bubble usually indicates that the lid and jar are not screwed together tightly or the delivery tube is plugged. If the tube cannot be cleared, it must be replaced.

Most of the newer bubble-type units have a pop-off type of high-pressure relief valve that is released if the pressure builds up to either 40 mm Hg or 2 psi. Pinch closed the small-bore tubing to build up pressure and test the pop-off valve. Feel for the gas to escape from the valve. Many units whistle to signal a gas leak. Do not use a unit whose pop-off valve does not open under pressure.

b. Nasal cannula

Current guidelines state that humidity does not need to be added to these devices if the flow is 4 L/min or less. However, some patients complain of nasal dryness and discomfort if the cannula's oxygen is not humidified. The physician and practitioner may believe that the patient's discomfort warrants the addition of a bubble-type humidifier. There is agreement that humidity should be added to flows of greater than 4 L/min. See Fig. 7-3 for a humidified nasal cannula setup.

c. Oxygen masks

It is not believed to be necessary to add humidity to any oxygen mask that has an oxygen flow of 4 L/min or less. Humidity should be added to any mask that has more than 4 L/min of oxygen added. This includes simple oxygen masks at higher flows, higher oxygen percentage air-entrainment masks, partial rebreathing masks, and non-rebreathing masks.

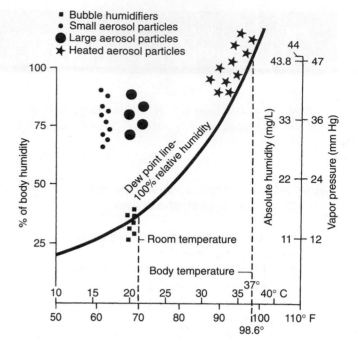

Fig. 7-1 Comparison of humidity content by bubble-type humidifiers and various nebulizers.

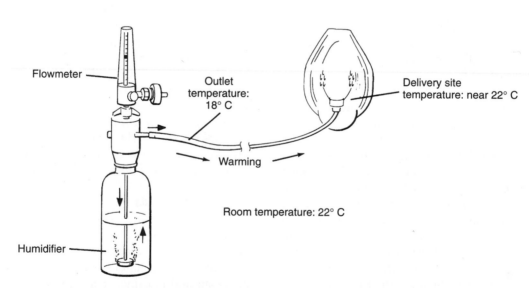

Fig. 7-2 Oxygen leaving outlet of the bubble-type humidifier is cooler than room temperature because of evaporation. Some warming toward room temperature occurs as the oxygen travels through the tubing to the patient. (From Scanlan CL: Humidity and aerosol therapy. In Scanlan CL, Spearman CB, Stoller JK, editors: *Egan's fundamentals of respiratory care,* ed 5, St Louis, 1990, Mosby.)

2. Humidity delivered through large-bore tubing

Most of these patients have had their upper airway bypassed by an endotracheal or tracheostomy tube. Because of this, they cannot humidify inspired gas in the normal manner. In some other cases, humidity is added because the patient is receiving dry medical oxygen. Therefore it is recommended that a heated humidifier be used with these patients. It should be set to deliver gas between 31° and 35° C to the patient and should be able to provide 80% to 100% RH in this temperature range. All of the following humidity and aerosol generating devices deliver the conditioned gas to the patient through large-bore (22-mm inner diameter [ID]) tubing.

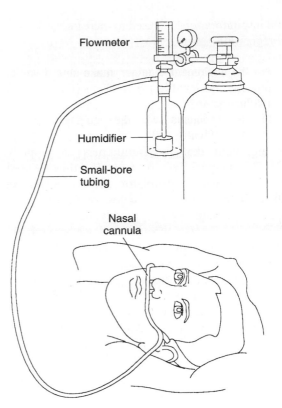

Flowmeter

Humidifier

Small-bore
tubing

Nasal
cannula

Fig. 7-3   Adult wearing a nasal cannula delivering oxygen humidified by a bubble-type humidifier. (From Guidelines for disinfection of home equipment, *Resp Care* 33:801-808, 1988.)

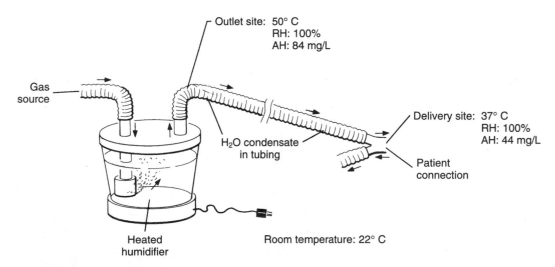

Outlet site: 50° C
RH: 100%
AH: 84 mg/L

Gas
source

H₂O condensate
in tubing

Delivery site: 37° C
RH: 100%
AH: 44 mg/L

Patient
connection

Heated
humidifier

Room temperature: 22° C

Fig. 7-4   Gases leaving outlet of heated humidifier are hot and saturated with water vapor. As cooling occurs in tubing, vapor condenses and absolute humidity (AH) decreases while relative humidity (RH) remains 100% (saturated). Note that almost half of the original vapor is "lost" to condensate in this example. (From Fink JB, Scanlan CL: Humidity and bland aerosol therapy. In Scanlan CL, Wilkins RL, Stoller JK, editors: *Egan's fundamentals of respiratory care*, ed 7, St Louis, 1999, Mosby.)

a. Large-volume humidifiers: cascade, wick, and passover-type

1. Get the necessary equipment for the procedure (Code: IIA1b) [Difficulty: An]

All of these humidifiers have an adjustable heater so that the water in the reservoir is at or greater than body temperature. This enables them to provide up to 100% of the patient's body humidity. It is necessary with all of these units to measure the temperature of the inspired gas near the patient. The gas temperature is usually kept the same as the patient's or a few degrees cooler (Fig. 7-4).

The Bennett Cascade is the most well known of these types of humidifiers (Fig. 7-5). It is most commonly used with a mechanical ventilator but can be used with other types of systems for delivering humidity with or without oxygen. Its basic principle of operation is an efficient bubble-type humidifier. The inspiratory gas must flow through the water for evaporation to occur. A variety of similar devices are now on the market.

The wick-type heated humidifier employs a wick, often made of sponge or paper, to soak up water for evaporation. The water, wick, or both are heated so that 100% RH can be delivered. These units are also used with mechanical ventilators or other systems, including air-entrainment devices. This is because they have very little resistance to the gas flowing through them as evaporation occurs.

Passover-type humidifiers simply have the patient's gas passing over the surface of a reservoir of hot water. They are sometimes called "hot pots." By themselves, these units are probably the least effective at humidifying gas. When they are used on ventilators, other features such as copper mesh

in a heated inspiratory tube are used to increase the surface area for evaporation.

2. **Put the equipment together, make sure it works properly, and identify any problems (Code: IIB1b) [Difficulty: An]**
3. **Fix any problems with the equipment (Code: IIB2b) [Difficulty: An]**

It is important that the humidifiers be properly assembled. This is especially important when they are used to humidify a mechanical ventilator. Any loose connections will result in an air leak and loss of tidal volume. Make sure that the water level is properly maintained.

As the heated gas passes through the large-bore tubing, there is some cooling. This results in condensation that must be drained out. Placing a water trap in the lowest point of the tubing drains the water and helps keep the tubing clear. Remember to continue to look periodically for water puffing or sloshing back and forth in the tubing. Make sure that any condensate is drained out of the tubing and thrown away. Do not drain the condensate back into

Fig. 7-5 Cascade humidifier. (From Scanlan CL: Humidity and aerosol therapy. In Scanlan CL, Spearman CB, Stoller JK, editors: *Egan's fundamentals of respiratory care,* ed 5, St Louis, 1990, Mosby.)

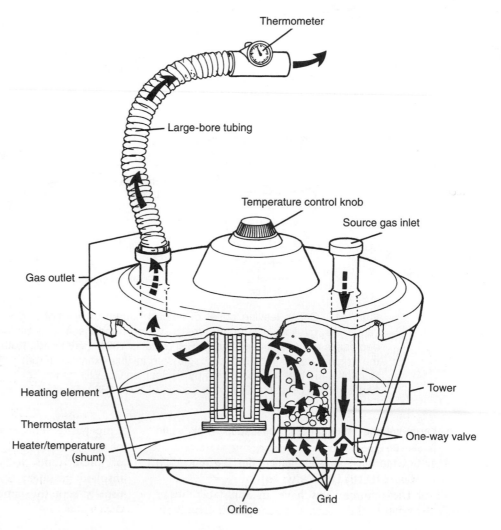

the water reservoir. This is because any microorganisms in the tubing or condensate could reproduce in the reservoir.

b. Heat-moisture exchanger

1. Get the necessary equipment for the procedure (Code: IIA1b) [Difficulty: An]

A heat moisture exchanger (HME) contains a highly absorbent material that is warmed and moistened when a patient's exhaled breath passes through it. The patient's next inspiration is warmed and humidified by the HME. In effect, the patient is rebreathing his or her own exhaled water vapor. These units are not as efficient as the previously described humidifiers and are not able to provide 100% of the body humidity to a patient.

There are many brands of HME but only two main types. The first type is designed to be added to the outer part of a tracheostomy tube. It has a 15-mm ID opening to attach to the tube; the other end of the HME is open to room air. They are small and convenient to use for many patients with a permanent tracheostomy and increase a patient's mobility. The second type is used with patients who require mechanical ventilation. The patient end of the HME is a 15-mm ID to attach to the endotracheal or tracheostomy tube. The other end of the HME has an opening to attach to the ventilator circuit. See Chapter 14 for more detail.

2. Put the equipment together, make sure it works properly, and identify any problems (Code: IIB1b) [Difficulty: An]

3. Fix any problems with the equipment (Code: IIB2b) [Difficulty: An]

Heat moisture exchangers typically come preassembled by the manufacturer. The 15-mm ID opening must be placed over the patient's endotracheal or tracheostomy tube. Secretions coughed into the HME present a significant problem because they can obstruct the flow of gas. This makes it difficult or impossible for the patient to breathe. The HME must be removed and discarded if it becomes obstructed. Replace it with a new one. Ideally, an HME should not be used with a patient known to cough out large amounts of secretions.

3. Nebulizers and related delivery systems

a. Ultrasonic nebulizers

1. Get the necessary equipment for the procedure (Code: IIA1c) [Difficulty: An]

Ultrasonic units are often chosen for delivering bland solutions to the lower airways because of the small particle size and the high output. Ultrasonic nebulizers work by converting electrical energy into very high frequency sound energy that creates aerosol particles. The frequency is vital because it results in a stable aerosol with a mean particle size that is about 3 μm in diameter. This is an ideal size to penetrate deeply into the lungs to the smallest

airways. The only control on these units is for amplitude (power) to control the aerosol output. The range is usually up to 3 to 6 mL/min depending on the model. This output is greater than most pneumatic nebulizers can produce. The aerosol can be carried to the patient by a built-in fan or by an outside oxygen source (Fig. 7-6). The patient's humidity deficit is minimized by the warm aerosol that is created.

The ultrasonic nebulizer should not be chosen for upper-airway aerosol deposition or for administering pharmacologically active medications such as bronchodilators, mucolytics, and antibiotics. These medications may not nebulize at the same rate as the saline diluent, which creates the risk of delivering a very concentrated dose at the end of the treatment. Some of the medications may also be mechanically broken down by the high-frequency vibration and made useless.

2. Put the equipment together, make sure that it works properly, and identify any problems (Code: IIB1c) [Difficulty: An]

3. Fix any problems with the equipment (Code: IIB2c) [Difficulty: An]

Always follow the manufacturer's instructions when setting the system up. Fig. 7-6 shows the common features, and Table 7-1 describes how to troubleshoot many common problems. It seems that many of the clinical difficulties have to do with keeping the proper fluid levels in the couplant chamber and the solution cup. If the sterile

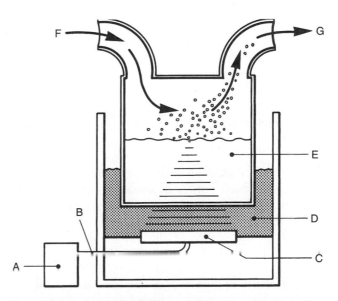

Fig. 7-6 Functional diagram of the ultrasonic nebulizer: *A,* electric current generator, *B,* cable, *C,* piezoelectric crystal, *D,* couplant chamber, *E,* solution cup, *F,* carrier gas inlet, and *G,* aerosol outlet . (From Barnes TA, editor: *Core textbook of respiratory care practice,* ed 2, St Louis, 1994, Mosby.)

TABLE 7-1	Ultrasonic Nebulizer Troubleshooting	
Symptom	**Possible problem**	**Suggested check**
Unit installed and connected as specified, but pilot light does not turn on when switch is turned to the "on" position	Electrical outlet defective Circuit breaker tripped Fuse blown	Check outlet with lamp or other appliance Reset the circuit breaker, or change fuse on the power switch; if the circuit breaker continues to trip or the fuse blows again, service is needed
Unit installed and connected as specified; power pilot light turns on, normal ultrasonic activity visible in nebulizer chamber, but no aerosol output occurs	Nebulizer chamber contaminated	Wash nebulizer chamber; decontaminate
Unit installed and connected as specified; power pilot light turns on, but little ultrasonic activity is visible in the nebulizer chamber, and aerosol output is low (even when on the no. 10 power setting)	Couplant water excessively aerated Nebulizer module and couplant water too cold Diaphragm distorted, permitting air bubbles to interfere with proper transmission of vibrational energy into the nebulizer chamber	Wait for deaeration Use warmer couplant water Check to see that diaphragm is properly shaped and installed; be sure the concave (recessed) side faces the interior of the chamber Clean couplant compartment and replace couplant water
Same as symptom described above but at a lower power setting	Power setting too low to start and establish nebulization	Turn output control knob to maximum power setting, then reduce to desired setting
Unit installed and connected as specified, and power pilot light turns on; "Add couplant" light is on, and no ultrasonic activity is visible in the nebulizer chamber	Insufficient couplant water	Add water to the couplant compartment
Unit installed and connected as specified, and power pilot light turns on; "Add couplant" light is off, but no ultrasonic activity is visible in the nebulizer chamber	Power supply overheated and its thermostatic control opened	The cooling air has been restricted, or cooling fins need cleaning; the switch will reset when the equipment returns to room temperature
Liquid reservoir filled and properly connected to nebulizer chamber, but chamber does not fill *(for continuous-feed system only)*	Foreign material or air bubbles in feed tubes Liquid level control in nebulizer chamber plugged with foreign material Air leaks at tube connection or reservoir cap	Flush the system Clean or flush the system Tighten all connections by pushing tubes into fittings

From Op't Holt T: Aerosol generators and humidifiers. In Barnes TA, editor: *Respiratory care practice*, St Louis, 1988, Mosby.

water in the couplant chamber is too low, the vibration cannot reach the solution cup, and no aerosol will be produced. If the saline level in the solution cup is either too low or too high, the vibrational energy will not focus properly on the surface of the saline solution, and no aerosol will be produced. Water should not be allowed to condense out and fill any low points in the large-bore tubing. If this were to occur, the ultrasonic particles would liquefy as the carrier gas is forced to pass through the condensate. The exiting gas would be humidified through evaporation but carry no aerosol particles. If the carrier gas is oxygen that is blended with air through an air-entrainment system, any backpressure might result in an increase in the oxygen percentage and a decrease in the total flow. Remember to always measure the oxygen percentage near the patient.

b. Large-volume, pneumatic nebulizers
1. Get the necessary equipment for the procedure (Code: IIA1c) [Difficulty: An]

Large-volume, pneumatically powered nebulizers all share the common feature of having a liquid reservoir of at least 250 mL. Commonly, they also entrain room air to increase the total gas flow. They share these common features:

a. All are powered by air or oxygen delivered through a flowmeter. As the gas flow drops, the aerosol output decreases.

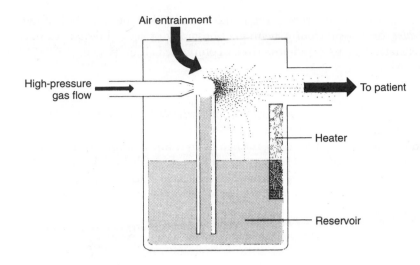

Fig. 7-7   Large volume, air-entrainment nebulizer. (From Shapiro BA, Kacmarek RM, Cane RD et al, editors: *Clinical application of respiratory care,* ed 4, St Louis, 1991, Mosby.)

b. All make use of Bernoulli's principle with a jet that is used to entrain liquid, room air, or both into the main gas flow.

c. All have a capillary tube that allows the liquid to flow *up* to the jet for nebulization. (Remember that with the bubble-type humidifiers, the oxygen flows *down* the capillary tube.)

d. All have a baffle that the aerosol is sprayed against to create a more uniform particle size.

Many, but not all, of the pneumatic nebulizers allow for a changeable inspired oxygen percentage. Provided that the jet is powered by oxygen, the air-entrainment ports can be opened up more to increase air entrainment (lowering the inspired oxygen percentage), or closed down to decrease air entrainment (raising the inspired oxygen percentage). The oxygen percentage usually can be varied from 35% to 100%. Remember always to analyze the inspired oxygen percentage near the patient because water in the aerosol tubing and backpressure decreases the entrained air and raises the oxygen percentage.

2. Put the equipment together, make sure that it works properly, and identify any problems (Code: IIB1c) [Difficulty: An]

3. Fix any problems with the equipment (Code: IIB2c) [Difficulty: An]

Most pneumatic nebulizers look similar to the bubble-type humidifiers. The key components include a large reservoir jar and a top with a DISS oxygen connector and capillary tube to the jet. These units allow for variable oxygen percentages. Keep the capillary tube and jet clear of debris, or the aerosol output will drop. Keep the air-entrainment ports open so that proper gas mixing occurs and the desired oxygen percentage is provided (Fig. 7-7). Heating of the water or aerosol or both is accomplished in one of the following ways:

a. A heated metal rod is immersed into the reservoir water through a port in the top of the nebulizer. A dial is used to control the temperature of the rod. The water temperature varies depending on how deep it is, so as the water level drops, the remaining water gets hotter. It is very important to measure the gas temperature near the patient and keep the water level stable to prevent burning the airway. The heated rod presents a risk of burns to a practitioner who accidentally touches it while it is still hot. It must be disinfected between patients and changed as often as the nebulizer is.

There are two other systems that are variations on the previously mentioned idea of directly heating the water in the reservoir jar. The first heats the water as it passes through the capillary tube. All have the advantage of a short warm-up time when compared with all of the other systems. Some units have an external temperature probe to place in the aerosol tubing. It acts as a servocontroller of the heating unit for better temperature regulation. Some types directly heat only a small amount of the reservoir water just before it is aerosolized.

b. A flexible heater is wrapped around the outside of the reservoir. A dial is used to control the temperature of the heater. The water temperature increases as the water level drops. Monitor the gas temperature near the patient for safety purposes.

c. A clip-on heating base plate can be added to special reservoir jars with a metal plate. These are preferable to the previously mentioned types because they ensure a constant temperature to the aerosol as the water level drops.

Heating the water or aerosol reduces the patient's humidity deficit and is usually done if the secretions are thick. See Fig. 7-1 for the location of the aerosol particles and their relationship with the dew point and the patient's body humidity.

4. Aerosol delivery systems

Large-bore tubing (also known as *aerosol tubing* or *corrugated tubing*) is needed to connect the aerosol generator with the patient. This tubing is 22 mm in internal diameter (ID).

a. Aerosol masks

The aerosol mask looks similar to the simple oxygen mask except that it has larger side ports for exhalation and has a 22-mm outer diameter (OD) adapter for the large-bore tubing to attach to (Fig. 7-8). This is often considered a low-flow oxygen mask because the ports are open to room air. Because of this, it is difficult to ensure that the patient receives the oxygen percentage that has been set. If the flow is high enough that aerosol mist can be seen flowing out of the side ports during an inspiration, little room air is being inspired. It is best to analyze the

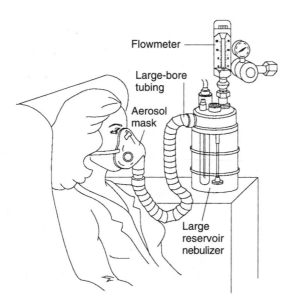

Fig. 7-8 Adult wearing an aerosol mask receiving supplemental oxygen and aerosol from a heated large-volume nebulizer. (From Guidelines for disinfection of home equipment, *Respiratory Care* 33:801-808, 1988.)

oxygen percentage inside the mask to be sure. Any of the previously mentioned humidity or aerosol devices can be used and powered by compressed air or oxygen.

b. Face tents

c. Tracheostomy masks/collars and Brigg's adapter/T-piece

Face tents, tracheostomy masks and collars, and Brigg's adapter (T-piece) are discussed in Chapter 6. Any of the previously mentioned humidity or aerosol devices can be used with them and powered by compressed air or oxygen.

🔲 EXAM HINT

Typically, there is an exam question covering troubleshooting problems with aerosol delivery equipment. Examples include but are not limited to: (1) incorrect water level in an ultrasonic so that no aerosol is produced; (2) plugged capillary line in a jet nebulizer so that no aerosol is produced; (3) missing baffle in a jet nebulizer so that no aerosol is produced; and (4) water in the large-bore tubing preventing aerosol from traveling through it. It is important to remember that with an oxygen-powered jet nebulizer system, the inspired oxygen percent increases if condensate water fills the low point of the aerosol tubing. This is because the backpressure on the jet and air-entrainment ports prevents room air from being drawn in. See Fig. 7-8.

---

5. Medication delivery systems
a. Small-volume, pneumatic nebulizers
1. Get the necessary equipment for the procedure (Code: IIA1c) [Difficulty: An]

A small-volume nebulizer (SVN) is designed to hold a relatively small volume of fluid (typically 3 to 5 mL) and to nebulize liquid medications such as bronchodilators, mucolytics, or antibiotics for inhalation. Either compressed air or oxygen can be used to generate the aerosol. These units operate under the same physical principles as the large-volume nebulizers described earlier.

Two different types of SVNs exist: mainstream and

Fig. 7-9 Mainstream type small-volume nebulizer for medications. (From Shapiro BA, Kacmarek RM, Cane RD et al, editors: *Clinical application of respiratory care,* ed 4, St Louis, 1991, Mosby.)

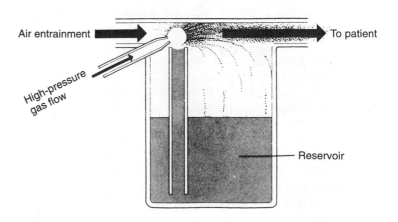

sidestream. *Mainstream nebulizers* are designed so that the main flow of gas to the patient flows through the aerosol as it is produced. A second high-pressure gas flow is used to power the jet to create the aerosol (Fig. 7-9). *Sidestream nebulizers* are designed so that the aerosol is produced out of the main flow of gas and added to it by the jet's gas flow (Fig. 7-10). Many manufacturers produce disposable medication SVN nebulizers for intermittent positive-pressure breathing (IPPB) circuits or handheld circuits. Most of these are the sidestream type. Select the nebulizer that produces a particle size that matches the therapeutic target.

See Fig. 7-11 for a typical handheld nebulizer circuit. The nebulizer can be powered by either air or oxygen. Typically, flows of 4 to 6 L/min are used to nebulize 3 to 5 mL of medication in about 10 minutes. The nebulizer

finger control allows the patient to power the nebulizer by covering the open hole in the "T." Uncovering the hole permits the gas to exit, and the medication is not nebulized and wasted. The reservoir tube serves to hold oxygen and medication for the next inspiration.

Practitioners face two possible risks when using SVNs. First, any aerosolized medications that escape into the room air may be inhaled. It is possible that the practitioner, or anyone else who happens be near, may have an allergic or other adverse reaction. Second, nebulized secretions from the patient's airway and lungs may be inhaled. This may place the practitioner or others at risk of acquiring a pulmonary infection from the patient. Although it is unlikely that many actual problems like this occur, it is a possibility. If either of these situations is a concern, a small-volume nebulizer with one-way valves and a down-

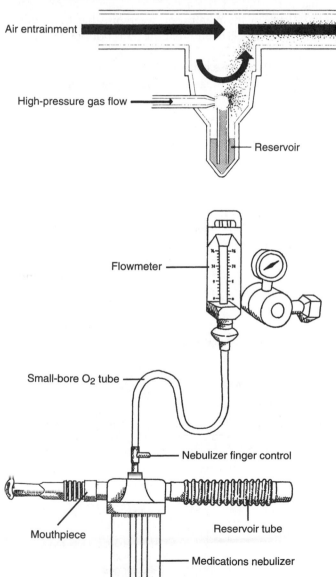

Fig. 7-10   Sidestream-type small-volume nebulizer for medications. (From Shapiro BA, Kacmarek RM, Cane RD et al, editors: *Clinical application of respiratory care,* ed 4, St Louis, 1991, Mosby.)

Fig. 7-11   Handheld small-volume nebulizer for medications with added components. (Adapted from Guidelines for disinfection of home equipment, *Respiratory Care* 33:801-808, 1988.)

stream particle filter should be used. This filter acts as a scavenging system and traps any exhaled aerosol droplets. (Fig. 7-12) A filtered SVN is recommended for use when nebulizing pentamidine isethionate (NebuPent). It, or a similarly filtered SVN, can be used for any other antibiotic or medication that should not contaminate the room air.

2. Put the equipment together, make sure that it works properly, and identify any problems (Code: IIB1c) [Difficulty: An]
3. Fix any problems with the equipment (Code: IIB2c) [Difficulty: An]

Most small-volume nebulizers consist of a medication reservoir and a top piece that contains a capillary tube and baffle. The top piece screws onto the reservoir and holds a mouthpiece and aerosol reservoir tube. Small-bore oxygen tubing connects the SVN to the flowmeter. If any small-volume nebulizer fails to generate an aerosol, make sure that the pieces are properly assembled and the capillary tube is not plugged with debris. Sometimes the capillary tube can be cleared by running it under water or pushing a needle through the channel. Make sure that the liquid in the reservoir is at the proper depth (typically 3 to 5 mL). Do not use a nebulizer that does not generate an aerosol.

b. Small particle aerosol generator
1. Get the necessary equipment for the procedure (Code: IIA1s) [Difficulty: An]
2. Fix any problems with the equipment (Code: IIB2t) [Difficulty: An]

The original small particle aerosol generator (SPAG) and newer SPAG II (Fig. 7-13) generate particles with a mass median aerodynamic diameter of 1.3 μm for alveolar deposition. They are used to nebulize the antimicrobial drug ribavirin (Virazole). The medication is used to treat the respiratory syncytial virus (RSV) that can cause a serious pneumonia in neonates.

Besides the SPAG unit with its nebulizer, 50 psi air and/or oxygen are needed to power the nebulizer and drying chamber. The SPAG is designed to deliver the aerosolized medication to an infant hood or other open system. Some practitioners have adapted the SPAG so that the medication can be delivered to infants on mechanical ventilators. This requires using a T-piece to connect the unit to the ventilator circuit and additional downstream filters to act as a scavenging system so the aerosolized medication does not foul the exhalation valve.

Check that an aerosol can be seen coming out of the delivery tube. Failure to generate an aerosol usually means that the nebulizer has a problem. Check for the proper fluid level in the medication reservoir, that the capillary tube is not blocked, and that the jet is not obstructed.

c. Metered dose inhalers

Metered dose inhalers (MDIs) are designed to dispense a premeasured amount of medication into the airway. Each activation increases the amount of medication that is taken by the patient. There are two main types of MDI: dry powder inhalers (DPIs) and chlorofluorocarbon (CFC) or hydrofluoroalkane (HFA)-powered inhalers.

1. Get the necessary equipment for the procedure (Code: IIA1s) [Difficulty: An]

Dry powder inhalers. DPIs dispense a dry medicinal powder into the patient's airways and lungs when inhaled.

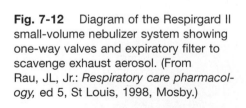

Fig. 7-12 Diagram of the Respirgard II small-volume nebulizer system showing one-way valves and expiratory filter to scavenge exhaust aerosol. (From Rau, JL, Jr.: *Respiratory care pharmacology,* ed 5, St Louis, 1998, Mosby.)

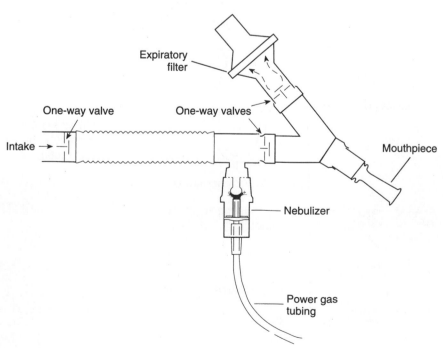

Relatively few drugs are currently available in DPI form. The drug manufacturer sells both the medication and the dispenser to the patient. The first two DPI medicines discussed here are held in a plastic capsule until released. The device is designed to open the capsule and allow it to be inhaled by the patient (Fig. 7-14).

The Spinhaler is used to pierce the gelatin capsule holding cromolyn sodium and dispense it into the patient's airway. As the patient inhales rapidly (a flow rate of at least 40 to 60 L/min is needed on any DPI), the plastic rotor blades spray the powder into the inhaled stream of air. The patient should inhale as deeply as possible and hold the breath for maximum deposition in the small airways. Care must be taken to hold the unit upright when the capsule is pierced and the powder is inhaled or it will spill. Cromolyn

sodium is used to prevent the onset of an asthma attack and is useless after an attack has begun.

The Rotahaler is designed to break in half a gelatin capsule containing a powdered form of albuterol or beclomethasone. Care must be taken with the Rotahaler to hold it horizontally after the capsule has been broken, or the medication will spill out. A fast inhalation with a breath hold is recommended to deliver the medication to the airways.

Multidose dispensers contain many doses of a medication within a drug reservoir (Fig. 7-14). A single dose is then loaded into the dispenser by the patient. A fast inhalation with breath hold is needed. These dispensers are more convenient to use than the single-dose units discussed previously. The following are currently available: Turbu-

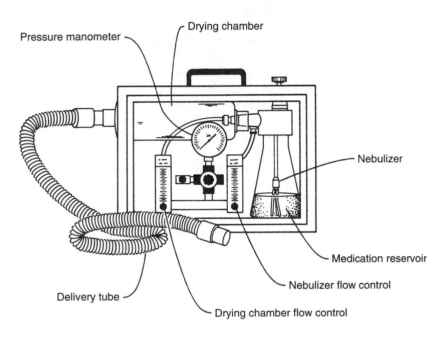

Fig. 7-13   Small-particle aerosol generator (SPAG) unit. (From Fink JB, Scanlan CL: Aerosol drug therapy. In Scanlan CL, Wilkins RL, Stoller JK, editors: *Egan's fundamentals of respiratory care,* ed 7, St Louis, 1999, Mosby.)

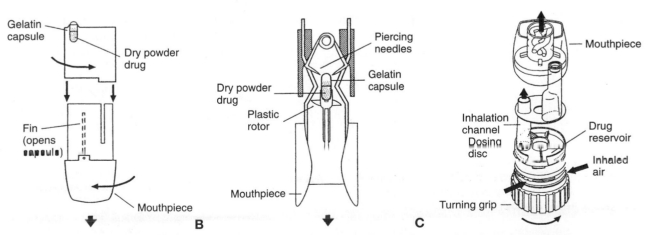

Fig. 7-14   Three types of dry powder inhaler (DPI). The Rotahaler **(A)** and Spinhaler **(B)** must have an individual medication capsule loaded for each inhalation. The Turbuhaler **(C)** has a drug reservoir that holds many doses of medication. (From Rau, JL, Jr.: *Respiratory care pharmacology,* ed 5, St Louis, 1998, Mosby.)

haler (terbutaline sulfate or budesonide), Rotadisk (albuterol or salmeterol), and Diskus (salmeterol). (See Chapter 8 for details on the medications.)

Some practice is needed in using the Spinhaler and Rotahaler units. The two main pieces must be unscrewed so that the capsule can be placed in the holding chamber. With the Spinhaler, the plastic slide must be moved up and down once to pierce the capsule. With the Rotahaler the mouthpiece is twisted around to break open the capsule. The medication is then forcefully inhaled. Unscrew both units to remove the empty capsule.

Chlorofluorocarbon (CFC- or hydrofluoroalkane (HFA)-powered inhalers. Many pharmaceutical companies have developed a CFC gas-powered metered dose inhaler (MDI). The available medications include sympathomimetic and anticholinergic bronchodilators, corticosteroid drugs, and an antibiotic. (See Chapter 8 for details on the medications.) All MDIs operate in the same way. They have several milliliters of medication and CFC or HFA contained inside a metal container with a built-in jet nozzle. The metering chamber is filled with medicine by tipping it over and back upright. A plastic actuator opens the jet when pressed into the container (Fig. 7-15). The patient can inhale the medication through the built-in mouthpiece. Also, there are adapters so that the medication can be sprayed into a mechanical ventilator circuit or through a bronchoscopy adapter to an endotracheal tube. A specific amount of medication is nebulized with each actuation of the device.

When assembling the MDI, make sure that the medication canister nozzle fits into the jet of the actuator. Patients should be instructed to use warm soapy water daily to wash the actuator out and keep the jet channel open.

d. Spacer and holding chamber for a metered dose inhaler

1. Get the necessary equipment for the procedure (Code: IIA1s) [Difficulty: An]

It has been shown that the addition to some sort of spacer or holding chamber between the actuator and the patient's mouth increases the amount of medication that is inhaled. These devices slow the aerosol down so that there is less impact on the back of the throat. This should result in fewer systemic side effects such as the risk of oral thrush (*Candidiasis* fungal infection) with an MDI-powered corticosteroid. Also, the patient with poor hand and breathing coordination wastes less medication.

A spacer is a simple open extension tube between the actuator and the patient. Its main advantage over inhaling directly from the MDI mouthpiece is that the aerosol plume expands and slows down so that more medication is inhaled (see Fig. 7-15). The patient should be told not to exhale through the spacer because any remaining medication will be blown out and wasted. There are spacers designed for use with a ventilator circuit when an MDI-based medication is to be given. A holding chamber holds the medication, as a spacer, but also has valves. These valves prevent the medicine from being exhaled out and allow the patient to inhale several times to get more medication. This is especially helpful for children or small adults with small tidal volumes. Some of the holding chambers have a built-in whistle that sounds if the patient is inhaling too quickly (see Fig. 7-16). Several types of spacers or holding chambers exist. Some spacers are designed to fit with only one actuator whereas others adapt to fit to any actuator. A face mask comes attached to some holding chambers so that pediatric patients or uncooperative adults can be given the medication.

Patients must be instructed to wash out their spacer or holding chamber on a daily basis. Warm, soapy water and a thorough rinsing are usually adequate for home use. However, a disinfecting liquid such as Cidex is preferable if the patient can afford it. Acetic acid (white vinegar) may also be used to save money.

MODULE B	Environmental devices

1. Incubators

a. Get the necessary equipment for the procedure (Code: IIA1j1) [Difficulty: R, Ap, An]

An incubator is indicated in the care of a sick newborn

Fig. 7-15 The effect of a spacer on aerosol particle size and velocity from a CFC-powered metered dose inhaler. (From Rau, JL, Jr.: *Respiratory care pharmacology,* ed 5, St Louis, 1998, Mosby.)

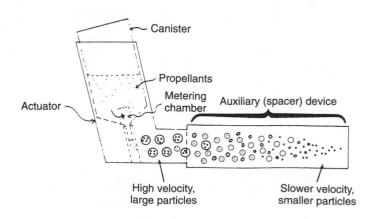

who needs an enclosed space for an isolated, controlled environment. See Fig. 7-17. (Some practitioners may refer to an incubator as an Isolette, which is a common brand of incubator.) Most incubators are used only in the neonatal or pediatric care units and are electrically powered through standard electrical outlets. However, there are some incubators designed to transport an infant between hospitals or within the hospital. They can make use of a standard electrical outlet but also feature self-contained batteries and oxygen tanks.

Traditionally, an incubator has been used to do four things for the infant: manage its temperature, manage its surrounding humidity, isolate it from the outside environment, and control its inspired oxygen percentage. An incubator does the first three tasks very well. However, precise oxygen delivery cannot be easily done for two reasons. First, these units have never been designed to

deliver an exact oxygen percentage. They have only two basic oxygen flow settings. The low-flow setting is intended to limit the infant to no more than 40% oxygen. On many units a red-colored plastic "flag" must be raised to deliver a higher flow of oxygen that may provide up to 80% or more oxygen. Second, whenever the side ports on the incubator are opened for patient care, the internal gases flow out and result in a lower oxygen percentage.

Because of these limits, it is *not* recommended that an incubator's built-in oxygen delivery system be used. Instead, it is recommended that the following components be assembled for precise oxygen delivery and humidity control: (1) an oxygen blender with flowmeter and small-bore oxygen tubing adapter (nipple); (2) small-bore oxygen tubing and adapter to connect the flowmeter to a cascade-type heated humidifier; (3) sterile, distilled water to fill the humidifier reservoir; (4) large-bore (aerosol) tubing

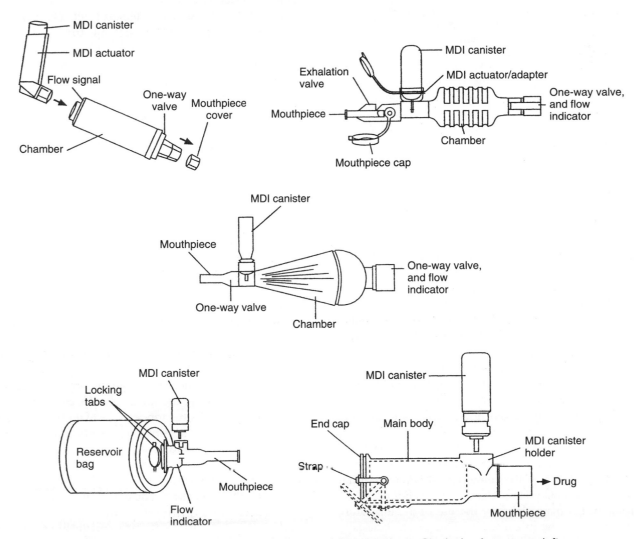

Fig. 7-16 Four types of MDI spacers and holding chambers. Clockwise from upper left: Monaghan Aerochamber, Aerosol Cloud Enhancer, InspirEase, and OptiHaler. (From Rau, JL, Jr.: *Respiratory care pharmacology,* ed 5, St Louis, 1998, Mosby.)

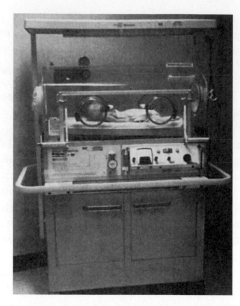

Fig. 7-17 An incubator used to control an infant's environment. The top structure is used to provide lighting. The incubator itself is made of clear Plexiglas so that the infant can be seen and has two closeable portholes on each side. These can be opened so that the caregiver can work with the infant. Controls below the infant are used to adjust the temperature, humidity, and possibly the oxygen percentage within the incubator. (From Scanlan CL, Heuer AL: Medical gas therapy. In Scanlan CL, Wilkins RL, Stoller JK, editors: *Egan's fundamentals of respiratory care,* ed 7, St Louis, 1999, Mosby.)

to direct the heated, humidified, high-percentage oxygen; (5) an oxygen hood (also called an oxyhood) to receive the humidified oxygen; (6) an oxygen analyzer to check the percentage inside the oxygen hood; and (7) a temperature probe to check the temperature of the heated humidified oxygen; place this into the large-bore tubing before it enters the incubator.

b. Put the equipment together, make sure that it works properly, and identify any problems (Code: IIB1j1) [Difficulty: R, Ap, An]

An incubator comes preassembled as a unit. Sterile, distilled water must be added if the built-in humidification system is used. This is not necessary if heated, humidified oxygen is given by an oxygen hood. Make sure that the temperature control, thermometer, and other systems on the incubator are working as directed by the manufacturer. The internal temperature of the incubator is usually kept between 36° and 36.5° C to maintain the infant in a neutral thermal environment (NTE). The desired NTE is set by the physician and is maintained by the use of a temperature sensor placed on the infant's skin. This sensor is usually placed on the abdomen and is connected to a servocontrol that automatically raises or lowers the temperature inside the incubator as needed.

If an oxygen hood is being used to deliver supplemental oxygen to the infant, the components previously listed must be properly assembled. Check the temperature of the humidified oxygen and check the oxygen percentage inside the oxygen hood near the infant's nose and mouth.

c. Fix any problems with the equipment (Code: IIB2j1) [Difficulty: R, Ap]

If the incubator is not maintaining the desired internal temperature or the internal humidification system is not working properly, follow the manufacturer's recommendations to repair or replace the entire unit. Make sure that the oxygen hood system is assembled properly, maintaining the desired gas temperature to maintain the infant's neutral thermal environment, and delivering the desired oxygen percentage. Adjust the cascade-type humidifier temperature or oxygen blender settings as needed.

2. Radiant warmers

a. Get the necessary equipment for the procedure (Code: IIA1j1) [Difficulty: R, Ap, An]

A radiant warmer is used to warm an infant who cannot be properly cared for inside an incubator. See Fig. 7-18. Typically these infants are very sick and require mechanical ventilation, require frequent medical procedures, or are receiving cardiopulmonary resuscitation.

b. Put the equipment together, make sure that it works properly, and identify any problems (Code: IIB1j1) [Difficulty: R, Ap, An]

A radiant warmer comes preassembled by the manufacturer. It uses infrared light to heat the infant and the area on which the infant is laid and cared for. A temperature sensor is placed onto the infant's skin, typically on the abdomen. The sensor uses a servomechanism so that the infant's skin temperature is used to either turn on or turn off the radiant warmer to maintain the infant's desired neutral thermal environment. This is usually between 36° and 36.5° C.

c. Fix any problems with the equipment (Code: IIB2j1) [Difficulty: R, Ap]

If the sensor and servo system are not properly calibrated or working, the infant may be either under- or overheated. Either situation can be dangerous because newborns are very sensitive to temperature changes. Replace a sensor or servo that is not working properly.

3. Aerosol (mist) tents

a. Get the necessary equipment for the procedure (Code: IIA1j2) [Difficulty: An]

The aerosol or mist tents are essentially like the oxygen tents discussed in Chapter 6. The main difference is that no supplemental oxygen is used because the patient does not need it. The top of the canopy can now be left open for

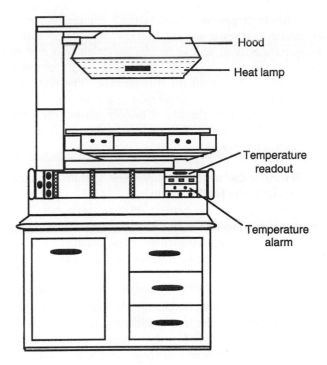

Fig. 7-18 Drawing of a radiant warmer used to warm an infant in an open setting. The heat lamp uses infrared light to warm the infant placed on the patient care area. (From *Respiratory care review perinatal/pediatric study guide*, Kettering, Ohio, RTS Publishing Company, 1996.)

better flow-through ventilation. Aerosol tents are sometimes used to treat an active infant with an upper respiratory tract problem such as laryngotracheobronchitis (LTB or pediatric croup). The tent is used because a small, active child will not keep an aerosol mask in place. A tent is not indicated for an older child or adult who will keep an aerosol mask in place that will easily provide the needed aerosol to the patient.

b. Put the equipment together, make sure that it works properly, and identify any problems (Code: IIB1j2) [Difficulty: An]

c. Fix any problems with the equipment (Code: IIB2j2) [Difficulty: An]

At least 10 L/min of compressed air should still be run through the nebulizer to make sure that there is no carbon dioxide buildup. The nebulizer or ultrasonic system should be cared for as described earlier to ensure that there is enough aerosol to treat the condition.

If the child has laryngotracheobronchitis, a cool aerosol is clinically preferred because it reduces airway edema. Never use so much aerosol that the child cannot be seen inside the tent. Also, be wary of fluid overloading the young patient who is in the tent for a prolonged period.

4. Scavenging systems

a. Get the necessary equipment for the procedure (Code: IIA1j3) [Difficulty: R]

A scavenging system is indicated in two clinical situations. The first is whenever a patient's therapeutic aerosol is vented into the room air and is potentially harmful to the respiratory therapist, other health-care professionals, or other patients or family members. The second is when a patient has an active *Mycobacterium tuberculosis* (TB) infection and is coughing.

In the first situation, a typical scavenging system consists of connecting aerosol tubing and a downstream filter that captures any excess medication the patient does not inhale. Currently it is recommended that this scavenging system be used whenever pentamidine isethionate (NebuPent) and ribavirin (Virazole) are nebulized. Fig. 7-12 shows the Respirgard II system used with NebuPent. There is no standardized system for capturing aerosolized Virazole. Commonly, one or two disposable, high-efficiency particulate air (HEPA) filters are added into the ventilator circuit before the exhalation valve. This prevents the exhalation valve from becoming clogged with medication and prevents the medication from being vented into the room air.

In the second situation, the patient with TB is kept in a negative airflow room, and airborne precautions are followed as described in Chapter 2. In addition, a HEPA filter is placed in the patient's room and all room air is drawn into the unit. The filter captures any TB bacilli that have been coughed out by the patient. This prevents the infection of anyone else.

MODULE C	Modify the patient's breathing pattern so that a medication is properly deposited (Code: IIIC2) [Difficulty: An]

1. Upper-airway deposition

Particles 10 µm or larger are more likely to impact on the upper airway (oropharynx, larynx, trachea, and mainstem bronchi) when the patient is coached to:
a. Inhale at a normal or faster speed. The flow should be greater than 30 L/min.
b. Inhale a normal tidal volume.
c. Breathe in a normal pattern.

2. Lower-airway and alveolar deposition

Particles 2 to 5 µm are more likely to deposit on the smaller airways (respiratory bronchioles) and in the alveoli when the patient is coached to:
a. Inhale at a slow speed. The flow should be less than 30 L/min.
b. Inhale an inspiratory capacity.
c. Hold the full breath in for 10 seconds if possible before exhaling.

Obviously, all patients will not be able to perform these techniques perfectly, but to the extent that they can, the medication will be deposited where it is needed and the treatment will be more effective.

 EXAM HINT

There is commonly one question that deals with recognizing that a patient is hyperventilating during a nebulizer treatment. Signs of hyperventilation include dizziness, lightheadedness, and tingling fingers. The patient should be told to breathe slower and less deeply.

MODULE D   Respiratory care plan

1. Participate in the development of the respiratory care plan [e.g., case management, development and application of protocols, disease management education] (Code: IC4) [Difficulty: An]

Be prepared to change the type of humidity and aerosol delivery system from among those discussed in this chapter based on the patient's condition. Review the indications, contraindications, uses, and limitations of the various systems.

The patient with a secretion problem should be helped by the addition of a bland aerosol or mucolytic medication and is better able to clear them out effectively. This should result in the patient feeling better, as well as having improved vital signs, oxygenation, breath sounds, and spirometry values. The use of a bland aerosol therapy can cause bronchospasm in some asthmatic patients. Patients with viscous, thick, dry secretions can have their airways occluded if aerosol therapy causes the secretions to take in water and swell. The patient must be able to cough out the thinned secretions, or suctioning equipment must be available to remove them.

In general, a cool humidity or aerosol system is used with patients with the following conditions:
1. Pediatric croup
2. Upper-airway irritation such as after extubation or a bronchoscopy procedure

In general, a body temperature humidity or aerosol system is used with patients with the following conditions:
1. Bypassed upper airway (endotracheal or tracheostomy tube)
2. Thick (viscous) secretions
3. Hypothermia
4. Neonate to maintain a neutral thermal environment

Neonates are sensitive to over hydration. Long-term aerosol therapy for them should be avoided or minimized. Adult patients with heart failure or pulmonary edema should also not be given long-term aerosol therapy. Instead, a Cascade-type humidifier can be used.

The adult patient who has thick secretions may be aided by long-term aerosol therapy of a dense mist at body temperature. The secretions are often liquefied and made easier to cough or suction out. An ultrasonic nebulizer is often used for this purpose. The child with croup is usually given a dense mist of a cool bland aerosol in a mist tent. This therapy is usually needed for only a few days. Be wary of fluid overload if the mist is needed for a longer period.

2. Interview the patient to determine sputum production (Code: IB6b) [Difficulty: An]

Find out from the patient approximately how much sputum is produced in a day. Also find out if certain times of the day are more productive or less productive. Try to relate this to breathing treatments, medications, activities, meals, and allergies.

3. Observe the patient for changes in sputum quantity and consistency (Code: IB1b) [Difficulty: An]

It is important to follow the patient's sputum quantity and consistency to know if the humidity or aerosol therapy is effective. Again, try to relate this to breathing treatments, medications, activities, meals, and allergies. It may be necessary to suggest a change in bland aerosol therapy administration based on the patient's condition. For example, change from normal saline to hypertonic saline for a sputum induction. See Chapter 8, Box 8-2, for information on the saline solutions used as mucolytics.

4. Auscultate the patient's breath sounds (Code: IB4a) [Difficulty: An]

Interpretation of breath sounds is discussed in Chapter 1. It should be expected that bland aerosol administration will result in the patient's secretions becoming thinner (less viscous) so that they can be coughed or suctioned out more easily. However, there are patients with a history of asthma who may react to inhaled saline solutions by developing bronchospasm.

 EXAM HINT

Past exams have had a question that deals with needing to stop aerosol therapy when a patient demonstrates reactive bronchospasm by the development of wheezing.

BIBLIOGRAPHY

AARC aerosol consensus statement. *Respir Care* 36:916-921, 1991.

AARC Clinical Practice Guideline: Selection of aerosol delivery device. *Respir Care* 37:891-897, 1992.

AARC Clinical Practice Guideline: Bland aerosol administration. *Respir Care* 38:1196-1200, 1993.

AARC Clinical Practice Guideline: Delivery of aerosols to the upper airway. *Respir Care* 39 (8):803-807, 1994.

Aloan CA, Hill TV: *Respiratory care of the newborn and child*, ed 2, Philadelphia, 1997, Lippincott Williams & Wilkins.

Barnes TA, editor: *Core textbook of respiratory care practice*, ed 2, St Louis, 1994, Mosby.

Barnhart SL, Czervinske MP: *Perinatal and pediatric respiratory care*, Philadelphia, 1995, WB Saunders Company.

Branson RD, Hess DR, Chatburn RL, editors: *Respiratory care equipment*, ed 2, Philadelphia, 1999, Lippincott Williams & Wilkins.

Fink JB: Humidity. In Fink JB, Hunt GE, editors: *Clinical practice in respiratory care*, Philadelphia, 1999, Lippincott-Raven.

Fink JB: Metered-dose inhalers, dry powder inhalers, and transitions, *Respir Care* 45:623-635, 2000.

Fink JB, Dhand R: Aerosol drug therapy. In Fink JB, Hunt GE, editors: *Clinical practice in respiratory care*, Philadelphia, 1999, Lippincott-Raven.

Fink JB, Scanlan CL: Aerosol drug therapy. In Scanlan CL, Wilkins RL, Stoller JK, editors: *Egan's fundamentals of respiratory care*, ed 7, St Louis, 1999, Mosby.

Fink JB, Scanlan CL: Humidity and bland aerosol therapy. In Scanlan CL, Wilkins RL, Stoller JK, editors: *Egan's fundamentals of respiratory care*, ed 7, St Louis, 1999, Mosby.

Hess DR: The delivery of aerosolized bronchodilator to mechanically ventilated intubated adult patients, *Respir Care* 35:399-404, 1990.

Hess DR: Nebulizers, principles and practice, *Respir Care* 45:609-622, 2000.

McPherson SP: *Respiratory Care Equipment*, ed 5, St Louis, 1995, Mosby.

Rau, Jr. JL: *Respiratory Care Pharmacology*, ed 5, St Louis, 1998, Mosby.

Scanlan CL, Heuer AL: Medical gas therapy. In Scanlan CL, Wilkins RL, Stoller JK, editors: *Egan's fundamentals of respiratory care*, ed 7, St Louis, 1999, Mosby.

Shapiro BA, Kacmarek RM, Cane RD et al, editors: *Clinical application of respiratory care*, ed 4, St Louis, 1991, Mosby.

Ward JJ, Hess D, Helmholz, Jr. HF: Humidity and aerosol therapy. In Burton GC, Hodgkin JE, Ward JJ, editors: *Respiratory care: a guide to clinical practice*, ed 4, Philadelphia, 1997, Lippincott-Raven.

Whitaker K: *Comprehensive perinatal & pediatric respiratory care*, ed 2, Albany, NY, 1997, Delmar.

White GC: *Equipment theory for respiratory care*, ed 3, Albany, NY, 1999, Delmar.

SELF-STUDY QUESTIONS

1. Ten minutes into a handheld nebulizer treatment to deliver albuterol (Proventil), the patient complains of dizziness and tingling fingers. What should be done?
   A. Advise the patient to breathe in the same pattern.
   B. Change the medication.
   C. Tell the patient to breathe more slowly.
   D. Advise the patient to breathe deeper and faster.
2. The respiratory therapist is helping to care for a 1-week-old infant with pneumonia. The infant has been placed into an incubator. The physician wants to know the best way to administer high humidity and 35% oxygen to the infant. What should be recommended?
   A. Send the desired oxygen percentage to a heated cascade-type humidifier to an oxyhood.
   B. Use the incubator's humidifier and the low oxygen setting on the unit.
   C. Place a 3 L/min nasal cannula on the infant and use the incubator's humidifier.
   D. Use the incubator's humidifier and the high oxygen setting on the unit.
3. The physician wants more aerosol inside the mist tent of a 3-year-old child. What would be the best way to do this?
   A. Cut a hole in the top of the tent.
   B. Close the hole on the top of the tent.
   C. Lower the temperature on the refrigeration unit.
   D. Increase the gas flow to the nebulizer.
4. Current clinical guidelines indicate that an incubator can be used for all of the following situations *except:*
   A. Isolate an infant.
   B. Provide a exact oxygen percentage.
   C. Control the temperature around an infant.
   D. Control the humidity level around an infant.
5. An entry-level respiratory therapist calls you when he has analyzed 40% oxygen to an infant inside an oxygen tent. This is despite his attempt to get the ordered 50% oxygen by setting the nebulizer's entrainment port at 60% and the oxygen blender to the nebulizer at 50%. What would you recommend?
   A. Increase the flow by 5 L/min.
   B. Set the blender to 100%.
   C. Check the accuracy of the oxygen analyzer.
   D. Set the entrainment port on the nebulizer to 100%.
6. A humidity or aerosol system delivering body temperature gas is used in all the following situations *except:*
   A. Patient with a tracheostomy.
   B. Twenty-month-old infant with laryngotracheobronchitis.
   C. COPD patient with thick secretions.
   D. Newborn receiving oxygen inside an oxygen hood.
7. A premature infant with respiratory distress syndrome is receiving mechanical ventilation, has a nasogastric tube, and has an umbilical artery catheter. What is the best way to maintain a neutral thermal environment for the infant?
   A. Place an oxygen hood over the infant's head.
   B. Put the infant inside an incubator and adjust the temperature based on the infant's rectal temperature.
   C. Place the infant under a radiant warmer with a skin temperature probe.
   D. Place the infant inside an incubator with a skin temperature probe.
8. While working as the supervising respiratory therapist in a large hospital, a variety of patients are your responsibility to manage. Under which of the following situations should a scavenging system be set up?
   I. Patient with active, untreated tuberculosis
   II. Patient receiving nebulized acetylcysteine (Mucomyst)
   III. Patient receiving nebulized ribavirin (Virazole)
   IV. Patient receiving nebulized pentamidine isethionate (NebuPent)
   A. I only
   B. III only
   C. I, III, and IV only
   D. II, III, and IV only
9. A T-piece is being used to deliver 40% oxygen and heated aerosol to the tracheostomy tube of an adult patient. While checking the patient's pulse oximeter reading, you notice that

it is only 88% and with each inspiration the aerosol cannot be seen coming from the end of the T-piece. What action would you recommend?

   I. Increase the oxygen flow to the nebulizer.

   II. Increase the delivered oxygen to 45%.

   III. Increase the temperature to the heated aerosol system.

   IV. Add 100 mL of aerosol tubing to the open end of the T-piece.

   V. Change the patient to a tracheostomy mask.

   A. I and II only

   B. I and IV only

   C. III and IV only

   D. II and V only

10. When doing patient rounds you notice that very little aerosol is going to a new patient's tracheostomy mask. Which of the following could be the problem?

   I. The water level is above the refill line on the nebulizer's reservoir jar.

   II. The nebulizer is not tightly screwed into the DISS connector on the flowmeter.

   III. The nebulizer jet is obstructed.

   IV. The water level is below the refill line on the nebulizer's reservoir jar.

   V. The capillary tube is obstructed.

   A. II, III, IV, and V only

   B. I and II only

   C. III and IV only

   D. III and V only

Answer Key

1. **C.** Rationale: The patient's signs and symptoms indicate hyperventilation. The easiest way to correct this situation is to have the patient breathe more slowly (and/or less deeply). If the patient continues to breathe in the same pattern the hyperventilation will continue. Although albuterol may cause tachycardia, it is unlikely to cause dizziness and tingling fingers in the patient. If the patient is advised to breathe deeper and faster the hyperventilation will get worse.

2. **A.** Rationale: A cascade-type humidifier can be adjusted to deliver the desired 35% oxygen to the patient at the desired temperature to meet the neutral thermal environment requirements. An oxyhood will deliver the oxygen and humidity to the infant's head and not be affected by the incubator portholes being opened for patient care. The incubator's low oxygen setting does not allow for a precise oxygen percentage to be delivered. It will probably provide about 40% oxygen but the percentage will drop when the portholes are opened. There is no way to know the oxygen percentage a 3 L/min nasal cannula will deliver to an infant. The incubator's high oxygen setting does not allow for a precise oxygen percentage to be delivered. It will probably provide about 80% oxygen but the percentage will drop when the portholes are opened.

3. **D.** Rationale: Increasing the gas flow on the nebulizer will increase the total amount of water that is nebulized and delivered to the mist tent. Mist tents are supposed to have a hole at the top of the tent canopy to allow the excess gas and aerosol to exit. Only oxygen tents, not mist tents, have the hole on the top of the tent canopy closed. This is to ensure that the oxygen tent has the highest possible oxygen percentage. Remember, a mist tent does not deliver supplemental oxygen. Lowering the temperature on the refrigeration unit will further cool the infant but will not affect the amount of aerosol delivered into the mist tent.

4. **B.** Rationale: Incubators are not able to provide an exact and adjustable oxygen percentage to an infant. The two oxygen flow settings are not adjustable to control the delivered oxygen percentage. In addition, when the portholes are opened for patient care, the internal gas leaks out and the oxygen percentage drops. Incubators are able to isolate an infant from the surrounding environment and control the temperature and humidity around the infant.

5. **D.** It is necessary to set the entrainment ports on the nebulizer to 100% source gas (50% blended oxygen) to prevent room air from being entrained. This way only 50% oxygen will power the nebulizer and be delivered into the oxygen tent. Increasing the flow to the nebulizer by 5 L/min will increase the flow through the nebulizer to increase aerosol production but will not change the oxygen percentage. Setting the blender to 100% oxygen will not close the air entrainment ports on the nebulizer. Therefore 60% oxygen will be delivered into the tent, not the ordered 50%. There is no indication that the oxygen analyzer is inaccurate. The problem is an incorrect equipment set up.

6. **B.** Rationale: An infant with laryngotracheobronchitis (LTB or croup) is usually best managed with a *cool*, bland aerosol. This helps to reduce the swelling in the large airways. Body temperature aerosol is delivered to a patient with a tracheostomy, thick (viscous) secretions, or a newborn in an oxygen hood to minimize the patient's humidity deficit.

7. **C.** Rationale: Placing the infant under a radiant warmer allows for adequate contact with the patient for its many necessary medical procedures. The skin temperature probe allows for the infant's temperature to be servocontrolled to prevent under or over heating. An oxygen hood will help to maintain the infant's head temperature but will not help with the rest of its body. Placing the infant inside an incubator will severely limit patient contact. It will be very difficult to maintain a steady temperature because the portholes are frequently opened. It will be difficult to try to maintain the incubator temperature based on occasional patient rectal temperature values. It would be acceptable to place the infant inside an incubator with a skin temperature probe if the unit could be kept closed. Unfortunately, this infant will need frequent contact for care and the portholes will need to be opened.

8. **C.** Rationale: A patient with active, untreated tuberculosis can infect other people. Therefore a HEPA filter must be set up in the patient's room as a scavenging system for trapping coughed out bacteria in the room air. It is currently recommended that the nebulized drugs ribavirin (Virazole) and pentamidine isethionate (NebuPent) be used with a scavenging system. This prevents the respiratory therapist or any one else from unintended inhalation. Although nebulized acetylcysteine (Mucomyst) does have a foul smell and can irritate the airways of an asthmatic patient, there are no current guidelines to administer it with a scavenging system.

9. **B.** Rationale: Increasing the oxygen flow to the nebulizer will better match the patient's inspired tidal volume. Also, adding 100 mL of aerosol tubing to the open end of the

T-piece will act as a reservoir to help to make sure that the patient only inhales 40% oxygen from the nebulizer. Enough flow and reservoir tubing should be used to make sure that aerosol can be seen exiting the end of the reservoir tubing during inspiration. This ensures that only humidified 40% oxygen is inhaled. There is no order or need to request an order to increase the delivered oxygen to 45% if these items are done. The patient's pulse oximeter reading is 88% because room air is being inhaled to dilute the set 40% oxygen. Increasing the temperature to the heated aerosol system will not affect the inspired oxygen percentage. There is no need to change the patient to a tracheostomy mask. It will not ensure that the patient gets 40% oxygen because it is an open system and the patient can inhale room air.

10. **A.** Rationale: Any of the following will result in less or no aerosol being delivered: (1) If the nebulizer is not tightly screwed into the DISS connector on the flowmeter the gas will leak and not go through the nebulizer. (2) If the nebulizer jet is obstructed, no aerosol will be created. (3) If the water level is *below* the refill line on the nebulizer's reservoir jar, no water will be drawn up the capillary tube to the jet and baffle; therefore no aerosol will be created. (4) If the capillary tube is obstructed, the water in the reservoir jar will not be drawn up to the jet and baffle. However, if the water level is *above* the refill line on the nebulizer's reservoir jar water, water will be drawn up the capillary tube to the jet and baffle. Aerosol will be generated if everything else if functioning normally.

8 Pharmacology

The examination content outline for the Written Registry Exam does not specifically list any pharmacology items. However, a review of all of the most recent versions of the exam has shown an average of 3 questions (3% of the exam) on pharmacology. The questions covered a wide variety of medications and their clinical uses.

1. Bronchodilators

The aerosolized bronchodilators are medications designed to relax the bronchial smooth muscles so that the airways dilate, airway resistance is reduced, and breathing is easier. The two groups of medications presented in the following discussion are widely given by respiratory therapists.

A xanthine agent is sometimes added to aid the breathing of a status asthmaticus patient who does not respond to optimum doses of the inhaled medications. Intravenous theophylline ethylenediamine (aminophylline) has been shown to be beneficial in these cases. However, it should be used with caution because it is difficult to regulate the proper serum level, and serious side effects can be seen with it.

a. Recommend and administer sympathomimetic agents

This group of medications is often called sympathomimetic amines, sympathomimetic bronchodilators, or beta-adrenergic bronchodilators. They have the effect of stimulating the body's sympathetic nerves, which results in bronchodilation and other effects. Patients with asthma are most effectively treated with drugs from this group.

A brief review of the autonomic nervous system aids in understanding how these (and the next group of medications) work and some side effects to watch for. The autonomic nervous system is not under voluntary control. It is an automatic system designed to regulate metabolism and the vital signs. It is made up of two branches: the sympathetic nervous system and the parasympathetic nervous system. The lungs, heart, and most other organs are innervated by both branches. The blood vessels in the mucous membranes are innervated only by the sympathetic branch. The parasympathetic nervous system is usually dominant and keeps the body functioning normally. The sympathetic nervous system is an "emergency" system that is dominant in times of great stress. It is sometimes called the "fight or flight" system. Adrenaline

(or epinephrine) is released by the adrenal glands in these emergencies. Adrenaline causes a number of effects, including the effect that many patients need: bronchodilation. The sympathetic nervous system has the following three different types of receptors that are located in different organs and are affected by adrenaline and related medications:

a. The a_1-receptors (alpha$_1$) are located in the blood vessels of the mucous membranes (and other tissues not of interest to us in this discussion). Vasoconstriction results when these receptors are stimulated.

b. The b_1-receptors (beta$_1$) are located in the heart. Tachycardia, increased stroke volume, and possibly dysrhythmias result when they are stimulated.

c. The b_2-receptors (beta$_2$) are located in the airways. Bronchodilation results when these are stimulated.

Aerosolized sympathomimetic bronchodilators are usually recommended under one of the three following situations:

Acute bronchospasm with severe shortness of breath. This patient is in need of rapid relief. Recommend a fast-acting medication such as albuterol. See Table 8-1 for information on peak onset times and duration for the various medications. Avoid drugs with unnecessary a_1- and b_1-effects or long onset and peak times.

Chronic but stable bronchospasm with moderate shortness of breath. These patients are in need of a dependable medication of longer duration. Recommend a medication such as salmeterol. This drug has a long onset time with a duration of up to 12 hours. It is important that the patient also have a prescription for a fast-acting drug in case of sudden bronchospasm. In addition, several newer medications come in oral as well as aerosol preparations. The oral forms are especially helpful when taken in the evening to help the patient get a good night's sleep. Table 8-2 lists information on the administration method, strength, and dosage for the sympathomimetic agents.

Treatment of the patient with laryngeal edema or bleeding from a bronchoscopy biopsy site. The laryngeal edema problem requires the administration of a medication that reduces the swelling of the mucous membrane of the larynx and epiglottis. If bleeding results from a biopsy during a bronchoscopy, the cut blood vessels must be made to constrict and clot. In both cases, racemic epinephrine (microNefrin, Vaponefrin, and Asthma-Nefrin) is the medication of choice because it stimulates alpha-1 receptors. This results in vasoconstriction of the mucosal and deeper blood vessels. Therefore the laryngeal edema swelling is reduced and biopsy bleeding stops.

TABLE 8-1	Receptor Preference and Basic Pharmacokinetics of the Beta-adrenergic Bronchodilators

Drug	Receptor	Onset (min)	Route	Peak (min)	Duration (hr)
CATECHOLAMINES					
Epinephrine	Alpha, beta	3-5	INH	5-20	1-3
		6-15	SC		
Isoproterenol	Beta nonspecific	2-5	INH	5-30	0.5-2
Isoetharine	Beta-2	1-6	INH	15-60	1-3
Bitolterol (colterol)	Beta-2	3-4	INH	30-60	5-8
NONCATECHOLAMINES					
Metaproterenol	Beta-2	1-5	INH	60	2-6
		15-30	PO		
Terbutaline	Beta-2	5-30	INH	30-60	3-6
		6-15	SC	30-60	1.5-4
		30	PO	120-240	4-8
Albuterol	Beta-2	15	INH	30-60	3-8
		30	PO	60-120	4-6
Pirbuterol	Beta-2	5	INH	30	5
Salmeterol	Beta-2	20	INH	180-300	12

INH, Inhalation; *PO,* orally; *SC,* subcutaneously.
From Rau JL Jr: *Respiratory care pharmacology,* ed 5, St Louis, 1998, Mosby.

TABLE 8-2	Dosages and Strengths Used for Various Methods of Administering Beta-adrenergic Bronchodilators

Drug	Brand names	Administration method	Strength	Dosage
Epinephrine	Adrenalin	Nebulizer	1:100 (1%)	0.25-0.5 mL qid
Racemic epinephrine	MicroNefrin	Nebulizer	2.25%	0.25-0.5 mL qid
	Vaponefrin			
	AsthmaNefrin			
Isoproterenol	Isuprel	Nebulizer	1:200 (0.5%)	0.25-0.5 mL qid
	Isuprel Mistometer	MDI	131 µg/puff	1-2 puffs qid
Isoetharine	Bronkosol	Nebulizer	1%	0.25-0.5 mL qid
	Bronkometer	MDI	340 µg/spray	1-2 puffs qid
Metaproterenol	Alupent	Nebulizer	5%	0.3 mL tid, qid
	Metaprel	MDI	0.65 mg/puff	2-3 puffs q4h
		Tablets	10, 20 mg	20 mg tid, qid
		Syrup	10 mg/5 mL	10 mg tid, qid
Terbutaline	Brethaire	MDI	0.2 mg/puff	2 puffs q4-6h
	Brethine	Injection	1 mg/mL	0.25 mg SC
	Bricanyl	Tablets	2.5, 5 mg	2.5 or 5 mg tid
Albuterol	Proventil	Nebulizer	0.5%	0.5 mL tid, qid
	Ventolin	MDI	90 µg/puff	2 puffs tid, qid
		DPI	200 µg/caps	1 caps, q4-6h
		Tablets	2 or 4 mg	2 or 4 mg tid, qid
		Extended release tablet	4 mg, 8 mg	q12h
		Syrup	2 mg/5 mL	2 or 4 mg tid, qid
Bitolterol (colterol)	Tornalate	MDI	0.37 mg/puff	2 puffs q8h
		Nebulizer	0.2%	1.25 mL tid or as ordered
Pirbuterol	MaxAir	MDI	0.2 mg/puff	2 puffs q4-6h
Salmeterol	Serevent	MDI	25 µg/puff	2 puffs q12h

DPI, Dry powder inhaler; *MDI,* metered dose inhaler; *SC,* subcutaneously.
From Rau JL Jr: *Respiratory care pharmacology,* ed 5, St Louis, 1998, Mosby.

Most of the medications listed in this section are chemically derived from adrenaline. They are somewhat different in their structures so that the desired effects and side (unwanted) effects vary. See Box 8-1 for the side effects of the sympathomimetic bronchodilators. Clinically, the most dangerous of these side effects are palpitations, tachycardia, and hypertension.

b. Recommend and administer anticholinergic agents

This group of medications works to promote bronchodilation by suppressing the action of the parasympathetic nervous system. This results in the sympathetic nervous system dominating and causing bronchial smooth muscle relaxation. The anticholinergic (also known as parasympatholytic) group has been found to be more effective in helping patients with chronic obstructive pulmonary disease (COPD), such as emphysema and chronic bronchitis, than patients with asthma. However, often it is best to treat COPD and asthma patients with medications from both the sympathomimetic and anticholinergic/parasympatholytic groups. A relatively new medication, Combivent, combines a sympathomimetic and an anticholinergic/parasympatholytic medication. See Table 8-3 for information on the parasympatholytic medications.

2. Antiinflammatory agents

a. Recommend the use of nonsteroidal antiinflammatory drugs (NSAIDS)

This general grouping includes several different types of over-the-counter medications. None are as powerful an antiinflammatory as the corticosteroid drugs, but some offer other clinical benefits:

1. acetylsalicylic acid (aspirin): antiinflammatory, mild analgesia, antipyretic, blocks platelet formation
2. ibuprofen (Advil, Motrin): antiinflammatory, mild analgesia, antipyretic,
3. antihistamine (Claritin): antiinflammatory

b. Recommend and administer corticosteroids

Corticosteroids affect the respiratory system in two ways. First, they potentiate the effects of the sympathomimetic agents. Second, they stop the inflammatory response seen in the airways of asthmatics after exposure to an

---

BOX 8-1	Clinically Observed Side Effects of Sympathomimetic Aerosolized Bronchodilators From the Most Commonly Seen to the Least Commonly Seen

Tremor: gentle, uncontrollable, involuntary muscle shaking
Palpitations and tachycardia: irregular heartbeats and fast heart rate
Headache
Increased blood pressure: possibly from both the alpha-1 effect on blood vessels and tachycardia
Nervousness and irritability
Dizziness
Nausea
Decreased PaO_2 level from a worsening of the ventilation/perfusion ratio

PaO₂, Partial pressure of O_2 in arterial blood.

TABLE 8-3 Strengths, Dosages, and Duration of Action for Aerosolized Anticholinergic Bronchodilators

Drug	Brand name	Strength	Dosage	Onset (min)	Peak (hr)	Duration (hr)
Atropine sulfate	Dey-Dose Atropine Sulfate					
	Adult	0.2% (1 mg/0.5 mL)	0.025 mg/kg tid, qid	15	0.5-1	3-4
	Child	0.5% (2.5 mg/0.5 mL)	0.05 mg/kg tid, qid			3-4
Ipratropium bromide	Atrovent	MDI: 18 µg/puff	2 puffs qid	15	1-2	4-6
		SVN: 0.02% strength	500 µg tid, qid	1-5		4-8
		Nasal spray: 0.03%	2 sprays/nostril bid, tid			
		0.06%	2 sprays/nostril tid, qid			
Ipratropium bromide + albuterol	Combivent	MDI: ipratropium, 18 µg/puff Albuterol, 90 µg/puff	2 puffs qid	15	1-2	4-6
Glycopyrrolate	Robinul*	0.2 mg/mL	1.0 mg tid, qid	15-30	0.5-1	6
Oxitropium bromide	Experimental agent	100 µg/puff	2 puffs qid	15	2	6-8

MDI, Metered dose inhaler; *SVN,* small-volume nebulizer.
*Available in injectable solution; used experimentally by aerosol.
From Rau JL Jr: *Respiratory care pharmacology,* ed 5, St Louis, 1998, Mosby.

allergen. This prevents mucosal edema from developing. The patient with chronic airflow obstruction such as mild asthma or asthmatic bronchitis should be given inhaled corticosteroids. When they are used as directed, there is little systemic (bodily) absorption. See Table 8-4 for specific strength and dosage information for the inhaled corticosteroids. The patient who is using any of these medications must gargle and rinse out his or her mouth after each use. If not, the patient runs the risk of developing a fungal infection of the mouth and throat.

The patient who is diagnosed with status asthmaticus should have systemic corticosteroids promptly given by the intravenous route. Examples of commonly used systemic corticosteroids include methylprednisolone (Medrol and Solu-Medrol), prednisone (Deltasone), prednisolone (Meticortelone and Delta-Cortef), cortisone (Cortone), and hydrocortisone (Cortef and Solu-Cortef). These drugs can be lifesavers if used properly. However, chronic use of large oral or intravenous doses can lead to serious systemic complications such as immunosuppression and adrenal gland insufficiency. If a patient has been taking systemic corticosteroids for an extended time, he or she should be gradually weaned off them after an inhaled corticosteroid has been started. It is dangerous to suddenly stop an oral or intravenous corticosteroid that has been used for a prolonged time.

3. Recommend and administer mucolytic or proteolytic agents

Acetylcysteine (Mucomyst) is a mucolytic drug that has been widely used with patients who have thick (viscous) mucus or mucous plugs. Because of its bad odor (rotten eggs) some patients may experience nausea and vomiting. Of greater concern is the stimulation of bronchospasm in some asthmatic patients. Because of this concern, it is often wise to either pretreat the patient with an aerosolized sympathomimetic bronchodilator or mix one with the acetylcysteine before it is nebulized for the patient. Any fast-onset bronchodilator can be used in the usual dose. Mucomyst is usually administered by handheld nebulizer or intermittent positive-pressure breathing (IPPB). Most adult patients are given 3 to 5 mL of the 20% solution or 6 to 10 mL of the 10% solution. The 20% solution is often diluted with an equal volume of normal saline solution. Direct instillation of 1 to 2 mL of the drug into the trachea also helps to liquefy secretions. The manufacturer recommends that all of the medication in a vial be used within 96 hours or be discarded. It should be stored in the refrigerator. A slightly purple color is commonly seen after the vial has been opened, but it can still be used safely.

Dornase alfa (Pulmozyme) is a proteolytic drug that has been approved for use in the treatment of patients with cystic fibrosis. It works by breaking up strands of DNA found in the secretions of these patients with a pulmonary infection. Usually a single daily dose of 2.5 mL of solution (containing 2.5 mg of dornase alfa) is inhaled by small-volume nebulizer. Store the drug in a refrigerator and protect it from strong light. It has no serious side effects.

4. Recommend and administer saline solutions

The various saline solutions (and sterile water) are known collectively as "bland" aerosols because they have no direct pharmacologic effect on the lungs and airways. However, when they are inhaled as an aerosol, a vagal nerve mediated reflex causes the bronchial/submucosal glands to release more watery secretions. Because of this action, a saline aerosol is commonly used to help liquefy secretions and induce a patient to cough out sputum.

TABLE 8-4   Corticosteroids Available by Aerosol for Oral Inhalation

Drug	Strength	Dose
Dexamethasone sodium phosphate (Decadron Respihaler)	84 µg/puff	Adults: 3 puffs tid or qid Children: 2 puffs tid or qid
Beclomethasone dipropionate (Beclovent, Vanceril) (Vanceril 84 µg double strength)	42 µg/puff	Adults: 2 puffs tid or qid Children: 1-2 puffs tid or qid
	84 µg/puff	Adults and children ≥6 years: 2 puffs bid
Triamcinolone acetonide (Azmacort)	100 µg/puff	Adults: 2 puffs tid or qid Children: 1-2 puffs tid or qid
Flunisolide (AeroBid)	250 µg/puff	Adults: 2 puffs bid Children: 2 puffs bid
Fluticasone propionate (Flovent)	44 µg/puff	>12 years: 2 puffs bid*
	110 µg/puff	88-220 µg bid, up to 440 µg bid†
	220 µg/puff	880 µg bid‡

*Recommended starting dose if on bronchodilators alone.
†If on inhaled corticosteroids previously.
‡If on oral corticosteroids previously.
From Rau JL Jr: *Respiratory care pharmacology*, ed 5, St Louis, 1998, Mosby.

5. Recommend the use of cardiac agents

There are many classes of medications that are used to treat heart conditions. It is beyond the scope of this book to discuss all of them. However, the following types are needed by many patients requiring respiratory care services.

a. Cardiotonic (positive inotropic) drugs

Positive inotropic agents are used to increase the contractility of the heart muscle. There are two classes of drugs that do this. Both are used in patients who have a weak or damaged myocardium. They increase the patient's myocardial contractility. This results in increased cardiac output, increased blood pressure, and increased urine output. The best-known, older group consists of cardiac glycosides and is commonly referred to as "digitalis." The cardiac glycosides increase the level of intramuscular sodium and calcium to increase the contraction of the heart muscle. Of these, Lanoxin (digoxin) is the preferred medication for a patient with congestive heart failure.

The newer group includes synthetic catecholamine agents. The catecholamine agents are similar to adrenaline and stimulate beta receptors in the heart. Dobutamine hydrochloride (Dobutrex) is used as a short-term agent in adult patients who have organic heart disease or who have had heart surgery. Its use results in an increase in contraction with only a minor increase in heart rate. Isoproterenol hydrochloride (Isuprel) is used to increase the heart rate and contractility in cases of heart block, congestive heart failure, or cardiac arrest. Epinephrine (Adrenaline) is used during a cardiac arrest to increase heart rate and contractility.

b. Antiarrhythmic drugs

Bradycardia is defined as a heart rate of less than 60 beats per minute in an adult at rest. If the patient has symptoms such as light-headedness or low blood pressure, the heart rate should be raised. Common medications that raise heart rate include atropine (atropine sulfate), isoproterenol (Isuprel), or epinephrine (Adrenaline chloride).

Tachycardia (a resting adult heart rate of greater than 100 beats per minute) and abnormal, fast heartbeats originating from the atria or ventricles are potentially very dangerous. Fast tachycardia and dangerous arrhythmias must be controlled with medications that slow down the heart's conduction system or suppress the generation of abnormal electrical signals. Common medications that do this include propranolol (Inderal), lidocaine (Xylocaine), and procainamide (Pronestyl). The arrhythmias and medications and other treatments for them are discussed in Chapter 10.

6. Recommend the use of vasoactive agents
a. Vasoconstrictors

Vasoconstrictors are medications that cause the peripheral blood vessels to constrict so that blood flow is reduced through them. Many medications do this by stimulating the alpha-1 (a_1) receptors on the vessels. There are three common clinical situations in which vasoconstrictors are used in the care of patients with cardiopulmonary problems.

1. Laryngeal edema or upper-airway edema

This type of problem requires the administration of a medication that reduces the swelling of the mucosa of the larynx, epiglottis, or tracheobronchial tree. Inhaled phenylephrine (Neo-Synephrine) or racemic epinephrine (microNefrin, Vaponefrin, Asthma-Nefrin) has been widely used for many years to treat upper-airway edema. Be aware that these drugs can also stimulate beta-1 (b_1) and beta-2 (b_2) receptors, so watch for signs of tachycardia.

2. Upper-airway procedure

Procedures in which the nasal passage must be entered with a medical instrument include nasotracheal intubation, passage of a fiber optic bronchoscope, and nasal surgery. Racemic epinephrine or phenylephrine is nebulized into the appropriate nostril. A so-called atomizer is often used for this purpose because it generates relatively large particles.

3. Hypotension

Hypotension is usually defined as a systemic blood pressure of less than 80 mm Hg in an adult and less than 70 mm Hg in a child. A pressure of less than this does not adequately perfuse the kidneys. Urine output drops dramatically or stops altogether. Cerebral blood flow is also greatly reduced. When hypotension is caused by vasodilation, as in allergic anaphylaxis, it usually has to be treated by inducing vasoconstriction. Hypotension from heart failure or a myocardial infarction often must also be treated with a vasoconstrictor. Common examples of medications that cause vasoconstriction to increase blood pressure include:

a. dopamine hydrochloride (Intropin)
b. norepinephrine (Levophed, Levarterenol)

The effects of dopamine are dose related. At relatively low doses, there is an increase in renal blood flow and urine output increases. There is no change in blood pressure. At medium doses, there is an increase in myocardial contractility and a progressive peripheral vasoconstriction. These effects raise the blood pressure without decreasing renal blood flow. At high doses, the total systemic vascular resistance further increases. However, renal blood flow and urine output both decrease. Current practice indicates that dopamine works best in patients with moderate hypotension. A patient who does not respond to dopamine probably needs norepinephrine (Levophed or Levarterenol) to raise the blood pressure. Any time a hypotensive patient is given a vasoconstricting agent, the blood pressure, peripheral blood flow, and urine output must be watched closely.

The prognosis is grim for patients who do not respond to these medications or for attempts to correct the underlying condition.

b. Vasodilators

Hypertension in the adult is defined as a blood pressure of greater than 140 to 150/90 mm Hg. The higher the blood pressure, the greater the strain on the heart. It also increases the risk of vessel rupture and stroke.

A wide variety of medications in a number of drug categories is used to reduce blood pressure. They range from diuretics to reduce blood volume, to calcium and sympathomimetic blockers that reduce heart rate and vasodilate, to angiotensin converting enzyme (ACE) inhibitors. Medications in these categories are used to treat moderate, chronic hypertension.

The patient in a hypertensive crisis (blood pressure greater than 200/120 mm Hg) must be treated quickly and effectively. The following medications are commonly given by the intravenous route to control severe hypertension:

a. nitroprusside (Nipride)
b. diazoxide (Hyperstat)
c. trimethaphan (Arfonad)

Nitroprusside is also given to reduce the afterload in a patient with left ventricular failure after a myocardial infarct. Any patient who is receiving a powerful vasodilator must have frequent blood pressure monitoring.

7. Recommend the use of diuretic agents

Diuretics are most commonly indicated in patients with edema or hypertension. Edema is usually a result of heart failure or fluid overload. Examples of diuretics used to treat these problems include:

a. furosemide (Lasix)
b. ethacrynic acid (Edecrin)
c. chlorothiazide (Diuril)

These are some of the most powerful diuretics in use today. They produce a rapid increase in urine output. They basically prevent the kidneys from retaining sodium (Na^+) so that water is excreted. A side effect of their use is a loss of potassium (K^+) through the kidneys.

Another category of diuretic is used in patients who have an increased intracranial pressure (ICP). The increased ICP is usually caused by cerebral edema from a head injury. Examples of medications used to treat an increased intracranial pressure include:

a. mannitol (Osmitrol)
b. sterile urea (Ureaphil, Urevert)

These medications have a large molecular weight and through osmosis "pull" fluid from the brain into the bloodstream. Because of this, they are sometimes called osmotic diuretics. When the medication crosses into the kidney it prevents the reabsorption of water and increases urine output.

☑ EXAM HINT

It is important that a patient receiving a drug such as Lasix be given replacement potassium (K+) to avoid dangerous hypokalemia. Review the normal potassium level listed in Chapter 1.

---

8. Recommend the use of antiinfective agents

The terms antiinfective, antibiotic, and antimicrobial refer to natural or synthetic chemicals that are toxic to bacteria and other microorganisms. Table 8-5 lists the most commonly found respiratory pathogens. Table 8-6 lists the antiinfective agent(s) and the spectrum of pathogens against which they are used.

TABLE 8-5 Common Respiratory Pathogens in Approximate Order of Frequency

	Gram Positive	Gram Negative	Cell Wall Deficient
Bacteria:	Streptococcus pneumoniae	Hemophilus influenzae	Mycoplasma
	Staphylococcus aureus*	Klebsiella pneumoniae	Acid-Fast
	Streptococcus faecalis (enterococcus)	Pseudomonas aeruginosa*	Mycobacterium tuberculosis*
		Serratia species*	
Viruses:			
	Rhinovirus	Varicella virus*	
	Adenovirus	Herpes simplex virus*	
	Respiratory syncytival virus	Cytomegalovirus*	
Fungi:			
	Candida albicans*	Histoplasma capsulatum (Ohio Valley)	
	Aspergillus species*	Coccidioides immitis (Southwest U.S.)	
	Pneumocystis carinii		
Protozoa:			
	Toxoplasma gondii*		
	Cryptosporidium*		

*Seen most frequently in debilitated or immunosuppressed hosts.

| TABLE 8-6 | Classification of Antibiotic Agents Commonly Used Against Pulmonary Infections |

Class or Group	Agents	Spectrum	Major toxicity
Penicillin	Penicillin G	Gram-positive organisms; *Staphylococcus aureus* often resistant	Allergy
Semisynthetic penicillins	Ampicillin, Omnipen	Gram-positive organisms, Gram negative *Haemophilus influenzae;* variable against gram-negative rods	Diarrhea and rash, especially with viral disease (mononucleosis)
	Oxacillin, Prostaphlin	Like penicillin, with antistaphylococcal effects	Allergy
	Carbenicillin, Geopen	Like penicillin, with antipseudomonas effects	Sodium overload-congestive failure
Cephalosporine	Cephalothin, Keflin	Like penicillin, with antistaphylococcal effects	Renal (usually not severe)
Aminoglycosides	Streptomycin	Primarily tuberculostatic	Vestibular, renal
	Tobramycin, TOBI *aeruginosa*	Pseudomonas lung infection in cystic fibrosis patients	Auditory, renal
	gentamicin, Garamycin	Gram-negative rods, including *Pseudomonas* and *Proteus*	Vestibular, renal
Macrolide	erythromycin, Erythrocin	Like penicillin (used in penicillin allergy); drug of choice for *Mycoplasma*	Gastrointestinal
Tetracyclines	tetracycline, Achromycin	Broad spectrum; useful against *Haemophilus* and *Mycoplasma* infections	Fungal overgrowth in bowel or vagina; hepatic with large IV doses
Chloramphenicol	Chloromycetin	Broad spectrum; used for *Haemophilus* if it is Ampicillin-resistant or if patient is allergic	Bone marrow
Antituberculosis agents	isonicotinic acid hydrazide (INH), Isoniazid	Used for both prophylaxis and treatment	Hepatic
	Ethambutol, Rifampin	Used for tuberculostatic therapy	Retinal (maculapathy), hepatic
Antifungal agents	ketoconazole, Nizoral	Major agent for systemic fungal disease	Gastrointestinal upset
	Amphotericin B	Major agent for systemic fungal disease	Renal, gastrointestinal
Antiviral agents	AZT, Retrovir	Stops reproduction in retroviruses. Used against HIV.	Anemia
	ribavirin, Virazole	Same spectrum, used against respiratory syncytial virus; experimental against HIV.	
Sulfonamides	pentamidine isethionate, NebuPent, Pentam 300	Prophylaxis against *Pneumocystis carinii*	Impaired renal and liver function
	trimethaprim and sulfamethoxazole, Bactrim	Used against *Pneumocystis carinii*	Impaired renal and liver function

EXAM HINT

Most Written Registry Exams have included one question asking the appropriate antiinfective agent to use to treat a respiratory pathogen. Usually this question covers the common bacteria, respiratory syncytial virus, or *Pneumocystis carinii.*

a. Antibacterial agents

There are many agents in this category used to treat the different types of pulmonary bacterial infections. This list is limited to the most commonly seen drugs and organism(s) they are used against:

1. penicillin (Penicillin G, Ampicillin, and so on.): used systemically against gram-positive bacteria.

2. gentamicin (Garamycin): used systemically and by aerosol against gram-negative bacteria. It has been given by small-volume nebulizer or IPPB.

3. tobramycin (TOBI): used by aerosol against the gram-negative bacteria *Pseudomonas* in children with cystic fibrosis. It is taken by metered dose inhaler.

4. isoniazid (INH): used systemically against *Mycobacterium Tuberculosis* (TB).

b. Antiviral agent: ribavirin

Ribavirin (Virazole) is most commonly used in the treatment of infants and young children who have bronchiolitis or pneumonia from the respiratory syncytial virus (RSV). Patients requiring treatment for their condition usually are very sick and have complicating factors such as prematurity or cardiopulmonary disease. They require the treatment course of 3 to 7 days of nebulization of the drug for 12 to 18 hours per day. Only the SPAG II (small particle aerosol generator) can be used for the procedure. This is because it is specifically designed to nebulize the 1- to 2-μm size particles needed to penetrate to the alveoli to kill the virus. Virazole is known to also be effective against influenza types A and B viruses and the herpes simplex virus.

c. Antipneumocystic agent: pentamidine isethionate

Pentamidine isethionate (NebuPent) has been approved for the prophylactic treatment of the fungal organism *Pneumocystis carinii*. Patients with impaired immune systems, such as those with acquired immunodeficiency syndrome (AIDS), are most likely to get *Pneumocystis carinii* pneumonia (PCP). Currently, these patients are given a single 300-mg dose of NebuPent mixed with 6 mL of sterile water once every 4 weeks through the Respirgard II nebulizer. (The AeroTech II unit may also be used.) Some patients must be pretreated with an inhaled bronchodilator to prevent bronchospasm before the NebuPent is inhaled. Do not mix the two medications in the Respirgard II or use the Respirgard II for any medication other than NebuPent. Mixing NebuPent with normal saline or a bronchodilator can result in a precipitation of the medications. When given by the inhalation route, there are few systemic side effects. There is also an intramuscular or intravenous form of pentamidine called Pentam 300. Bactrim (trimethoprim and sulfamethoxazole) is preferred over systemic pentamidine because there are fewer and less-serious side effects.

9. Recommend the use of sedative agents

Sedatives are medications that affect the brain to induce calming in a patient who can be either simply anxious or very agitated and uncooperative. Examples of when a patient should be given a sedative include: (1) when he or she is struggling against a necessary intubation or the mechanical ventilator so that his or her condition worsens, (2) he or she is displaying self-destructive behavior because of a drug reaction, and (3) before a medical procedure for so-called conscious sedation. The effects on the patient are dose related. Low to moderate doses calm the patient. Higher doses induce sleep. There are three different groupings of these types of medications. The most widely used are the benzodiazepines because they have fewer side effects, fewer drug interactions, and are less likely to cause addiction than the barbiturate drugs. In addition, the benzodiazepine agents can be pharmacologically reversed. The barbiturates are widely used during general anesthesia to rapidly induce sleep. Commonly used examples of these types of medications include:

a. Benzodiazepine minor tranquilizers: midazolam (Versed), diazepam (Valium), chlordiazepoxide (Librium), alprazolam (Xanax), triazolam, (Halcion), flurazepam (Dalmane)
b. Nonbarbiturate sedative-hypnotics: ethchlorvynol (Placidyl), meprobamate (Miltown), glutethimide (Doriden), chloral hydrate (Noctec)
c. Barbiturate sedative-hypnotics: pentobarbital sodium (Nembutal), secobarbital sodium (Seconal), phenobarbital (Luminal), thiopental (Pentothal)

The benzodiazepine antagonist drug flumazenil (Romazicon) is indicated in the reversal of benzodiazepine agents such as Valium, Librium, and so forth. Patients who are unconscious usually quickly awaken after the proper dose of Romazicon is given. Watch the patient for signs of seizure activity related to the rapid reversal of the benzodiazepine medication. Furthermore, the patient should be observed for 2 hours in case resedation occurs. If it does, Romazicon can be given again.

10. Recommend the use of analgesic agents

Analgesics are medications that control or block pain after injury or a surgical procedure. Morphine is indicated to control the pain of a myocardial infarct and to vasodilate the patient with pulmonary edema. In addition, pain-relieving agents, when given in large enough doses, induce sleep. The patient who is both in pain and agitated may be treated with a combination of an analgesic and a sedative, for example, moderate doses of morphine and Valium. The two drugs potentiate each other. Or the physician may decide to give the patient only morphine at a larger dose. Examples of commonly used analgesics include:

a. morphine sulfate injection (Morphine Sulfate) or tablets (Duramorph SR)
b. codeine phosphate (Methylmorphine)
c. hydromorphone (Dilaudid)
d. meperidine (Demerol)
e. propoxyphene (Darvon)

Patients receiving sedatives or analgesics must be closely monitored. Both can cause respiratory center depression if given in great enough doses. This may be used to help control an agitated patient breathing out of phase with a ventilator. However, a spontaneously breathing patient may hypoventilate and even experience apnea and death. Another concern with these agents is that morphine and these other medications can become habit forming or addictive if used for a prolonged period of time.

The narcotic antagonist drug naloxone (Narcan) counteracts the effects of narcotic agents such as morphine, heroin, and codeine. Narcan does *not* reverse benzodiazepine or barbiturate drugs. Remember that the patient who received an accidental overdose of morphine given to control pain will feel pain again when Narcan is given to reverse the overdose.

11. Recommend the use of neuromuscular blocking agents

Neuromuscular blocking agents are used to cause a

pharmacologic paralysis. These medications block nerve transmission from reaching skeletal (voluntary) muscles. Complete paralysis follows. They are used most commonly as part of balanced anesthesia before major thoracic or abdominal surgery. These drugs are also used in the intensive care unit to stop a patient from fighting against an intubation or to prevent the patient from struggling against the mechanical ventilator. All are given intravenously and act rapidly. Obviously, in all these cases the patient must use a manual resuscitator or ventilator. Examples of the commonly used neuromuscular blocking agents include:

a. Depolarizing blocker: succinylcholine chloride (Anectine, Quelicin)
b. Nondepolarizing blockers: pancuronium bromide (Pavulon) (preferred drug), vecuronium bromide (Norcuron), gallamine triethiodide (Flaxedil), atracurium besylate (Tracrium)

The nondepolarizing blockers such as Pavulon are preferred for their longer duration of action. Although all these agents induce complete paralysis of all voluntary muscles, they have little or no effect on the involuntary muscles or autonomic nervous system. Some patients may have a minor, passing change in heart rate and blood pressure. Remember that they are able to hear, feel pain, and are completely awake and alert to their surroundings. Care must be taken to sedate the patient for anxiety and give analgesics for pain. Talk to the patient normally and move the patient periodically to prevent pressure sores.

The nondepolarizing neuromuscular blocker agents can be reversed so that the patient can breathe and move again. These intravenous medications include neostigmine bromide (Prostigmin) (preferred) and edrophonium (Tensilon). It should be noted that these reversing agents cause an outpouring of oral and bronchial secretions. Atropine is given to prevent this. The reversing agents have no effect on the depolarizing neuromuscular blocker succinylcholine chloride. Patients given this drug usually regain movement within 15 minutes after the medication is stopped.

12. Recommend the use of surfactant agents

Surfactant has been approved for the prevention or treatment of infant respiratory distress syndrome (RDS) in premature neonates. These neonates have immature lungs that lack natural surfactant. As a result, they develop atelectasis. These four surfactant agents have been approved for instillation into the airways to treat this problem and are widely used:

a. colfosceril palmitate, cetyl alcohol, and tyloxapol (Exosurf)
b. beractant (Survanta)
c. poractant alfa (Curosurf)
d. calfactant (Infasurf)

Dosages for all of the medications are based on the infant's weight. Be prepared to make rapid changes in the neonate's mechanical ventilator settings as the lungs rapidly become more compliant.

MODULE B Drug dosage calculations (math review)

The National Board for Respiratory Care (NBRC) Examination Content Outline does not specifically list drug dosage calculations. However, previous Written Registry Examinations have included one calculation.

The problems will be easier to solve by remembering the following:
1. One millimeter = 1 cc = 1 gram (g) of water (mass)
2. Most drug doses are listed in milligrams instead of grams. Convert grams to milligrams by moving the decimal point three places to the right (the same as multiplying by 1000). For example: 0.5 g = 500 mg.
3. Know how to interconvert fractions, decimal fractions, and percentages. For example: 1:100 = 1/100 = 0.01 = 1%.

One common way to solve any drug dosage calculation is by the creation of a proportional problem. To do this the drug concentration must be converted into a fractional form. The proportional problem can then be set up to solve for the unknown. For example:
1. How much active ingredient is in 0.5 mL of Bronkosol?

A 1% (1:100) drug concentration means that there is 1 part of active ingredient in 100 parts of the solution. Or there is 1 mL or g of active ingredient in 100 mL or g of the solution. This can be set up in the following proportion:

$$\frac{1 \text{ mL active ingredient}}{100 \text{ mL total solution}} = \frac{\text{unknown active ingredient or } x}{0.5 \text{ mL solution}} \text{ (cross multiply)}$$

$100\ x = 0.5$ mL (Divide both sides of the equation by 100.)

$x = 0.005$ mL $= 0.005$ g $= 5$ mg of active ingredient

2. How much active ingredient is in 0.25 mL of Alupent? Alupent is 5% active ingredient.

A 5% drug concentration means that there are 5 parts of active ingredient in 100 parts of the solution. So there are 5 mL or g of active ingredient in 100 mL or g of the solution. This can be set up in the following proportion:

$$\frac{5 \text{ mL active ingredient}}{100 \text{ mL total solution}} = \frac{\text{unknown active ingredient or } x}{0.25 \text{ mL solution}} \text{ (cross multiply)}$$

$100\ x = 1.25$ mL (Divide both sides of the equation by 100.)

$x = 0.0125$ mL $= 0.0125$ g $= 12.5$ mg of active ingredient

Thus it can be seen that the amount of active ingredient can be calculated if the drug concentration is given in either a fractional or percentage form.

The next two examples deal with calculating the volume of medication needed to deliver a desired amount of active ingredient. With these types it is necessary to convert to consistent units, usually converting grams to milligrams. For example:

3. How much 0.5% Proventil is needed to give a patient 2.5 mg of active ingredient by small-volume nebulizer?

A 0.5% (1:200) drug concentration means that there is 1 part of active ingredient in 200 parts of the solution. Or there is 1 mL or g of active ingredient in 200 mL or g of the solution. This converts to 1000 mg/200 mL. Set up the following proportion:

$$\frac{1000 \text{ mg active ingredient}}{200 \text{ mL total solution}} = \frac{2.5 \text{ mg}}{x \text{ mL solution}} \text{ (cross multiply)}$$

500 mL = 1000 x (Divide both sides of the equation by 1000.)

x = 0.5 mL of Proventil should be given.

4. How much 4% Xylocaine is needed to give a patient 100 mg of active ingredient by handheld nebulizer before a bronchoscopy?

A 4% drug concentration means that there are 4 parts of active ingredient in 100 parts of the solution. So there is 4 mL or g of active ingredient in 100 mL or g of the solution. This converts to 4000 mg/100 mL. Set up the following proportion:

$$\frac{4000 \text{ mg active ingredient}}{100 \text{ mL total solution}} = \frac{100 \text{ mg}}{x \text{ mL solution}} \text{ (cross multiply)}$$

10,000 mL = 4000 x (Divide both sides of the equation by 4000.)

x = 2.5 mL of Xylocaine should be given.

Thus the volume of medication needed to deliver a given amount of active ingredient can be calculated if the drug concentration is given in either a fractional or percentage form.

MODULE C Respiratory care plan

1. **Participate in the development of the respiratory care plan [e.g., case management, development and application of protocols, disease management education] (Code: IC4) [Difficulty: An]**

The respiratory therapist should be able to determine if the patient is having cardiopulmonary problems. Review, if needed, the information presented earlier in the book that deals with bedside assessment, blood gases, pulmonary function tests, and advanced cardiopulmonary monitoring.

Many treatment protocols require the practitioner to count the patient's heart rate before, at least once during, and after an aerosolized bronchodilator is given. This is because of the risk of tachycardia. It is generally acceptable to count for 30 seconds and multiply by 2 for 1 minute's count. Record the various heart rates. The heart rhythm can be determined as the pulse is measured. A stethoscope can be used to be verify an abnormality. A common policy is to stop the treatment if the patient's pulse increases by more than 20% from the initial level.

Listen for a reduction in wheezing after the administration of an aerosolized bronchodilator as proof that it has been effective at reducing bronchospasm. If the patient is being given an aerosolized bronchodilator for bronchospasm, it is expected that the patient's spirometry results will move toward more normal values as the bronchospasm is reduced. The two most important bedside spirometry values to follow are the peak flow and forced expiratory volume in 1 second (FEV_1). A 15% to 20% improvement in either one or both after the inhalation of an aerosolized bronchodilator indicates (1) the medication works, and (2) the patient has reversible bronchospasm. A patient with stable asthma may be given a drug such as cromolyn sodium (Intal) or nedocromil sodium (Tilade) by inhalation to prevent a future asthma attack. Remember that these drugs are not to be used *during* an asthma attack. Listen for a reduction in airway secretions after a productive cough. The mucolytics should help make the secretions less thick.

If the patient's condition does not improve after the administration of the prescribed medication, there may be another problem. A chest radiograph might help to clarify the situation. Most patients gladly tell you if their breathing is easier after the delivery of the proper medication. It is just as important to know when the patient does *not* feel any better. Possibly the medication does not work, or the dose is insufficient. Stop a breathing treatment any time the patient appears to have had an allergic reaction to a medication. Tell the patient's physician and ask for further orders.

📇 EXAM HINT

Although the NBRC has not listed respiratory center stimulants as testable, their use has been questioned on the Written Registry Exam. Remember that the correct course of treatment to stimulate the breathing of a premature infant is to administer the drug theophylline (aminophylline) or caffeine.

2. **Make a recommendation to change the dosage or concentration of an aerosolized medication**

Bronchodilators. Make a recommendation to decrease the amount of medication if the patient is having serious side effects such as tachycardia or palpitations. Make a recommendation to increase the amount of medication if the asthmatic patient's bronchospasm is not reversed and there are no adverse side effects. The current guidelines on the pharmacologic management of asthma list the medications that should be used depending on how the patient's asthmatic condition is categorized. All asthmatic patients should have an inhaled, short-acting, rapid-onset beta-adrenergic bronchodilator. The medication albuterol (Proventil, Ventolin, Xopenex) is widely used for quick relief. For persistent asthma, several additional medications are taken for long-term control. These include an inhaled corticosteroid (beclomethasone, triamcinolone), an inhaled long-acting beta-adrenergic bronchodilator (salmeterol), and a preventative agent (cromolyn sodium or zafirlukast). The most severe persistent asthmatics also require a corticosteroid medication by syrup or pill and sustained-release theophylline. It is recommended that the National Institutes of Health guidelines, as listed in the bibliography, be reviewed for complete information.

Mucomyst or saline solutions. Make a recommendation to increase the amount of medication if the patient's secretions are still too viscous to cough out or suction and there are no adverse side effects to the medication. Make a recommendation to decrease the amount of medication if the patient's secretions are watery enough for expectoration or suctioning or if there are side effects to the drug like bronchospasm.

3. Change the dilution of a medication used in aerosol therapy

The various saline solutions and sterile water are known collectively as "bland" aerosols because they have no direct pharmacologic effect on the lungs and airways. They are used to increase the volume of liquid in a small-volume nebulizer after the medication has been added. Most of these nebulizers work most efficiently when they hold about 3 to 5 mL of liquid. Usually normal saline solution (0.9% sodium chloride) is added.

Adding little or no saline to the medication results in the patient inhaling a very concentrated solution or causes the nebulizer to malfunction. The nebulizer aerosolizes the medication within a few minutes. The patient should quickly feel the beneficial effects of the treatment. However, depending on the nature of the medication, the patient might find it to be quite irritating to the airway. Coughing or bronchospasm can result. Side effects, such as tachycardia, should be watched for with sympathomimetic agents because the medication enters the bloodstream so quickly.

The more saline that added, the less concentrated the solution will be. The nebulizer takes longer to aerosolize the medication because of the added volume. Relief of symptoms therefore takes longer. However, it is less likely to irritate the airway. Side effects with sympathomimetic agents can be less severe because the drug is given over a longer period. However, remember that increasing the amount of saline makes no difference on the total amount of medication that is in the nebulizer for the patient. Tachycardia or other side effects may still be seen if the total amount of medication is given.

| BOX 8-2 | Saline Solutions Used as Mucolytics |

NORMAL SALINE SOLUTION, 0.9% SALINE
Direct instillation into the airway:
Infants may be given about 1 mL several times before suctioning
Adults may be given about 3-5 mL several times daily before suctioning
Aerosol: most medication nebulizers hold 3-5 mL that is nebulized several times daily
Miscellaneous:
Usually is well tolerated because it is isotonic to the body
Particle size is fairly stable as nebulized

HYPOTONIC SALINE SOLUTION, 0.45% SALINE
Direct instillation into the airway: same as with normal saline solution
Aerosol: same as with normal saline solution; many practitioners use this concentration in ultrasonic nebulizers
Miscellaneous: particles tend to shrink because of evaporation, which results in smaller particles than nebulized that are closer to isotonic; impaction is more likely in the smaller airways

HYPERTONIC SALINE SOLUTION, 1.8%-20% SALINE
Aerosol: some practitioners use a large-reservoir nebulizer with a heater to generate the aerosol
Hypertonic saline solution is most commonly used to induce a cough and sputum sample for cytology (lung cancer) or fungal or mycobacteria (tuberculosis) culture; it should not be used for a general bacteria culture because the high salt concentration inhibits the growth of most bacteria
Miscellaneous:
Particles tend to enlarge because of the absorption of water vapor, which results in larger particles than nebulized that are closer to isotonic; impaction is more likely in the upper airway
This concentration is the most likely to cause bronchospasm in asthmatic patients, because it is the farthest from isotonic and, therefore, the most irritating

---

Saline-only aerosol treatments, as for an induced sputum, are more effective at higher concentrations of saline. See Box 8-2 for complete information on the saline solutions.

BIBLIOGRAPHY

AARC clinical practice guideline: surfactant replacement therapy, *Respir Care* 39(8):824-829, 1994.

Au JP, Ziment I: Drug therapy and dosage adjustment in asthma, *Respir Care* 31:415-418, 1986.

Bills GW, Soderberg RC: *Principles of pharmacology for respiratory care,* ed 2, Albany, NY, 1998, Delmar.

Howder CL: Cardiopulmonary pharmacology: a handbook for respiratory practitioners and other allied health personnel, ed 2, Baltimore, 1996, Williams & Wilkins.

Malmeister M: Pharmacology associated with respiratory care. In Fink JB, Hunt GE, editors: *Clinical practice in respiratory care,* Philadelphia, 1999, Lippincott-Raven.

McLaughlin AJ, Levine SR: *Respiratory care drug reference,* Gaithersburg, MD, 1997, Aspen.

National Institutes of Health: *Practical guide for the diagnosis and management of asthma,* Publication number 97-4053, October 1997.

Physicians' Desk Reference, ed 52, Montvale, NJ, 1998, Medical Economics.

Rau JL: *Respiratory care pharmacology,* ed 5, St Louis, 1998, Mosby.

Tashkin DP: Dosing strategies for bronchodilator aerosol delivery, *Respir Care* 36:977-988, 1991.

Witek TJ: *Pharmacology and therapeutics in respiratory care,* Philadelphia, 1994, WB Saunders Company.

Ziment I: Drugs used in respiratory care. In Burton GG, Hodgkin JE, Ward JJ, editors: *Respiratory care: a guide to clinical practice,* ed 4, Philadelphia, 1997, Lippincott-Raven.

SELF-STUDY QUESTIONS

1. You are called to help assess a premature neonate. The patient is having difficulty breathing and respiratory distress syndrome is suspected. You would recommend all of the following *except:*
   A. flumazenil (Romazicon)
   B. beractant (Survanta)
   C. calfactant (Infasurf)
   D. proactant alpha (Curosurf)

2. A 2-month-old infant has periods of apnea that result in bradycardia and cyanosis. What medication should be recommended to treat the apnea periods?
   A. lidocaine (Xylocaine)
   B. neostigmine (Prostigmin)
   C. theophylline (Aminophylline)
   D. isoetharine (Bronkosol)

3. A 35-year-old patient has AIDS and was previously treated for *Pneumocystis carinii* pneumonia. What can be used to prevent the infection from reoccurring?
   A. Trimethoprim and sulfamethoxazole (Bactrim) by pill
   B. Pentamidine (NebuPent) by nebulizer
   C. Tobramycin (TOBI) by metered dose inhaler
   D. Amphotericin B by intravenous catheter

4. A mechanically ventilated patient who has been paralyzed with a neuromuscular blocking agent should be given a sedative agent for what reason?
   A. To sustain the paralysis
   B. To control pain
   C. To keep the patient synchronized with the ventilator
   D. To relieve the patient's anxiety

5. A patient had a bronchoscopy procedure and biopsy taken of a suspected lung tumor. Following the biopsy there is uncontrolled bleeding. What would you recommend to control the bleeding?
   A. Instill epinephrine through the bronchoscopy at the site of the bleeding.
   B. Administer heparin by intravenous line.
   C. Nebulize albuterol (Proventil) by small-volume nebulizer.
   D. Administer lidocaine (Xylocaine) by intravenous line.

6. A 10-year-old boy with cystic fibrosis has been having recurrent episodes of *Pseudomonas aeruginosa* pneumonia. What should be recommended to prevent this from happening?
   A. Instill pentamidine (Pentam) into the trachea by way of a suction catheter.
   B. Administer pentamidine (NebuPent) once a month by small-volume nebulizer.
   C. Isonicotinic acid hydrazide (Isoniazid) should be taken twice a week for six months.
   D. Tobramycin (TOBI) should be taken by metered dose inhaler every other month.

7. A patient has developed sepsis from an infected surgical wound and is in shock. What is the most effective way to raise her blood pressure?
   A. Administer an intravenous diuretic such as furosemide (Lasix).
   B. Give her oral digitalis (Lanoxin).
   C. Give her intravenous dopamine (Intropin).
   D. Administer one unit of packed red blood cells.

8. Your 48-year-old patient has large amounts of thick secretions related to chronic bronchitis from smoking. There is no sign of infection. What should be administered to help manage the secretion problem?
   A. salmeterol (Serevent)
   B. dornase alpha (Pulmozyme)
   C. normal (0.9%) saline
   D. acetylcysteine (Mucomyst)

9. A home-care patient with asthma has finished her standard dose of albuterol (Ventolin). After waiting 15 minutes he performs a peak flow measurement, which shows 65% of his personal best. What should be recommended to the physician?
   A. Decrease the dose of albuterol.
   B. Add an intravenous corticosteroid to the patient's medications.
   C. Maintain the present therapy.
   D. Increase the dose of albuterol.

10. A 14-year-old patient with cystic fibrosis and a pulmonary infection has many thick secretions. What should be recommended to help manage the secretion problem?
    I. Nebulize acetylcysteine (Mucomyst)
    II. Intravenous fluticasone (Flovent)
    III. Nebulize dornase alpha (Pulmozyme)
    IV. Intravenous flumazenil (Romazicon)
    A. I and III only
    B. I and II only
    C. III and IV only
    D. I, III, and IV only

11. An adult patient is panicking and fighting against the mechanical ventilator. All of the following may be used to control the patient on the ventilator *except:*
    A. flumazenil (Romazicon)
    B. pancuronium bromide (Pavulon)
    C. succinylcholine (Anectine)
    D. morphine sulfate (Duramorph)

12. A 4-month-old pediatric patient has chronic lung disease secondary to recovering from infant respiratory distress syndrome (RDS). The patient now has pneumonia caused by respiratory syncytial virus and is on a mechanical

ventilator. What can be given to improve the patient's condition?

A. Intravenous racemic epinephrine (microNefrin)
B. Ribavirin (Virazole) by SPAG II nebulizer
C. Intratracheal beractant (Survanta)
D. Cromolyn sodium (Intal) by small-volume nebulizer

Answer Key

1. **A.** Rationale: Flumazenil (Romazicon) is used to reverse the effects of the benzodiazepine-type sedative agents (Valium, Versed). There is no indication that the patient had been given a sedative. The other three drugs (Survanta, Infasurf, Curosurf) are used in surfactant replacement therapy in neonates with respiratory distress syndrome.

2. **C.** Rationale: Theophylline (Aminophylline) is known to be a respiratory center stimulant in infants and will stimulate breathing. This should help to prevent the apnea spells. Xylocaine is a local anesthetic agent. It is used to numb an injury or stop cardiac arrhythmias such as premature ventricular contractions (PVC). Prostigmin is used to reverse the paralyzing effects of the nondepolarizing neuromuscular blocking agents like Pavulon. Bronkosol is a fast acting sympathomimetic bronchodilator. It does not simulate breathing.

3. **B.** Rationale: NebuPent is given by small volume nebulizer once every 4 weeks as a preventative agent for *Pneumocystis carinii* pneumonia. Bactrim is the preferred medication to treat an actual *Pneumocystis carinii* pneumonia infection. TOBI is given by MDI to treat a cystic fibrosis patient with *Pseudomonas aeruginosa* pneumonia. Amphotericin B is given by intravenous catheter to treat systemic fungal infections that do not respond to oral antiinfective therapy.

4. **D.** Rationale: A sedative agent will have a calming effect on a patient anxious about being unable to move or communicate while paralyzed on the ventilator. A sedative will not control pain or sustain a pharmacologic paralysis. Although a high enough dose of a sedative will put a patient to sleep and therefore prevent "fighting" the ventilator, that is not its primary purpose. In addition, if the patient is pharmacologically paralyzed, there is no need for any other medication to control the patient's breathing efforts.

5. **A.** Rationale: Epinephrine has vasoconstricting properties (as well as properties causing bronchodilation and tachycardia) and should help to stop bleeding at the biopsy site. Intravenous heparin is contraindicated because it increases clotting time and will likely increase the bleeding. Albuterol (Proventil) is a very effective bronchodilator, but has no effect on peripheral blood vessels. Lidocaine (Xylocaine) is used to stop cardiac arrhythmias, but has no effect on peripheral blood vessels.

6. **D.** Rationale: Tobramycin (TOBI) has been approved by the Food and Drug Administration (FDA) to prevent the development of *Pseudomonas aeruginosa* pneumonia in cystic fibrosis patients. Pentamidine (Pentam or NebuPent) has been approved by the FDA to prevent the development of *Pneumocystis carinii* pneumonia, not *Pseudomonas aeruginosa* pneumonia. Isoniazid (INH) is used to prevent or treat a *Mycobacterium tuberculosis* (TB) infection.

7. **C.** Rationale: Intravenous dopamine (Intropin) will act as a vasoconstrictor and raise her blood pressure until the infection can be controlled by an antibiotic. Oral digitalis (Lanoxin) is given to maintain heart function in a patient with chronic heart failure. Although it will increase this patient's cardiac output, it is not the preferred medication to use to treat a problem of vasodilation secondary to sepsis. Packed red blood cells will help to raise the patient's blood pressure by raising intravascular volume. However, one unit is not enough to have a clinically significant effect. The most effective solution is to constrict the patient's blood vessels with Intropin to restore normal blood pressure.

8. **D.** Rationale: Acetylcysteine (Mucomyst) is very effective at decreasing the viscosity (thickness) of mucoid secretions. Dornase alpha (Pulmozyme) is not indicated in this patient because purulent (infected) secretions with DNA strands are not present. Normal (0.9%) saline has been shown helpful in decreasing the thickness of pulmonary secretions. However, it is not as effective as acetylcysteine (Mucomyst).

9. **D.** Rationale: Increasing the dose of albuterol should improve the patient's bronchodilation and result in an improved peak flow. Because the patient's peak flow is only 65% of personal best, the albuterol dose should not be maintained or decreased. Adding an intravenous corticosteroid to the patient's medications would require the home care patient to travel to the physician's office for injections. This is not a practical solution. In addition, there is no clear indication that intravenous corticosteroids are needed at this time.

10. **A.** Rationale: Nebulize acetylcysteine (Mucomyst) and dornase alpha (Pulmozyme) to decrease the viscosity (thickness) of mucoid and purulent secretions. Fluticasone (Flovent) is an inhaled corticosteroid; it has no effective on secretions. Flumazenil (Romazicon) is used to reverse the effects of the benzodiazepine-type sedative drugs like Valium or Versed. It has no effect on pulmonary secretions.

11. **A.** Rationale: Flumazenil (Romazicon) is used to reverse the effects of benzodiazepine-type sedative agents (Versed, Valium). Rather than calming a patient, Romazicon is used to reverse the effects of oversedation. Pancuronium bromide (Pavulon) and succinylcholine (Anectine) are medications used to paralyze a patient. This will certainly result in the patient's breathing being controlled by the ventilator. Morphine sulfate (Duramorph) is given to control pain and will have a secondary benefit of sedating the patient if enough is given.

12. **B.** Rationale: Ribavirin (Virazole) is given to stop the reproduction of respiratory syncytial virus (RSV). It is given by the SPAG II nebulizer. Racemic epinephrine (MicroNefrin) is a vasoconstricting drug and is given by small volume nebulizer to shrink edematous mucous membranes of the upper airway. Intratracheal beractant (Survanta) is given to a premature neonate with RDS. It would not be needed in this older patient who has recovered from the condition. Cromolyn sodium (Intal) is given by small-volume nebulizer to prevent the onset of asthma. It is not effective against RSV.

9 Bronchopulmonary Hygiene Therapy

A review of the most recent Written Registry Exams has shown an average of three questions (3% of the exam) on bronchopulmonary hygiene therapy.

MODULE A | **Teach the patient proper coughing techniques and coach him or her to cough productively (Code: IIIB3) [Difficulty: An]**

Ideally, the patient is taught proper coughing techniques before surgery. If not, teach them postoperatively:
  a. Minimize traction or tension on the incision, to decrease the pain, by placing either your hands or the patient's hands on both sides of the incision. A pillow also can be held against the incision by the practitioner or patient.
  b. Instruct the patient to breathe two or three times in through the nose and out through the mouth.
  c. Instruct the patient to take in as deep a breath as possible and to perform a normal cough.
  d. If the patient cannot cough normally because of pain, a serial or huff cough can be performed.

Teach the patient with obstructive airways disease the following cough techniques:
  a. Avoid an ineffective, shallow, hacking cough.
  b. Position the patient in a sitting position, bent slightly forward, with feet on the floor or supported. The patient who must lie in bed can be positioned on the preferred side with the legs flexed at the knees and hips.
  c. Instruct the patient to perform a midinspiratory cough.
    1. Breathe two or three times in through the nose and out through the mouth.
    2. Breathe in to a comfortable volume larger than the tidal volume but not as deeply as possible.
    3. Briefly hold the breath.
    4. Cough hard or perform a serial cough at relatively low flows. This should help to raise secretions without causing airway collapse.
    5. Squeezing the knees and thighs together at the instant of coughing helps to increase the airflow and volume.

Coaching is important because patients in pain or suffering from chronic lung disease tend to be uncooperative and do not try hard. Give positive reinforcement when the patient does well. Correct any problems the patient is having following the instructions. Demonstrations are often useful so that the patient can copy a good example.

MODULE B | **Modify the postural drainage therapy**

 EXAM HINT

Although the postural drainage therapy positions are not listed as testable on the Written Registry Exam, they should be reviewed in preparation for questions that ask about making position changes based on the patient's condition. Expect a question about identifying the need to stop postural drainage resulting from patient intolerance. Usually this involves having a patient sit up if he or she is having a problem while in a head-down position.

1. **Change the length of time of the treatment (Code: IIIC5) [Difficulty: An]**
   Lung segments should generally be drained for 3 to 15 minutes. If the patient is tolerating the position and secretions are still being cleared, the position can be held longer. Stop the treatment if the patient is showing any signs of intolerance.

   It is generally recommended that the total time of the procedure be no longer than 30 to 40 minutes. This is because the patient may become exhausted by the various position changes. If this is the case, the practitioner must select the worst segments to be drained first. It may take several drainage sessions to drain all of the involved segments.

2. **Change the treatment techniques used (Code: IIIC5) [Difficulty: An]**
   Be prepared to modify the postural drainage, percussion, and vibration procedures, depending on how the patient tolerates them. For example:
1. Some patients will not tolerate certain positions, especially head down, because of pain or shortness of breath. Watch for hypoxemia, elevated blood pressure, tachypnea, or tachycardia as signs of poor tolerance.
2. Percussion rate, pressure, and hand position may need to be modified, depending on the patient's tolerance, chest size, and secretion clearance.
3. It may not be possible to percuss or vibrate female patients in the right middle lobe and left lingular positions because of breast tissue.
4. Hypoxemia should be prevented with supplemental oxygen in those patients who need it. Pulse oximetry can be performed before and during the procedure to monitor the patient's oxygen saturation.
5. Cardiac patients should have their heart rate, heart

rhythm, and blood pressure monitored. Check the heart rate before the procedure and with each position change.

6. Postoperative or trauma patients may not tolerate certain positions or percussion or vibration because of pain.

7. Patients with copious secretions that cannot be coughed out should not be put in a compromising situation. Suctioning equipment must be available. This situation may include patients who are not alert or who have a tracheostomy.

8. Very obese patients may not tolerate any head-down positions because of increased shortness of breath.

3. Organize the sequence of drainage positions and treatment techniques (Code: IIIC5) [Difficulty: An]

There are differences of opinion as to the sequence in which the segments should be drained. Some authors state that an apices-to-bases approach is better, whereas others state that a bases-to-apices pattern is preferred. It makes sense to take an apices-to-bases approach for a first treatment when all lobes are to be drained. This pattern gives the patient time to get used to the whole procedure. It may also be safer because the practitioner can evaluate the patient through a sequence of positions that progresses from the least to the most stressful.

If the patient is known to tolerate all positions without any difficulties and the lower lobes are the worst in terms of secretions, choose to drain the lower lobes first. If time permits, work up through the middle lobe and lingular to the upper lobes.

4. Change the postural drainage therapy position based on the patient's response (Code: IIIC5) [Difficulty: An]

It may be found during the treatment that the patient's secretions are more effectively drained if he or she is repositioned in a position different than what would seem to be the ideal angle. It may be that the patient's airway anatomy is different than what is expected. Patients with chronic lung disease such as cystic fibrosis or bronchiectasis often know what positions and angles are best for draining their own lungs. Follow their advice if it produces good results.

Some patients may not tolerate being properly placed because their underlying lung or heart disease is aggravated by the unnatural body position. This is most commonly seen in the head-down positions used to drain the lower lobes. Watch for signs of hypoxemia and shortness of breath. The patient may have to be put in a better-tolerated but less-desirable position. As long as there is some downward angle to the bronchus, mucus will drain. Each patient must be evaluated on an individual basis.

5. Modify postural drainage therapy equipment: percussors and vibrators (Code: IIIC5) [Difficulty: An]

The terms *percussor* and *vibrator* are sometimes used interchangeably. There are several manufacturers who produce either electrically or pneumatically powered percussors and vibrators. Some are large enough to be wheeled into the patient's room. Obviously, electrically powered units need a standard electrical outlet for power and the pneumatically powered units need to be plugged into a 50-psi oxygen or air source.

Pediatric units must be smaller to accurately focus on the much smaller target area of the infant's chest. They are battery powered. Some practitioners find that an electric toothbrush with padded bristles works very well. Manual percussion of infants can be aided by using soft rubber palm cups that come in several pediatric sizes.

Some electrically powered units use a rubber belt and different-sized wheels to change gears and produce several vibration rates. Others electrically vary the motor speed to change the vibration rate. Some pneumatically driven units can have their percussion force and rate varied.

General Physiotherapy has recommended the following percussion rates for its models:

a. Less than 20 cycles per second for a large adult
b. Twenty to 30 cycles per second for an average adult
c. Greater than 30 cycles per second for small adults and children

It is important to remember that there is no consensus on the ideal percussion/vibration rate to use with any patient. It seems reasonable to use whatever rate is tolerated by the patient and results in the most effective mobilization of secretions.

Some adult percussors and vibrators come with a variety of patient contact pads. Select the one that best fits the patient's chest area that needs to be percussed. For example, a flat pad is used over a broad area of the patient's back whereas a U-shaped pad is used around the patient's side.

MODULE C	Positive expiratory pressure (PEP) therapy

📋 EXAM HINT

Expect one question on positive expiratory pressure (PEP) therapy. This may cover the equipment needed, indications for the procedure, or adjustment of PEP therapy settings.

Positive expiratory pressure (PEP) therapy involves having a spontaneously breathing patient exhale against a fixed-orifice resistor to create expiratory pressures between 10 and 20 cm water. It is also called PEP mask therapy because many pediatric patients use a face mask to deliver the pressure to the airways. Box 9-1 lists indications for its use. In patients with air trapping resulting from small airways disease, PEP therapy seems to act like pursed lips breathing to keep the small airways

BOX 9-1	Indications for Positive Expiratory Pressure Therapy

To reduce air trapping in patients with emphysema, bronchitis, and asthma

To prevent or reverse atelectasis

To help mobilize retained secretions in patients greater than 4 years old who have cystic fibrosis, chronic bronchitis, bronchiectasis, or bronchiolitis obliterans

To maximize the delivery of aerosolized medications, such as bronchodilators, in patients receiving bronchial hygiene therapy

BOX 9-2	Relative Contraindications to Positive Expiratory Pressure Therapy

Untreated pneumothorax

Intracranial pressure greater than 20 mm Hg

Active hemoptysis

Recent trauma or surgery to the skull, face, mouth, or esophagus

Patient with asthma attack or acute worsening of chronic obstructive pulmonary disease who cannot tolerate increased work of breathing

Acute sinusitis or epistaxis

Tympanic membrane rupture or other known or suspected middle ear pathology

Nausea

BOX 9-3	Hazards or Complications of Positive Expiratory Pressure Therapy

Pulmonary barotrauma

Increased intracranial pressure

Myocardial ischemia or decreased venous return to the heart

Increased work of breathing

Air swallowing that can lead to vomiting

Discomfort from mask or skin breakdown from the mask pressure

Claustrophobia

from collapsing. This allows the trapped alveolar gas to be more completely exhaled. Patients with atelectasis or who are at risk for developing atelectasis respond well to PEP therapy. It seems that PEP pushes air through the pores of Kohn of open alveoli into adjacent areas of atelectasis to force the alveoli open. The other indications are discussed next.

Box 9-2 lists relative contraindications to PEP therapy. There are no absolute contraindications. Box 9-3 lists hazards and complications of PEP therapy. These should be weighed against the benefits to the patient when making the recommendation to start PEP therapy. Other considerations include the patient's history of pulmonary disease that has responded to postural drainage therapy, ineffective cough to clear retained secretions, breath sounds indicating secretions, and chest radiograph findings of infiltrates.

1. **Positive expiratory pressure (PEP) therapy equipment**
   a. **Get the necessary PEP mask for the procedure (Code: IIA1k) [Difficulty: R, Ap, An]**

   The PEP mask should be transparent, flexible, and fit the patient's facial contours so that no air will leak out as

the pressure is increased. The following equipment is needed for PEP therapy as shown in Fig. 9-1:
   a. Appropriate size PEP mask or mouthpiece and nose clips, or universal airway (elbow) adapter for attachment to an endotracheal or tracheostomy tube
   b. Expiratory resistor
   c. Pressure manometer calibrated in cm water
   d. Small-bore oxygen tubing to connect the expiratory resistor to the pressure manometer
   e. Basin and tissues to collect and dispose of sputum
   f. Gloves, mask, goggles, and gown for the practitioner

The following *additional* equipment is needed to deliver an aerosolized medication as shown in Fig. 9-1:
   a. Small-volume nebulizer
   b. T-piece and female adapter to connect the nebulizer to the expiratory resistor
   c. Large-bore aerosol tubing to act as medication reservoir

   b. **Assemble, check for proper function, and identify any problems with the PEP mask (Code: IIB1k) [Difficulty: R, Ap, An]**

   As shown in Fig. 9-1, the component pieces must be properly put together. Make sure that all connections are airtight. If a leak is present, the desired PEP goal will not be reached or maintained. In addition, if an air leak is present it may be felt or a high-pitched sound may be heard. If a nebulizer is added for aerosolizing medications, ensure that it works properly. Connect the small-volume nebulizer into the system as shown. Add the medication and run a flow of oxygen or air at 4 to 6 L/min through the nebulizer (as is customary).

   c. **Alter the PEP therapy equipment (Code: IIIC5) [Difficulty: An]**

   Be prepared to adjust the expiratory resistance to meet the clinical goal of PEP therapy. The Resistex unit has four fixed orifice settings to choose from. The orifice diameters are 4 mm, 3.5 mm, 3 mm, and 2.5 mm interior diameter. The PEP mask made by Astra Meditec uses a series of differently sized pediatric endotracheal tube

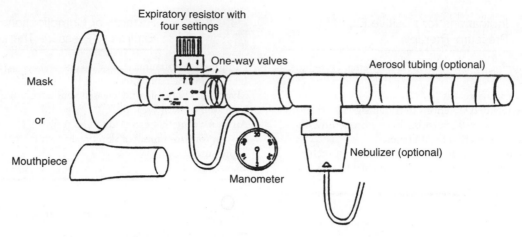

Fig. 9-1   Positive expiratory pressure (PEP) mask components. The basic PEP assembly requires a transparent mask or mouthpiece, expiratory resistor (this shows the Resistex), and pressure manometer with connecting oxygen tubing. If a nebulized medication is added, the following are also needed: small-volume nebulizer with T-piece, oxygen tubing to flowmeter, and large-bore tubing for an aerosol reservoir. (From Malmeister MJ, Fink JB, Hoffman GL et al: Positive-expiratory-pressure mask therapy: theoretical and practical considerations and a review of the literature, *Respir Care* 36(11):1218–1229, 1991.)

BOX 9-4	Steps in Performing Positive Expiratory Pressure (PEP) Therapy

1. Put the equipment together as shown in Fig. 9-1.
2. Have the conscious patient sit up straight, rest elbows on a table, and hold the PEP mask comfortably but tightly over the nose and mouth. The patient may use a mouthpiece and nose clips if preferred.
3. The patient should inhale a deeper-than-normal breath, but not to total lung capacity, by using the diaphragm. The unconscious patient will only inhale a tidal volume breath.
4. The conscious patient should exhale to functional residual capacity fast enough to generate 10-20 cm H_2O in the manometer. Have the patient look at the pressure manometer to judge how fast to exhale. The unconscious patient will exhale passively but still benefit by the increased baseline pressure.
5. The patient should have an expiratory time about three times longer than inspiratory time (an inspiratory:expiratory ratio of 1:2 to 1:4 is acceptable). This can be accomplished by changing the expiratory resistor and/or having the patient change the force of exhalation.
6. Between 10 and 20 proper PEP breaths should be performed.
7. The patient should now perform two or three "huff" type coughing efforts to raise secretions.
8. Repeat steps 2 to 7 between four and eight times (for about 10-20 min) for a full PEP treatment.

Patients in the intensive care unit can perform PEP therapy as often as every hour or as little as every 6 hr. They should be reevaluated for treatment effectiveness every 24 hr.

Patients in the acute-care or home-care settings can perform PEP therapy from two to four times/day. The acute-care patient should be reevaluated every 72 hr; the home-care patient can be evaluated at longer intervals or when a change in pulmonary status occurs.

adapters. They are fitted into an adapter through which the patient exhales. With either unit, the patient should be started out with the largest opening to breathe out through.

d. Fix the PEP mask equipment (Code: IIB2k) [Difficulty: R, Ap, An]

Any leaks in the system will prevent the PEP goal from being reached. Tighten any loose connections. If the one-way valves are put together backwards, the patient will inspire against a resistance instead of exhaling against it. Observe the one-way valves in use and ask the patient if he or she finds it easy to inhale but more difficult to exhale. Move the valves to their proper positions if incorrectly placed. If no mist is seen coming from the nebulizer, check the capillary tube or baffle for an obstruction; clear it by running tap water or a sterile needle through it. See Chapter 7 if necessary for more information on fixing problems with small-volume nebulizers.

2. Instruct and encourage the patient to perform PEP therapy (Code: IIIB3) [Difficulty: An]

The patient must be old enough to understand instructions and able to perform the procedure. Box 9-4 lists the steps in performing a proper PEP therapy treatment. PEP therapy has proven effective in helping patients with chronic, copious amounts of secretions. Primarily this includes children 4 years of age or older with cystic fibrosis. It also helps any patient with chronic bronchitis, bronchiectasis, or bronchiolitis obliterans. Clinical evidence indicates that the PEP dilates the small airways so that air is able to get past obstructing secretions. This fills the alveoli and, on expiration, tends to force the secretions into the larger airways for coughing or suctioning out.

PEP therapy seems also to increase the effectiveness of inhaled aerosolized bronchodilators. As shown in Fig. 9-1, the PEP system can be joined with a small-volume nebulizer. The slowed exhalation during PEP breathing should promote better deposition of medication in the small airways.

3. Alter the treatment duration and PEP therapy techniques as needed (Code: IIIC5) [Difficulty: An]

Be prepared to adjust the expiratory resistance to meet the clinical goal of PEP therapy. Initially, the pressure or resistance to exhalation should be kept low. As the training continues, the resistance or pressure the patient breathes against can be increased. The goals are to maintain a positive expiratory pressure of 10 to 20 cm water with an I:E ratio of about 1:3. If the pressure is too high or the expiratory time too long, the patient will likely become fatigued. If the orifice is too large, the pressure will not be high enough to be of any benefit. The patient will probably become tired if the total treatment time lasts longer than 20 minutes.

During the treatment, ask the patient if he or she feels dyspnea, pain, or chest discomfort. Also monitor the patient's breath sounds, blood pressure, heart rate, and breathing pattern rate. Monitor oxygenation by pulse oximetry, mental clarity, and skin color. Evaluate sputum for quantity, color, odor, and viscosity. Be prepared to stop the treatment if necessary.

4. Coordinate the sequence of therapies to modify bronchial hygiene (Code: IIIC5) [Question difficulty: An]

Coordinate PEP therapy with effective "huff" cough techniques, postural drainage therapy (PDT), and/or aerosolized medication delivery. As listed in Box 9-4, PEP breaths should be alternated with huff coughs to clear secretions. Huff coughs are not full, deep coughs; rather, they are performed as follows:

a. Have the patient inhale a slow, deep breath but not to total lung capacity.
b. Hold the breath in for 1 to 3 seconds.
c. Perform several quick, forced exhalations with an open epiglottis.
d. Small children may be taught to say "huff" with each quick exhalation. It may also help to have the young patient perform a "chicken breath" by flapping his or her arms against the sides of the chest during the exhalation.

PDT may be used before or after PEP therapy or it may be alternated with PEP therapy to help in the removal of secretions. Likewise, aerosolized medications may be inhaled before or simultaneously with PEP therapy.

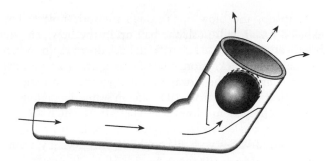

Fig. 9-2 Cross-section through a Flutter valve showing the flow of exhaled gas raising the steel ball. (From Scanlan CL, Wilkins RL, Stoller JK: *Egan's fundamentals of respiratory care,* ed 7, St Louis, 1999, Mosby.)

Bronchodilators and mucolytic agents should be very helpful with PEP therapy to mobilize secretions.

MODULE D   High-frequency airway oscillation

1. Flutter valve

a. Get the necessary equipment for the procedure (Code: IIA1l) [Difficulty: R, Ap]

The Flutter valve (Fig. 9-2) is a pipe-shaped device with a steel ball nesting loosely inside the bowl. The Flutter valve has been used with cystic fibrosis patients to help them loosen up their secretions. It is believed that the high-frequency oscillations of backpressure on the airway caused by the fluttering steel ball help to dislodge thick (viscous) secretions.

b. Put the equipment together, make sure it works properly, and identify any problems (Code: IIB1l) [Difficulty: R, Ap]

The Flutter valve comes preassembled by the manufacturer. There should be a perforated cap over the bowl to keep the ball from falling while letting exhaled air escape.

c. Fix any problems with the equipment (Code: IIB2l) [Difficulty: R, Ap]

The patient needs to keep the Flutter valve in the proper position with the perforated cap in the upright position. This keeps the patient's exhaled air blowing though the device to push up the steel ball. If a patient should cough secretions into the unit, it will become clogged. Air will not flow through it. Try clearing the obstruction with a cotton swab or by running warm water through the unit.

2. Instruct the patient in the use of the Flutter valve and encourage its use (Code: IIIB3) [Difficulty: An]

Because of its simplicity, small children as well as adults can be instructed in its use. The patient is taught to take a deeper than usual breath, hold the Flutter valve with the cap up, and blow out through the mouthpiece. The exhaled breath will push the ball up in the bowl, air will briefly escape, and the ball will fall back down again. When the ball falls back, more pressure is exerted against the patient's airway. The airway pressure generated during the exhalation will vary from 10 to 25 cm water depending on how fast the patient blows out. The rate at which the ball flutters up and down is about 15 Hz (hertz or cycles per second) and varies with the angle of the bowl. Typically, the patient repeats the maneuver for 10 to 20 breaths. The patient should then perform two or three huff-type coughs. The cycle of Flutter valve exhalations and huff coughs is repeated four to eight times. Total treatment time should not be longer than 20 minutes. If inhaled bronchodilator or mucolytic medications are ordered for the patient, they should be taken before the Flutter valve treatment.

3. Instruct the patient in the use of the intrapulmonary percussive ventilation device and encourage its use (Code: IIIB3) [Difficulty: An]

Intrapulmonary percussive ventilation (IPV) has been advocated for patients with diffuse patchy atelectasis or retained secretions. It has been used most widely and successfully with cystic fibrosis patients to help them mobilize secretions. It is believed that the high respiratory rate and airway pressures achieved with IPV help to dilate the airways so that any retained secretions are loosened. In addition, as the small airways are "splinted" open by continuous positive airway pressure (CPAP), air is pulsed past secretions so that they can be coughed out. Currently, the Percussionaire IPV-1 and IPV-2 are the only units that perform intrapulmonary percussive ventilation. See Fig. 9-3. They have several controls that enable the patient

and therapist to determine the inspiratory time, delivered pressure, rate of delivered breaths, and level of CPAP. Both IPV units also deliver nebulized medications. A source gas of 50 psi oxygen or air is needed to power the unit. The following are recommendations for initial IPV settings:

1. Begin therapy with a source pressure of 30 psi. The range is 20 to 50 psi.
2. Set a respiratory rate that is comfortable for the patient. The range is 100 to 225 percussive cycles/min (1.7 to 3.75 Hz).
3. If medication is ordered, place it into the reservoir and turn on the nebulizer.
4. CPAP may be left off initially. Up to 30 cm water are available.

The patient should be instructed to place the mouthpiece into his or her mouth and push the thumb button to deliver percussive breaths. The goal is to have the patient inhale the percussive breaths (with nebulized medication) for 5 to 10 seconds. This delivers breaths at the set rate and causes an increase in the baseline pressure (CPAP). When the thumb button is released, the percussive breaths stop and the patient can exhale. The patient can then repeat the process as often as desired. Between percussive breaths, the patient can continue to inhale the aerosolized medication through the small-volume nebulizer. The total IPV treatment time should not be longer than 20 minutes.

4. Instruct the patient in the use of the high-frequency chest wall oscillation (HFCWO) device and encourage its use (Code: IIIB3) [Difficulty: An]

Currently, the only available high-frequency chest wall oscillation (HFCWO) device is the ABI Vest (Fig. 9-4). It

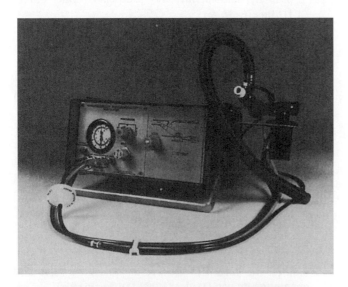

Fig. 9-3 The Percussionaire IPV-2 intrapulmonary percussive ventilator with air hoses and medication small-volume nebulizer with mouthpiece. (Courtesy Percussionaire, Sandpoint, ID.)

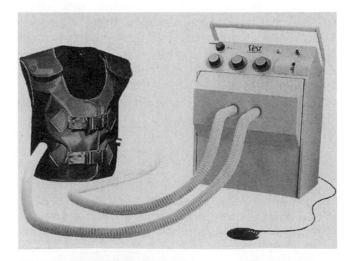

Fig. 9-4 The ABI Vest high-frequency chest wall oscillation device with its pumping and control unit, air hoses, inflatable vest, and foot control. (Courtesy American Biosystems, St. Paul, MN.)

consists of a nonstretchable inflatable vest that covers the entire torso and an electrically powered pumping and control system. The controls allow an adjustable air pulse rate between 5 Hz that produces a vest pressure of 28 mm Hg and 25 Hz, which produces a vest pressure of 39 mm Hg. HFCWO has been found to help cystic fibrosis patients mobilize retained secretions. It is believed that the pressure on the outside of the chest is transmitted internally to increase expiratory airflow and push secretions from small to larger airways.

The patient should be instructed to sit up during the treatment, put on the inflatable vest, and connect the two air hoses between the vest and the pump outlets. Currently, the recommendation is to have the patient set whatever oscillation rate results in the greatest production of secretions. Common sense indicates that it is appropriate to start at the lowest rate and pressure and progress to a faster rate and higher pressure as the patient tolerates. Treatments typically last 30 minutes and can be repeated up to six times per day. This procedure cannot be used in a patient with a chest wall injury such as broken ribs.

| MODULE E | Instruct the patient in autogenic drainage and encourage its use (Code: IIIB3) [Difficulty: An] |

Autogenic drainage (AD) is a form of directed lung expansion and coughing technique that can be taught to most cystic fibrosis children who are at least 4 years old. (The various coughing techniques for patients with an acute secretion problem or COPD were covered earlier.) With AD, the patient is taught the following:
1. Sit up straight.
2. Phase 1 breathing starts with a large inspiratory capacity breath followed by a series of shallow breaths. This is supposed to unstick peripheral secretions. There should be no coughing.
3. Phase 2 breathing involves larger than tidal volume breaths. This is to help collect mucus in the medium-size airways. There should be no coughing.
4. Phase 3 breathing involves progressively larger tidal volumes approaching the inspiratory capacity. This should move the mucus into the larger airways.
5. A series of huff-type coughs are now performed to remove the secretions.

| MODULE F | Respiratory care plan |

1. Participate in the development of the respiratory care plan [e.g., case management, development and application of protocols, disease management education] (Code: IC4) [Difficulty: An]

The procedures discussed earlier are primarily used with cystic fibrosis or chronic bronchitis patients. All have been shown to help in the mobilization of secretions. However, each patient may find that one procedure works better than another. Be prepared to make recommendations to change the type of procedure as well as how each procedure is conducted. In addition, other respiratory care procedures such as oxygen therapy and inhaled bronchodilators and mucolytic medications may have to be modified as the patient's condition warrants.

Make a recommendation for a chest radiograph to find specific areas for postural drainage therapy. A white shadow on a chest radiograph over what should be normal lung may indicate areas of atelectasis or infiltrates that can be targeted for treatment. Repeat chest radiographs should be performed to look for an improvement in the lungs. The resolution may be either slow or dramatic, depending on the original problem and how it responds to the various treatments used on it.

The American Association for Respiratory Care (AARC) Clinical Practice Guideline recommends that the following be evaluated to determine if postural drainage therapy (PDT) is needed:
1. Postural drainage therapy is usually not indicated if an optimally hydrated patient is coughing out less than 25 mL/day with the procedure.
2. A dehydrated patient should have apparently ineffective PDT continued for at least 24 hours after the patient is rehydrated. The combination of rehydration and PDT may help mobilize previously viscous secretions.
3. PDT is not indicated in a patient who is producing greater than 30 mL of secretions per day if the treatments do not increase the sputum production. This is because the patient is already able to cough out the sputum effectively.

PEP therapy has been indicated in patients who have retained secretions that are difficult to cough out. Raise or lower the PEP level to help the patient without causing fatigue or complications. If PEP therapy does not increase the amount of sputum produced per day in a patient who already produces more than 30 mL, PEP may not be needed. It does not make sense to continue an ineffective treatment.

2. Note the patient's response to therapy (Code: IIIA1c) [Difficulty: An]

Ask the patient how he or she feels before, during, and after the treatment. For any of the preceding procedures, be prepared to measure the patient's blood pressure, heart rate, and respiratory rate before, during, and after a change in therapy. Minor changes (<20%) can be expected. The patient's breath sounds should be auscultated before the treatment begins to determine which segments are normal or have secretions. Auscultate each segment after the treatment and the patient has coughed. Listen for air moving into formerly silent areas or areas that are cleared of secretions. The patient's oxygenation should improve as secretions and mucous plugs are removed and atelectatic areas open up.

Postural drainage therapy should not be performed for at least 1 hour after a patient has eaten. This is to help minimize the chances of nausea and vomiting from the head-down positions.

3. Observe the patient for changes in sputum production and consistency (Code: IIIA1c) [Difficulty: An]

See the preceding discussion. All of these procedures should increase the patient's production of secretions if they are present.

BIBLIOGRAPHY

AARC clinical practice guideline: Directed cough, *Respir Care* 38(5):495-499, 1993.

AARC clinical practice guideline: Use of positive airway pressure adjuncts to bronchial hygiene therapy, *Respir Care* 38(5):516-521, 1993.

AARC clinical practice guideline: Postural drainage therapy, *Respir Care* 36:1418-1426, 1991.

Branson RD, Hess DR, Chatburn RL: *Respiratory care equipment*, ed 2, Philadelphia, 1999, Lippincott Williams & Wilkins.

Campbell TC, Ferguson N, McKinlay RGC: The use of a simple self-administered method of positive expiratory pressure (PEP) in chest physiotherapy after abdominal surgery, *Physiotherapy* 72(10):498-500, 1986.

Eid N, Buchheit J, Neuling M et al: Chest physiotherapy in review, *Respir Care* 36(4):270-282, April 1991.

Eubanks DH, Bone RC: Comprehensive respiratory care, ed 2, St Louis, 1990, Mosby.

Fink JB: Volume expansion therapy. In: Burton GC, Hodgkin JE, Ward JJ, editors: *Respiratory care: a guide to clinical practice*, ed 4, Philadelphia, 1997, Lippincott-Raven.

Fink JB: Bronchial hygiene therapy and lung expansion. In: Fink JB, Hunt GE, editors: *Clinical practice in respiratory care*, Philadelphia, 1999, Lippincott-Raven.

Frownfelter DL: Chest physical therapy and airway care. In Barnes TA, editor: *Core textbook of respiratory care practice*, ed 2, St Louis, 1994, Mosby.

Hess DR, Branson RD: Chest physiotherapy, incentive spirometry, intermittent positive-pressure breathing, secretion clearance, and inspiratory muscle training. In Branson RD, Hess DR, Chatburn RL, editors: *Respiratory care equipment*, ed 2, Philadelphia, 1999, Lippincott Williams & Wilkins.

Hill KV: Bronchial hygiene therapy. In Aloan CA, Hill TV, editors: *Respiratory care of the newborn and child*, ed 2, Philadelphia, 1997, Lippincott-Raven.

Hoffman GL, Cohen NH: Positive expiratory pressure therapy, *NBRC Horizons* 19(2):1-7, 1993.

Johnson NT, Pierson DJ: The spectrum of pulmonary atelectasis: pathophysiology, diagnosis, and therapy, *Respir Care* 31(11):1107-1120, 1986.

Malmeister MJ, Fink JB, Hoffman GL et al: Positive-expiratory-pressure mask therapy: theoretical and practical considerations and a review of the literature, *Respir Care* 36(11):1218-1229, 1991.

Oberwaldner PT, Johannes CE, Zach MS: Forced expirations against a variable resistance: a new chest physiotherapy method in cystic fibrosis, *Pediat Pulmonol* 2(6):358-367, 1986.

Scanlan C, Myslinski MJ: Bronchial hygiene therapy. In Scanlan CL, Wilkins RL, Stoller JK, editors: *Egan's fundamentals of respiratory care*, ed 7, St Louis, 1999, Mosby.

Scott AA, Koff PB, Airway care and chest physiotherapy. In Koff PB, Eitzman D, Neu J, editors: *Neonatal pediatric respiratory care*, ed 2, St Louis, 1993, Mosby.

Shapiro BA, Kacmarek RM, Cane RD et al, editors: *Clinical application of respiratory care*, ed 4, St Louis, 1991, Mosby.

Sobush DC, Hilling L, Southorn PA: Bronchial hygiene therapy. In Burton GC, Hodgkin JE, Ward JJ, editors: *Respiratory care: a guide to clinical practice*, ed 4, Philadelphia, 1997, Lippincott-Raven.

White GC: *Equipment theory for respiratory care*, ed 3, Albany, NY, 1999, Delmar.

Wojciechowski WV: Incentive spirometers, secretion evacuation devices, and inspiratory muscle training devices. In Barnes TA, editor: *Core textbook of respiratory care practice*, ed 2, St Louis, 1994, Mosby.

SELF-STUDY QUESTIONS

1. A patient who is being instructed in positive expiratory pressure (PEP) therapy complains that it is taking too long to breathe out. What would you do?
   A. Tell the patient to blow out harder.
   B. Change the expiratory resistance to a larger-diameter orifice.
   C. Change the expiratory resistance to a smaller-diameter orifice.
   D. Increase the flow of oxygen to the system.

2. A 10-year-old cystic fibrosis patient has large amounts of secretions. He cannot tolerate postural drainage therapy because of nausea that results when he is tipped head down. Aerosolized bronchodilators and mucolytic agents are at optimal doses. What else could be recommended?
   A. Add heliox to the aerosolized medication delivery system.
   B. Intubate and begin mechanical ventilation.
   C. Add autogenic drainage.
   D. Add CPAP at 10 cm water.

3. A 56-year-old patient has been in the Trendelenburg position for 10 minutes receiving percussion and vibration. She develops tachycardia and dyspnea. Which of the following should the respiratory therapist do?
   A. Continue for 5 minutes with gentle percussion.
   B. Turn the patient to the other side.
   C. Give the patient oxygen.
   D. Have the patient sit up.

4. A 12-year-old patient with cystic fibrosis has had PEP therapy started at 5 cm water. After a few minutes of use the patient fails to cough productively. What should be done now?
   A. Increase the PEP level to 10 cm water.
   B. Increase the PEP level to 15 cm water.
   C. Change to incentive spirometry.
   D. Discontinue the treatment.

5. After several days of receiving postural drainage and percussion therapy to all lobes in the left lung, the patient's

chest radiograph shows improvement except for the left lower lobe. What position should he now be placed in for postural drainage?

- A. Right side down with the head of the bed down 30 degrees
- B. Right side down with the bed flat
- C. Left side down with the head of the bed down 30 degrees
- D. Flat on his back with the bed flat and a pillow beneath the knees

6. A physician has ordered PEP therapy with albuterol. All of the following are needed to start the treatment *except:*
   - A. Variable orifice resistor
   - B. Pressure manometer
   - C. Bedside spirometer
   - D. Nebulizer with reservoir

7. The patient benefits from using the Flutter valve by which of the following?
   - I. Increased transpleural pressure
   - II. Airway vibrations
   - III. Increased intrapleural pressure
   - IV. Rapid variation in airway pressure
   - A. I and II only
   - B. II and III only
   - C. III and IV only
   - D. II and IV only

8. A 48-year-old female has had her gall bladder removed. What is most effective in preventing postoperative atelectasis?
   - A. Blow bottles
   - B. PEP therapy
   - C. Mechanical chest percussor
   - D. Inspiratory muscle training

9. A patient is being started on high-frequency chest wall oscillation (HFCWO) to help mobilize secretions. Which of the following instructions should the patient be given for the initial treatment?
   - I. Lie on the side with the most secretions.
   - II. Sit up straight.
   - III. Set the controls at a low rate and pressure.
   - IV. Set the controls at a high rate and pressure.
   - V. Set the unit for maximum nebulization during inspiration.
   - A. II and III only
   - B. I and III only
   - C. II, IV, and V only
   - D. I, III, and V only

10. Intrapulmonary percussive ventilation (IPV) has been ordered for a patient with cystic fibrosis. Which of the following is true of the procedure?
    - I. The pressure will dilate the airways.
    - II. The high cycling rate will liquefy the secretions.
    - III. The negative pressure generated will pull secretions into the larger airways.
    - IV. The percussive breath should be taken for 5 to 10 seconds.
    - V. The CPAP level should be set at 15 cm water initially.
    - A. I and II only
    - B. III and IV only
    - C. I and IV only
    - D. III, IV, and V only

11. A patient is using the Flutter valve and coughs productively.

Later, the patient tries to use the device but finds that no air will go through it. What should be done?

- A. Have the patient breathe in harder.
- B. Check for an obstruction.
- C. Remove the steel ball to reduce the backpressure.
- D. Have the patient blow out harder.

12. A mechanical percussor is ordered to assist with secretion clearance in a patient receiving postural drainage therapy. The patient is positioned to drain the posterior basal segments of both lower lobes. The percussor is activated and applied to the patient's lower back. After a minute the patient complains of skin discomfort. What should the respiratory therapist do?

- A. Have the patient sit up.
- B. Apply oxygen and check the pulse oximeter value.
- C. Increase the speed on the percussor.
- D. Change to another type of pad on the percussor.

Answer Key

1. **B.** Rationale: By changing the expiratory resistance to a larger diameter orifice the patient will be able to exhale more quickly. See Fig. 9-1. Telling the patient to blow out harder will increase the pressure within the system. This could increase the patient's discomfort. Changing the expiratory resistance to a smaller diameter orifice will further increase the expiratory time not decrease it. Although a PEP system can have oxygen added to it to power the nebulizer, there is no mention of one in the question. In addition, the use of supplemental oxygen to a nebulizer does not have any effect on the expiratory time of the patient.

2. **C.** Rationale: A child of 10 can usually be taught autogenic drainage. This procedure enables the patient to inspire deeply and cough more effectively. Heliox has not been used in the routine management of patients with cystic fibrosis. It has been used in the short-term management of patients with a fixed large airway obstruction and in patients with status asthmaticus. The patient's condition is not serious enough to justify starting CPAP or intubation and mechanical ventilation. There is no mention of respiratory failure at this time.

3. **D.** Rationale: The patient should sit up because tachycardia and dyspnea are definite indications of intolerance of the head down position. It could be dangerous for the patient to continue in the head down position for even 5 more minutes. The treatment should be stopped and the patient should sit up rather than being turned to the other side. Give the patient supplemental oxygen only if needed after having the patient sit up and finding that he or she is hypoxic.

4. **A.** Rationale: It is reasonable to increase the PEP level from 5 to 10 cm water. Have the patient try this moderately increased pressure for several minutes and evaluate the effectiveness of the patient's cough effort. The PEP level should not be increased to 15 cm water unless 10 cm water has been shown to be ineffective. Incentive spirometry is indicated for atelectasis or the prevention of atelectasis. It is not indicated for secretion clearance as is PEP therapy. It is too early in the treatment to determine that PEP therapy should be discontinued.

5. **A.** Rationale: To drain the left lower lobe, the patient must be placed with the right side down on the bed and the head of the bed down 30 degrees. The other positions will not

properly drain the left lower lobe. Review the postural drainage positions if needed.

6. **C.** Rationale: A bedside spirometer is not needed because the patient's exhaled volume does not need to be measured. In addition, a spirometer cannot be connected to the unit for volume measurement. All of the other listed items are needed. The variable orifice resistor is needed to set the level of expiratory resistance. A pressure manometer is needed to determine that the expiratory pressure is kept in the 10 to 20 cm water range. A small volume nebulizer with reservoir is needed to deliver the albuterol.

7. **D.** Rationale: The Flutter valve is designed to cause rapid airway vibrations. These vibrations result in a rapid variation in airway pressure. This results in the airways rapidly dilating and then contracting to their resting diameter. These changes seem to loosen up secretions so that they can be coughed out more easily by the patient. Neither increased transpleural pressure or increased intrapleural pressure have any effect on the mobilization of secretions.

8. **B.** Rationale: PEP therapy will increase end expiratory lung pressure. This should increase alveolar volume and prevent the development of atelectasis. Blow bottles are no longer in use because they have been shown to not be effective in the management of atelectasis. A mechanical chest percussor can be used with postural drainage therapy to help mobilize secretions. However, it does not have any benefit in preventing atelectasis. Inspiratory muscle training is beneficial in patients with chronic obstructive lung disease because they are usually deconditioned. This should be part of a general conditioning program. However, inspiratory muscle training has no direct effect on atelectasis and should not be confused with use of an incentive spirometer.

9. **A.** Rationale: The patient must sit up straight because the vest is ridged. To work best it should have even contact with the patient's entire chest wall. This would not happen if the patient were lying on a side. It is best to have the patient start at the lowest rate and pressure to gain confidence in the unit and not risk injury. The HFCWO unit does not have a nebulizer.

10. **C.** Rationale: During IPV, the percussive breath should be taken for 5 to 10 seconds to dilate the airways. This dilation allows air to get past secretions so that a large breath is taken in and the secretions can be coughed out. Although the cycling rate during IPV is high, it will not liquify the secretions. IPV delivers positive pressure breaths, not negative pressure breaths. Initially the CPAP should be set at zero. A higher value may be set later if needed.

11. **B.** Rationale: It is likely that the patient coughed secretions into the unit. Check for an obstruction. If one is present, it must be cleaned out. A cotton swab or warm running water should clear out any secretions. The Flutter valve is designed to be blown out through, not breathed in through. It is not an incentive spirometer device. Removing the steel ball from the device will prevent it from working as intended. If the patient blows out hard the obstruction may be blown deeper into the unit.

12. **D.** Rationale: Try another type of pad on the percussor to determine if it is more comfortable for the patient. A flat one is probably be best for the lower back. The patient is not having a reaction to the head down position and does not need to sit up. There is no indication that the patient is hypoxic. Increasing the speed on the percussor is likely to increase the skin irritation.

A review of the most recent Written Registry Exams has shown an average of nine questions (9% of the exam) on cardiac monitoring and cardiopulmonary resuscitation.

MODULE A   Cardiac monitoring

1. Review the results of previous electrocardiogram tests from the patient's chart (Code: IA1g) [Difficulty: An]

A patient who has been admitted for a suspected myocardial infarction (MI) or other serious cardiac condition has probably had an electrocardiogram (ECG) performed. Review the interpretation report to find out if there is a cardiac problem. If the patient did have an MI, he or she will have had a series of ECGs performed to follow its progress and response to treatment.

2. Recommend an electrocardiogram for additional patient data (Code: IA2g) [Difficulty: An]

An ECG is indicated if the patient is suspected of having cardiac problems. Symptoms such as syncope, angina pectoris, sudden crushing chest pain, shortness of breath, or unstable heart rate and blood pressure point to a heart problem. An ECG is indicated to document the nature of the cardiac problem or rule out the heart as a source of the symptoms.

☞ EXAM HINT

There are usually one or two questions that require the respiratory therapist to recognize possible signs of a myocardial infarction and recommend either ECG monitoring or the performance of a diagnostic 12-lead ECG.

3. Recommend an echocardiogram for additional patient data (Code: IA2g) [Difficulty: An]

An echocardiogram is a noninvasive ultrasound procedure used to evaluate the structure and function of the heart. With it, high-frequency sound waves are sent through the chest wall to bounce off heart structures and give a visual image. General indications for the test include evaluation of heart wall motion (to look for decreased movement indicating a myocardial infarction or cardiomyopathy), evaluation of the heart valves (to look for defects), evaluation of the heart during stress testing (to look for decreased heart wall movement indicating decreased blood flow through a clogged coronary artery), and to identify pericardial fluid.

A transesophageal echocardiogram (TEE) makes use of a long, flexible ultrasonography probe that is placed into the distal esophagus or proximal stomach. A TEE has been shown to give better cardiac images in patients who are obese or who have chronic obstructive pulmonary disease (COPD). General indications for the test include the aforementioned indications, to differentiate between intracardiac and extracardiac masses and tumors, to diagnose a dissecting thoracic aneurysm, and to intraoperatively monitor patients at risk for myocardial ischemia (coronary artery bypass grafting, carotid artery procedures, and major thoracic or abdominal artery procedures). Patients with known esophageal abnormalities or recent esophageal surgery should not have a TEE performed.

4. Electrocardiography devices
a. Cardiac electrodes
1. Get the necessary equipment for the procedure (Code: IIA1p) [Difficulty: An]
2. Put the equipment together, make sure that it works properly, and identify any problems (Code: IIB1p) [Difficulty: An]
3. Fix any problems with the equipment (Code: IIB2p) [Difficulty: R, Ap, An]

Cardiac electrodes, or leads, pick up the electrical signal from a heart contraction and conduct it to the electrocardiogram machine. There are several different types of leads that are distinguished by their placement on the patient and how long they are used.

The first type of lead is used for a period of hours or days for basic rhythm monitoring or Holter monitoring. They are usually called *chest leads* (or *chest electrodes*) and consist of four parts: (1) a conducting wire coated with an electrically neutral plastic, (2) an adapter at one end of the wire that plugs into the ECG machine, (3) a different adapter at the opposite end of the wire that attaches to a patient electrode, and (4) the patient electrode (Fig. 10-1). Conducting jelly is added to the surface of the electrode to reduce the skin's resistance to the heart's electrical signal. An adhesive ring holds the electrode tightly to the skin. The conducting wire snaps or clips onto the back of the electrode. Typically, three of these chest leads are used for rhythm monitoring. Holter monitoring involves using chest leads and long-term precordial leads.

The second type of cardiac electrodes is often used for only a few minutes during a diagnostic electrocardiogram.

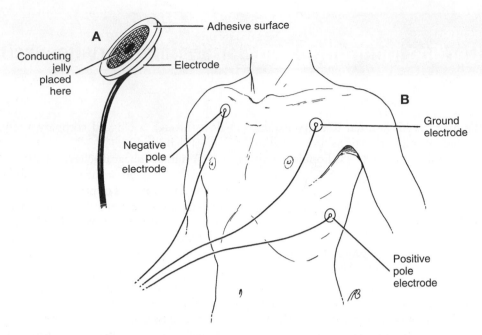

Fig. 10-1   A, Close-up of the features of a prepackaged monitoring electrode or lead. **B,** Standard electrode placements for lead II monitoring. This results in the traditional-looking ECG waveform with upright P, QRS, and T waves. (Note: The electrodes are often labeled as right arm (RA) instead of negative pole, left arm (LA) instead of ground electrode, and left leg (LL) instead of positive electrode.) (From Eubanks DH, Bone RC: *Comprehensive respiratory care,* ed 2, St Louis, 1990, Mosby.)

They come in two sets of electrodes for different placements. Limb leads come as a group of four with one for each limb (Fig. 10-2). Precordial leads came in a group of six and are placed on the chest in the positions shown in Fig. 10-3. Long-term precordial leads must be used for a Holter monitor. A conducting and adhesive jelly is used to reduce the skin's resistance and to hold the lead in place. The limb leads are longer and they may need to be held in place by a rubber strap. With all types of cardiac leads, bad skin contact, dried conducting jelly, or a disconnected wire results in a distorted or absent electrical signal.

b. **Electrocardiograph**

1. **Get the necessary equipment for the procedure (Code: IIA1p) [Difficulty: An]**
2. **Put the equipment together, make sure that it works properly, and identify any problems (Code: IIB1p) [Difficulty: An]**
3. **Fix any problems with the equipment (Code: IIB2p) [Difficulty: R, Ap, An]**

Twelve-lead ECG test for diagnostic purposes. A 12-lead ECG test requires a machine capable of receiving electrical input from the four limb leads and six precordial leads (see Figs. 10-2 and 10-3). The operator can manually select the combinations needed to get the 12 different combinations for a 12-lead ECG tracing or they can be done automati-

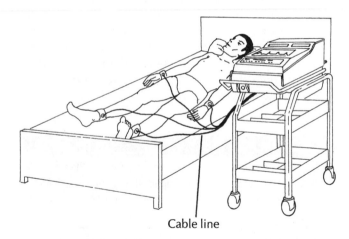

Cable line

Fig. 10-2   Limb electrodes or leads properly placed on all four of the patient's limbs. Make sure that the right leg lead is placed on the right leg, the right arm lead is placed on the right arm, and so forth. The electrode cables are then plugged into the electrocardiograph machine to record the ECG tracings. (From Eubanks DH, Bone RC: *Comprehensive respiratory care,* ed 2, St Louis, 1990, Mosby.)

cally. The various electrocardiogram combinations are printed out on ECG paper. Modern units also store the patient's information on a self-contained computer.

Basic bedside rhythm monitoring. A bedside rhythm monitoring unit usually receives input from only three or

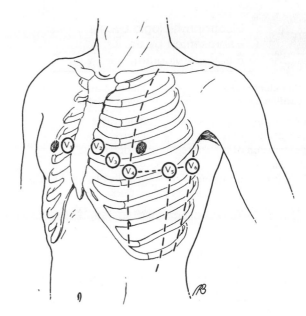

Fig. 10-3   Proper placement of the six precordial leads. (See Table 10-1 for a description of the locations.) (From Eubanks DH, Bone RC: *Comprehensive respiratory care,* ed 2, St Louis, 1990, Mosby.)

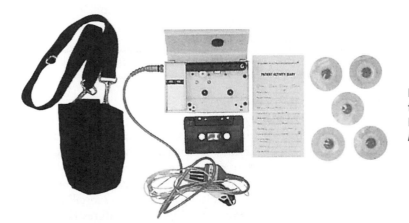

Fig. 10-4   Holter monitoring system for ambulatory electrocardiography. (From Pagana K, Pagana TJ: *Mosby's manual of diagnostic and laboratory tests,* St Louis, 1998, Mosby.)

four chest leads. That collective signal is sent to an oscilloscope (video display terminal) for a real-time display of the patient's rhythm. These ECG machines have several additional features. They continuously display the patient's heart rate. High and low heart rate alarm settings can be set. If the high or low setting is reached, an audible and visual alarm is triggered. The patient's heart rhythm can be recorded on ECG paper manually by pushing a record button or automatically when an alarm setting is reached. These units are often seen mounted at the patient's bedside in the intensive care unit.

Cardiopulmonary resuscitation cart. Cardiopulmonary resuscitation (CPR) "crash" carts have electrocardiographs and oscilloscopes mounted on them. These are connected to the defibrillator. This allows for synchronous defibrillation (cardioversion). Crash carts have other features that are similar to those seen on bedside rhythm monitoring units. Portable versions of these units are used when the patient must be transported. They operate by battery power when unplugged from the wall electrical outlet.

Holter monitoring. Holter monitoring involves recording a patient's complete ECG for 1 to 3 days through the use of a portable, battery-powered monitor. In addition, the patient keeps a diary of any episodes of chest pain, dyspnea, and so forth. The whole system includes the recording device, magnetic tape to record the patient's ECG, a set of chest leads (and precordial leads if needed), a carrying bag for the recording device, and a patient activity diary (see Fig. 10-4).

Successful ECG monitoring requires that the right electrodes be chosen, put together properly, attached to the patient as indicated, and connected to the correct ECG machine. Any errors will result in an electrical signal that is distorted or absent. Recheck all patient electrodes and wire connections if a problem is seen.

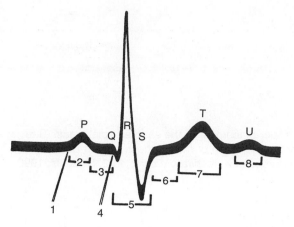

Fig. 10-5 Sequence of electrical events of the cardiac cycle during normal sinus rhythm. (See Table 10-2 for the description of each event.) (From Phillips RE, Feeney MK: *The cardiac rhythms: a systematic approach to interpretation,* ed 3, Philadelphia, 1990, WB Saunders.)

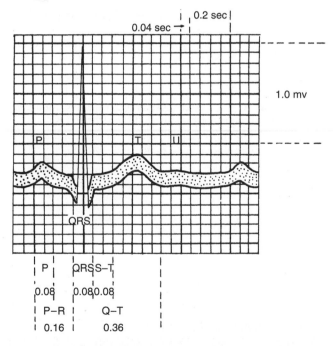

Fig. 10-6 Timing of the electrical events of the cardiac cycle during normal sinus rhythm. (From Spearman CB, Sheldon RL, Egan DF: *Egan's fundamentals of respiratory therapy,* ed 4, St Louis, 1982, Mosby.)

5. Begin electrocardiogram monitoring (Code: IB9a and IC1b) [Difficulty: An]

Holter monitoring is done to diagnose noncritical patients with a suspected cardiac problem. Because the patient will be mobile for at least 1 day, the limb leads are placed on the upper and lower chest area. Precordial leads are placed normally. The patient wears a tight-fitting undershirt or netlike dressing to keep the leads in place. The patient cannot bathe while the leads are on.

TABLE 10-1	Electrophysiologic Events Represented by the Electrocardiogram
Sequential electrical events of the cardiac cycle	**Electrocardiographic representation**
1. Impulse from the sinus node	Not visible
2. Depolarization of the atria	P wave
3. Depolarization of the atrioventricular node	Isoelectric
4. Depolarization of the atria	Usually obscured by the QRS complex
5. Depolarization of the ventricles	QRS complex
a. Intraventricular septum	a. Initial portion
b. Right and left ventricles	b. Central and terminal portions
6. Quiescent state of the ventricles immediately after depolarization	ST segment: isoelectric
7. Repolarization of the ventricles	T wave
8. Afterpotentials following repolarization of the ventricles	U wave

From Phillips RE, Feeney MK: *The cardiac rhythms: a systematic approach to interpretation,* ed 3, Philadelphia, 1990, WB Saunders.

Emergency electrocardiogram monitoring is done on any patient with a serious cardiopulmonary problem. If there is a possibility that the patient will experience serious changes in heart rate or rhythm, he or she should be continuously monitored. In this case, use bedside rhythm monitoring. This unit should have an oscilloscope for viewing the rhythm and additional features for counting the heart rate, setting high and low heart rate alarms, and recording the rhythm on standard ECG paper for a permanent record.

The most common chest electrode pattern used for rhythm monitoring is called *lead II*. The three chest electrodes are placed as shown in Fig. 10-1, *B*. The negative (right arm, RA) electrode is on the right upper chest. The positive (left leg, LL) electrode is placed on the left lateral chest. The ground (left arm, LA) electrode is placed on the left upper chest. With this electrode configuration, known as Einthoven's triangle, the heart's electrical signal is followed as it flows from the right atrium to the left ventricle. This results in the so-called normal ECG tracing with upright P, R, and T waves as shown in Figs. 10-5 and 10-6. Table 10-1 shows the sequential electrical events of the normal cardiac rhythm that corresponds with Fig. 10-5.

6. Perform an electrocardiogram (Code: IB9a and IC1b) [Difficulty: An]

To determine the patient's cardiac diagnosis, it is necessary to perform a 12-lead ECG. This test involves the

TABLE 10-2 Standard Electrocardiogram Leads

	Leads	Positive electrode		Negative electrode
Bipolar	1. I	Left arm	and	Right arm
	2. II	Left leg	and	Right arm
	3. III	Left leg	and	Left arm
Unipolar	4. aV_R	Right arm		
	5. aV_L	Left arm		Central terminal*
	6. aV_F	Left leg		
Precordial	7. V_1	Right of sternum in 4th intercostal space (4th ICS)		
	8. V_2	Left of sternum in 4th ICS		
	9. V_3	Midway between V_2 and V_4		Central terminal*
	10. V_4	Midclavicular line in 5th ICS		
	11. V_5	Midway between V_4 and V_6		
	12. V_6	Lateral chest in 5th ICS		

aV, Augmented voltage; *ICS*, intercostal space.

*The *central terminal* is a combination of electrode potentials, producing a summation effect. This serves as the single negative or *indifferent* electrode. The specific combination of electrodes for each lead is automatically determined in the lead selector switch. (From Phillips RE, Feeney MK: *The cardiac rhythms: a systematic approach to interpretation,* ed 3, Philadelphia, 1990, WB Saunders.)

use of an electrocardiograph machine with heat-sensitive ECG recording paper, four limb leads, and six precordial leads (see Figs. 10-2 and 10-3). Table 10-2 describes the locations of the precordial leads and the positive and negative electrode combinations that are used to record the heart's electrical signal through the 12 different leads. Each lead individually records the heart's electrical activity, but does so from a different position in relation to the heart. These 12 leads give the physician a three-dimensional impression of how the cardiac conduction system and the myocardium are functioning. Abnormal functioning can be diagnosed. Review the normal anatomy and physiology of the heart and its conduction system if necessary.

Clinical experience is important in performing a diagnostic ECG. Improper placement of the precordial or limb leads can easily result in a misleading ECG tracing and a misdiagnosis. For example, reversing the arm leads causes the QRS to be reversed in lead I. Technical errors in grounding the patient and not keeping the patient still during the ECG also result in useless tracings because of electrical interference and an unstable baseline.

7. Interpret the results of the electrocardiogram (Code: IC2b and IB10a) [Difficulty: An]

Before discussing ECG interpretation, it is important to understand how ECG paper is designed so that the heart's electrical signal traced on it can be understood. This special paper is heat sensitive and, after exiting the ECG machine, shows a black line from the heated stylus. Fig. 10-7 shows the grid markings on the paper and how to interpret the ECG tracing for voltage and time. Each large square box is 5 mm in height and represents 0.5 millivolts (mV) of the heart's electrical force. The large square box is divided into five smaller boxes that are 1 mm in height and

represent 0.1 mV. Timing of the ECG tracing is determined by the speed with which the paper passes under the heated stylus. Normally, this is 25 mm per second. At this speed, each large square box is .20 seconds, and each of the five small boxes is .04 seconds. There are 300 large boxes in 1 minute's time (.20 seconds × 300 = 60 seconds).

The following 10 features should be examined in every electrocardiogram:

1. Heart rate
2. Rhythm
3. P wave
4. PR interval
5. QRS interval
6. QRS complex
7. ST segment
8. T wave
9. QT interval
10. U wave

The systematic evaluation of these factors usually results in a clear understanding of the patient's cardiac function. All of these factors are discussed and illustrated in this chapter.

The *heart rate* can be most accurately found by counting it for 1 minute; however, this time-consuming method is not always practical. An approximate heart rate can be quickly found. First, find a heartbeat tracing in which the R wave is on a heavy vertical line. Then count the number of large boxes between this first R wave and the next R wave (see Fig. 10-8 for an example). Approximate heart rates can be estimated as follows:

Two large boxes = 150 beats per minute (300 divided by 2)

Three large boxes = 100 beats per minute (300 divided by 3)

Four large boxes= 75 beats per minute (300 divided by 4)

Five large boxes = 60 beats per minute (300 divided by 5)

Six large boxes = 50 beats per minute (300 divided by 6)

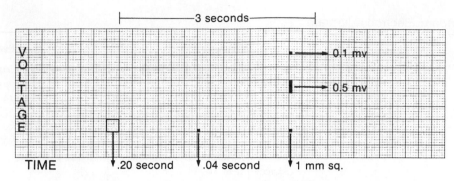

Fig. 10-7 ECG paper with added details on how to interpret time and voltage. (From Patel JM, McGowan SG, Moody LA: *Arrhythmias: detection, treatment, and cardiac drugs,* Philadelphia, 1989, WB Saunders.)

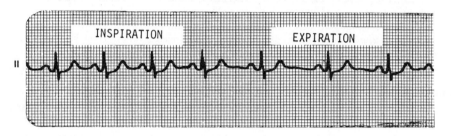

Fig. 10-8 Sinus arrhythmia showing slightly increased heart rate during inspiration and slightly decreased heart rate during exhalation. (From Goldberger AL: *Clinical electrocardiography: a simplified approach,* ed 6, St Louis, 1999, Mosby.)

Obviously, the normal cardiac rhythm must be understood to distinguish it from the abnormal rhythms. The normal adult's cardiac rhythm is usually called *normal sinus rhythm* (NSR) and has these characteristics:

a. Heart rate between 60 and 100 beats per minute while at rest.

b. Rhythm that varies by no more than ±10% between QRS complexes.

c. P wave before every QRS complex and upright in lead II.

d. A QRS complex follows every P wave.

e. Proper timing of the components of the ECG rhythm. 10-2.

Fig. 10-6 shows the normal timing of the components of the ECG tracing.

a. Abnormal cardiac rhythms

The following list of abnormal cardiac rhythms (usually called arrhythmias or dysrhythmias) includes many of those that are commonly encountered in clinical practice. It is beyond the scope of this text to discuss all possible arrhythmias. Instead, those that are either frequently seen and/or dangerous are described. Each of the following cardiac irregularities is: (a) defined, (b) exemplified, (c) described, (d) discussed in terms of its clinical

significance, and (e) accompanied by a treatment (if any) description.

1. Arrhythmias with a sinoatrial node origin

The following three arrhythmias all originate from the sinoatrial (SA) node. The electrical signal follows the normal pathway and results in contraction of both atria and ventricles, as expected. They are distinguished from normal sinus rhythm by the differences in rate and regularity of the impulses.

Sinus arrhythmia. This arrhythmia is characterized by normal complexes, but is a heart rate that varies with the respiratory cycle (see Fig. 10-8 for an example). Notice how the QRS complexes are closer together on inspiration than on expiration. This is because the increased venous return to the heart during inspiration causes the heart to fill more quickly so that the pulse rate quickens. The opposite rhythm effect is sometimes seen with a patient on a mechanical ventilator. No cardiac treatment is needed. The mechanically ventilated patient should have every attempt made to lower the intrathoracic pressure.

Sinus tachycardia. Sinus tachycardia in the adult is defined as a heart rate of more than 100 beats per minute while at rest. All complexes are normal, and the rate is

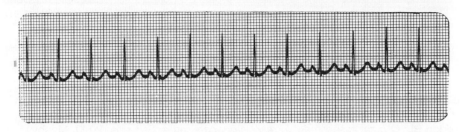

Fig. 10-9   Sinus tachycardia. (From Goldberger AL: *Clinical electrocardiography: a simplified approach,* ed 6, St Louis, 1999, Mosby.)

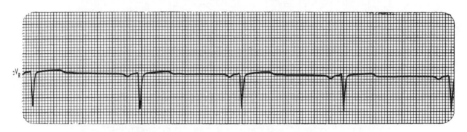

Fig. 10-10   Sinus bradycardia. (From Goldberger AL: *Clinical electrocardiography: a simplified approach,* ed 6, St Louis, 1999, Mosby.)

seldom more than 140 (see Fig. 10-9 for an example). Causes include caffeine, anxiety, fever, pain, or hypotension. Correction of the problem results in the heart rate decreasing to the normal range. Cardiac drugs are not needed.

Sinus bradycardia. Sinus bradycardia is defined as a heart rate of less than 60 beats per minute while at rest (see Fig. 10-10). All complexes remain normal. This is commonly seen in well-trained athletes during rest and in patients receiving digitalis or morphine. Cardiac drugs are not needed.

If sinus bradycardia is associated with a myocardial infarct, it may result in fainting or congestive heart failure (pulmonary edema). The patient must be treated not only for the heart attack but also to increase the heart rate. Atropine with or without isoproterenol (Isuprel) is commonly used to speed up the heart rate. A pacemaker is needed if the patient does not respond to medications and continues to have symptoms.

2. Arrhythmias with an abnormal atrial origin

The following three arrhythmias originate in either one or both atria from a source other than the SA node. The electrical signal travels through the atria, which results in their contraction. It then moves on to the atrioventricular (AV) node and the ventricles, which contract normally. All of these arrhythmias result in faster than normal atrial

contraction and often in a faster than normal ventricular contraction.

Paroxysmal atrial tachycardia. Paroxysmal atrial tachycardia (PAT) (also known as paroxysmal supraventricular tachycardia [PSVT]) is a series of three or more premature atrial contractions. It is characterized by a heart rate between 140 and 250 beats per minute with an average rate of 180. The ECG tracing will show a normal QRS complex after each P wave. See Fig. 10-11. Notice the abnormal origin of the P wave seen during the PAT episode. The recommended term for any abnormal origin to a heartbeat is *focus.* The term *foci* refers to more than one abnormal site to a heartbeat.

Patients with long runs of PAT usually complain of a sudden onset of pounding or fluttering in the chest. This is often associated with breathlessness, weakness, and angina pectoris in patients with coronary artery disease. Because of these problems, long runs of PAT must be treated. Treatment usually progresses in the following sequence: (1) give a sedative, (2) stimulate the vagus nerve by rubbing the carotid sinus (see Fig. 10-12), (3) give propranolol (Inderal) or a similar medication, and (4) perform synchronized cardioversion. (This last procedure is described in Chapter 17.) Obviously, if the patient responds to one treatment method there is no need to go on to the next.

Atrial flutter. Atrial flutter is characterized by a single, fast, abnormal atrial focus that fires at a rate of about 250 to

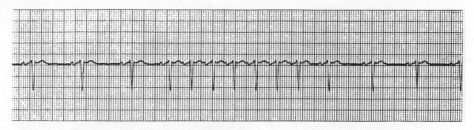

Fig. 10-11 A short run of paroxysmal trial tachycardia (PAT). Although a short run is probably not dangerous, a long run should be treated. (From Wilkins RL, Krider SJ, Sheldon RL: *Clinical assessment in respiratory care,* ed 4. St Louis, 2000, Mosby.)

ATRIAL FLUTTER

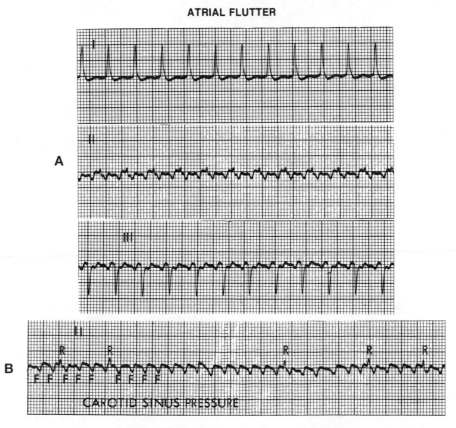

Fig. 10-12 Two examples of atrial flutter. **A,** Note the variable appearance of the flutter waves in different leads. This example shows a 2:1 ratio between atrial contractions and ventricular contractions. **B,** This shows how the ventricular rate is decreased after carotid sinus pressure is applied. The "F" letterings show flutter waves from a single focus. The "R" letterings mark R waves when the electrical signal traveled through the AV node to stimulate the ventricles. (From Goldberger AL: *Clinical electrocardiography: a simplified approach,* ed 6, St Louis, 1999, Mosby.)

350 beats per minute. This rate is so fast that the AV node does not pass all of them along to the ventricles. On an ECG, a ratio between the fast flutter waves and the QRS complex is seen. Usually this ratio is 2:1, but it may be 3:1, 4:1, or more. (See Fig. 10-12 for several example ECG tracings of atrial flutter.) As with PAT, the fast ventricular rate found in atrial flutter is not well tolerated. An attempt must be made to suppress the abnormally fast atrial focus.

Carotic sinus pressure, digoxin (Lanoxin), or synchronized cardioversion are the preferred treatments to slow down the heart rate.

Atrial fibrillation. This condition is identified by the variably shaped fibrillation waves and the irregular spacings between the QRS complexes. Each focus is seen on the ECG as a separately shaped wave. As with atrial flutter, the AV node does not pass the electrical current from each

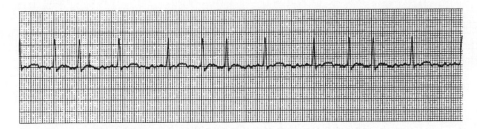

Fig. 10-13 Atrial fibrillation. Note the variable shapes to the fibrillation waves indicating their different origins. Also note how the distances between the R waves change considerably. This depends on when an electrical signal from the atria passes through the AV node to the ventricles. (From Wilkins RL, Krider SJ, Sheldon RL: *Clinical assessment in respiratory care,* ed 4, St Louis, 2000, Mosby.)

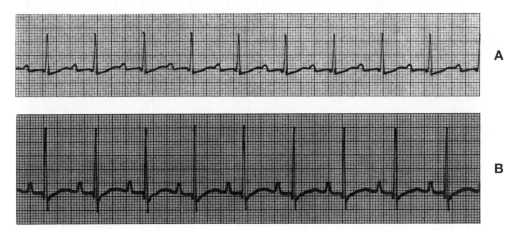

Fig. 10-14 First-degree AV block results in a PR interval that is longer than the normal interval of five small blocks or .20 seconds. ECG strip **A** shows a PR interval of 0.30 seconds. ECG strip **B** shows a PR interval of 0.24 seconds. (From Wilkins RL, Krider SJ, Sheldon RL: *Clinical assessment in respiratory care,* ed 4, St Louis, 2000, Mosby.)

fibrillation wave through to the ventricles. However, with atrial fibrillation, the ratio is not set, and there is variable spacing between the QRS complexes and an inconsistent rate (see Fig. 10-13). Patients with atrial fibrillation do not completely empty their ventricles. Often, this results in the formation of blood clots that become pulmonary or cerebral emboli. Digitalis and synchronized cardioversion usually are effective treatments. Heparin or coumadin may be added to prolong the blood's clotting time.

3. Arrhythmias with an atrioventricular node origin

Both of the following arrhythmias originate in an abnormal atrioventricular (AV) node. The patient may or may not have a normal SA node, atria, and ventricles.

Atrioventricular (AV) block. AV block is most commonly caused by digitalis toxicity, arteriosclerosis, or myocardial infarction. The latter two may result in scarring, inflammation, or edema. These causes slow down or prevent the transmission of the electrical signal from the SA node through the AV node and to the ventricles. *First-degree* AV block is seen with an increased PR interval of at least .20

seconds. Each P wave is followed by a normal QRS complex (see Fig. 10-14). It does not require any treatment. *Second-degree* AV block results in some P waves being blocked out completely with no ventricular response. This more serious condition comes in two different variations. Wenckebach (also known as Mobitz type I) is characterized by a progressively longer PR interval until a P wave is not conducted through at all. Then the cycle starts over again and continues to repeat itself. (See Fig. 10-15 for examples.) Medications such as atropine or isoproterenol may be used to increase the heart rate. Mobitz type II is seen on the ECG as a rhythm in which the PR interval is normal for those that result in a QRS complex, but some P waves are completely blocked (see Fig. 10-16). The ratio between those P waves that conduct and those that are blocked off may be 2:1, 3:1, or 4:1. Mobitz type II is a sign of severe conduction system disease. The usual treatment is to place a cardiac pacemaker into the patient. *Third-degree* AV block is also known as complete heart block (see Fig. 10-17). No P waves are conducted through to the ventricles. The ventricles beat about 40 times per minute based on the

WENCKEBACH (MOBITZ TYPE I) SECOND-DEGREE AV BLOCK

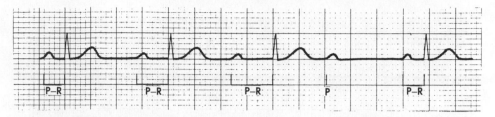

P–R   P–R   P–R   P   P–R

WENCKEBACH (MOBITZ TYPE I) SECOND-DEGREE AV BLOCK

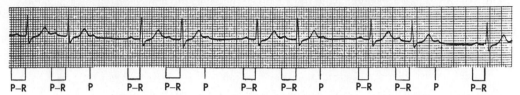

P–R   P–R   P   P–R   P–R   P   P–R   P–R   P   P–R   P–R   P   P–R

Fig. 10-15 Two examples of Wenckebach (Mobitz type I) second-degree AV block. Note how the PR interval progressively lengthens with each beat until one P wave is not conducted through at all. The cycle then repeats itself. (From Goldberger AL: *Clinical electrocardiography: a simplified approach,* ed 6, St Louis, 1999, Mosby.)

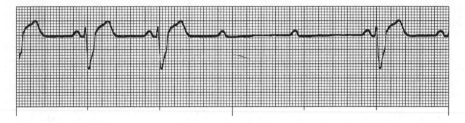

Fig. 10-16 Mobitz type II second-degree heart block. Note how some P waves are conducted through the AV node with a resulting QRS complex and other P waves are not conducted. (From Aehlert B: *ECG's made easy,* St Louis, 1995, Mosby.)

THIRD-DEGREE (COMPLETE) AV BLOCK

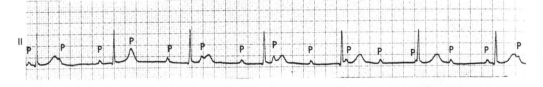

THIRD-DEGREE (COMPLETE) AV BLOCK

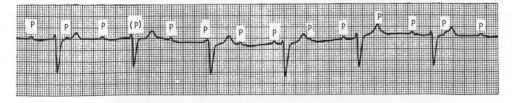

Fig. 10-17 Two examples of third-degree (complete) heart block. Both show P waves that have no relationship with the QRS complexes. The top example has QRS complexes of the normal width indicating that the AV junction is acting as the pacemaker. The bottom example has QRS complexes that are wider than normal because the ventricles are being paced from below the AV junction. Instead, an idioventricular pacemaker is determining the patient's heart rate. (From Goldberger AL: *Clinical electrocardiography: a simplified approach,* ed 6, St Louis, 1999, Mosby.)

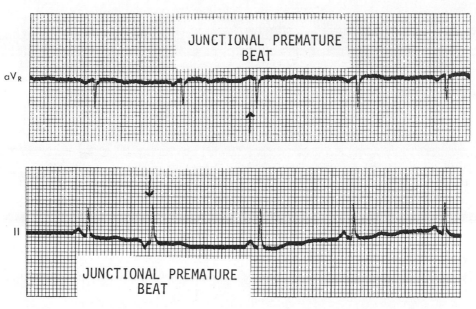

Fig. 10-18 Two ECG tracings of junctional premature beats. They are from the same patient but from different leads. The arrows point out retrograde P waves of opposite polarity from normal. (From Goldberger AL, Goldberger E: *Clinical electrocardiography,* St Louis, 1981, Mosby.)

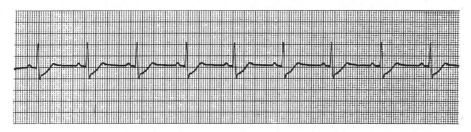

Fig. 10-19 An ECG tracing showing ST segment depression. This is usually caused by myocardial hypoxia and can lead to a myocardial infarction if not promptly treated. (From Wilkins RL, Krider SJ, Sheldon RL: *Clinical assessment in respiratory care,* ed 4, St Louis, 2000, Mosby.)

intrinsic rate of the bundle of His and Purkinje fibers. Obviously, a heartbeat this slow is not normal or healthy. Patients have no stamina and frequently faint. A cardiac pacemaker must be placed into these patients.

Junctional premature beats. A junctional premature beat is also known as a premature AV nodal contraction (PNC), nodal beat, or junctional beat (see Fig. 10-18). This arrythmia involves the atrioventricular node sending out a premature electrical signal and becoming the primary pacemaker instead of the SA node. The ventricles contract normally with the expected QRS complex.

4. Arryhthmias with a ventricular origin

Myocardial infarction. A myocardial infarction (MI) or acute myocardial infarction (AMI), commonly known as a heart attack, is an occlusion of a coronary artery that results in the death of some segment of the heart muscle. Often, the patient with partial or complete coronary artery occlusion has symptoms of shortness of breath, central chest pain, pain that radiates down the left arm or up the left side of the neck, or a feeling of stomach upset. If an ECG is performed, it may show ST segment depression as a sign of myocardial hypoxia (Fig. 10-19). If the patient is properly treated, an MI may be prevented by opening the blocked artery.

Often, however, the patient comes to the hospital too late, and an MI with heart damage is present. If the damaged area is large enough, the heart fails to pump adequately and the patient dies. A smaller infarct weakens the heart. In addition, the damaged or dying tissue acts as an abnormal focus for the arrhythmias discussed next. The series of ECG changes that occurs during the acute stage of an MI and as the heart heals are shown in Fig. 10-20 and are listed here:

1. The initial ECG may be normal. This happens about 15% of the time. The patient should be

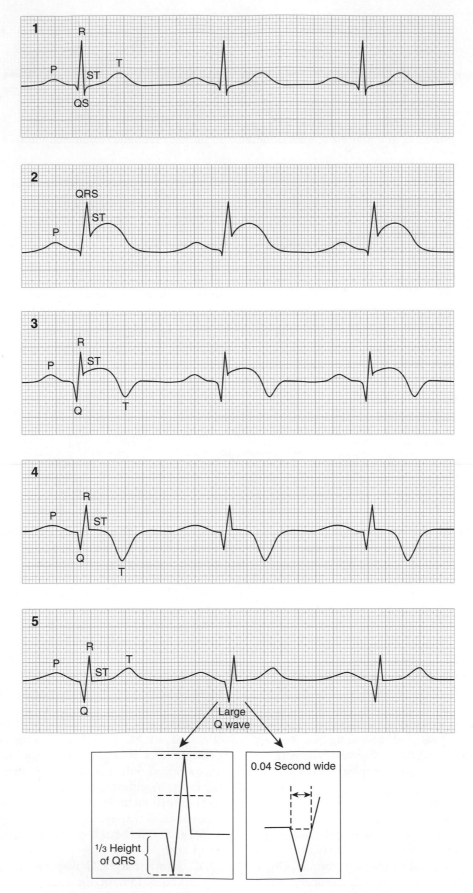

Fig. 10-20 The sequence of ECG rhythms commonly seen following a myocardial infarction. See the text for a description of each step in the sequence.

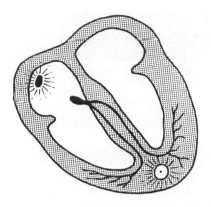

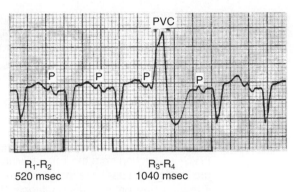

R_1-R_2
520 msec

R_3-R_4
1040 msec

Fig. 10-22   PVCs cause a fully compensatory pause. Note that the interval between the two sinus beats that surround the PVC (R3 and R4 in this case) is exactly two times the normal interval between the sinus beats R1 and R2. Notice that the P waves come on time, except that the third P wave is interrupted by the PVC and therefore does not conduct normally through the AV junction. The next (fourth) P wave also comes on time. The fact that the sinus node continues to pace despite the PVC results in the fully compensatory pause. (From Goldberger AL: *Clinical electrocardiography: a simplified approach,* ed 6, St Louis, 1999, Mosby.)

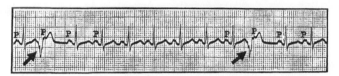

Fig. 10-21   Premature ventricular contraction *(arrows)* is detected when an impulse is propagated from a ventricular focus before the next normal beat is due. The QRS complex is commonly widened and not preceded by a P wave. A longer than usual (compensatory) pause follows. Retrograde activation of the atria may occur following a premature contraction, or the normal sinus P waves may continue. The sinus P waves following the PVC are blocked by conduction system refractoriness. (From Stein E: *Clinical electrocardiography: a self-study course,* Philadelphia, 1987, Lea & Febiger.)

admitted for observation and cardiac enzyme studies if symptoms are present.

2. The first sign of an MI is an elevated ST segment. This occurs within a few hours of the injury.
3. Next the T wave inverts. This happens within hours to days of the infarct.
4. The ST segment returns to the normal baseline position within days to weeks.
5. After a period of weeks to months, the T wave becomes upright again. A lasting ECG change is an enlarged Q wave as shown.

Premature ventricular contraction. A premature ventricular contraction (PVC) is an abnormal, fast contraction of the ventricles that originates from a focus below the AV node (see Fig. 10-21). This is usually a sign of a diseased or hypoxic ventricle. Pathologic causes include arteriosclerotic heart disease or MI. An example of an isolated PVC is shown in Fig. 10-22 and has these traits:

1. It is premature and happens before the normal heartbeat.
2. There is no P wave.
3. The QRS complex is bizarre looking and more than .12 seconds wide.
4. The T wave is inverted.
5. Usually, there is a fully compensatory pause before the next normal heartbeat.

A single PVC is not dangerous unless it originates during the T wave, when the heart is especially vulnerable to electrical stimulation. Then it can cause ventricular fibrillation. Patients with PVCs should be watched more closely and probably treated when their PVCs are seen more frequently than 1 in 10 beats, seen in groups of two or three, or seen in multiple configurations. For example, two different-looking PVCs mean that there are two different ventricular foci firing prematurely (Fig. 10-23). Bigeminy is when every second beat is a PVC; trigeminy is when every third beat is a PVC. Dangerous PVCs must be rapidly treated. Lidocaine (Xylocaine) is given intravenously if the heart rate is more than 60 beats per minute. If that does not work, procainamide hydrochloride (Pronestyl) is added.

Ventricular tachycardia. Ventricular tachycardia (VT or V tach) is a serious consequence of untreated premature ventricular contractions (see Fig. 10-24). VT is defined as a series of three or more consecutive PVCs. Runs of VT may be fairly short or prolonged. The rate counted during VT is between 110 and 250 beats per minute. Cardiac output falls dramatically during this arrhythmia. If the patient has a stable blood pressure, VT is treated with lidocaine as an antiarrhythmic. Synchronized cardioversion is needed if the lidocaine is ineffective. If the VT is sustained and the patient is unresponsive, pulseless, hypotensive, or in pulmonary edema, unsynchronous cardioversion is necessary. If left untreated, VT usually progresses to either ventricular flutter (see Fig. 10-25) or ventricular fibrillation (discussed next). Ventricular flutter looks similar on the ECG to VT except that the rate is usually faster and the rhythm less regular. Its treatment is the same as VT and, if left untreated, will progress to ventricular fibrillation. Both

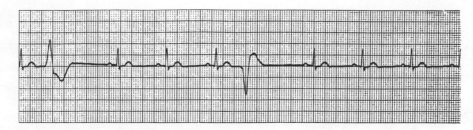

Fig. 10-23 An ECG tracing showing multifocal premature ventricular contractions (PVCs). Counting from the left, after the normal beat, note that the next beat and sixth beat are PVCs. Because they look different they do not originate at the same abnormal focus. Therefore the patient has multifocal PVCs. This dangerous situation should be quickly corrected. (From Wilkins RL, Krider SJ, Sheldon RL: *Clinical assessment in respiratory care,* ed 4, St. Louis, 2000, Mosby.)

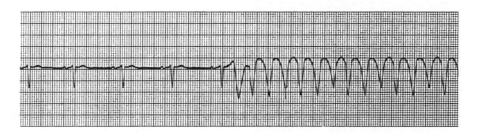

Fig. 10-24 ECG tracing showing normal sinus rhythm that suddenly converts to ventricular tachycardia. This can happen if a premature ventricular contraction occurs early in the heart's repolarization process and is called the R-on-T phenomena. If ventricular tachycardia is not treated promptly, it will deteriorate into ventricular flutter or ventricular fibrillation. (From Wilkins RL, Krider SJ, Sheldon RL: *Clinical assessment in respiratory care,* ed 4, St Louis, 2000, Mosby.)

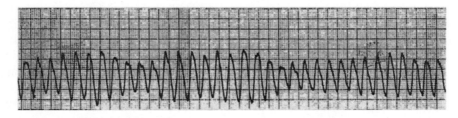

Fig. 10-25 Example of an ECG showing ventricular flutter. If this arrhythmia is not treated promptly it will deteriorate into ventricular fibrillation. (From Kacmarek RM, Mack CW, Dimas S: *The essentials of respiratory care,* ed 3, St Louis, 1990, Mosby.)

of these arrhythmias originate from a single fast ventricular focus as shown in Fig. 10-21.

Ventricular fibrillation. Ventricular fibrillation (VF or V fib) is caused when multiple, fast ventricular foci are firing (see Fig. 10-26 for the electrical pathways). When several ventricular foci are firing in an uncoordinated manner, the rhythm is chaotic and without any pattern. There is virtually no cardiac output. The patient is pulseless and without any blood pressure. This is a true medical emergency. If not treated immediately, brain death will occur within minutes. CPR must be started to provide oxygen to the brain. The treatment of choice for VF is defibrillation as quickly as possible. No attempt is made to synchronize the electrical shock. Fig. 10-27 shows the usual position of the defibrillator paddles. It is hoped that with prompt CPR efforts and electrical defibrillation, the patient's heartbeat will return to normal sinus rhythm (Fig. 10-5).

Ventricular asystole. Ventricular asystole (or asystole) occurs when there is no cardiac electrical signal and no myocardial activity. The ECG tracing shows a flat line, indicating that there is no cardiac electrical activity. The presence of this arrythmia is ominous. When seen after a full attempt at CPR, it indicates a nonfunctioning heart.

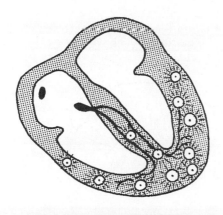

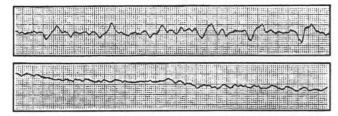

Fig. 10-26 Multiple disorganized contractions of the ventricles characterize ventricular fibrillation and represent cardiac arrest. It may be of sudden onset or may follow premature ventricular contractions, ventricular tachycardia, or ventricular flutter. (From Stein E: *Clinical electrocardiography: a self-study course,* Philadelphia, 1987, Lea & Febiger.)

The patient will almost assuredly die. Some physicians may elect to defibrillate the patient in asystole in an attempt to generate some sort of rhythm. Because of the dire consequences of ventricular asystole, it is wise to double-check all the equipment. This includes the ECG leads or defibrillator paddles being used to check the rhythm, all electrical connections, and the functioning of the ECG monitor to be sure that there is no technical error.

☞ EXAM HINT

There may be an ECG tracing. Usually it is of ventricular fibrillation. The situation usually requires knowing that the arrhythmia is life threatening and requires CPR or defibrillation as necessary.

MODULE B	Cardiopulmonary resuscitation (CPR) equipment

1. Manual resuscitator (bag-valve)
a. Get the necessary equipment for the procedure (Code: IIA1d) [Difficulty: An]

The first consideration when deciding which manual resuscitator to select is the size of the patient. Although the

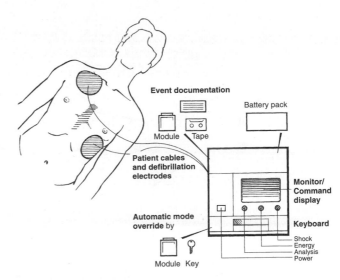

Fig. 10-27 Schematic drawing of automated external defibrilator and its attachment to the patient. (Modified from Cummins RO: *Advanced cardiac life support,* Dallas, 1994, American Heart Association.)

volume of the reservoir bag and the tidal volume expelled from it vary among the types of bags, there are three basic sizes. An infant or newborn unit typically has a reservoir bag volume of about 250 mL. A pediatric unit usually has a reservoir bag volume of about 250 to 500 mL, and an adult unit typically has a reservoir bag volume of 1500 to 2000 mL. In addition to all of these reusable units, there are a number of disposable units that are thrown away after one patient use. They also come in comparable infant, pediatric, and adult reservoir bag volumes.

Any unit should deliver 100% oxygen at the flow rate of 15 L/min. An oxygen reservoir system must be added to the basic unit to achieve these oxygen percentages. The valve to the patient must be clearable within 20 seconds if it becomes fouled by vomitus, sputum, or blood.

Neonatal and pediatric units must have a pressure-release (pop-off) valve that opens at 40 cm H_2O pressure. The pressure may be adjustable. If an adult unit has a pressure release valve, it must have an override system that is easy to operate.

b. Put the equipment together, make sure that it works properly, and identify any problems (Code: IIB1d) [Difficulty: An]

Fig. 10-20 shows line drawings of a complete set of Laerdal infant, pediatric, and adult manual resuscitators. The following steps should be taken when the function of a manual resuscitator is evaluated:

1. Squeeze and release the bag to see if the nonrebreathing valve and air/oxygen reservoir intake valve open and close properly.
2. Feel the air leave the outlet port of the nonrebreathing valve when the bag is squeezed.

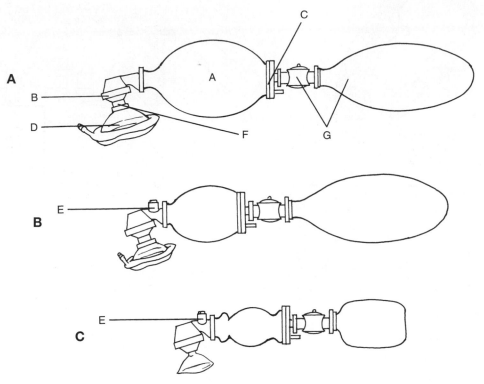

Fig. 10-28   A, Adult Laerdal resuscitator. **B,** pediatric Laerdal resuscitator. **C,** infant Laerdal resuscitator. These features are found on all modern units: *A,* self-filling reservoir bag; *B,* elation valve that does not jam at an oxygen flow of 15 L/min or in subfreezing temperatures (it must be clearable of debris within 20 seconds); *C,* intake valve for adding draw room air or supplemental oxygen into the reservoir bag; *D,* transparent mask that easily conforms to the patient's face; *E,* pressure-relief (pop-off) valve that is set to open at 40 cm water; *F,* standard 15 mm ID/22 mm OD connector for the endotracheal tube or face mask; *G,* oxygen enrichment/reservoir system. In addition, some units have an adjustable positive end-expiratory pressure (PEEP) valve (not shown) attached to the elation valve. (From Eubanks DH, Bone RC: *Comprehensive respiratory care,* ed 2, 1990, St Louis, Mosby.)

3. Occlude the outlet port and squeeze the bag. No gas should leak out. If present, the pop-off valve should open at the correct pressure.
4. The face mask should fit onto the 22-mm outer diameter (OD) fitting and have its cushion properly inflated.

c. Fix any problems with the equipment (Code: IIB2d) [Difficulty: An]

Check for a reversed or improperly seated one-way valve if the gas does not enter or exit the unit as it should. In clinical use, mucus, vomitus, and blood can foul the nonrebreathing valve system and must be cleared within 20 seconds. Do this by disconnecting the unit from the patient, aiming the adapter into a neutral area, and squeezing the bag to blow out the obstruction. Replace a unit that cannot be promptly cleared.

2. Mouth-to-valve mask resuscitator
a. Get the necessary equipment for the procedure (Code: IIA1d) [Difficulty: An]

The following are important considerations when selecting the best device for the victim:
1. The mask must fit the victim's face so that there is no air leak. There should be infant, child, and adult sizes available.
2. The mouthpiece should be designed so that it fits only one way into the mask. Some units include a short length of aerosol tubing between the mouthpiece and mask for greater flexibility.
3. The one-way (nonrebreathing) valve should be designed to ensure that all of the rescuer's breath is directed into the victim, and the victim's exhaled breath is vented to room air rather than back at the rescuer. Some units include a bacteria

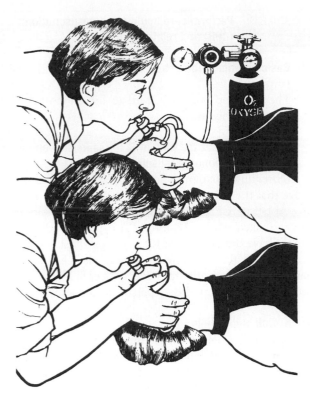

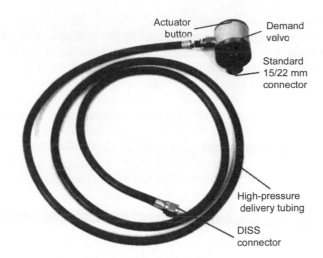

Fig. 10-30 Features of a pneumatic resuscitator with high-pressure hose. (From Scanlan CL: Emergency life support. In Scanlan CL, Spearman CB, Sheldon RL, editors: *Egan's fundamentals of respiratory care,* ed 5, St Louis, 1990, Mosby.)

Fig. 10-29 Proper positioning to use a mouth-to-valve mask resuscitator. The top rescuer has added supplemental oxygen to the device. The bottom rescuer is ventilating without the use of added oxygen. (Courtesy Laerdal Medical Corporation, Armonk, NY.)

filter in the one-way valve between the rescuer and victim.

4. It should be possible to add supplemental oxygen through a T-piece or nipple on the mask. This is important for hospital or ambulance use. If a T-piece is added, it must be designed to easily fit between the mouthpiece and face mask. An oxygen administration nipple should have a cap over it when not in use to prevent any leakage of the delivered breath.

b. Put the equipment together, make sure that it works properly, and identify any problems (Code: IIB1d) [Difficulty: An]

Mouth-to-valve resuscitators are relatively simple devices. Most have only two or three pieces: a face mask, a mouthpiece with a one-way valve, and possibly an oxygen T-piece (Fig. 10-29.) The "male" and "female" connections are designed to fit together in only one way. When they are properly assembled, there should be no air leaks when the breath is delivered to the victim.

c. Fix any problems with the equipment (Code: IIB2d) [Difficulty: An]

If the breath cannot be delivered, check the one-way valve to make sure that it has not been put together backward. Reverse it, if necessary, and ventilate the victim's airway. Keep the oxygen nipple on the mask or T-piece capped off if it is not being used. Air will leak out during the delivered breath if the cap is left off the nipple.

3. Pneumatic (demand-valve) resuscitator
a. Get the necessary equipment for the procedure (Code: IIA1d) [Difficulty: An]

The two most commonly available pneumatic (gas-powered) resuscitators are the Robertshaw demand valve and Hudson's elder valve (Fig. 10-30). An advantage of these types of units over manual resuscitators is that they are easier to operate. One hand can be used to activate the actuator/manual control button for an extended period of time without fatigue. The patient outlet has a standard 15-mm ID/22-mm OD connector. It fits any endotracheal tube adaptor or face mask. The operator delivers tidal volume gas to the patient as long as the button is pressed or until the pressure limit is reached. This may be set as high as 60 cm of water. If possible, select a unit that delivers a constant flow rate of less than 40 L/min (to minimize gastric insufflation) and that gives an audible alarm if the pressure limit is reached. Because of the factors of variable inspiratory time and pressure limiting, the delivered tidal volume varies with the patient's changing pulmonary condition. This is a drawback of these units compared with the manual resuscitators. Clinical experience is needed to use either type of pneumatic resuscitator to safely deliver an appropriate tidal volume to most patients.

A variation on the pneumatic resuscitator is the demand valve. With it, the spontaneously breathing patient can trigger a breath similar to how the assist mode operates on a mechanical ventilator. The breath is delivered until the pressure preset by the rescuer is reached or the patient makes an expiratory effort. If the patient should become apneic, the rescuer can depress the actuator button to deliver a tidal volume.

b. Put the equipment together, make sure that it works properly, and identify any problems (Code: IIB1d) [Difficulty: An]

Pneumatic resuscitators come preassembled by the manufacturer. The only additional piece of equipment is a length of high-pressure oxygen hose with a female diameter-index safety system (DISS) connector at both ends. Screw one end of the hose to the inlet of the demand valve as shown in Fig. 10-30. The other end of the hose is then screwed onto either a reducing valve or regulator connected to the hospital's central oxygen source or a flowmeter connected to an oxygen cylinder. Turning on the flowmeter to maximum or inserting the reducing valve into the central oxygen source conducts pure oxygen at 50 psig to the unit. The demand valve reduces this pressure to its working pressure (up to 60 cm of water).

When it is properly assembled and the oxygen source is opened, you should feel gas escape from the outlet port when the actuator/manual control button is pushed. The gas flow should stop when the button is released. By attaching a test lung to the outlet port and starting a breath, you can see that the test lung fills during inspiration and cycles off when the pressure limit is reached. Make sure that the unit properly cycles on and off.

c. Fix any problems with the equipment (Code: IIB2d) [Difficulty: An)

The following types of problems can be encountered with demand valve units:
1. Foreign body obstruction of the control valve. Remove the unit from the patient, point it into a neutral area, and depress the actuator/manual control button to blow the obstruction clear. Do not use a unit that cannot be cleared of an obstruction or will not cycle on and off properly.
2. A gas leak can be heard or felt. Search out and tighten the loose connection to seal the leak and deliver 50 psig of oxygen pressure to the unit.

EXAM HINT

Usually there is an exam question that deals with a malfunctioning manual resuscitator, mouth-to-valve resuscitator, or demand valve resuscitator. Often, the question involves using the ventilating device without the patient's chest rising. Fixing the problem can involve clearing an obstruction or properly assembling a one-way valve.

MODULE C	Perform cardiopulmonary resuscitation (CPR) and related functions

1. Basic cardiac life support (Code: IIID1a) [Difficulty: An]

The key steps of basic cardiac life support (BCLS) include the following:

a. Establish that the patient is unresponsive and needs cardiopulmonary resuscitation

Observing a patient who *appears* to be dead does not prove that the patient needs CPR. Clinical death must be proved before CPR is begun. Adults should be tapped or gently shaken while shouting, "Are you okay?" Infants should have the bottom of their feet gently slapped while shouting, "Wake up!" The rescuer can also clap his or her hands together loudly to wake a sleeping infant. CPR should never be started on a person who does not need it.

b. Call out for help

Call out for help if the victim does not respond to any attempts at arousal. The second rescuer should be told to call in the cardiac arrest team. Many hospitals have a cardiac arrest button in each patient's room. If this is the case, the first rescuer can push the button while calling out for help. Dial 911 if the victim is found at home.

c. Open the airway

The head-tilt/chin-lift maneuver is the procedure of choice for opening the airway of all victims except those with a known or suspected cervical (neck) spine injury. The victim is gently positioned on his or her back. In an adult, the head is firmly pushed back with one hand, and the jaw is pulled upward with the fingers of the other hand (Fig. 10-31). In an infant, it is not necessary to tilt the head

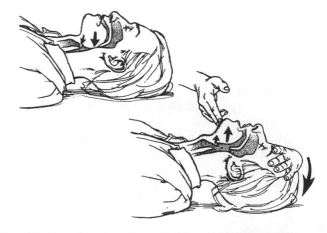

Fig. 10-31 Opening the adult's airway. *Top,* Airway obstruction produced by the tongue and epiglottis. *Bottom,* Relief by head-tilt/chin-lift method. (From Standards and guidelines for cardiopulmonary resuscitation [CPR] and emergency cardiac care [ECC], *JAMA* 268: 2186, 1992.)

back beyond a neutral position. Children may need to have the head pushed back slightly beyond neutral.

The jaw-thrust maneuver is the procedure of choice for opening the airway of all victims with a known or suspected cervical spine injury. The rescuer's elbows are rested on the ground, and the hands are placed on either side of the victim's jaw. Lifting of the jaw usually opens the airway and eliminates the need to tilt the head back. See Fig. 10-32 for the adult maneuver.

Any obstruction that can be seen in the mouth or throat should be removed. The cross-finger technique can be used to open the mouth wide enough so that a finger or suction device can be inserted to remove a blockage (Fig. 10-33). An oral airway should be used only in an unconscious patient to keep the tongue from falling back and blocking the airway.

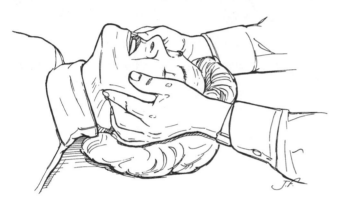

Fig. 10-32   Opening the adult's airway by the jaw-thrust method. (From Watson MA: Cardiopulmonary resuscitation, in Barnes TA, editor: *Respiratory care practice,* St Louis, 1988, Mosby.)

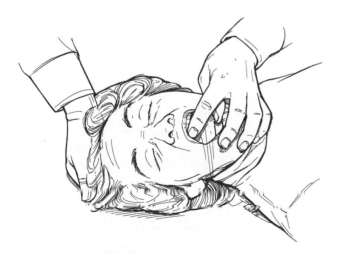

Fig. 10-33   The cross-finger method of opening the victim's mouth to look for an obstruction. (From Watson MA: Cardiopulmonary resuscitation, in Barnes TA, editor: *Respiratory care practice,* St Louis, 1988, Mosby.)

d. Determine that the patient is not breathing

The rescuer places his or her face close to the victim's face to *look* for rising and falling of the chest, *listen* for victim's movement, and *feel* any air movement from the victim's breathing (Fig. 10-34). This should be done for 3 to 5 seconds to be sure that the patient is really apneic and not just breathing slowly.

e. Ventilate the patient
1. Mouth-to-mouth breathing

The first rescuer should begin mouth-to-mouth breathing as soon as possible if there is no spontaneous breathing by the victim once the airway is opened. No matter the age of the victim, there must be an effective seal between the rescuer and the victim. The adult victim's nose must be pinched closed; often the infant's nosed can be blocked by the cheek of the rescuer. The mouth of the rescuer can cover both the nose and mouth of an infant. Alternative methods of ventilation include mouth to nose and mouth to stoma (Fig. 10-35).

In an adult, two breaths large enough to raise the victim's chest should be given. An adequate volume of 800 mL and up to 1200 mL may be given. Blow into the victim's mouth for 1 to 1.5 seconds. This is to ensure a large enough volume without having to use much pressure. Keeping the ventilating pressure as low as possible minimizes the risk of forcing air into the stomach. Ensure that the victim exhales completely by watching the chest fall and feeling the air escape against your cheek. Rescue

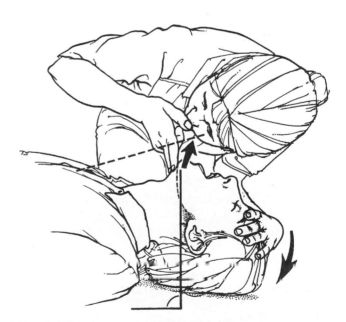

Fig. 10-34   Determining breathlessness by looking, listening, and feeling. (From Standards and guidelines for cardiopulmonary resuscitation [CPR] and emergency cardiac care [ECC], *JAMA* 268: 2187, 1992.)

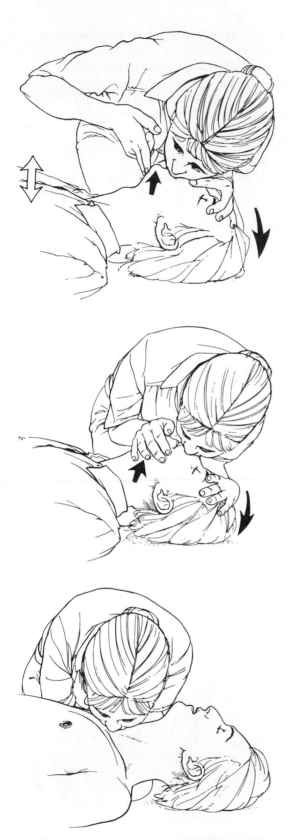

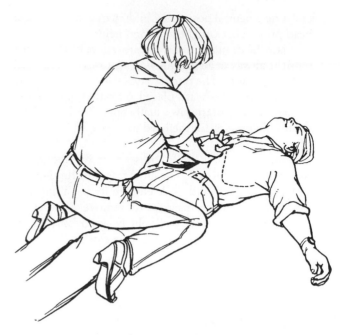

Fig. 10-36 Administering the Heimlich maneuver to an unconscious adult victim of an airway obstruction. (From Standards and guidelines for cardiopulmonary resuscitation [CPR] and emergency cardiac care [ECC], *JAMA* 268: 2193, 1992.)

breathing should be performed at a rate of 10 to 12 times/min (every 6 seconds) if the victim has a pulse but is apneic.

In a child, two breaths large enough to raise the victim's chest should be given. A child obviously needs less volume than an adult. All of the same considerations apply as in the adult. Rescue breathing should be performed at a rate of 20/min (every 3 seconds) in an infant and 15/min (every 4 seconds) in a child.

If the victim's airway cannot be ventilated, reposition the head and attempt to ventilate again. Failure to ventilate a second time means that the victim has an obstructed airway. The following steps should be taken:

Unconscious adult obstructed airway maneuvers

a. Position the victim on his or her back.

b. Perform the Heimlich maneuver (also known as abdominal thrusts) several times if needed. This is done by kneeling astride the victim, placing the heel of one hand midline on the abdomen slightly above the navel, but well below the xiphoid process. The other hand is placed on top, and both are quickly thrust upward toward the chest (Fig. 10-36). The markedly obese or obviously pregnant victim can have chest thrusts performed on them. The rescuer's hands should be placed on the lower half of the sternum as with cardiac compressions. Several compressions should be performed slowly but similarly to a cardiac compression.

Fig. 10-35 Adult mouth-to-mouth, mouth-to-nose, and mouth-to-stoma ventilation. (From Standards and guidelines for cardiopulmonary resuscitation [CPR] and emergency cardiac care [ECC], *JAMA* 268: 2188, 1992.)

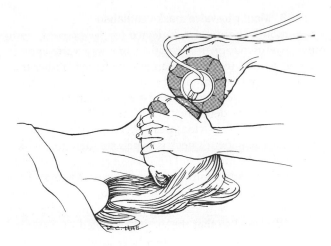

Fig. 10-38 Ventilation of an adult with a manual resuscitation bag and mask. (From Eubanks DH, Bone RC: *Comprehensive respiratory care,* ed 2, St Louis, 1990, Mosby.)

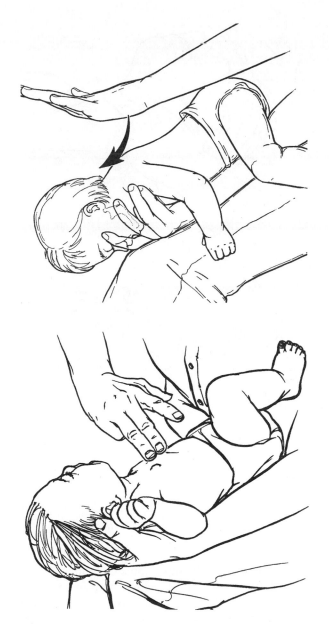

Fig. 10-37 Administering back blows and chest trusts to an infant victim of an obstructed airway. (From Standards and guidelines for cardiopulmonary resuscitation [CPR] and emergency cardiac care [ECC], *JAMA* 268: 2258, 1992.)

c. Attempt to clear out any foreign body with a finger sweep. First, grasp the victim's tongue and jaw between your thumb and fingers, and lift the jaw open. Next, insert the index finger of the other hand along the inside of the victim's cheek and down the back of the throat so as to hook and remove food, gum, dentures, and so on.

Unconscious child (1 year old and older) obstructed airway maneuvers

a. Position the victim on his or her back.
b. Heimlich maneuver: Same as the adult maneuver but

with up to five thrusts performed if needed. Chest thrusts are not used.

c. Finger sweep: Same as the adult, except that the index finger is inserted only when a foreign body has been seen. Blindly inserting the index finger may push a foreign body further down the throat.

Unconscious infant obstructed airway maneuver

a. The infant is straddled over the rescuer's forearm. The infant's jaw and head are held by the rescuer's hand. The infant's head should be lower than the body. Five firm back blows are delivered between the shoulder blades with the heel of the rescuer's other hand (Fig. 10-37).

b. The infant is sandwiched by the rescuer's other arm and the head and body are supported and turned to a supine position. The head should remain lower than the body. Five chest thrusts are performed in the same location and manner as cardiac compressions but at a slower rate. Steps 1 and 2 can be done by placing the infant on the rescuer's lap.

c. Same as step 3 in the unconscious child mentioned earlier.

2. Manual resuscitator (bag-valve)

A manual resuscitator should be used during hospital-based CPR as soon as one is available. The resuscitation mask must be held to the victim's face so that there is no air leak during the forced inspiration (Fig. 10-38). An assistant can hold the mask tightly to the face so that the rescuer who is pumping the resuscitation bag can use both hands. This has been shown to produce a larger tidal volume. The valve adapter fits directly over the tube adapter for victims who have endotracheal of tracheostomy tubes. Rescue breathing continues with the previously mentioned considerations for volume and rate.

3. Mouth-to-valve mask ventilation

A mouth-to-valve mask device (or *pocket mask*) combines a resuscitation mask with a one-way valve mouthpiece. It is used to ventilate an apneic patient rather than perform mouth-to-mouth breathing. Concerns about protecting the rescuer from patient infections such as acquired immunodeficiency syndrome (AIDS) and hepatitis have lead to their widespread acceptance. As shown in Fig. 10-29, the patient's neck is hyperextended, the mask is applied over the mouth and nose to get an airtight seal, and the rescuer breathes into the mouthpiece. It is best if the rescuer is positioned at the victim's head so that the chest can be seen to rise with each delivered breath. The one-way valve is designed so that the victim's exhaled gas is vented out to the room air. Some units have a nipple adapter so that supplemental oxygen can be added to the delivered breath. Simply attach oxygen tubing between the nipple and oxygen flowmeter and turn the flowmeter on to the manufacturer's recommended flow. It is best if these devices are replaced by a manual resuscitator as soon as possible.

f. Add supplemental oxygen (Code: IIIB4c) [Difficulty: An]

The victim should be given 100% oxygen as soon as possible. There is no contraindication for giving pure oxygen during a resuscitation effort. This can be done easily if a manual resuscitator is used to ventilate the victim. Most modern units are capable of giving 100% oxygen if the oxygen flow is high enough and a reservoir is added. Some older units can give supplemental oxygen at some percentage less than 100%. These are still better than using room air, but should be replaced as soon as possible with a unit capable of delivering 100% oxygen.

g. Determine pulselessness

The carotid pulse is felt for in all victims except children younger than 1 year. The carotid pulse is found by gently feeling with two or three fingers in the groove between the larynx and the sternocleidomastoid muscle on either side of the neck (Fig. 10-39). Check for 5 to 10 seconds to be sure that the victim is pulseless and not just bradycardiac. An infant younger than 1 year should have the pulse felt in the brachial artery; the carotid artery is difficult to find in such young children because they have short, chubby necks.

The femoral pulse can be felt for as an alternative site in victims in the hospital who are wearing few clothes. Once the CPR team has arrived and two-person CPR is instituted, the femoral pulse may be most accessible for monitoring the pulse and the effectiveness of the chest compressions.

h. Perform external chest compressions

The absence of a pulse confirms a cardiac arrest. Blood must be pumped by external chest compressions of the

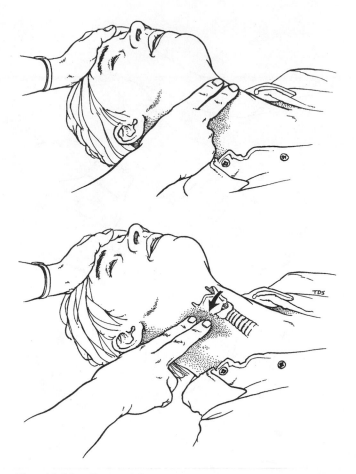

Fig. 10-39 Determining pulselessness by checking the carotid pulse of an adult. (From Standards and guidelines for cardiopulmonary resuscitation [CPR] and emergency cardiac care [ECC], *JAMA* 268: 2189, 1992.)

heart. The victim must be supine on a hard surface. A CPR backboard is placed behind a victim who is in bed.

In adults and large children or those more than 8 years old, the heel of the rescuer's hand is placed over the lower half of the sternum. This is found by placing the middle finger of one hand in the notch where the ribs meet the sternum, placing the index finger next to it, and placing the other hand next to the finger. The first hand is placed over it, the elbows are locked, and the shoulders are directly over the hands. This creates the most efficient pumping action (Fig. 10-40). The rescuer pivots from the hips, with half of the time spent pumping down and half of the time releasing pressure. The hands should always touch the victim's chest. The sternum must be compressed 1.5 to 2.0 inches (3.8 to 5.0 cm) in an average adult. The compression rate should be between 80 and 100/min.

In a child 8 years old or younger, hand position is found as in the adult. The child's sternum must be compressed with *one* hand to a depth of 1 to 1.5 inches (2.5 to 3.8 cm). Half of the time should be spent on compression and half on relaxation. The rate should be 100/min to achieve a rate of 80/min between ventilations.

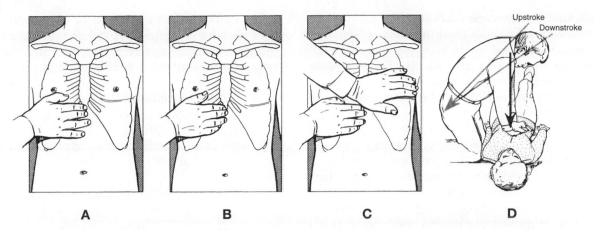

Fig. 10-40   Cardiac compression of an adult. **A,** locate tip of xiphoid process. **B,** place two fingertips at xiphoid process. **C,** place palm of other hand on sternum next to fingers. **D,** arm and body positions for cardiac compression. (From Barnes TA, editor: *Respiratory care practice,* St Louis, 1988, Mosby.)

In an infant, two or three fingers are placed over the middle of the sternum one finger width below an imaginary line drawn between the nipples (Fig. 10-41). The child's sternum must be compressed to a depth of 0.5 to 1 inch (1.3 to 2.5 cm). Half of the time should be spent on compression and half on relaxation. The rate should be at least 100/min.

The steps for one- and two-person CPR follow.

1. Adult one-rescuer CPR:
  a. Assess the victim's need for CPR.
  b. Call out for help.
  c. Open the airway.
  d. Assess the victim's lack of breathing.
  e. Give two rescue breaths.
  f. Assess the victim's lack of a pulse.
  g. Perform 15 chest compressions at a rate of 80 to 100/min. Count them out as "one and, two and, three and . . ."
  h. Reopen the airway and give two breaths.
  i. Repeat this cycle (15:2 ratio) a total of four times.
  j. Check the victim's carotid pulse from 5 seconds. If it has not returned, give two breaths and continue with compressions.
  k. If the pulse has returned, check on the return of breathing. If it has not returned, give 12 breaths/min.
  l. If CPR is continued, check for the return of a heartbeat and breathing every few minutes.

2. Adult two-rescuer CPR:
  a. Perform steps a to f as in one-rescuer CPR.
  b. The first rescuer performs five chest compressions at a rate of 80 to 100/min. Count them out as "one and, two and, three and. . . ."
  c. The second rescuer gives one breath during a 1.5- to 2-second pause between sets of compressions.

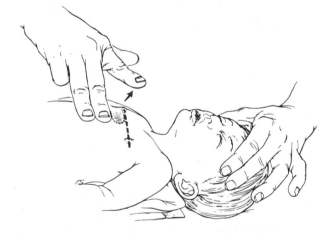

Fig. 10-41   Locating the proper finger position for chest compressions on an infant. (From Standards and guidelines for cardiopulmonary resuscitation [CPR] and emergency cardiac care [ECC], *JAMA* 268: 2256, 1992.)

  d. Repeat this cycle (5:1 ratio) several times.
  e. The second rescuer calls for a 5-second pause after 1 minute and checks for the return of pulse or breathing.
  f. Provide breathing, circulation, or both as needed. If CPR is continued, check for the return of a heartbeat and breathing every few minutes.
  g. Switch positions whenever one rescuer becomes tired. Make the switch at the end of a cycle, check the victim for a return of pulse or breathing, and continue as needed.

3. Infant and child one- and two-rescuer CPR:
  a. Perform steps a to f as described in one-rescuer CPR.
  b. In either case, a rescuer performs sets of five chest compressions. These are delivered at a rate of at least

100/min to deliver at least 80 compressions/min between ventilations. Count them out as "one and, two and, three and . . . ."

c. One breath is given during a 1- to 1.5-second pause between sets of compressions.

d. Repeat this pattern (5:1 ratio) for about 1 minute (20 cycles).

e. The second rescuer calls for a 5-second pause and checks for the return of pulse or breathing.

f. Provide breathing and/or circulation as needed. If CPR is continued, check for the return of a heartbeat and breathing every few minutes.

g. Switch positions whenever one rescuer becomes tired. Make the switch at the end of a cycle, check the victim for a return of pulse or breathing, and continue as needed.

 EXAM HINT

Past exam questions have focused on basic cardiac life support procedures. However, there have been occasional advanced CPR questions. Discussion of key advanced CPR procedures is included here and in other areas of this text.

2. Advanced cardiac life support (Code: IIID1b) [Difficulty: An]

It is beyond the scope of this text to present advanced cardiac life support (ACLS) in detail. The following items relate to procedures that are important in the care of adult, pediatric, and neonatal patients needing advanced resuscitation.

a. Make a recommendation for an arterial blood gas measurement (Code: IA2e) [Difficulty: An]

Blood for arterial blood gas (ABG) determination is usually drawn in any hospital-based CPR effort. It should not be done at the expense of time that should be spent starting effective ventilations and chest compressions or defibrillating the heart. The blood gas values give important information on the patient's oxygenation and whether the patient is acidotic. Changes in the ventilation efforts and medications such as bicarbonate are based on information from the arterial blood gases.

The femoral site is usually the best to draw from in a CPR situation. This is because it is the largest artery and easiest to hit. Also, it is far enough from the chest that blood can be drawn without interfering in the chest compression efforts.

b. Interpret the results of arterial blood gas analysis (Code: IB10c and IC2e) [Difficulty: An]

The full discussion of ABG interpretation is presented in Chapter 3. During a CPR attempt the key things to look for are the patient's PaO_2 and $PaCO_2$, because they relate

to the adequacy of ventilations and chest compressions. If the patient has an acidotic pH and a normal or low $PaCO_2$ the patient has an uncorrected metabolic acidosis. Intravenous sodium bicarbonate is indicated.

c. Endotracheal intubation

Oral endotracheal intubation is usually performed during a CPR attempt. See Chapter 11 for a complete discussion of endotracheal tubes, intubation equipment, and the process of performing intubation.

d. Make the recommendation to defibrillate the patient

Defibrillation sends a specific amount of direct electrical current (DC) through the patient's chest wall and heart. Its purpose is to stimulate the entire cardiac muscle and electrical system so that the source of an abnormal signal will be suppressed. The sinoatrial (SA) node usually then takes over as the normal pacemaker. A more complete discussion of defibrillation is presented in Chapter 17.

As discussed earlier, synchronized defibrillation (cardioversion) should be performed under the following circumstances: atrial flutter, paroxysmal atrial tachycardia, atrial fibrillation, and ventricular tachycardia unless the patient is pulseless, unresponsive, hypotensive, or in pulmonary edema.

Unsynchronized defibrillation should be performed under the following circumstances: ventricular fibrillation or ventricular tachycardia when the patient is pulseless, unresponsive, hypotensive, or in pulmonary edema. Some physicians may also administer a cardiac shock to a patient in ventricular asystole.

 EXAM HINT

There is usually one question that requires the therapist to identify the indications for defibrillation and recommend the procedure.

e. Recommend medications during an emergency

According to the most recent guidelines, bicarbonate (sodium bicarbonate) should be used, if at all, only after all other CPR procedures have been instituted. Bicarbonate may then be used if a diagnosis has been made and the patient has a preexisting metabolic acidosis, hyperkalemia, or tricyclic or phenobarbitol overdose. Bicarbonate may also be beneficial if the patient has been in prolonged arrest or if CPR has been performed for an extended time.

When used, bicarbonate should be given initially at a dose of 1 mEq/kg; a half dose is then given every 10 minutes. If available from arterial blood gas results, use the calculated base deficit or bicarbonate concentration as a guideline for giving more bicarbonate. Do not completely correct the base deficit to avoid accidentally making the patient alkalotic.

Other cardiac and blood pressure medications are

discussed in Chapter 8. Be prepared to recommend any of those medications as indicated.

f. Recommend the instillation of medications through the endotracheal tube during an emergency situation

Cardiac medications should be instilled down the endotracheal tube when a resuscitation attempt is underway and the patient does not have a functional central or peripheral intravenous (IV) line. The following medications may be instilled into all patients: lidocaine, epinephrine, and atropine. In addition, naloxone may be given to pediatric patients. Adults should be given a dose 2 to 2.5 times the normal intravenous amount. The medication should be diluted by adding 10 mL of normal saline or distilled water. Pediatric patients should be given a dose that is 10 times the normal IV amount. It should be diluted with 1 to 2 mL of normal or half normal saline.

> **EXAM HINT**
>
> There is usually one question that requires either the recommendation that CPR drugs be given through the endotracheal tube or the medications that can be given by this route. There is usually one question that requires the interpretation of ABG results during a CPR attempt to identify a metabolic acidosis and the administration of intravenous sodium bicarbonate to correct the situation.

---

g. Instill the ordered medication down the endotracheal tube

The following steps for instillation are recommended:
1. Disconnect the manual resuscitator from the endotracheal tube and stop the chest compressions.
2. Pass a suction catheter or feeding tube past the distal tip of the endotracheal tube.
3. Quickly inject the drug solution down the catheter.
4. Withdraw the suction catheter.
5. Reconnect the manual resuscitator to the endotracheal tube and give the patient several deep breaths. This helps to force the medication down to the alveolar level or causes aerosolization so that there is faster absorption.
6. Resume chest compressions and ventilation.

h. Observe the size of the patient's pupils and their reaction to light

Normally the pupils react to a light being shined into them by constricting. The pupils dilate within 30 to 40 seconds after cardiac arrest and do not constrict normally when the brain is hypoxic. If CPR is being done properly to deliver oxygen to the brain, the pupils should constrict normally. Fixed (nonreactive) and dilated pupils are an ominous sign. Even if the heart can be restarted, the brain has probably suffered irreversible damage.

There are several conditions in which the pupils do not react as expected. The pupils remain constricted if the victim has received morphine sulfate or other opiates. The pupils are dilated if the victim has received atropine, quinidine, or epinephrine. Hypothermia also causes the pupils to dilate.

i. Recommend capnography to evaluate the adequacy of resuscitation

The general discussion of capnography was presented in Chapter 5. If quickly available, capnography can be used to help confirm that the endotracheal tube is properly located in the trachea. It is also helpful if the patient is being transported or the endotracheal tube is being repositioned. The presence of exhaled carbon dioxide confirms that the tube is properly positioned in the trachea. In addition, there is clinical evidence that monitoring the exhaled carbon dioxide level during a CPR attempt is helpful in evaluating the patient's response. In general, if chest compressions and assisted ventilation are effective, carbon dioxide is removed from the tissues and circulated to the lungs for exhalation. If the CPR efforts are ineffective, little exhaled carbon dioxide is measured.

3. Pediatric advanced life support (Code: IIID1c) [Difficulty: An]

The general steps and procedures related to pediatric advanced life support (PALS) are covered in this chapter, Chapter 8, and Chapter 11.

4. Neonatal resuscitation program (Code: IIID1d) [Difficulty: An]

A neonatal resuscitation program (NRP) provides training in resuscitating a newborn at birth in the delivery room. In addition to the basic and advanced CPR steps discussed in this chapter and Chapters 8 and 11, the person trained in NRP is prepared to perform the following:
  a. Dry the newborn and keep it warm.
  b. Suction the airway to remove amniotic fluid and meconium.
  c. Evaluate the newborn to determine the need for 100% oxygen, bag-mask ventilation, intubation, and chest compressions.

It is beyond the scope of this text to cover all aspects of ACLS, PALS, and NRP training. The bibliography lists helpful sources of information.

> **EXAM HINT**
>
> Historically, the NBRC has had one question on basic cardiac life support. However, every opportunity should be taken to learn the advanced CPR procedures such as life-threatening arrhythmia recognition, intubation, and defibrillation.

MODULE D	**Respiratory care plan**

1. Participate in the development of the respiratory care plan [e.g., case management, development and application of protocols, disease management education] (Code: IC4) [Difficulty: An]

It is critically important that the respiratory therapist be able to recognize the need to start CPR procedures. This chapter's discussion should be helpful in preparing for this possibility.

BCLS, ACLS, PALS, and NRP are all cardiopulmonary resuscitation-related protocols. CPR should be started, adjusted, and terminated based on these protocols and the patient's recovery.

The practitioner should make a recommendation to the physician to stop a procedure being performed as an adjunct to CPR if the patient is suffering an adverse reaction to it. For example, bag and mask ventilation may force air into the stomach; recommend intubation. Always notify the physician of any change in the patient's condition or if there is a complication to any CPR-related procedure.

BIBLIOGRAPHY

AARC clinical practice guideline: Resuscitation in acute care hospitals, *Respir Care* 38(11):1179-1188, 1993.

AARC clinical practice guideline: Defibrillation during resuscitation, *Respir Care* 40(7):744-748.

AARC clinical practice guideline: Management of airway emergencies, *Respir Care* 40(7):749-760.

Abedin Z, Conner RP: *12 lead ECG interpretation: the self-assessment approach*, Philadelphia, 1989, WB Saunders.

Aehlert B: *ECGs Made Easy*. St Louis, 1995, Mosby.

Aloan CA, Hill TV, editors: *Respiratory Care of the Newborn and Child*, ed 2, Philadelphia, 1997, Lippincott-Raven.

Andreoli KG, Fowkes VH, Zipes DP, et al: *Comprehensive cardiac care*, St Louis, 1979, Mosby.

Barnes TA, editor: Core *textbook of respiratory care practice*, ed 2, St Louis, 1994, Mosby.

Barnhart SL, Czervinske MP: *Perinatal and pediatric respiratory care*, Philadelphia, 1995, WB Saunders Company.

Branson RD, Hess DR, Chatburn RL, editors: *Respiratory care equipment*, ed 2, Philadelphia, 1999, Lippincott Williams & Wilkins.

Burton GC, Hodgkin JE, Ward JJ, editors: *Respiratory care: a guide to clinical practice*, ed 4. Philadelphia, 1997, Lippincott-Raven.

Butler HH: How to read an ECG, *RN Magazine* 35-45, Jan 1973.

Butler HH: How to read an ECG, *RN Magazine* 49-61, Feb 1973.

Butler HH: How to read an ECG, *RN Magazine* 50-59, March 1973.

Cairo JM, Pilbeam SP: *Mosby's respiratory care equipment*, ed 6, St Louis, 1999, Mosby.

Davis D: *Differential diagnosis of arrhythmias*, Philadelphia, 1991, WB Saunders.

Emergency Cardiac Care Committee and Subcommittee, American Heart Association: Guidelines for cardiopulmonary resuscitation and emergency cardiac care, *JAMA* 268(16):2184-2281, 1992.

Eubanks DH, Bone RC: *Comprehensive respiratory care*, ed 2, St Louis, 1990, Mosby.

Fink JB, Hunt GE, editors: *Clinical practice in respiratory care*, Philadelphia, 1999, Lippincott-Raven.

Goldberger AL, Goldberger E: *Clinical electrocardiography*, ed 4, St Louis, 1995, Mosby.

Harwood R: *Exam review and study guide for perinatal/pediatric respiratory care*. Philadelphia, 1999, FA Davis Company.

Hess D, Goff G, Johnson K: The effect of hand size, resuscitator brand, and use of two hands on volumes delivered during adult bag-valve ventilation, *Respir Care* 34:805-810, 1989.

Hurst JM, Branson RD, Davis K Jr et al: Cardiopulmonary resuscitation. In Burton GG, Hodgkin JE, Ward JJ: *Respiratory care: a guide to clinical practice*, ed 3, Philadelphia, 1991, JB Lippincott.

Kacmarek RM, Mack CW, Dimas S: *The essentials of respiratory care*, ed 3, St Louis, 1990, Mosby.

Madama VC: Safe mouth-to-mouth resuscitation requires adjunct equipment, caution, *Occupat Health Safety* 60(1):56-64, 1991.

Marriott HJL: *Practical electrocardiography*, ed 7, Baltimore, 1983, Williams & Wilkins.

Pagana K, Pagana TJ: *Mosby's manual of diagnostic and laboratory tests*. St Louis, 1998, Mosby.

Patel JM, McGowan SG, Moody LA: *Arrhythmias: detection, treatment, and cardiac drugs*, Philadelphia, 1989, WB Saunders.

Phillips RE, Feeney MK: *The cardiac rhythms: a systematic approach to interpretation*, ed 3, Philadelphia, 1990, WB Saunders.

Scanlan CL, Wilkins RL, Stoller JK, editors: *Egan's fundamentals of respiratory care*, ed 7, St Louis, 1999, Mosby.

Scanlan CL: Emergency life support. In Scanlan CL, Spearman CB, Sheldon RL, editors: *Egan's fundamentals of respiratory therapy*, ed 5, St Louis, 1990, Mosby.

Shapiro BA, Kacmarek RM, Cane RD, et al, editors: *Clinical application of respiratory care*, ed 4, St Louis, 1991, Mosby.

Standards and guidelines for cardiopulmonary resuscitation (CPR) and emergency cardiac care (ECC). *JAMA* 268:2171-2295, 1992.

Stein E: *Clinical electrocardiography*, Philadelphia, 1987, Lea & Febiger.

Sweetwood HM: *Clinical electrocardiography for nurses*, Rockville, MD, 1983, Aspen Systems.

Wilkins RL, Krider SJ, Sheldon RL: *Clinical Assessment in Respiratory Care*, ed 3, St Louis, 1995, Mosby.

Whitaker K: *Comprehensive perinatal & pediatric respiratory care*, ed 2, Albany, NY, 1997, Delmar.

White GC: *Equipment theory for respiratory care*, ed 3, Albany, NY, 1999, Delmar.

SELF-STUDY QUESTIONS

1. A normal sinus rhythm can be identified by:
   - I. A resting rate of 60 to 100 beats per minute in an adult
   - II. A P wave before every QRS complex
   - III. A regular rhythm
   - IV. A QRS complex after every P wave
   - V. An upright T wave in lead II
   - A. II and IV only
   - B. II, III, and IV only
   - C. I, II, III, and V only
   - D. I, II, III, IV, and V only

2. Your ventilator-dependent patient is set up for routine ECG monitoring. Because of refractory hypoxemia, the physician orders 10 cm water of positive end-expiratory pressure (PEEP). Shortly after the PEEP therapy is added, you notice that the patient has developed sinus arrhythmia. Which of the following is the best course of action to follow?
   A. Recommend the administration of atropine.
   B. Recommend synchronized cardioversion.
   C. Recommend decreasing the PEEP from 10 to 5 cm water.
   D. Make a record of the rhythm and inform the nurse and physician of your observation.
3. Electrocardiogram monitoring is important with an intensive care unit in all of the following situations *except:*
   A. If it is used to evaluate peripheral perfusion.
   B. The patient has an electrolyte disturbance.
   C. The patient has a history of arrhythmias.
   D. The patient is being given a rapid infusion of potassium.
4. Following an exercise routine a 59-year-old male experiences sudden chest pain with shortness of breath. ECG monitoring in the Emergency Department reveals the following rhythm strip. What should the respiratory therapist recommend?

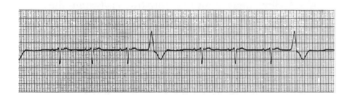

(Wilkins RL, Krider SJ, Sheldon RL: *Clinical assessment in respiratory care,* ed 4, St Louis, 2000, Mosby.)

   I. Synchronized cardioversion
   II. 12-lead ECG
   III. Defibrillation
   IV. Administer oxygen
   V. Angioplasty
   A. I and V only
   B. II and IV only
   C. II, III and IV
   D. I, II, IV, and V only
5. A mouth-to-valve resuscitation device is being used on an apneic patient. The respiratory therapist delivers a breath, but the patient's chest does not rise. What should be done next?
   A. Begin chest compressions.
   B. Request a lateral neck radiograph.
   C. Check the valve for proper position.
   D. Perform abdominal thrusts.
6. Which of the following medications can be administered down the endotracheal tube during a CPR attempt?
   I. Epinephrine
   II. Potassium chloride
   III. Atropine
   IV. Lidocaine
   A. I only
   B. II and III only
   C. I and IV only
   D. I, III, and IV only

7. Two respiratory therapists respond to a cardiopulmonary arrest call and begin CPR procedures on an adult patient. On looking at the ECG monitor, the following rhythm strip is seen. What should be recommended in this situation?

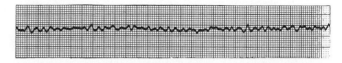

(Goldberger AL, Goldberger E: *Clinical electrocardiography,* ed 4, St Louis, 1995, Mosby.)

   A. Defibrillate the patient.
   B. Increase the oxygen flow to the manual resuscitation bag and mask.
   C. Change ventilation and chest compression duties.
   D. Intubate the patient.
8. CPR steps have been underway for 15 minutes when an arterial blood gas sample is drawn and sent off for analysis. The following results are obtained with 100% oxygen being used to ventilate the patient:
   pH   6.97
   $PaCO_2$ 30 torr
   PaO_2 210 torr
   HCO_3^- 8 mEq/liter
   What should the therapist recommend at this time?
   A. Decrease the oxygen percentage.
   B. Decrease the respiratory rate.
   C. Administer intravenous sodium bicarbonate.
   D. Add mechanical dead space to the manual resuscitator.
9. During a CPR attempt on a 50-year-old patient, the respiratory therapist successfully intubates the patient and begins ventilating with a manual resuscitator. The physician is unable to start an IV line. How should the CPR drugs be given?
   A. Intraosseous injection
   B. Endotracheal instillation
   C. Intracardiac injection
   D. Nasal spray
10. A 59-year-old patient is brought to the hospital with a complaint of sudden, severe substernal chest pain and dyspnea. What is the initial thing that the respiratory therapist should recommend?
   A. Begin ECG monitoring.
   B. Draw an arterial blood gas sample.
   C. Get a chest radiograph.
   D. Get a capnometer value.
11. Defibrillation should be done immediately in which of the following patient situations?
   A. Second degree heart block
   B. Atrial flutter
   C. Pulseless ventricular tachycardia
   D. Sinus tachycardia

Answer Key

1. **D.** Rationale: All of the listed options are found in the normal sinus rhythm. See the text for the discussion, Fig. 10-5 for a tracing, and Table 10-1 for a review if necessary.

2. **D.** Rationale: Sinus arrhythmia is shown in Fig. 10-8. Review the associated discussion if needed. In a patient receiving mechanical ventilation and PEEP, it is possible to put too much pressure on the heart, which reduces venous return. If the returning blood volume is decreased, the cardiac output will also decrease. The patient should be monitored and key people informed. It is too early to decide if the PEEP level is too high and should be reduced. The physician should be consulted before making any change. Atropine will increase the patient's heart rate and is not indicated in this situation. There is no indication that the patient has an arrhythmia that requires synchronized cardioversion.

3. **A.** Rationale: ECG monitoring will not provide any useful information about peripheral perfusion. The patient could have a normal heart rhythm and have altered perfusion. Electrolyte disturbances, especially the potassium (K^+) level, can alter the heart's electrical conduction system. It is wise to monitor a patient with a known history of arrhythmias in case they return. Fast or excessive infusion of potassium can lead to serious arrhythmias that justify ECG monitoring.

4. **B.** Rationale: The rhythm strip shows two identical premature ventricular contractions (PVCs). This, combined with the patient's history of sudden chest pain and shortness of breath, suggest a heart problem. A 12-lead ECG is indicted for the physician to be able to determine the patient's cardiac condition. Oxygen is indicated for the shortness of breath. In addition, the oxygen will help the heart if it is hypoxic. The patient's condition is not life threatening and there is no need for either synchronized cardioversion or defibrillation. A cardiac catheterization procedure is needed to identify any coronary artery blockages before angioplasty is indicated.

5. **C.** Rationale: It is easy and quick to check the valve for proper position. Fix the valve if necessary and attempt to ventilate the patient again. Because the patient's pulse has not yet been checked, there is not yet an indication that chest compressions are needed. Getting a lateral neck radiograph will greatly delay (probably fatally) ventilating the patient. There is not yet an indication that the patient needs abdominal thrusts to clear an airway obstruction. It the patient cannot be ventilated by the fixed mouth-to-valve resuscitation device, check for an obvious obstruction in the mouth or throat. Reposition the head and attempt to ventilate again. If the patient still cannot be ventilated, then perform abdominal thrusts.

6. **D.** Rationale: Current ACLS guidelines state that atropine, epinephrine (both for bradycardia) and lidocaine (to suppress ventricular arrhythmias) can be given via the endotracheal tube during a CPR attempt if the patient does not have a functioning intravenous line. Potassium chloride can be given only intravenously.

7. **A.** Rationale: The rhythm strip shows ventricular fibrillation. The best way to treat this dangerous arrhythmia is to immediately defibrillate the patient. All of the other listed options are reasonable in a CPR attempt when appropriate. However, they are all secondary to treating the patient's ventricular fibrillation.

8. **C.** Rationale: Interpretation of the patient's ABG results shows hyperventilation with a metabolic acidosis. Intravenous sodium bicarbonate should be given to correct the patient's acidosis. It is appropriate to keep the patient's PaO_2 at 210 torr during the CPR attempt to try to oxygenate the brain. Decreasing the respiratory rate or adding mechanical dead space to the manual resuscitator will result in the patient's carbon dioxide rising and a further lowering of the pH.

9. **B.** Rationale: Current ACLS guidelines state that atropine, epinephrine, and lidocaine can be given via the endotracheal tube during a CPR attempt if the patient does not have a functioning intravenous line. Intraosseous (within the bone) injection of CPR drugs is approved for neonatal resuscitation attempts. Intracardiac injection of CPR drugs should be tried only if the endotracheal drug route is unsuccessful. Currently CPR drugs are not given by nasal spray.

10. **A.** Rationale: The patient's symptoms indicate a cardiac problem. It is wise to quickly begin ECG monitoring in case the patient has an arrhythmia. An arterial blood gas sample can be drawn after ECG monitoring is started. A chest radiograph can also be done after ECG monitoring is started. A capnometer value to check the patient's exhaled carbon dioxide value is not indicated at this time.

11. **C.** Rationale: Pulseless ventricular tachycardia is a life-threatening arrhythmia. See Fig. 10-24. If the rate is so fast that a pulse cannot be felt, the cardiac output and blood pressure will be very low. The patient must be defibrillated as soon as possible to restore normal sinus rhythm. Second degree heart block is treated with drugs or a pacemaker to speed up the heart rate. Atrial flutter and sinus tachycardia are fast, but not lifethreatening, arrhythmias that are first treated with medications to slow down the heart rate.

11 Airway Management

A review of the most recent Written Registry Exams has shown an average of six questions (6% of the exam) on airway management.

MODULE A | **Care for the following artificial airways and equipment to maintain a patent airway**

---

1. Properly position the patient to maintain a patent airway and minimize hypoxemia (Code: IIIB1d) [Difficulty: An]

Positioning of the head to open the airway is discussed in Chapter 10. Briefly, use the head tilt-chin lift maneuver to hyperextend the neck of an adult, and slightly extend the neck of a child to open the airway. You can place a small pad behind the neck and head to put the patient in the "sniff position." Always keep the head in line with the body. If the patient has a known or suspected cervical spine injury, the neck cannot be hyperextended. Instead, open the airway with the jaw-thrust maneuver. Keep the head in line with the body.

The patient may be supine during the airway-opening procedures just mentioned. Frequently, however, the patient is positioned with the head and body elevated. An unconscious patient is less likely to vomit and aspirate in either the Fowler's or semi-Fowler's position. The combination of either of these body positions and the head and neck hyperextended into the sniff position will probably keep the airway open, minimize the risk of aspiration of vomitus, and minimize the patient's work of breathing (WOB). This should help to minimize hypoxemia.

2. Humidify an artificial airway (Code: IIIB1b) [Difficulty: An]

Patients with an endotracheal or tracheostomy tube in place should ideally be provided 100% relative humidity at body temperature. If not, secretions in the airway may dry and result in mucous plugs. Patients with an oropharyngeal or nasopharyngeal airway may also be given supplemental humidity by a simple aerosol mask to help prevent drying of secretions. See Chapter 7 for a complete discussion of humidity and aerosol therapy and administrative devices.

3. Oropharyngeal airways
a. Get the necessary equipment (Code: IIA1f1) [Difficulty: An]

The oropharyngeal airway (or bite block) is made of plastic that is hard enough to withstand any patient's biting force. This airway is indicated in two situations. First, it is used in an unconscious, supine patient who is experiencing upper airway obstruction because the tongue is falling back and blocking the oropharynx. Second, the oropharyngeal airway is used in a patient who is unconscious and biting down hard when having a seizure. This can cause injury to the patient or pinch off an oral endotracheal tube if one is present.

A properly sized and placed oropharyngeal airway lifts the tongue forward from the posterior portion of the oropharynx to keep a patent airway and make suctioning oral secretions easier. An oropharyngeal airway is poorly tolerated in a conscious patient and can cause gagging and even vomiting. Oropharyngeal airways come in a variety of sizes from infant to adult. The proper size is found by holding the airway against the patient's face with the flange against the lips. The end of the airway should reach the angle of the jaw (Fig. 11-1). Too large an airway can block the oropharynx by extending past the tongue. Too small an airway can push the tongue back into the oropharynx rather than pulling the tongue forward as it should. Fig. 11-2 shows a properly placed and sized oropharyngeal airway.

A number of manufacturers make oropharyngeal airways, which fall into two basic types: hollow center and I-beam (Fig. 11-3).

1. Hollow center

Hollow center types have an oval or rectangular shape in cross section and are hollow in the center. A suction catheter can be easily placed through the hollow center so that the back of the throat can be cleared of secretions. Some types have an outer tube that can be attached by a practitioner to provide a mouthpiece for rescue breathing. If rescue breathing must be performed, it is probably more effective to ventilate with a mask and manual resuscitator when one becomes available.

2. I-beam

I-beam types are shaped like an I-beam in cross section. A suction catheter can easily be guided along the groove on either side of the I-beam to the back of the throat so that secretions can be cleared out.

b. Put the equipment together, make sure that it works properly, and identify any problems (Code: IIB1f1) [Difficulty: An]

Most oropharyngeal airways are single units. There is nothing to assemble. There are some hollow-center types that have an attachable outer part. The outer part is

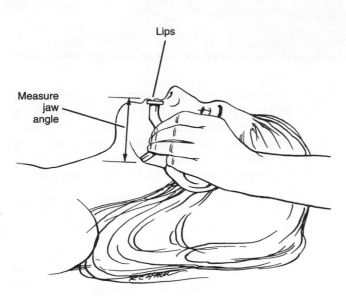

Fig. 11-1 Procedure for measuring the proper size of the oropharyngeal airway. (From Eubanks DH, Bone RC: *Comprehensive respiratory care,* ed 2, St Louis, 1990, Mosby.)

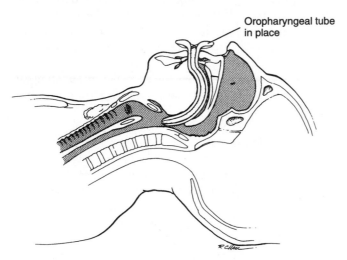

Fig. 11-2 Cross section through the head showing the proper position of an oropharyngeal airway. (From Eubanks DH, Bone RC: *Comprehensive respiratory care,* ed 2, St Louis, 1990, Mosby.)

snapped onto the oropharyngeal airway when the practitioner must perform rescue breathing. It has a wide flange so that the lips can be covered and sealed to prevent a leak.

c. Fix any problems with the equipment (Code: IIB2f1) [Difficulty: An]

Make sure that the channel in the hollow-center types is patent. If a unit is plugged by secretions, blood, or a foreign substance, the patient cannot breathe through the

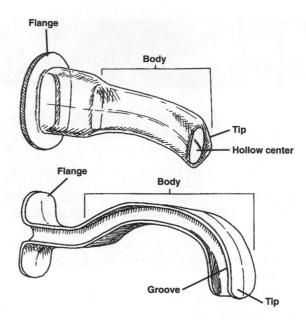

Fig. 11-3 Close-ups of hollow and I-beam types of oropharyngeal airways.

opening. A suction catheter cannot be passed through either. Remove an airway that the patient cannot breathe through.

d. Insert the correct oropharyngeal airway (Code: IIIB1a) [Difficulty: An]

There are two widely used methods to insert an oropharyngeal airway.

1. First method

a. Open the patient's mouth with the cross-finger technique. Insert the airway backward into the patient's mouth until it reaches the palate. Some authors recommend inserting it past the uvula.

b. Twist the airway 180 degrees, and insert it the rest of the way until the tongue is supported by the curved body.

c. The flange should rest at the lips (Fig. 11-4).

2. Second method

a. Open the patient's mouth with the cross-finger technique. Insert the airway into the mouth with the curved body rotated toward a cheek.

b. Twist the airway 90 degrees, and insert it the rest of the way so that the tongue is supported by the curved body.

c. The flange should rest at the lips.

4. Nasopharyngeal airways

a. Get the necessary equipment (Code: IIA1f1) [Difficulty: An]

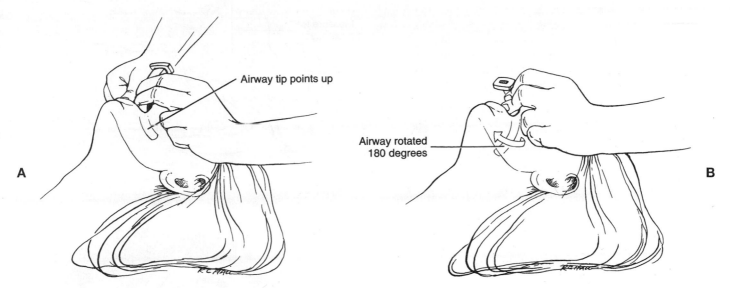

Fig. 11-4 Procedure for inserting an oropharyngeal airway. **A,** Airway is placed with the tip pointing toward the palate. **B,** Airway is rotated 180 degrees to support the tongue. (From Eubanks DH, Bone RC: *Comprehensive respiratory care,* ed 2, St Louis, 1990, Mosby.)

Nasopharyngeal airways (also known as nasal airways, nasal trumpets, or nasal stints) are made of a relatively soft and pliable plastic or rubber. This decreases the chances of damaging the delicate mucous membranes of the nose and nasopharynx. A nasopharyngeal airway is often used in a supine patient to ensure a patent airway by pushing the tongue forward off of the posterior portion of the oropharynx. The nasopharyngeal airway is probably not as effective in keeping the tongue forward as the oropharyngeal airway. However, it is better tolerated in a semiconscious or alert patient.

It is also commonly used to provide a secure channel through which to pass a suction catheter or bronchoscope. The nasopharyngeal airway protects the patient's mucous membranes from the trauma of repeatedly passed catheters. Another use is in a patient with trauma to the jaw or in a patient with seizures with a tightly closed jaw. In these cases an oropharyngeal airway cannot be used. The nasopharyngeal airway can be passed into the patient's oropharynx to push the tongue forward and maintain an airway.

Several manufacturers make the two basic types of nasopharyngeal airways, the *blunt tip* and the *beveled tip.* The beveled-tip types come with right-sided and left-sided cut bevels. If possible, get the airway with the bevel cut that opens toward the patient's oropharynx (toward the nasal septum). For example, if the airway is going to be inserted into the left naris, the bevel should be cut on the right side of the tube so that it is open to the patient's oropharynx. If you were inserting the tube into the right nostril, you would want the bevel cut on the left side of the tube.

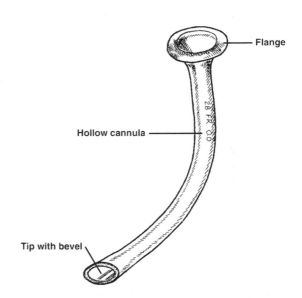

Fig. 11-5 Typical nasopharyngeal airway.

See Fig. 11-5 for a close-up of a nasopharyngeal airway. All nasopharyngeal airways have a flange that fits up close to the patient's nostril. This prevents the entire tube from being pushed into the patient. All nasopharyngeal airways have a cannula with a channel for breathing or suctioning through. Nasopharyngeal airways come in a variety of sizes for adults. They can be properly sized by measuring from the tip of the nose to the tragus of the ear and adding 2 to 3 cm (Fig. 11-6).

Fig. 11-6 Procedure for measuring the proper size of the nasopharyngeal airway. (From Eubanks DH, Bone RC: *Comprehensive respiratory care,* ed 2, St Louis, 1990, Mosby.)

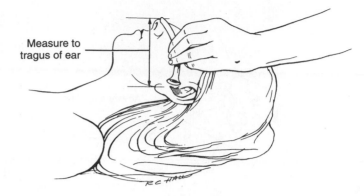

Measure to tragus of ear

b. Put the equipment together, make sure that it works properly, and identify any problems (Code: IIB1f1) [Difficulty: An]

c. Fix any problems with the equipment (Code: IIB2f1) [Difficulty: An]

All nasopharyngeal airways are made up of a single piece. There is nothing to assemble. Make sure that the tube is not plugged by dried secretions, blood, or a foreign body. If plugged, the patient cannot breath through it, and a suction catheter cannot be passed through it. Remove a plugged nasopharyngeal airway.

d. Insert the correct nasopharyngeal airway (Code: IIIB1a) [Difficulty: An]

The following steps are used for nasopharyngeal airway insertion:

1. Select the most patent nostril. Check the patient's chart for a history of a broken nose, deviated septum, or current head cold. Interview the conscious patient to see whether one nostril is more open than the other. Place your finger in front of the patient's nostrils to feel which one has greater airflow. Avoid forcing the airway into a nostril and nasal passage that may be damaged by the procedure.
2. Lubricate the properly sized airway with a sterile, water-soluble lubricant such as K-Y jelly. Place the lubricant on a sterile, 4 x 4-in gauze pad, and then smear it over the length of the airway.
3. Tell the patient what you are going to do.
4. Gently place the airway into the nostril. It should be directed straight back parallel to the hard palate. Stop if you feel any resistance. Try a different angle if resistance is felt. Do not force the airway. Try the other nostril if necessary.
5. Check the placement by looking into the patient's mouth with a flashlight and tongue depressor. A properly placed nasopharyngeal airway can be seen in the oropharynx and extends behind the tongue (Figs. 11-7 and 11-8).
6. Secure the airway by sticking a safety pin through the flange and taping the pin to the bridge of the patient's

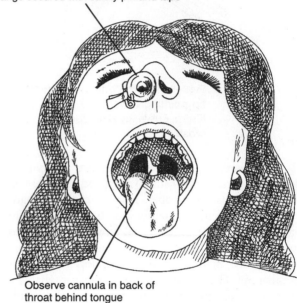

Flange secured with safety pin and tape

Observe cannula in back of throat behind tongue

Fig. 11-7 Proper position of the nasopharyngeal airway behind the tongue can be determined by looking into the mouth. The tube is also secured by placing a safety pin through the flange and taping it to the cheek.

nose or cheek (see Fig. 11-7). This helps prevent the airway from being accidentally pulled out or pushed in.

7. Rotate the airway to the other nostril, if possible, on a regular basis. This helps prevent ulceration of the mucous membrane. Some authors recommend rotation at least every 48 hours, whereas others recommend rotation at much shorter time intervals.

5. Tracheostomy tubes

a. Get the necessary equipment (Code: IIA1f3 and IIIB1a) [Difficulty: An]

The tracheostomy tube offers the same uses as the endotracheal tube such as maintaining a secure airway, providing a direct suctioning route to the lungs, preventing aspiration, and assuring a safe route to provide mechanical ventilation. In addition, it is placed in the patient who has

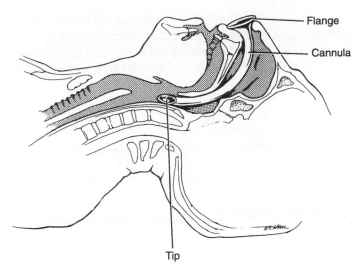

Flange
Cannula
Tip

Fig. 11-8 Cross section of head showing the proper position of the nasopharyngeal airway. (From Ellis PD, Billings DM: *Cardiopulmonary resuscitation: procedures for basic and advanced life support,* St Louis, 1980, Mosby.)

an upper airway obstruction or facial trauma that makes intubation impossible. A tracheostomy tube is often placed in a patient who requires long-term mechanical ventilation or who needs a permanent artificial airway. In the long term, a tracheostomy is said to be more comfortable than an endotracheal tube, even though it requires a surgical procedure. An additional advantage of a tracheostomy tube over an endotracheal tube is that it allows the patient to eat and drink.

These tubes come in a variety of sizes for patients of all ages from neonate to adult. See Table 11-1 for tracheostomy tube sizes based on patient age. Most modern tracheostomy tubes are constructed of a hard polyvinyl chloride (PVC) plastic and have a high-volume, low-pressure cuff. Some specialty tubes are made of silver, rubber, or latex. The older, silver tubes have a cuff that may be removed. Specific information on three types of tubes is given in the following text.

b. Put the equipment together, make sure that it works properly, and identify any problems (Code: IIB1f3) [Difficulty: An]

The following are commonly seen examples of tracheostomy tube styles:

1. Standard tracheostomy tube

The majority of patients have a standard tube placed after the tracheostomy procedure. Refer to Fig. 11-9 for these features of a typical tracheostomy tube:

a The cannula is the airway through which the patient breathes. The proximal end is outside of the patient's stoma and attached to an adjustable flange. The angle of the flange can be adjusted so that the distal end of the cannula fits properly into the patient's trachea. Soft, cloth tracheostomy tie strings are tied to the ends of the flange. The loose ends are tied behind the patient's neck to hold the tube in place. The distal end of the cannula

TABLE 11-1	Endotracheal and Tracheostomy Tube Sizes Based on Patient Age*		
Age	ID (mm)	Approximate OD (mm)	Fr size (OD)
NEWBORN			
<1000 g	2.5	4.0	12
1000-2000 g	3.0	5.0	14
2000-3000 g	3.5	5.5	16-18
3000 g to 6 mo old	3.5-4.0		
PEDIATRIC			
18 mo	4.0	6.0	18
3 yr	4.5	6.5	20
5 yr	5.0	7.0	22
6 yr	5.5	8.0	24
8 yr	6.0	9.0	26
ADULT			
16 yr	7.0	10.0	30
Normal-sized woman	7.5-8.0	11.0	32-34
Normal-sized man	8.0-8.5	12.0	34-36
Large adult	9.0-10.0	13.0-14.0	38-42

ID, Internal diameter; *OD*, outer diameter; *Fr*, French.
*Two notes: First, it is important to always use the largest tube that can be placed into the patient without causing any harm during the intubation. This is because the larger the ID of the tube, the less airway resistance it causes. Be prepared to insert a tube that is one size larger or smaller than anticipated based on individual variances. Second, the mathematical relationship between the OD in millimeters and Fr size can be easily calculated. The Fr size is determined by multiplying the OD in millimeters by 3. The OD in millimeters is found by dividing the Fr size by 3.

has a small area where radiopaque material is imbedded. As with an endotracheal tube, this allows the end of the cannula to be seen on a chest radiograph. The cuff is a high residual volume, low-pressure type. Air is put into and taken out of the cuff by an inflation tube with a pilot balloon and one-way valve.

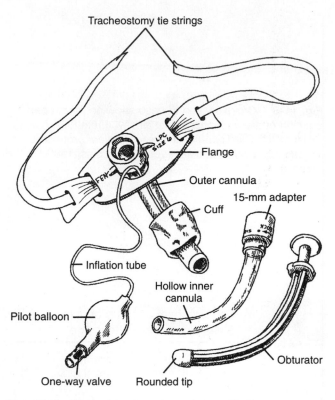

Tracheostomy tie strings

Flange

Outer cannula

15-mm adapter

Cuff

Inflation tube

Hollow inner cannula

Pilot balloon

Obturator

One-way valve   Rounded tip

Fig. 11-9 Typical tracheostomy tube with its component parts and features.

b. The obturator is slid into the outer cannula's opening before it is inserted into the patient's stoma. The obturator has a rounded end that protrudes from the end of the cannula. This prevents any tissue trauma during the insertion. The obturator is removed as soon as the cannula is in place.

c. An inner cannula is slid into the outer cannula's opening and locked into place with a clockwise twist. This completes the airway. The proximal end has a standard 15-mm outer diameter (OD) adapter so that all respiratory care equipment fits onto it. The distal end is flush with the end of the outer cannula. Some practitioners believe that the inner cannula should be periodically removed and cleaned so that secretions do not build up. Other practitioners believe that this is unnecessary if the airway is properly humidified and suctioning is performed as needed.

2. Fenestrated tracheostomy tube

A fenestrated tube is often placed in a patient who can breathe spontaneously and who is being considered for a complete removal of the tracheostomy tube. If the patient does well with this tube, it can probably be removed safely. If the patient has difficulty, the plug can be removed, the inner cannula can be replaced, and the patient's airway can be suctioned or mechanically ventilated.

Refer to Fig. 11-10 when reviewing these features of the fenestrated tracheostomy tube:
a. The outer cannula has an opening called the fenestration (Dutch for window). The rest of the cannula, cuff, inflation tube, and flange are the same as already discussed.
b. The inner cannula functions as discussed earlier. When it is in place, the tube functions as the standard model does.
c. The outer cannula plug is used to prevent the patient from breathing through the proximal end of the tube. The plug does not cover the fenestration; therefore the patient is able to breathe through the upper airway. The patient can now talk and cough out any secretions.

EXAM HINT

A standard tracheostomy tube should be replaced with a fenestrated tube when a patient is improving and can breathe spontaneously (off of the ventilator) for an extended period of time. Remove the inner cannula so that the patient can breathe through the upper airway. Replace the inner cannula when mechanical ventilation is resumed.

---

3. Speaking tracheostomy tube

Refer to Fig. 11-11 when reviewing these features of the speaking tracheostomy tube:
a. The cannula is the standard type except that an additional tube has been added to carry a compressed gas through a hole in the back of the cannula. This gas flows up through the vocal cords and allows the patient to speak. The voice is not as strong as normal but is still a great help to the patient's psychologic well-being. The patient can still be mechanically ventilated and suctioned, and can eat and drink as usual.
b. A Y-connector is added to the compressed gas tube. Usually about 4 to 6 L/min of compressed air or oxygen are set by a flowmeter to run to the Y. Closing off the other opening in the Y with a finger diverts the gas into the patient's larynx for speaking. A little experimentation with flows helps the patient find the flow that works best for speaking.

c. Fix any problems with the equipment (Code: IIB2f3) [Difficulty: An]

Most tubes have cuffs that must be inflated before insertion into the patient to make sure that the cuff is sealed and the one-way valve does not leak. Do not use a tube with a leaking cuff or leaking one-way valve. Make sure that the obturator, inner cannula, and plug all fit properly into the outer cannula. They all should easily snap into place and be easily removable. Check this before inserting the tube into the patient.

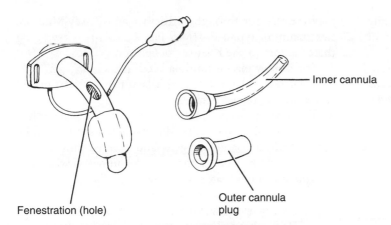

Fig. 11-10   Fenestrated tracheostomy tube with its component parts and features. (From Eubanks DH, Bone RC: *Comprehensive respiratory care,* ed 2, St Louis, 1990, Mosby.)

Inner cannula

Fenestration (hole)

Outer cannula plug

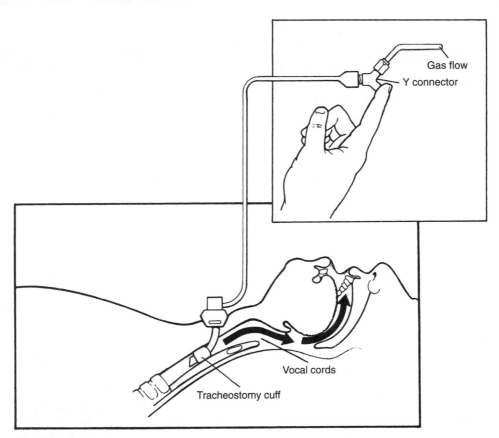

Gas flow

Y connector

Vocal cords

Tracheostomy cuff

Fig. 11-11   Pitt tracheostomy tube permits the patient to speak. Note its special feature that directs outside gas flow past the vocal cords. (From Simmons KF: Airway care. In Scanlan CL, Spearman CB, Sheldon RL, editors: *Egan's fundamentals of respiratory care,* ed 5, St Louis, 1990, Mosby.)

EXAM HINT

The following things can plug the lumen of the cannula: (1) Secretions or foreign matter. (2) A cuff that has herniated or slipped over the end of the tube. (3) Placement of the tip of the tube into the subcutaneous tissues. Initially, attempt to suction to remove any obstruction. If the catheter cannot be inserted beyond the tube and the patient is having respiratory distress, the tube must be removed and replaced.

---

6. Tracheostomy buttons

a. Get the necessary equipment (Code: IIA1f3) [Difficulty: An]

A tracheostomy button is a hard plastic tube that is placed into the patient's stoma to keep it open after the tracheostomy tube has been removed. The patient is able to eat, talk, and cough normally. Yet, in case the patient has difficulty or needs a breathing treatment, the airway can be reestablished quickly. In general, the patient sizes for tracheostomy buttons match the sizes for tracheostomy tubes listed in Table 11-1. Information on two types of buttons is given in the following text.

b. Put the equipment together, make sure that it works properly, and identify any problems with it (Code: IIB1f3) [Difficulty: An]

Refer to Fig. 11-12 when reviewing these features of the tracheostomy button:

1. The hollow outer cannula has a slightly flared proximal end. This keeps the button from slipping entirely into the patient. The distal end is flanged and split into several flexible "grippers."
2. A closure plug fits into the outer cannula and snaps into the flexible grippers on the end of the outer cannula. This seals the button so that the patient breathes through the upper airway.
3. A hollow inner cannula can be inserted into the outer cannula instead of the plug. This inner cannula has a standard 15-mm OD so that a T-piece/Briggs adapter or other respiratory care equipment can be attached if needed. The patient can also be suctioned.
4. Spacers of various widths are used to make sure that the inner cannula is placed at the right depth. The end of the tube should enter the trachea but not obstruct it. See the airway picture in Fig. 11-12 for the proper position.

Special tracheostomy buttons are used with patients who are not to breathe in through their upper airway but may breathe out through it. Kistner and Passey-Muir are two common types. Refer to Fig. 11-13 when reviewing these features of the Kistner tracheostomy tube:

1. The hollow plastic cannula keeps the stoma open. The distal end is flanged so that it is not likely to be pulled out of the trachea accidentally.
2. The proximal end of the cannula is capped with a one-way valve. The valve allows the patient to breathe in room air or an oxygen- and aerosol-enriched gas source. Expiration is through the upper airway. The patient can talk, eat, and cough normally.

c. Fix any problems with the equipment (Code: IIB2f3) [Difficulty: An]

Make sure that all component pieces of these tracheostomy buttons fit together properly and can be easily disconnected if necessary. The cannula must be kept clear of any secretions, blood, or foreign debris. A suction catheter should be passable through the hollow opening in the cannula. If the button is obstructed and the patient is having trouble breathing through the upper airway, the button should be removed and replaced with another button or a tracheostomy tube.

7. Get a laryngeal mask airway (Code: IIA1f5) [Difficulty: R, Ap, An]

A laryngeal mask airway (LMA) is used by an anesthesiologist to provide a way to ventilate an anesthetized patient without placing an endotracheal tube. The

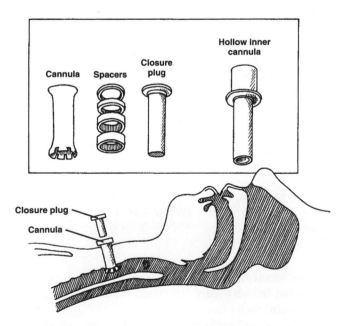

Fig. 11-12 Typical tracheostomy button properly positioned in patient. Insert shows its component parts.

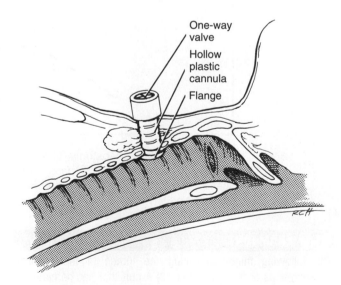

Fig. 11-13 Kistner tracheotomy button. (From Eubanks DH, Bone RC: *Comprehensive respiratory care*, ed 2, St Louis, 1990, Mosby.)

LMA comes in six sizes. The appropriate size depends on the weight of the patient. LMAs range from size 1 to size 5. Size 1 is for children under 6.5 kg, size 2½ for children from 20 to 30 kg, size 4 for an average adult of 70 to 80 kg, and size 5 for an adult more than 80 kg. As seen in Fig. 11-14, the distal end of the LMA has a cuff that surrounds and seals the larynx when it is inflated. The proximal end of the attached tube has a standard adapter for ventilation with a manual resuscitator or an anesthesia machine. The LMA does not absolutely protect against aspiration and tidal volume gas can leak if mechanical ventilation pressures greater than about 20 cm H_2O are needed. In these situations, an appropriately sized endotracheal tube may be inserted through the LMA into the patient's trachea to provide a more secure airway and assure consistent tidal volume delivery.

8. Get an esophageal obturator airway (Code: IIA1f5) [Difficulty: R, Ap, An]

An esophageal obturator airway, and its variations, is designed to be placed into the esophagus of an unconscious adult patient. There are four different types that provide the same two functions: to ensure a stable airway for artificial ventilation and to prevent vomiting and aspiration. See Box 11-1 for the indications for these tubes

and a comparison with an endotracheal tube. Because the four airway types have different features, an illustration and brief explanation of each follow.

Esophageal obturator airway (EOA). The original EOA is shown in Fig. 11-15 and is a modified adultsize endotra-

---

BOX 11-1 Indications, Contraindications, Advantages, and Disadvantages of the Various Esophageal Obturator Airway Devices

---

GENERAL INDICATIONS

Emergency personnel are not trained in endotracheal intubation.

Attempted endotracheal intubation has not been successful.

Patient is apneic, without reflexes, and unconscious.

GENERAL CONTRAINDICATIONS

Endotracheal intubation can be performed.

Patient is responsive with an intact gag reflex.

Patient is less than 16 years old or less than 5 feet tall.

Esophageal obturator device would be needed for more than 1 to 2 hours.

Patient is known to have esophageal trauma, pathology, or to have ingested a corrosive substance.

ORIGINAL ESOPHAGEAL OBTURATOR AIRWAY (EOA) ADVANTAGES

Rapid control of the airway.

Can be inserted into the patient in an awkward position without the head or neck being hyperextended.

Prevents the insufflation of gas into the stomach during bag-mask ventilation.

Prevents the movement of stomach contents into the pharynx.

ESOPHAGEAL GASTRIC TUBE AIRWAY (EGTA) ADVANTAGES

All of the above.

The stomach can be emptied.

ESOPHAGEAL-TRACHEAL COMBITUBE (ETC) AND PHARYNGEAL TRACHEAL LUMEN (PTL) AIRWAY ADVANTAGES

All of the above.

The stomach can be emptied.

The patient can be ventilated whether the tube is placed into the esophagus (as intended) or trachea.

Prevents aspiration of blood from the upper airway.

DISADVANTAGES OF THE ESOPHAGEAL OBTURATOR DEVICES

Accidental and unrecognized tracheal intubation by the EOA or EGTA tubes.

Possibility of upper airway tear and hemorrhage during tube insertion.

Incomplete airway or face mask seal resulting in air leak during ventilation.

The airway cannot be reliably kept open.

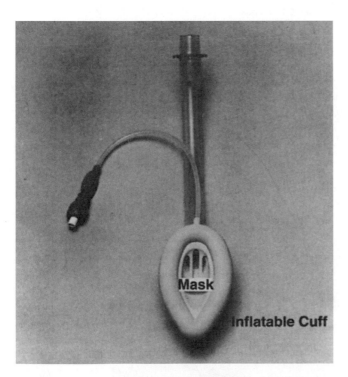

Fig. 11-14 Laryngeal mask airway (LMA). It features an inflatable mask that creates a seal around the patient's larynx. The proximal end of the tube can be connected to a resuscitation bag, anesthesia machine, or mechanical ventilator. (From Intavent International SA, Henley-on-Thames, England.)

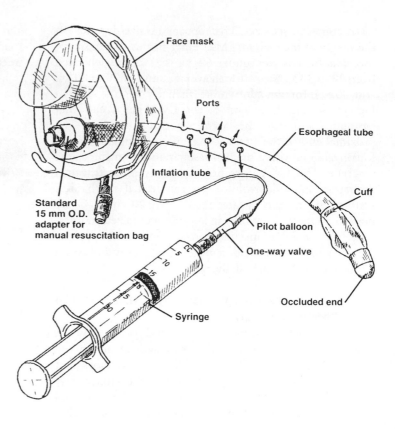

Fig. 11-15 An original esophageal obturator airway (EOA) with its component parts and features. Note the occluded end of the endotracheal tube, the ports cut into the tube, and the face mask designed only for this unit. A standard resuscitation face mask does not fit onto the adapter on the end of the endotracheal tube. (From Sills JR: *Respiratory care certification guide,* ed 1, St Louis, 1991, Mosby.)

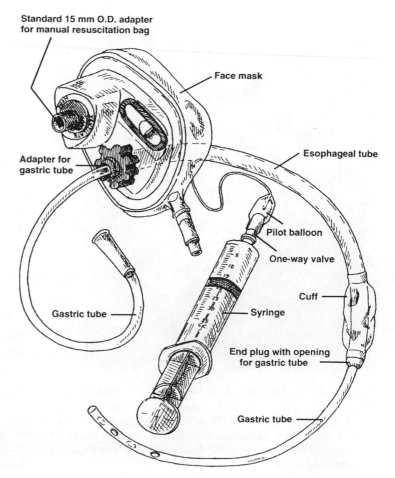

Fig. 11-16 An esophageal gastric tube airway (EGTA) with its component parts and features. Note the gastric tube to empty the patient's stomach and the face mask designed only for this unit. A standard resuscitation face mask does not fit onto the adapter on the end of the endotracheal tube. (From Sills JR: *Respiratory care certification guide,* ed 1, St Louis, 1991, Mosby.)

cheal tube. The distal end of the tube has been plugged and ports have been cut into the tube. When the tube is inserted into the patient's esophagus, the cuff inflated, and the special face mask sealed on the patient's face, the patient can be ventilated with a manual resuscitation bag. The ventilated gas exits the ports and enters the patient's lungs.

Esophageal gastric tube airway (EGTA). The EGTA is similar in function to the EOA except that the patient's stomach contents can be removed. As seen in Fig. 11-16, a gastric (Levine) tube can be inserted through the esophageal tube and into the patient's stomach.

Pharyngeal tracheal lumen airway. The pharyngeal tracheal lumen (PTL) is shown in Fig. 11-17. It consists of two endotracheal tubes, one having a bite block wrapped around its distal end. With a PTL, the patient can be ventilated whether the tube is placed into the esophagus or into the trachea. After insertion, the rescuer blows into the mouthpiece to inflate the cuff on the endotracheal tube and to inflate a larger cuff around the

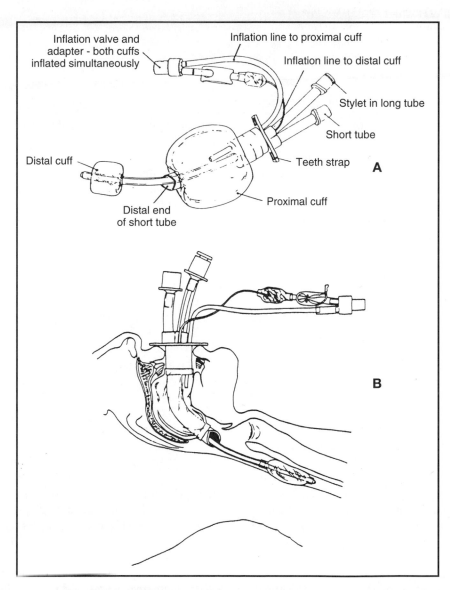

Fig. 11-17   Pharyngeal tracheal lumen (PTL) airway. **A,** Shows PTL with its distal cuff (in esophagus or trachea) and proximal cuff (in pharynx) inflated. The patient can be ventilated through either the long tube or short tube depending on the placement of the distal end of the long tube. **B,** Shows intended placement of the long tube into patient's esophagus. When both cuffs are inflated, the patient will be ventilated through the short tube. (From Moore EE, Mattox KL, Feliciano DP: *Trauma,* Norwalk, CN, 1991, Appleton & Lange. Reproduced with the permission of the McGraw-Hill Companies.)

Fig. 11-18 Esophageal-tracheal Combitube (ETC) with its components and features. Note the two lumens of the ETC with its distal cuff (in patient's esophagus or trachea) and proximal cuff in patient's pharynx, and perforations between the two cuffs that allow ventilation through the esophageal port. Depending on placement of the tube in the esophagus (as intended) or trachea, the patient can be ventilated through the esophageal or tracheal port when both cuffs are inflated. (From Blosser SA, Stauffer JL: *Clin Chest Med,* 17:355-378, 1996.)

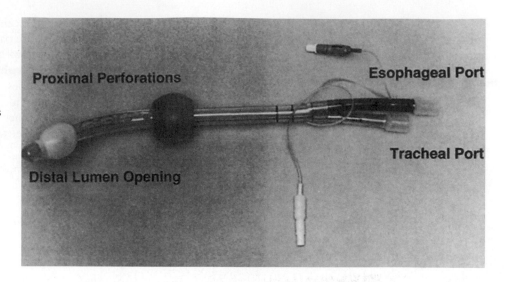

bite block. The cuff on the endotracheal tube seals the esophagus (or trachea) and the larger cuff seals the pharynx. Depending on the placement of the endotracheal tube into the esophagus (as intended) or the trachea, the patient can be ventilated through the appropriate endotracheal tube.

Esophageal-tracheal combitube. The esophageal-tracheal combitube (ETC) is shown in Fig. 11-18 and is a double-lumen tube. With the ETC, the patient can be ventilated whether the tube is placed into the esophagus or trachea. Its two cuffs are individually inflated to seal the esophagus (or trachea) and pharynx. Depending on the placement of the endotracheal tube into the esophagus (as intended) or the trachea, the patient can be ventilated through the appropriate tube lumen.

Clinical experience with the four types of esophageal obturator airways is highly recommended because they do not operate like standard endotracheal tubes.

9. Intubation equipment: laryngoscope and blades
a. Get the necessary equipment (Code: IIA1f4) [Difficulty: An]

The laryngoscope is made up of two basic parts: a handle and a blade. The most commonly seen handle is made of stainless steel; some newer units are made of plastic. The handle contains two C-cell batteries to power the light source in the blade. They all have a common base with a hooking bar so that the blades can be attached (Figs. 11-19 and 11-20).

Blades come in a variety of sizes from pediatric to adult. They all have a common hook so that they can be snapped and locked in place on the handle. The stainless steel handles use stainless steel blades. The newer plastic handles use plastic blades. The two different sets of handles and blades are not interchangeable. The blades come in two different shapes. The Miller blades are straight and MacIntosh blades are curved (see Fig. 11-19). The

intubating person may specify a particular style of blade as well as blade size.

b. Put the equipment together, make sure that it works properly, and identify any problems (Code: IIB1f4) [Difficulty: An]

See Fig. 11-20 for the steps in fastening the blade to the handle:
1. Hold the handle in the left hand and the blade in the right hand.
2. Place the hook on the blade over the hooking bar on the base of the handle.
3. Pull the blade down so that it snaps into place on the handle. The handle and blade should fit together at a 90-degree angle.
4. Make sure that the light bulb in the stainless steel blade is tight.

c. Fix any problems with the equipment (Code: IIB2f4) [Difficulty: An]

The light source shines when the handle and blade are properly connected because an electrical circuit has been completed. Failure of the light source to shine may result from any of the following problems:
1. The handle and blade are not properly connected and snapped into place. Disconnect them by performing the opposite motions and reconnect them properly.
2. There are cross-connected stainless steel and plastic components. Stainless steel handles go only with stainless steel blades, and plastic handles go with plastic blades.
3. The batteries are low, as shown by the bulb failing to glow or glowing with a yellow instead of a white light. Unscrew the cap from the handle. Replace the old batteries with two new C-cell batteries. When reassembled, the bulb should glow with a white light.
4. The batteries are not placed properly. The positive poles

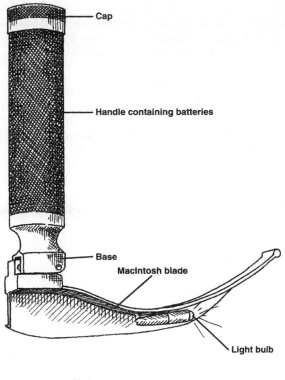

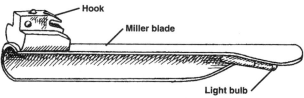

Fig. 11-19 Laryngoscope handle with a MacIntosh (curved) blade attached. A Miller (straight) blade is shown below for comparison. Note component parts and features.

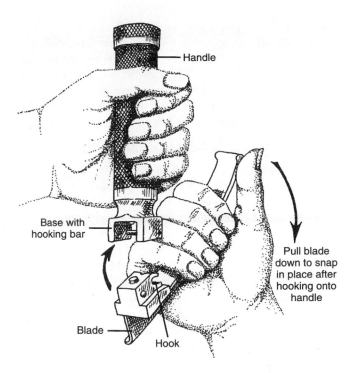

Fig. 11-20   Motions to attach a laryngoscope to a handle.

(+) must be toward the base of the handle, and the negative poles (−) must be toward the cap of the handle. When reassembled, the bulb should glow with a white light.

5. The lightbulb in the stainless steel blade is loose or defective. Tighten the lightbulb by turning it clockwise. It should light up if it was just loose. Unscrew and throw away a defective lightbulb. Replace it with a lightbulb of the same size. When reassembled, the bulb should glow with a white light. The newer plastic laryngoscopes use a fiberoptic bundle as the light source. There is no lightbulb to tighten or replace.

Besides the laryngoscope handle and blades, there are a number of additional items that are typically needed to ensure a smooth, safe intubation procedure. These are listed in Box 11-2.

> **EXAM HINT**
>
> Know how to trouble shoot and fix a malfunctioning laryngoscope and blade.

BOX 11-2	Equipment for Oral and Nasal Intubation

Pediatric and adult laryngoscope handles with batteries
Straight and curved pediatric and adult laryngoscope blades
Variety of nasal and oral endotracheal tubes
Water-soluble, sterile lubricant
Metal stylet
Magill forceps for nasal intubation
Hemostat
Tongue depressors
Oropharyngeal airways
Bite block
Nasopharyngeal airways
10-mL syringe with three-way stopcock
Manometer to measure intracuff pressure
Tape or tube-restraining device
Yankauer or other oral suction device
Sterile suction catheter for tracheal suctioning
Stethoscope for listening to breath sounds

10. Oral and nasal endotracheal tubes

a. Get the necessary equipment (Code: IIA1f2 and IIIB1a) [Difficulty: An]

An endotracheal tube is the best emergency device for maintaining a secure airway. It also provides a direct suctioning route to the lungs and prevents aspiration. Mechanical ventilation can easily be provided through it. An endotracheal tube is meant to be a temporary airway; however it can be kept in patients for weeks if necessary. Virtually all endotracheal tubes used clinically now are made of pliable plastic. Always select a tube that has a large residual volume and low pressure cuff unless there is a specific reason not to do so. For the most part, oral and nasal endotracheal tubes can be used interchangeably. The nasal endotracheal tube is longer and more curved than an oral endotracheal tube. The greater curve of the nasal tube should result in less pressure on the nasal mucosa. An anesthesiologist requests a nasal tube if he or she is going to place it by the nasal route. Oral tubes are used in the majority of patients.

The tubes come in sizes from 4-mm OD through 14-mm OD so that patients of all ages and sizes can be intubated. The OD size increments are 0.5 mm. The thickness of the outer wall of the tube varies from 0.5 to 1 mm, which results in a reduction of the inner diameter (ID) of the tube by about 1 to 2 mm. Table 11-1 lists the approximate ID of an endotracheal tube to place into a patient based on age. It is common practice to refer to the size of endotracheal tube (or tracheostomy tube) needed by its ID. Once the tube is properly placed into the patient, the excess tube, beyond 3 to 4 cm past the teeth, should be cut off. This reduces the airway resistance and mechanical dead space.

Most endotracheal tubes have the standard features

shown in Fig. 11-21. There are a number of specialty endotracheal tubes that can be found in limited use. They all share the same characteristics except for some special feature. These tubes are worth considering if available.

1. Pediatric endotracheal tubes

Pediatric endotracheal tubes come in two basic types. One type has a constant diameter. During intubation, the tube should be inserted until the black mark about 2 cm from the tip is at the vocal cords. The second type has a body with a relatively wide proximal part that narrows at the distal end. The design is supposed to allow the smaller diameter tip to be passed through the vocal cords but prevent the wide "shoulder" from passing into the trachea. Both types of tube end with a single opening with a bevel cut (see Fig. 11-22). It is recommended that children less than 8 years of age have a tube without a cuff.

2. Armored tubes

Armored tubes have a steel spring coiled through them. An advantage of the armored tubes over regular tubes is that they do not collapse if the patient bites down. Furthermore, the tube may be prebent for shape and does not kink like a plastic tube might.

3. Preformed tubes

Preformed tubes have been preshaped for better patient comfort and security. One style has a forward bend so that the tube can be taped to the chin. There is also a pediatric tube with a bend. This type may be taped to the forehead.

4. Guidable (trigger) tubes

Guidable tubes have a wire embedded within the wall of the tube (see Fig. 11-23). When the ring at the proximal end is pulled, the distal tip is flexed up to shorten the radius

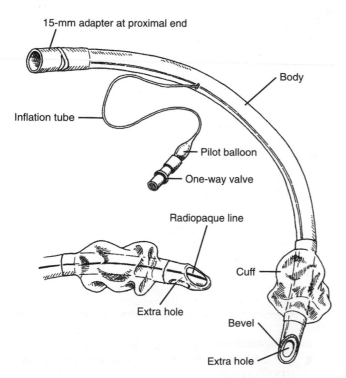

15-mm adapter at proximal end

Inflation tube

Body

Pilot balloon

One-way valve

Radiopaque line

Cuff

Extra hole

Bevel

Extra hole

Fig. 11-21 Typical, modern endotracheal tube with its component parts. Insert shows important features found at the distal end of the tube.

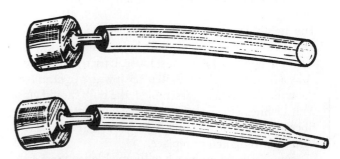

Fig. 11-22 Comparison of the two different types of pediatric endotracheal tubes. The top type of tube is made by several manufacturers and has a uniform diameter. The bottom tube is made by Cole and features a narrowing of the distal tip to pass through the vocal cords. Note that neither has a cuff. (From Burgess WR, Chernick V: *Respiratory therapy in newborn infants and children*, ed 2, New York, 1986, Thieme.)

of the curve. This allows the tube to be directed into the anterior trachea. Guidable trigger tubes make it easier to intubate a patient with an anterior larynx or to perform a blind nasal intubation.

5. Double-lumen endotracheal tubes

Double-lumen endotracheal tubes are used to allow independent lung ventilation. A double-lumen tube is also used during special procedures performed on one lung such as bronchoscopy, bronchoalveolar lavage, lobectomy, and pneumonectomy. The other lung may be mechanically ventilated to maintain the patient's blood gas values (see Fig. 11-24). An adapter can be added to join the two proximal ends of the channels together so that a single ventilator can be used to ventilate both lungs. The Carlens tube is used to preferentially intubate the left bronchus. The White tube is used to preferentially intubate the right bronchus (see Fig. 11-25 for both). Robertshaw makes tubes for either right or left bronchial intubation.

Several limitations are inherent in all double-lumen tubes. First, they can be used only on adults because the smallest size is 8-mm OD. Second, the small internal diameter of the two lumens results in a high airway

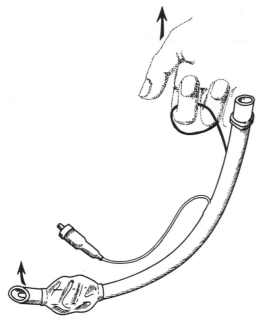

Fig. 11-23 Guidable or "trigger" type endotracheal tube. A wire is embedded within the wall of the tube. When the ring at the proximal end is pulled, the distal tip is flexed up to shorten the radius of the curve. This allows the tube to be directed into an anterior trachea. (Modified from Heffner JE: *Respir Manage* 19(3):53, 1989.)

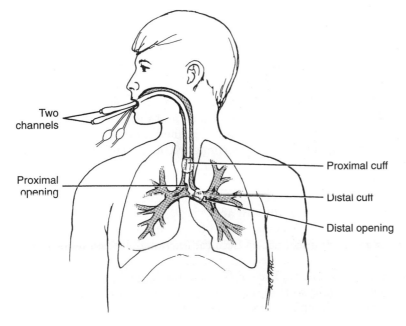

Two channels

Proximal opening

Proximal cuff

Distal cuff

Distal opening

Fig. 11-24 Double-lumen endotracheal tube properly positioned in patient so that both lungs can be independently ventilated or suctioned, or have special procedures performed. (From Eubanks DH, Bone RC: *Comprehensive respiratory care,* ed 2, St Louis, 1990, Mosby-Year Book.)

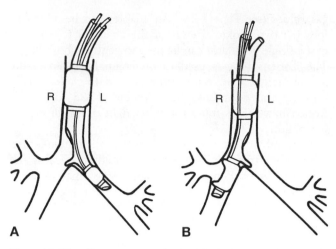

Fig. 11-25 Two types of double-lumen endotracheal tubes. **A,** Carlens tube; its distal tube enters left mainstem bronchus. **B,** White tube; its distal tube enters right mainstem bronchus. Note how both tubes have a cuff that seals the trachea and a cuff that seals a bronchus. Each has its own inflation tube, pilot balloon, and one-way valve. (From Miller RD, editor: *Anesthesia,* New York, 1981, Churchill Livingstone.)

resistance. Third, a much smaller than normal suction catheter must be used to remove any tracheal secretions.

EXAM HINT

Know the special clinical uses of a double-lumen endotracheal tube.

EXAM HINT

Know the proper size of endotracheal or tracheostomy tube to use for an adult. A question may ask you to select the appropriate size tube.

---

b. Put the equipment together, make sure that it works properly, and identify any problems (Code: IIB1f2) [Difficulty: An]

Refer to Fig. 11-21 for these components of a standard endotracheal tube:

1. The hollow curved body is the main part of the tube through which the patient can breathe, or a suction catheter can be placed. The OD and ID size are printed on the side of the tube. Make sure that the central channel is not plugged by dried secretions, blood, or a foreign body.
2. The proximal end is left outside of the patient's nose or mouth. An adapter with a 15-mm-OD equipment connector is inserted into the tube. The other end of the

adapter narrows and is individually sized to fit snugly into the ID of the endotracheal tube. The adapters cannot be cross-fitted to different sizes of endotracheal tubes.

3. The distal end is inserted into the patient's trachea. The tip is cut with either a right- or left-sided bevel. The bevel cut creates an oval-shaped opening that is less likely to become plugged with secretions than is a round opening. An extra hole (the Murphy eye) is cut in the tube on the opposite side of the bevel.
4. A line of radiopaque material is imbedded in the tube from the tip back to the cuff. It is seen as a white line on the chest radiograph showing the location of the tube's tip in the trachea (see the insert in Fig. 11-21).
5. A cuff (balloon) is located a few centimeters from the tip of the tube. It is blown up with air to seal the trachea so that mechanical ventilation can be performed and aspiration is prevented. Most modern tubes have a large residual volume, low-pressure cuff.

  Note: All tubes with a 5-mm OD or greater have cuffs. Smaller neonatal and pediatric tubes are available with or without a cuff.

6. A cuff-filling inflation tube is connected about half way down the tube. The proximal end is left out of the patient's mouth, and the distal end goes to the cuff so that it can be inflated and deflated. A pilot balloon that inflates and deflates with the cuff is found in the middle of the capillary tube or connected with the one-way valve at the distal end. The one-way valve has an end that connects to any syringe. When the syringe is disconnected, the one-way valve seals to prevent the air in the cuff from escaping.
7. With a double-lumen endotracheal tube, each lumen has its own 15-mm adapter, cuff, one-way valve, pilot balloon, and inflation tube to inflate the cuff. As with traditional endotracheal tubes, both cuffs should be test-inflated. They should hold the air without a leak and then be easily deflated. One additional piece of equipment, a plastic Y, can be used with a double-lumen tube. The plastic Y can be used to connect together the proximal ends of both tubes. Both 15-mm adapters are removed and one branch of the Y is inserted into each of the proximal ends of the tubes. The open end of the Y has a 15-mm adapter so that it can be connected to a ventilator or oxygen source.

c. Fix any problems with the equipment (Code: IIB2f2) [Difficulty: An]

The cuff(s) should be inflated and the syringe should be disconnected from the one-way valve before the tube is placed in the patient. This ensures that the system works properly. The cuff(s) should hold the air. Do not use any tube with a leaking cuff or leaking one-way valve. Deflate the cuff before placing the tube into the patient.

BOX 11-3	Indications and Contraindications for Oral Endotracheal Intubation

GENERAL INDICATIONS FOR ENDOTRACHEAL INTUBATION

Provide a secure, patent airway
Provide a route for mechanical ventilation
Prevent aspiration of stomach or mouth contents
Provide a route for suctioning the lungs
Use general anesthesia

INDICATIONS FOR ORAL INTUBATION

Fastest, easiest method to secure the airway
Simpler, less invasive method cannot ensure an open airway

CONTRAINDICATIONS FOR ORAL INTUBATION

Cervical spine injury such that the patient's neck cannot be hyperextended
Lower facial injury
Oral surgery

BOX 11-4	Complications of Endotracheal Intubation

GENERAL COMPLICATIONS

Reflex laryngospasm
Perforation of the esophagus or pharynx
Esophageal intubation
Bronchial intubation
Reflex bradycardia
Tachycardia or other arrhythmias from hypoxemia
Hypotension
Bronchospasm
Aspiration of tooth, blood, gastric contents, laryngoscope bulb
Laceration of pharynx or larynx
Nosocomial infection
Vocal cord injury
Laryngeal or tracheal injury from the tube or the excessive cuff pressure

COMPLICATIONS OF THE ORAL ROUTE

Cervical spine injury
Tooth trauma from the blade being pulled back
Eye trauma from the handle or the operator's hand

COMPLICATIONS AFTER EXTUBATION

Reflex laryngospasm
Aspiration of stomach contents or oral secretions
Sore throat
Hoarseness
Laryngeal edema (postintubation croup)

MODULE B	Perform endotracheal intubation (Code: IIIB1a) [Difficulty: An]

Oral endotracheal intubation is the recommended procedure for securing the airway during an emergency such as a CPR attempt. In uncomplicated cases, the patient can be quickly intubated with an apneic period of no more than 20 seconds. This procedure is explained for a team of two respiratory therapists. It is difficult, if not impossible, for a single therapist to perform this important task without placing the patient at great risk. Usually the therapist who intubates is considered the leader and the other therapist acts as the assistant. Therapists must feel comfortable in both roles. See Box 11-3 for a list of indications and contraindications for oral intubation and Box 11-4 for a list of complications.

Steps in an emergency oral endotracheal intubation include the following:

1. Prepare the patient. The assistant should:
   a. Place the head and neck in the sniff position.
   b. Ventilate the patient with 100% oxygen by a face mask and manual resuscitator or demand valve.
2. The intubator should put on a surgical mask, goggles, and clean gloves on both hands, and then perform the following.
3. Prepare the endotracheal tube.
   a. Select the proper endotracheal tube (see Table 11-1 for the recommended tube sizes based on age). If time permits, the next smaller and larger tube size should also be selected.
   b. Inflate the cuff with a 10- or 20 mL syringe. Remove the syringe from the one-way valve. Make sure that it holds the air and then deflate the cuff completely.
   c. Lubricate the last few centimeters of the endotracheal tube with a water-soluble lubricant.
   d. Lubricate a stylet with the sterile water-soluble lubricant. Place the stylet into the tube so that the natural curve of the tube is maintained. The tip of the stylet should not go past the end of the tube (Fig. 11-26). Some practitioners may prefer not to use a stylet. Many believe that the stylet offers the advantage of being able to bend the tube to match the patient's anatomy if a second attempt is needed.
4. Prepare the laryngoscope and blade.
   a. Select a laryngoscope handle.
   b. Select a laryngoscope blade. The blades come in several sizes from pediatric to adult. There are two main classes of blades: straight and curved (see Fig. 11-19). The straight blades (Miller is a common brand) are designed to lift the epiglottis to expose the tracheal opening. The curved blades (MacIntosh is a common brand) are designed to fit into the vallecula (between the base of the tongue and the epiglottis). As the blade is lifted, the epiglottis is raised and the tracheal opening can be seen. Personal experience

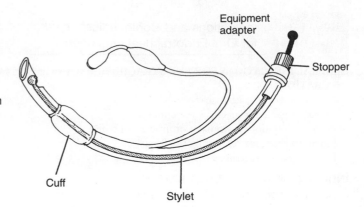

Fig. 11-26 Stylet with stopper properly placed in standard endotracheal tube to maintain its curved shape. (From Eubanks DH, Bone RC: *Comprehensive respiratory care,* ed 2, St Louis, 1990, Mosby.)

and training leads the practitioner to select between the two styles.

   c. Attach the blade to the handle (see Fig. 11-20). Make sure that the light bulb shines brightly.

5. The intubator should tell the assistant to stop ventilating the patient and stand clear so that an intubation can be attempted. The assistant should check his or her watch to silently count off 20 seconds. The intubator should be told when 20 seconds has passed so that the patient can be reventilated if the intubation is proving to be difficult.

6. Open the victim's mouth as widely as possible without using force. Remove any dentures or foreign material. Suction out any saliva, blood, or vomitus.

7. Grasp the laryngoscope handle in the left hand. Carefully advance the blade between the teeth or gums along the right side of the mouth. Move the tongue to the left side of the mouth to allow a clear view of the oropharynx (see Fig. 11-27). Advance the blade along the base of the tongue until the epiglottis is seen.

8. With a *straight blade:*
   a. Advance the blade so that it barely passes the epiglottis.
   b. Do not advance the blade too far or it will enter the esophagus or trachea.
   With a *curved blade:*
   a. Advance the blade tip into the vallecula.
   b. Lift the blade tip into this space.

9. With either blade, lift the laryngoscope handle and blade toward the patient's chest at a 45-degree angle (see Fig. 11-28). The straight blade lifts the epiglottis. The curved blade lifts the soft tissues of the vallecula and the epiglottis lifts with them. Do *not* pull back on the patient's upper teeth. If needed, tell the assistant to put downward pressure on the patient's larynx.

10. The vocal cords and glottis should be clearly seen (see Fig. 11-29).

11. Tell the assistant to place the endotracheal tube into your right hand.

12. Place the tube into the patient's mouth and trachea. In

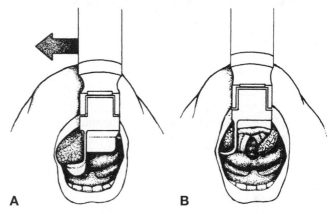

Fig. 11-27 Proper placement of the laryngoscope blade to move the patient's tongue. **A,** Proper placement of the laryngoscope blade to the right of the patient's tongue to move it to the left. This should give a clear view of the glottis. **B,** Tongue partially obstructs the view if it is not moved to the left. (From Shapiro BA et al: *Clinical application of respiratory care,* ed 4, St Louis, 1991, Mosby.)

the adult, the proximal end of the cuff should be placed 3 to 4 cm past the vocal cords (Fig. 11-30). In children less than 6 months, with an uncuffed endotracheal tube, place the end of the tube about 1 cm past the vocal cords.

13. Hold the tube in place.

14. Withdraw the laryngoscope blade.

15. Tell the assistant to inflate the cuff. Place about 10 mL of air into the cuff (of an adult's tube) so that some resistance can be felt. The cuff pressure can be measured and adjusted later.

16. Pull out the stylet (if used).

17. The assistant should ventilate the patient with the manual resuscitator bag or a demand valve.

18. The intubator should listen to both lung fields in the upper lobes and bases. Bilateral breath sounds should be heard.

19. If the breath sounds are equal and bilateral, the

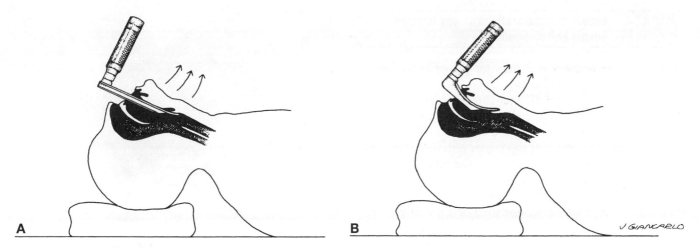

Fig. 11-28 Proper use of the laryngoscope blade to expose the larynx by lifting the glottic structures. Note how the lifting is at a 45-degree angle toward the patient's chest. *Never* pull back on the blade against the teeth. **A,** A straight blade is used to lift the epiglottis to expose the trachea. **B,** A curved blade is used to lift soft tissues of the vallecula to expose the trachea. (From Shapiro BA et al: *Clinical application of respiratory care,* ed 4, St Louis, 1991, Mosby.)

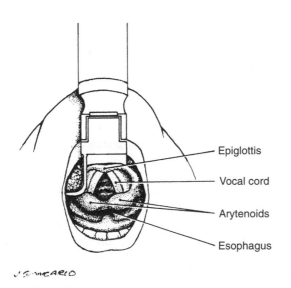

Fig. 11-29 Major anatomic features that can be seen when epiglottis is lifted. Opening to trachea can be seen between vocal cords. (From Shapiro BA et al: *Clinical application of respiratory care,* ed 4, St Louis, 1991, Mosby.)

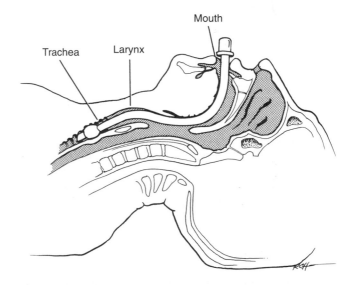

Fig. 11-30 Oral endotracheal tube properly positioned within the trachea. (From Eubanks DH, Bone RC: *Comprehensive respiratory care,* ed 2, St Louis, 1990, Mosby.)

assistant can secure the tube in place with tape or a tube holder. If the breath sounds are unequal or absent on one side, the tube has been placed into a bronchus (usually the right mainstem). The cuff should be deflated and the tube then withdrawn 1 to 2 cm in an adult, less in a child. The cuff should be reinflated and breath sounds listened to again. When the breath sounds are equal, the tube can be secured.

20. If no breath sounds are heard, listen over the stomach area. If air is heard bubbling into the stomach, the tube has been placed into the esophagus. Immediately remove the tube. Ventilate the patient and prepare to attempt reintubation with a new endotracheal tube.

The practitioner should only perform those procedures for which he or she has been trained. If the patient cannot be intubated with the standard equipment and procedure, an anesthesiologist or trained physician should be called in. Be prepared to assist as necessary.

MODULE C	Ensure that the artificial airway is properly placed and maintained

1. Palpate the endotracheal tube for proper placement (Code: IB2b) [Difficulty: An]

Often the endotracheal tube can be palpated in an infant as it is being inserted through the larynx. This is because the laryngeal structures are so pliable. Feeling the tube being inserted through the larynx indicates that it is properly located within the trachea. If the tube cannot be palpated through the larynx, it has probably been inserted into the esophagus. It is more difficult to use this technique with confidence in adults because their laryngeal structures are stiffer.

2. Auscultate the patient's breath sounds and interpret any changes (Code: IB4a and IIIA1k) [Difficulty: An]

Respiratory efforts without breath sounds indicate that a complete obstruction exists in the patient's airway. Inspiratory or expiratory stridor or wheezing indicate that a partial obstruction exists in the patient's airway. Listen for stridor over the larynx and wheezing over the major airways. The restoration of the normal airway should result in the return of normal breath sounds over all areas of both lung fields (unless there is another, unrelated problem).

It is especially important to check for bilateral breath sounds after an endotracheal tube has been placed. If the tube has been inserted too far, it usually enters the right mainstem bronchus because it comes off of the trachea at a less acute angle than the left mainstem bronchus. No breath sounds are heard over the left lung field. If both lung fields cannot be auscultated, at least listen to the right apical area. This one site can be checked because the segmental bronchus to the right upper lobe comes off of the right mainstem bronchus in such a way that if the right mainstem bronchus is intubated, the upper lobe segmental bronchus will be blocked.

3. Exhaled carbon dioxide detector

a. Get the necessary equipment (Code: IIA1n1) [Difficulty: An]

An exhaled carbon dioxide detector can be placed on an endotracheal tube to monitor the proper placement of the endotracheal tube. This is often done if a patient is being transported and there is a possibility of the tube being dislodged. A disposable unit such as the Easy Cap end-tidal CO_2 detector may be selected (Fig. 11-31). The Easy Cap comes in a neonatal/pediatric size for infants less than 15 kg and a standard size for larger children and adults. Its carbon dioxide indicator changes color from dark purple to yellow when CO_2 is exhaled through it. Another choice is the MiniCAP III CO_2 Detector. It is a reusable item that has a mainstream type of infrared carbon dioxide detector. The unit is powered by a battery pack. Its

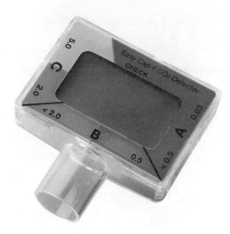

Fig. 11-31 Easy Cap $ETCO_2$ detector. This disposable device comes in adult and pediatric sizes and is able to detect exhaled carbon dioxide. Color change from dark purple to yellow indicates exhaled CO_2 to confirm tracheal placement of endotracheal tube or effective efforts at cardiopulmonary resuscitation. (From Nellcor, Hayward, CA.)

light-emitting diode signals the presence of carbon dioxide with each exhalation. A capnograph should be selected if it is necessary to get a more accurate CO_2 reading. Its general function and the interpretation of capnography tracings was discussed in Chapter 5.

b. Put the equipment together, make sure that it works properly, and identify any problems (Code: IIB2n1) [Difficulty: An]

The Easy Cap comes as a single unit within a sealed foil container. Before using it, match the initial purple color of the indicator with the purple color labeled CHECK on the product dome. Do *not* use an Easy Cap unit whose color is not the same or darker than that on the product dome. Remove both caps from the patient and circuit connector ports. The Easy Cap is then attached to the patient's endotracheal tube by its 15-mm ID connector port. The Easy Cap's 15-mm OD circuit end is connected to the manual resuscitator to ventilate the patient. If a heat and moisture exchanger is used, it should be placed between the patient's endotracheal tube and the Easy Cap and manual resuscitator. The Easy Cap should not be used with a heated humidifier or nebulizer because too much humidity affects its accuracy. The MiniCAP III has a disposable adapter that connects the mainstream CO_2 detector to the patient's endotracheal tube. The adapter has a 15-mm ID end for attachment to the endotracheal tube and a 15-mm OD end to which the manual resuscitator can be attached. The assembly and operation of a capnograph is discussed in Chapter 5. Review it if necessary.

c. Fix any problems with the equipment (Code: IIB2n1) [Difficulty: An]

Because the Easy Cap comes as a self-contained single piece unit, there is nothing to repair. The following items can contaminate the Easy Cap and cause a patchy yellow or white discoloration of the indicator: stomach contents, mucus, pulmonary edema fluid, and intratracheal epinephrine. The color does not change with the breathing cycle and it should be throw away. The caps over the two connector ports must be removed to attach the Easy Cap to the endotracheal tube and manual resuscitator. The 15-mm ID patient connector port fits only over the endotracheal tube adapter. The 15-mm OD circuit connector port fits only into the manual resuscitator or demand-valve adapter. The adapter is the only removable part in the MiniCAP III. It fits only in one direction into the CO_2 detection unit. The other end of the adapter fits only into a manual resuscitator outlet. Troubleshooting with a capnograph was presented in Chapter 5.

4. Make the recommendation for an upper airway and chest radiograph, as needed, to help determine the patient's condition (Code: IA2b) [Difficulty: An]

A chest radiograph should always be taken to confirm the location of a newly placed endotracheal or tracheostomy tube. The chest radiograph should be repeated if there has been a significant change in the patient's condition or if the tube has been pulled back or pushed deeper into the trachea. A chest radiograph also confirms the presence and location of an opaque foreign body in the airway. Metallic objects, stones, and coins can be clearly seen. Less radiopaque objects can be barely seen, if at all. The chest radiograph also detects a pneumothorax related to the tracheostomy procedure or other pulmonary conditions. If needed, an upper airway radiographic examination can be performed to look for a foreign body or to check the position of the tracheostomy tube.

5. View the upper airway or chest radiograph to see the position of the endotracheal or tracheostomy tube (Code: IA1e and IB7c) [Difficulty: An]

All modern endotracheal and tracheostomy tubes contain a strip of radiopaque material near the distal tip of the tube. This is easily noticed as the white line seen on the chest radiograph and confirms the location of the tip of the tube in the airway (see Fig. 11-21. The ideal location of the tip of the endotracheal tube is the middle third of the trachea. When the tube is positioned properly, it is less likely for the tip to be pushed into the carina when the patient bends his or her head forward or for the cuff to hit the vocal cords if the patient's head is bent back. Both endotracheal and tracheostomy tubes should be positioned midline within the trachea. They

should not be twisted laterally because the tip can cause damage to the tracheal wall.

6. Identify the placement of the endotracheal tube by any available means (Code: IIIB1e) [Difficulty: An]

Review the previous discussions if needed. Some limitations exist in the use of an Easy Cap carbon dioxide detector. It should not be used during mouth-to-mouth resuscitation, to detect right mainstem bronchus intubation, to detect hypercarbia, or to determine the placement of an esophageal obturator airway.

The esophageal detection device (EDD) is able to show that the endotracheal tube has been placed within an airway by pulling a small sample of gas from the patient's lungs. If the endotracheal tube has been accidentally put into the esophagus, the deflated bulb will stay collapsed. See Fig. 11-32. A limitation of the EDD is that it inflates whether the endotracheal tube is placed into the trachea or either mainstem bronchus. Remember to auscultate for bilateral breath sounds.

EXAM HINT

Be prepared to determine the proper placement of the endotracheal tube by palpation of the neck, auscultation of bilateral breath sounds, detection of exhaled carbon dioxide, observation of bilateral symmetrical chest movement on inspiration, or visualization of the tip of the tube on a chest radiograph.

---

7. Ensure that the endotracheal or tracheostomy tube stays properly positioned (Code: IIIB1a) [Difficulty: An]

The endotracheal tube body has centimeter marks placed on it starting at the distal end and finishing at the proximal end. Check and record the centimeter mark present at the patient's teeth or gums. The average adult's distance from the midtrachea to the teeth is about 23 to 25 cm. The practitioner can tell if the tube has been accidentally pulled out a little or pushed further into the patient by looking at the current centimeter mark. If the tube is intentionally adjusted, the new centimeter mark should be checked and recorded.

A wide variety of handmade, as well as manufactured, devices are available to secure the endotracheal tube in the correct position. Fig. 11-33 shows one way to make a tube holder from adhesive tape. This is flexible when the patient moves and is inexpensive. Tincture of benzoin can be applied to the patient's cheeks to make the tape hold more securely without tearing the skin. An oropharyngeal airway may or may not be needed.

The manufactured tube holders are made of plastic with cloth ties and usually include a built-in bite block. Make sure that it is sized properly to the patient's mouth. Too large a bite block can injure the tongue, lips, and

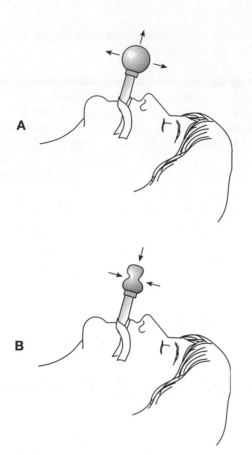

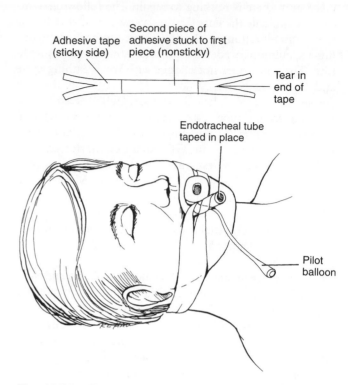

Fig. 11-32 Esophageal detection device (EDD). This squeeze bulb device is attached to proximal end of patient's endotracheal tube and air is squeezed out. **A,** Shows reinflation of bulb with air from patient's lungs when the endotracheal tube has been properly placed. **B,** Shows that the bulb fails to reinflate when the endotracheal tube has been accidentally placed into the patient's esophagus. (From Scanlan C, Simmons K: Airway management. In Scanlan CL, Wilkins RL, Stoller JK, editors: *Egan's fundamentals of respiratory care,* ed 7, St Louis, 1999, Mosby.)

Fig. 11-33 Taping the endotracheal tube to secure it in the airway. (From Eubanks DH, Bone RC: *Comprehensive respiratory care,* ed 2, St Louis, 1990, Mosby.)

mouth. Watch for a gag reflex. This type of holder is useful in the patient who is prone to seizures.

8. Change the position of the endotracheal or tracheostomy tube (Code: IIIB1a and IIIC6a) [Difficulty: An]

As mentioned earlier, an endotracheal tube is ideally located within the middle third of the trachea. Check the chest radiograph for positioning. If the tube is too high within the trachea, it may be pulled up through the vocal cords if the patient's head is hyperextended. An air leak may be heard at the larynx if the patient is using a mechanical ventilator. In this case, the cuff should be deflated and the tube inserted deeper into the trachea.

Conversely, if the tip of the tube is inserted too deeply into the trachea, it may be pushed into a mainstem

bronchus if the patient's head is moved toward the chest. In this situation no breath sounds would be heard in the opposite lung (usually the left). The cuff should be deflated and the tube pulled up into the middle third of the trachea. Reinflate the cuff after the tube is repositioned. A chest radiograph should be taken to confirm the tube's position after it has been moved.

A tracheostomy tube should be positioned so that the flange is snug against the base of the neck and the outer cannula is within the trachea. If pulled out too far, the cuff may be seen at the stoma. An air leak may be heard or secretions may be seen to bubble out of the stoma. Correct the problem by deflating the cuff, inserting the tube so that the flange is against the base of the neck, and reinflating the cuff.

EXAM HINT

There is usually a question that deals with understanding that the lack of breath sounds over the left lung indicates that the endotracheal tube has been placed into the right mainstem bronchus. The tube must be withdrawn to the trachea.

9. Cuff pressure manometers

a. Get the needed cuff pressure manometer (Code: IIA1n1) [Difficulty: An]

b. Put the equipment together, make sure that is works properly, and identify any problems with it (Code: IIB1n1) [Difficulty: An]

A cuff pressure manometer is a device that is designed to measure the air pressure within an endotracheal or tracheostomy tube cuff. When a tracheal tube is first inserted, the volume of air that is injected into the cuff should be measured and charted. After that, if more air is inserted or any air is removed from the cuff it should be measured and recorded in the chart. A number of manufactured units are available for measuring cuff pressure. The Cufflator is discussed here because it is widely used. This system consists of a pressure gauge calibrated in centimeters of water, a hand-pumped reservoir, internal one-way valve, pressure release valve, and adapter to fit into the one-way valve on the cuff inflating tube. A three-way stopcock can be added to the one-way valve adapter. This can be used to prepressurize the system before attaching it to the patient's one-way valve on the cuff inflating tube (Fig. 11-34). The pressure in the cuff can be measured as air is added by squeezing the hand pump or as air is removed by the pressure release valve. The volume of air added or removed cannot be measured.

A second system can be "homemade," although it is also commercially available. It consists of a 5- to 10-mL syringe, a three-way stopcock, and a pressure gauge (either millimeters of mercury or centimeters of water). The syringe and pressure gauge are attached to two of the ports on the stopcock. The third port on the stopcock is connected to the one-way valve on the cuff inflating tube. When the stopcock handle is opened to all three ports, the pressure throughout the system and the cuff are the same. Air can be added or removed with the syringe. The pressure gauge shows the system and cuff pressure as the air volume is adjusted (Fig. 11-35). One advantage of this system over the Cufflator is that the volume of air that is added or subtracted can be measured. This system can also be prepressurized so that its pressure matches the pressure anticipated in the cuff.

c. Fix any problems with the equipment (Code: IIB2n1) [Difficulty: An]

With any of these systems, it is necessary to keep airtight connections. If the pressure drops unexpectedly, an air leak will be noticed. Tighten the connections to create a seal so that the pressure is maintained.

10. Keep an endotracheal or tracheostomy tube cuff properly inflated

a. Determine tracheal tube cuff volume and pressure (Code: IB9h) [Difficulty: An]

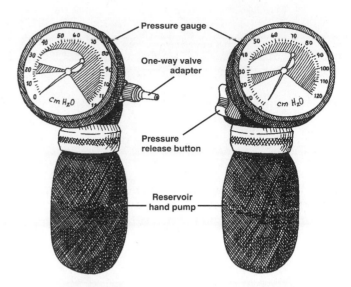

Fig. 11-34 Cufflator device used to measure cuff pressure with its component parts.

All of the adult and larger pediatric endotracheal and tracheostomy tubes have a cuff for sealing the airway. Most brands of modern tubes have cuffs that are designed to have a relatively large reservoir volume that fills at a relatively low pressure. The soft, flexible balloon seals the airway by having a large surface area that conforms to the shape of the trachea. There are two slightly different ways to inflate the cuff and maintain a safe cuff pressure. Both methods can be used only with patients on a positive-pressure ventilator.

1. Minimal leak

a. Connect the cuff pressure measuring device (see earlier discussion) to the one-way valve on the cuff inflating tube.

b. Listen with a stethoscope over the patient's larynx.

c. Inflate or deflate the cuff as necessary while listening for an air leak.

d. Stop changing the air volume when a minimal leak is heard at the peak airway pressure in the breathing cycle. The tidal volume should still be delivered except for this minor leak.

e. Note the cuff pressure when the minimal leak was heard. Note the cuff volume, if possible.

f. Disconnect the cuff pressure measuring device.

g. It may be necessary to add more volume and pressure to the cuff if the leak gets worse when the peak airway pressure increases.

2. Minimal occluding volume

The purpose is to find the cuff pressure that results in *no leak* at the cuff when the patient's airway pressure is greatest. The following are the steps in the procedure:

a. Connect the cuff pressure measuring device (see

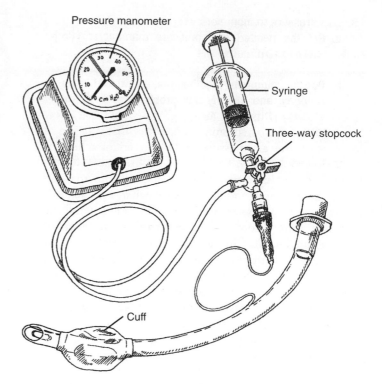

Fig. 11-35 Cuff measuring device made from pressure manometer, three-way stopcock, and 10-mL syringe.

earlier discussion) to the one-way valve on the cuff inflating tube.

b. Listen with a stethoscope over the patient's larynx.

c. Inflate or deflate the cuff as necessary while listening for an air leak.

d. Stop changing the air volume when no leak is heard at the peak airway pressure in the breathing cycle.

e. Note the cuff pressure when the seal was heard. Note the cuff volume, if possible.

f. Disconnect the cuff pressure measuring device.

g. It may be necessary to add more volume and pressure to the cuff if a leak results when the peak airway pressure increases.

This discussion relates only to those tubes that must be actively filled with air and have variable intracuff pressures. Several manufacturers have developed endotracheal and tracheostomy tubes that have built-in cuff pressure limitations. Follow the manufacturer's guidelines when inflating these cuffs. This discussion would not be complete without mentioning the recent manufacture of systems designed to raise the cuff pressure to match the peak airway pressure of a patient using a mechanical ventilator. A tube connects the inspiratory circuit to the one-way valve on the cuff inflating tube. As a positive-pressure breath is delivered, the pressure in the circuit is also applied to the patient's cuff. There should be no loss of tidal volume. When the patient exhales and the airway pressure drops to normal, the cuff pressure also drops back to its normal level.

b. Maintain tracheal tube cuff volume and pressure (Code: IIIA1j and IIIB1a) [Difficulty: An]

It is commonly recommended that the cuff pressure be monitored at least every 8 hours or whenever air is taken out of or put into the cuff.

c. Interpret the tracheal tube cuff volume and pressure (Code: IB10h) [Difficulty: An]

All manufacturers (except Kamen-Wilkenson) have designed cuffs that must be actively filled with air by way of a one-way valve and syringe. These cuffs have greater than atmospheric pressure within them. That pressure is placed against the wall of the trachea. The greater the pressure on the wall of the trachea, the greater the disruption of normal lymphatic and blood flow. Shapiro et al state that a patient with a normal blood pressure (120/80 mm Hg) has the following effects at these cuff pressures:

1. Lymphatic flow blockage occurs at pressures greater than 5 mm Hg (8 cm H_2O). Edema of the tracheal mucosa results.

2. Capillary blood flow blockage occurs at pressures greater than 18 mm Hg (24 cm H_2O). Venous (and lymphatic) drainage stops as a result.

3. Arterial blood flow blockage occurs at pressures greater than 30 mm Hg (42 cm H_2O). Arterial (and lymphatic and capillary) flow stops as a result.

In general, the clinical goal is to keep the cuff pressure as low as possible to make sure that the circulation through the tracheal wall is normal. Based on Shapiro et al, it seems reasonable to try to keep the cuff pressure no greater than 15 mm Hg (21 cm H_2O). This holds true for all normotensive patients. Hypertensive patients may be able to tolerate higher cuff pressures than normotensive patients before blood flow to the tracheal tissues is stopped. Hypotensive patients suffer from the loss of blood flow to the tracheal wall at lower cuff pressures than those previously listed.

d. Inflate and deflate the cuff as indicated (Code: IIIC6c) [Difficulty: An]

A spontaneously breathing patient must have the cuff inflated to prevent the aspiration of oral secretions into the lungs. In general, keep the pressure at about 15 mm Hg (21 cm H_2O), as discussed earlier. It may be necessary to keep a higher cuff pressure in a mechanically ventilated patient. However, Shapiro and associates recommend that if the cuff pressure must be greater than 20 mm Hg, the endotracheal or tracheostomy tube is too small. Ideally, the tube should be replaced with a larger one. However, some patients are too unstable to tolerate reintubation of their airways and must simply have the cuff pressure increased temporarily.

It is clear that a cuff pressure greater than the patient's mucosa capillary pressure prevents the flow of blood through the area covered by the cuff. Tissue ischemia (hypoxemia) results. If the ischemia is severe enough, tissue necrosis follows. The higher the cuff pressure and the longer the high cuff pressure is maintained, the greater the likelihood of tissue necrosis. If the necrosis is circumferential (all the way around) to the trachea, tracheal stenosis may occur. Tracheal stenosis is found when the diameter of the trachea is narrowed because of scar tissue buildup after the normal mucosa and underlying tissues have died. The patient's airway is permanently narrowed and, if serious, must be surgically corrected. Another severe complication of high cuff pressures and tracheal necrosis is the development of a tracheoesophageal fistula. This is an opening between the trachea and esophagus. This is more likely when the patient also has a nasogastric tube in place. The fistula permits food to pass into the airway and lungs, causing pneumonia. Mechanical ventilation is more difficult because of the air leak from the lungs to the esophagus. Surgical repair of the fistula is required.

EXAM HINT

There is usually a question that deals with adjusting a cuff pressure to a safe level of no more than 20 mm Hg or making a recommendation to replace a tracheal tube that is too small and requires too high a cuff pressure. A small endotracheal tube should also be replaced with a larger one if a patient cannot wean from the ventilator because of the high airway resistance created by the smaller tube.

MODULE C **Change a tracheal tube**

---

1. Change the endotracheal tube (Code: IIIC6a) [Difficulty: An]

There are usually only two reasons to replace a patient's endotracheal tube. First, the tube should be changed if it is too small and the cuff must be overfilled to seal the airway. Excessive pressure results in damage to the tracheal wall as previously discussed.

Second, the tube should be replaced if the cuff is leaking or ruptured and the airway cannot be sealed. The patient may be reintubated by the procedure described earlier. Or, a tube changing stylet may be used (Fig. 11-36). The stylet is a hollow, flexible plastic tube that can be bent and holds its shape. It has a center mark and 1 cm markings counting out to each end. These are to help keep the proper depth for inserting the replacement endotracheal tube. It can be used on an endotracheal tube that is at least 7.5 mm outer diameter. The procedure for changing the endotracheal tube with a tube changing stylet includes the following:

a. Obtain the needed equipment: replacement endotracheal tube and one that is a size smaller, 10-mL syringe to inflate the cuff, sterile gloves, goggles, and sterile water-soluble lubricant. Make sure the cuff inflates and deflates properly.

b. Tell the patient what you are going to do. Put on the gloves and goggles.

c. Remove the patient's oxygen equipment.

d. Suction the secretions from the patient's trachea and oral pharynx.

e. Reoxygenate and ventilate the patient.

f. Place some lubricant on the outside of the stylet.

g. Remove the oxygen equipment and pass the stylet through the endotracheal tube into the patient's trachea.

h. Insert it to about the same depth as marked on the distal end of the endotracheal tube. For example, if the distal end of the endotracheal tube is 22 cm, insert the tube changer to 22 cm.

i. Deflate the cuff on the endotracheal tube.

j. While holding the distal tip of the tube changer in place, pull the defective endotracheal tube over the tube changer and out of the patient.

k. Advance the new endotracheal tube over the stylet. Hold the distal end of the stylet and push the new tube into the patient to the same depth mark on the stylet as the old tube had been.

l. Hold the endotracheal tube in place and remove the stylet.

m. Ensure that the tube has been placed into the trachea to the proper depth by listening for bilateral breath sounds.

n. Inflate the cuff to a safe pressure.

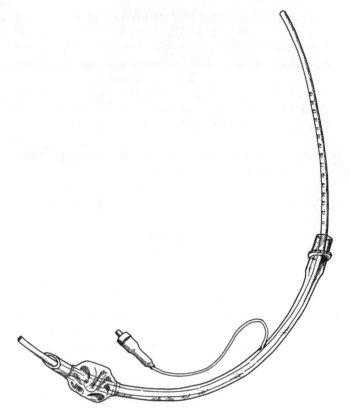

Fig. 11-36 Endotracheal tube changer (guide) inserted through an endotracheal tube. The JEM 400 unit can be inserted through a tube that is 7.5-mm ID or larger. The tube changer is used to aid in replacement of an esophageal obturator airway or a defective endotracheal tube with a functional endotracheal tube. See text for how to use the tube changer instead of traditional intubation equipment. (Modified from Heffner JE: *Respir Manage* 19(3):53, 1989.)

o. Secure the tube in place and note the depth marking at the patient's teeth or gums.

p. Obtain a chest radiograph.

A defective one-way valve or severed cuff inflating tube may not necessarily lead to a reintubation; often it can be bypassed. This is done by slipping a small diameter needle (usually about 21 gauge) into the inflating tube, attaching a three-way stopcock to the hub of the needle, and screwing a 10-cc syringe into one of the stopcock ports (Fig. 11-37). The cuff pressure can be measured by attaching a pressure manometer to the other port on the stopcock. Air can be added by the 10-cc syringe and the pressure measured simultaneously (Fig. 11-38). There is now a commercially available system to bypass a severed cuff inflating tube.

2. Change the tracheostomy tube (Code: IIIC6a and IIIB1a) [Difficulty: An]

A tracheostomy tube may have to be changed because of a ruptured cuff or because of another problem. In addition, patients with a permanent tracheostomy have the tube changed on a routine schedule as part of the tracheostomy care. These two different situations are discussed separately.

a. Emergency tube change

Several things can cause the clinical emergency of obstruction such as the cuff herniating over the end of the

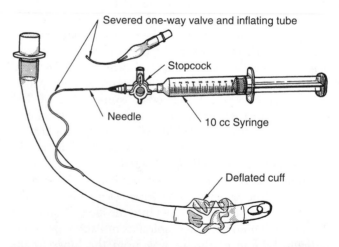

Fig. 11-37 Emergency system for inflating the cuff when the one-way valve and inflating tube are severed. (From Sills JR: *Respir Care* 31:199-201, 1986.)

tube, a mucus plug blocking the lumen, or the end of the tube forced into the tracheal tissues. Unfortunately, these problems cannot be seen from the outside. If the patient is in acute respiratory distress and an obstruction is suspected, attempt to pass a suction catheter. Failure to pass it beyond the end of the tube confirms the obstruction. A rapid clinical decision has to be made to choose the best action. The tube should be removed if the obstruction is

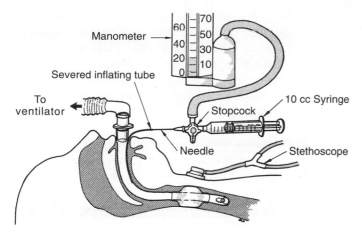

Fig. 11-38   Measuring intracuff pressure as the cuff is reinflated with an emergency system. The stethoscope is used to listen for the presence of a leak at the larynx. (From Sills JR: *Respir Care* 31:199-201, 1986.)

complete and the patient cannot breathe. A spontaneously breathing patient can continue to breathe through the stoma. An apneic patient must be temporarily ventilated with mouth-to-stoma breaths. As rapidly and carefully as possible another tracheostomy tube should be inserted. This usually results in a patent airway. If loose tracheal mucosa is blocking the airway, an endotracheal tube must be inserted past the tissue and deeper into the trachea. Call the physician as soon as possible to evaluate the patient's condition.

b. Routine tube change

If possible, the tube should not be changed until several days after a fresh tracheostomy procedure. This allows time for the stoma site to form granulomatous tissue as it begins to heal. The site is then less likely to bleed as the tube is changed. When the tracheostomy tube is changed it is usually part of the tracheostomy wound care. The following are typical steps in changing the tracheostomy tube:

1. Gather the necessary equipment: a new tracheostomy tube of the same size and the next size smaller, its inner cannula, its obturator, tracheostomy tie strings to secure the tube in the patient (see Fig. 11-9), a sterile 4- x 4-in gauze pad, sterile scissors, a 10-mL syringe to inflate the cuff, sterile water-soluble lubricant, sterile gloves, and goggles. Make sure the cuff inflates and deflates properly.
2. Put on the gloves and goggles.
3. Maintaining sterile technique, make sure the obturator easily fits into and comes out of the tracheostomy tube.
4. Cut a slit into the center of the gauze pad.
5. Apply some lubricant to the tip of the tracheostomy tube.
6. Tell the patient what you are going to do.
7. Remove the oxygen and/or aerosol from the patient.
8. Suction the patient's trachea. Reoxygenate the patient.
9. Untie the tracheostomy strings.
10. Deflate the cuff.
11. Remove the 4- x 4-in gauze pad.
12. Remove the tracheostomy tube by pulling it in a curved motion toward the patient's chest.
13. Inspect the tracheostomy opening for signs of infection such as redness, pus, or swelling. Report signs of infection to the nurse or physician.
14. Carefully insert the new tracheostomy tube with obturator into the stoma. The motion should be opposite that used to remove the original tube. Make sure not to force the tube into the tissues of the trachea.
15. Remove the obturator and insert the inner cannula. Lock it in place.
16. Give the patient oxygen and/or aerosol as before the tube change.
17. Inflate the cuff to a safe pressure.
18. Listen for bilateral breath sounds.
19. Slide the new 4- x 4-in gauze pad around the tube so that the slit fits around it.
20. Tie the tracheostomy tie strings behind the patient's neck.

MODULE D   **Extubate the patient (Code: IIIB1c) [Difficulty: An]**

Extubation should be performed only by trained personnel and under the proper conditions to ensure the patient's safety. See Box 11-5 for a list of complications that can occur after extubation.

1. Endotracheal tube

The generally recommended steps in extubation include the following:

a. Evaluate the patient's cardiopulmonary status. The reason(s) for the tube being placed should be corrected. The most recent blood gas results should be acceptable. Tracheal secretions should be minimal and not so thick that they cannot be coughed out by the patient. Bedside spirometry results

BOX 11-5	Complications After Extubation

ENDOTRACHEAL TUBE REMOVAL
Laryngospasm
Regurgitation and aspiration of stomach contents
Aspiration of saliva
Sore throat
Dysphagia
Postintubation laryngeal edema (croup)
Hoarseness from vocal cord edema or paralysis

TRACHEOSTOMY TUBE REMOVAL
Difficult tube removal from a tight stoma
Granuloma or scar at the stoma
Unhealed, open stoma

CUFF-RELATED COMPLICATIONS
Granuloma
Tracheomalacia
Tracheal stenosis
Tracheal web formation
Tracheoesophageal fistula
Arterial fistula

should show an acceptable tidal volume, vital capacity, and maximal inspiratory pressure.

b. Inform the patient about the removal of the tube and the follow-up care that is needed.

c. The patient's inspired oxygen percentage may be kept the same or increased prior to the extubation. If increased, it should be done at least 5 to 10 minutes before the tube is removed.

d. Suction the trachea until all secretions are removed.

e. Suction the oral pharynx to remove all saliva. Be prepared to suction out additional oral secretions and mucus after extubation.

f. In rapid succession:
   1. Give a deep sigh breath.
   2. Deflate the cuff. Cut the inflation tube to the cuff to ensure its collapse.
   3. Pull out the tube when the lungs are full.
   Alternatively, in rapid succession:
   1. Give a deep sigh breath.
   2. Place a suction catheter through the tube into the trachea. This works best with a self-contained catheter and sheath system.
   3. Deflate the cuff. Cut the inflation tube to the cuff to ensure its collapse.
   4. Pull out the tube when the lungs are full.
   5. Apply suction as the tube is withdrawn.

g. Have the patient cough vigorously to remove any secretions.

h. Apply a cool, bland aerosol by face mask with the previous amount of oxygen.

i. Monitor and evaluate the patient every 30 minutes for several hours. Encourage deep breathing and coughing. Check the vital signs. Measure pulse oximetry or arterial blood gases after 20 minutes. Listen to the breath sounds and larynx. Inspiratory stridor is a sign of laryngeal edema. Be prepared to nebulize racemic epinephrine (Vaponephrine) if needed. Be prepared to reintubate the patient if necessary.

2. **Tracheostomy tube**
   a. Follow steps a through g from the previous list.
   b. Depending on the physician's order, do one of the following:
      1. Apply a bland aerosol by tracheostomy mask to the stoma site with the previous amount of oxygen.
      2. Cover the stoma site with a sterile 4- x 4-in dressing. Tape it in place. Apply a bland aerosol by face mask with the previous amount of oxygen.
      3. Monitor and evaluate the patient every 30 minutes for several hours. Encourage deep breathing and coughing. Check the vital signs and breath sounds. Measure pulse oximetry or arterial blood gases after 20 minutes. Be prepared to reintubate the patient if necessary.
      4. Routine stoma care to ensure healing usually includes the following each shift:
         aa. Remove the dressing. Inspect the stoma for signs of infection such as pus, redness, and swelling.
         bb. Clean the stoma site with hydrogen peroxide on a sterile gauze pad.
         cc. Apply antibiotic ointment to the stoma site.
         dd. Reapply a sterile dressing.

MODULE E	Respiratory care plan

1. **Participate in the development of the respiratory care plan [e.g., case management, development and application of protocols, disease management education] (Code: IC4) [Difficulty: An]**

The indications or uses for the various airways are listed with the information on that airway. In general, the airway should be removed when it is no longer needed. Typically, an oropharyngeal airway should be removed from a patient who has regained consciousness. A nasopharyngeal airway should be removed if the patient no longer needs it as an airway or for a suctioning route. Endotracheal and tracheostomy tubes can be removed when the patient does not need mechanical ventilation or a suctioning route, is no longer in danger of aspiration, or does not need a permanent artificial airway.

Effective communication is important for good patient care. The conscious patient with an endotracheal tube or tracheostomy is unable to speak. Alternative ways to communicate must be provided. Examples include alphabet boards and picture boards for pointing, and pencil and paper for notes. Head nods for yes and no and lip reading are often used. It is important that questions are worded so that they can be answered with a *yes* or *no*. Avoid questions that require a lengthy written answer unless the patient seems ready and willing to do so.

It is not possible to predict how a patient may react to the placement of an artificial airway or its prolonged need. Some patients react with relief and relax when the WOB is reduced. Others may become angry at the limitations imposed on them. Still others may become depressed. Be prepared to deal with these reactions or changes in the patient's emotional response to this very stressful situation.

BIBLIOGRAPHY

AARC Clinical Practice Guideline: Management of respiratory emergencies, *Respir Care* 40:749, 1995.

AARC Clinical Practice Guideline: Removal of the endotracheal tube, *Respir Care* 44:85, 1999.

American Heart Association Emergency Cardiac Care Committee and Subcommittees: Guidelines for cardiopulmonary resuscitation and emergency cardiac care: adult advanced cardiac life support, *JAMA* 268:2199, 1992.

Dantzker DR, MacIntyre NR, Bakow ED: *Comprehensive respiratory care,* Philadelphia, 1995, WB Saunders.

Durbin CG: Artificial airways. In Cairo JM, Pilbeam SP, editors: *Mosby's respiratory care equipment,* ed 6, St Louis, 1999, Mosby.

Eubanks DH, Bone RC: *Comprehensive respiratory care,* ed 2, St Louis, 1990, Mosby.

Frownfelter DL: Chest physical therapy and airway care. In Barnes TA, editor: *Core textbook of respiratory care practice,* ed 2, St Louis, 1994, Mosby.

Heffner JE: Managing difficult intubations in critically ill patients, *Respir Manage* 19(3):53, 1989.

Hess DR, Branson RD: Airway and suction equipment. In Branson RD, Hess DR, Chatburn RL, editors: *Respiratory care equipment,* ed 2, Philadelphia, 1999, Lippincott Williams & Wilkins.

JEM 400 Endotracheal Tube Changer (product literature guide), Instrumentation Industries Inc, Bethel Park, Penn.

Kovac AL: Dilemmas and controversies in intubation, *Respir Manage* 21(4):77, 1991.

Levitzky MG, Cairo JM, Hall SM: *Introduction to respiratory care,* Philadelphia, 1990, WB Saunders.

Lewis RM: Airway care. In Fink JB, Hunt GE, editors: *Clinical practice in respiratory care,* Philadelphia, 1999, Lippincott-Raven.

Plevak DJ, Ward JJ: Airway management. In Burton GC, Hodgkin JE, Ward JJ, editors: *Respiratory care: a guide to clinical practice,* ed 4, Philadelphia, 1997, Lippincott-Raven.

PressureEasy Cuff Pressure Controller, ReviveEasy PtL Airway, and Endotracheal/Trach Tube Pilot Tube Repair Kit (product literature), Respironics, Inc, Monroeville, PA.

Roth P: Airway care. In Aloan CA, Hill TV, editors: *Respiratory care of the newborn and child,* ed 2, Philadelphia, 1997, Lippincott-Raven.

Scanlan C, Simmons K: Airway management. In Scanlan CL, Wilkins RL, Stoller JK, editors: *Egan's fundamentals of respiratory care,* ed 7, St Louis, 1999, Mosby.

Shapiro BA et al, editors: *Clinical application of respiratory care,* ed 4, St Louis, 1991.

Sills JR: An emergency cuff inflation technique, *Respir Care* 31:199, 1986.

Sills JR: *Respiratory care certification guide,* ed 1, St Louis, 1991, Mosby.

Whitaker K: *Comprehensive perinatal & pediatric respiratory care,* ed 2, Albany, NY, 1997, Delmar.

White GC: *Equipment theory for respiratory care,* ed 3, Albany, NY, 1999, Delmar.

SELF-STUDY QUESTIONS

1. A 30-year-old unconscious patient who had been involved in an automobile accident is brought into the emergency department of a small, rural hospital. A cervical spine injury is suspected and the attending physician wants recommendations for an airway that can be placed without hyperextending the patient's neck. What should the respiratory therapist recommend as best for this patient?
   A. ETC.
   B. Nasopharyngeal airway.
   C. Oropharyngeal airway.
   D. Double-lumen endotracheal tube.

2. A 59-kg (130-lb) woman must be intubated to initiate mechanical ventilation. What size tube should be used?
   A. 6.0-mm ID.
   B. 7.0-mm ID.
   C. 8.0-mm ID.
   D. 9.0-mm ID.

3. A hospitalized patient rapidly develops ventilatory failure because of an accidental overdose of morphine sulfate for pain control. The preferred way to quickly provide a safe, secure airway is to:
   A. Place an oropharyngeal airway.
   B. Hyperextend the patient's neck into the sniff position.
   C. Place a nasal endotracheal tube.
   D. Place an oral endotracheal tube.

4. Following a successful CPR attempt a patient with an oral endotracheal tube is placed on a mechanical ventilator in the Intensive Care Unit. The respiratory therapist notices that the exhaled CO_2 monitor is appropriately changing color with each breath cycle. The patient's breath sounds are present on the right side but diminished on the left side. What is the most likely cause of this situation?
   A. Left-sided pneumothorax.
   B. Right bronchial intubation.
   C. Malfunctioning exhaled CO_2 monitor.
   D. Delivered tidal volume is too small.

5. A 2-year-old child admitted with severe croup has just been extubated after 2 days with an oral endotracheal tube. The child is given oxygen and aerosolized water through a heated large volume nebulizer. Thirty minutes later, mild inspiratory stridor is heard over the child's throat area. What should be done *first*?
   A. Deliver nebulized racemic epinephrine.
   B. Reintubate the child.

C. Perform a cricothyrotomy.

D. Perform a tracheostomy.

6. A 55-year-old, 77-kg (170-lb) male patient has been returned from the operating room with a fresh tracheostomy. The respiratory therapist determines the cuff pressure on the 6.0 mm ID tracheostomy tube to be 35 mm Hg. The ventilator is delivering a tidal volume of 750 mL and returning a tidal volume of 650 mL and a leak can be heard at the tracheostomy site. What should be done?

A. Increase the tidal volume by 100 mL.

B. Increase the cuff pressure to seal the trachea to stop the tidal volume leak.

C. Replace the tracheostomy tube with one that is 8.5 mm ID.

D. Deflate the cuff enough to reduce the cuff pressure to 15 mm Hg.

7. An intubated and mechanically ventilated adult patient has been returned to the long-term care unit after being transported to the radiology department for an abdominal radiograph examination. The respiratory therapist observes that the patient's trachea is midline. However, the patient's left chest area does not rise with inspiration as much as the right chest area. The endotracheal tube is at the 28-cm mark at the patient's teeth. What should be done now?

A. Check the abdominal radiograph for signs of vomiting and aspiration.

B. Pull the endotracheal tube back about 4 cm.

C. Check the patient's end-tidal carbon dioxide level.

D. Deliver a larger tidal volume breath to inflate the left lung better.

8. A conscious patient is recovering from Guillain-Barré syndrome and is able to breathe spontaneously off of the mechanical ventilator for several hours. She currently has a standard 7.5 mm ID tracheostomy tube. To help her weaning process but to enable her to be ventilated at night, what should be done?

A. Remove the tracheostomy tube when she is off of the ventilator.

B. Substitute a speaking-type tracheostomy tube.

C. Replace the current tracheostomy tube with one that is 6.0 mm ID.

D. Substitute a fenestrated tracheostomy tube.

9. A patient who suffered facial burns and smoke inhalation has recovered enough to be extubated. Although the patient is receiving 40% oxygen with a bland aerosol, significant inspiratory stridor is noticed within 15 minutes. Following the inhalation of a vasoconstricting medication the patient's breath sounds are improved. Thirty minutes later the patient's SpO_2 is 80% and the inspiratory stridor is more serious. The patient is very anxious and is pulling off the oxygen mask. What should the respiratory therapist recommend to best manage the patient's problem?

A. Draw an arterial blood gas value.

B. Increase the patient's oxygen to 50%.

C. Intubate the patient.

D. Administer a sedative medication.

10. Placement of an esophageal obturator airway is indicated in all of the following situations *except:*

A. The patient has swallowed acid in a suicide attempt.

B. The patient is a 6-foot-tall adult.

C. The patient is unconscious.

D. Endotracheal intubation attempts have not been successful.

11. All of the following may be used to help determine the position of an endotracheal tube:

I. End-tidal carbon dioxide monitoring.

II. An esophageal detection device (EDD).

III. Laryngeal palpation during tube insertion.

IV. Neck and chest radiographs.

V. Observation of bilateral chest movement.

A. I, III, and IV only.

B. II, IV, and IV only.

C. I, II, III, and V only.

D. I, II, III, IV, and V.

12. A respiratory therapist replaces a patient's tracheostomy tube with another one of the same size and inflates the cuff with 5 mL of air as was done previously. Immediately, the patient has difficulty breathing and no air can be felt coming from the tube. What could be the problem?

A. The tip of the tube has been placed into the subcutaneous tissues.

B. The patient has closed her epiglottis over the trachea.

C. More air must be added to the cuff to form a seal.

D. The tube has been placed into the esophagus by accident.

Answer Key

1. **A.** Rationale: The ETC can be placed through the patient's mouth with the head in a neutral position. The patient can be ventilated whether the tip of the tube enters the esophagus, as intended, or the trachea. A nasopharyngeal airway and oropharyngeal airway holds the tongue off of the back of the throat but does not provide a secure airway. A double-lumen endotracheal tube may be needed only if the patient had unilateral lung problems and needed independent lung ventilation. There is no indication for these measures in this patient.

2. **C.** Rationale: An adult woman normally has an 8.0 (or 7.5) mm ID endotracheal tube placed into her. Review Table 11-1 for the recommended sizes of endotracheal and tracheostomy tubes for patients of all sizes.

3. **D.** Rationale: In an emergency situation it is fastest and easiest to place an oral endotracheal tube into most patients. A safe and secure airway can be assured within 20 to 30 seconds. An oropharyngeal airway only keeps the tongue from blocking the back of the throat. It does not provide a safe, secure airway. Hyperextending the patient's neck into the sniff position opens the airway but does not secure it from possible dangers such as vomiting and aspiration. Placing a nasal endotracheal tube requires an anesthesiologist and special equipment. This delay is unnecessary when oral endotracheal intubation can be done by a trained respiratory therapist.

4. **B.** Rationale: Right bronchial intubation is indicated by the presence of the patient's breath sounds on the right side but diminished on the left side. There is no direct evidence of a left-sided pneumothorax. The exhaled CO_2 monitor is functioning properly because it is supposed to change color (from dark purple to yellow when exposed to exhaled carbon dioxide) during the breathing cycle. Even a small tidal volume should deliver equal air to both lungs and result in equal breath sounds over both lungs.

5. **A.** Rationale: A mild case of stridor is first treated by nebulizing the vasoconstricting medication racemic epinephrine. This usually results in enough constriction of the throat's mucous membrane blood vessels to dilate the airway and correct the stridor. If this does not work, the patient may need to be intubated. A cricothyrotomy is only done only to create an emergency airway opening if the patient's upper airway is obstructed by a foreign body or trauma. A tracheostomy is only done only if a long-term surgical airway opening is needed. This patient certainly does not need either of the latter two solutions to his or her problem.

6. **C.** Rationale: Because the cuff pressure is so high on the small tracheostomy tube, it is best to replace the tube with one that is 8.5 mm ID. This is the correct size for an adult man. Increasing the tidal volume by 100 mL may deliver a larger tidal volume or it may just increase the leak around the tracheostomy tube. The real problem is a tube that is too small for the patient's trachea. It is unsafe to increase the cuff pressure to seal the trachea to stop the tidal volume leak. Although the increased pressure overinflates the cuff to stop the leak, the circulation is cut off from the patient's tracheal mucosa and the mucosa can die. It is unsafe to deflate the cuff enough to reduce the cuff pressure to 15 mm Hg because the patient's tidal volume leak can worsen.

7. **B.** Rationale: An adult patient usually has the proximal end of the tube at the 23- to 25-cm mark at the teeth for a midtracheal tube tip position. This, and the observation that the left side of the patient's chest is not moving as much as the right side, indicates that the tube has been pushed down into the right mainstem bronchus. The best thing to do is reposition the tube by suctioning the patient's airways and throat, deflating the cuff, withdrawing the tube about 4 cm, and reinflating the cuff. Of course, check for bilateral breath sounds, confirm a safe cuff pressure, and get a chest radiograph to complete the procedure. There is nothing to be gained by checking the abdominal radiograph because signs of vomiting and aspiration are not seen on it. Pneumonitis can be seen on a chest radiograph but not on an abdominal radiograph because an abdominal radiograph does not include the chest. Checking the patient's end-tidal carbon dioxide level demonstrates exhaled CO_2. However, this is not specific enough for this situation because the right lung can give off the gas even if the left lung is not ventilated. Delivering a larger tidal volume breath does not inflate the left lung any better because the endotracheal tube has been pushed down the right mainstem bronchus.

8. **D.** Rationale: Substituting a fenestrated tracheostomy tube for the standard tube allows her to breathe spontaneously through the upper airway when the inner cannula is removed. This allows her to talk, which can have a very positive emotional impact on the patient. It is probably going too far to remove the tracheostomy tube when she is off of the ventilator. This necessitates removing the tube, covering the stoma, and reinserting the tube later in the day. This can lead to damage to the tracheal tissue. In additional, if the patient's condition suddenly deteriorates while the tracheostomy tube is removed, no secure airway is available. Although a speaking-type tracheostomy tube allows her to speak while on the ventilator, it does not enable her to breathe through her upper airway when she is off of the ventilator as a fenestrated tube allows. Replacing the current 7.5 mm ID tracheostomy tube with one that is 6.0 mm ID greatly increases the patient's WOB. This can tire her out and delay her recovery.

9. **C.** Rationale: The patient should be reintubated because of the serious nature of the inspiratory stridor that is unresponsive to the inhaled vasoconstricting drug (racemic epinephrine), the low SpO_2 value, and the combative nature of the patient. An arterial blood gas value is not necessary because the SpO_2 value of 80% confirms hypoxemia. Getting the ABG sample and waiting for the results only delays the necessary intubation. Increasing the patient to 50% oxygen helps relieve the hypoxemia. However, once the patient is intubated and can breathe adequately, the SpO_2 value should increase to a safe level on the previous 40% oxygen. It could be very dangerous to administer a sedative medication to this patient. Sedating the patient further reduces the patient's ability to breathe through the narrowed airway.

10. **A.** Rationale: An EOA should not be placed into a patient who has swallowed acid because the tube will cause further damage to the esophagus. An EOA is designed for patients who are at least 5 feet tall. A shorter individual may have the tip of the tube enter the stomach instead of staying within the esophagus as intended. A patient must be unconscious to tolerate an EOA because it passes through the throat and can stimulate a gag reflex in a conscious person. Endotracheal intubation provides a more secure airway that an EOA. Therefore if trained personnel were available to insert either tube, an EOA should be used only after endotracheal intubation has been unsuccessful.

11. **D.** Rationale: All of these may be used, along with listening for bilateral breath sounds, to confirm the location of the endotracheal tube. An end-tidal carbon dioxide monitoring system (capnograph) or disposable carbon dioxide detector such as the Easy Cap may be used to detect exhaled carbon dioxide. If the tube is placed within the esophagus, no carbon dioxide will be found. An EDD can be attached to the endotracheal tube. After the bulb has been squeezed, it inflates with air from the patient's lungs if the tube is within a major airway. See Fig. 11-32. Laryngeal palpation during tube insertion allows the tube to be felt as it passes through the larynx. Remember that these three methods differentiate only between airway and esophageal intubation. They do not detect a tube that has been inserted too deeply and has entered a mainstem bronchus (usually the right). A neck and chest radiograph shows the tube entering the larynx and its tip within the trachea (or a bronchus). Observation of bilateral chest movement is valuable because equal movement correlates with tracheal intubation and ventilation of both lungs.

12. **A.** Rationale: If the tip of the tracheostomy tube has been placed into the subcutaneous tissues the patient will not be able to ventilate at all. The tube must be immediately withdrawn. Because the tracheotomy site is below the larynx, it does not matter if the patient has closed her epiglottis over the trachea. She still can breathe through the tracheostomy tube. It is unlikely that the new cuff requires any more air than the previous one. Even if this were the case, the patient should still be able to breathe through the tube. It should not be possible to place a tracheostomy tube into a patient's esophagus.

12 Suctioning the Airway

A review of the most recent Written Registry Exams has shown an average of two questions (2%) on suctioning the airway.

MODULE A   Suctioning devices

1. Oropharyngeal suction devices

a. Get the necessary equipment for the procedure (Code: IIA1g) [Difficulty: An]

Oropharyngeal suctioning is considered a clean (not sterile) procedure. The suctioning device is packaged sterile but may be used more than once. A Yankauer suction catheter is widely used. It is made of hard plastic and has an angled catheter to reach into the back of the mouth. There may be one large opening or several medium-sized openings at the tip of the catheter. The openings are large enough to permit easy suctioning of saliva, food, or vomit. Some handles include a thumb control valve so that suction can be applied to the tip only when wanted. Covering the opening with a thumb creates a vacuum at the tip for suctioning the patient's mouth (Fig. 12-1). The Yankauer may be discarded when no longer needed or sterilized for use with another patient.

A flexible plastic or rubber catheter can also be used. It should be the largest diameter possible to reduce its chance of becoming plugged. The opening at the catheter tip should be cut straight (perpendicular) across instead of at an angle. There should not be any side openings (Fig. 12-2). The catheter is discarded when no longer needed.

b. Put the equipment together, make sure that it works properly, and identify any problems (Code: IIB1g) [Difficulty: An]

The catheters just mentioned are single pieces with nothing to assemble. They must be attached to a vacuum source by a length of soft rubber tubing. With clean gloves on both hands, attach the Yankauer, plastic, or rubber catheter to the vacuum tubing. The vacuum must be applied to the tip of the catheter for oral secretions to be removed. Check for a vacuum at the tip by any of the following methods:

1. Listen for the sound of air being drawn into the tip.
2. Put the tip into a container of sterile water. Close the thumb control opening. The water must be drawn up the catheter.
3. Place a clean-gloved hand over the tip if no water is

available. Close the thumb control opening. The glove should be attracted to the catheter.

c. Fix any problems with the equipment (Code: IIB2g) [Difficulty: An]

Failure to have a vacuum at the catheter tip can mean:

1. The vacuum is not turned on. Check the following:
   a. Some centralized vacuum systems have a single dial that turns the system off and on and sets the vacuum level. Other centralized vacuum systems have an on and off switch and a dial for the vacuum level.
   b. Freestanding vacuum systems must be plugged into a working electrical outlet. The on and off switch must be turned on. The simpler systems have a preset vacuum level. Variable vacuum levels can be set with a dial in the more sophisticated systems.
2. The system is not sealed, so the vacuum is lost to the atmosphere. Check the following:
   a. Make sure that the rubber vacuum tubing fits tightly over the connectors on the catheter and on the vacuum system.
   b. Make sure that the catheter and vacuum tubing are not cracked or cut. Replace a Yankauer, plastic, or rubber catheter or vacuum tubing that is defective.
   c. Close the thumb control if it has been left open.
   d. Check the central or freestanding vacuum system to make sure that the secretion collection bottle is sealed properly.
3. The system is blocked, and no vacuum can get through to the tip. Check the following:
   a. Check for a pinch in the vacuum tubing or soft catheter.
   b. Check for a blockage in the catheter or vacuum tubing. Try to suction some sterile water to clear the blockage into the secretion collection bottle. Replace the catheter, or vacuum tubing, or both if the blockage cannot be cleared.
   c. Empty out a collection bottle that is full.

2. Suction catheters

Suctioning catheters are intended for removing secretions and foreign material from the trachea. They come sterile and individually packaged. It is highly recommended that the outer diameter (OD) of the catheter be no more than one half the inner diameter of the airway that it is passing through. This guideline is intended to minimize the obstruction to the airway so that the patient can still breathe around the catheter.

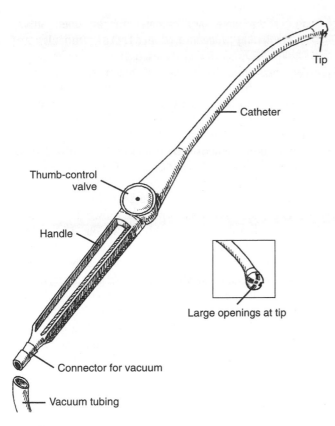

Fig. 12-1 Features of Yankauer suction catheter.

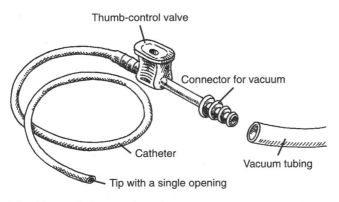

Fig. 12-2 Features of suction catheter with cross-cut tip.

See Table 12-1 for the recommended suction catheter sizes for the various endotracheal or tracheostomy tubes.

	TABLE 12-1	Recommended Suction Catheter French Sizes for the Various Endotracheal and Tracheostomy Tube Sizes*

Age	ID* of tube sizes (mm)	Suction catheter size (Fr)
NEWBORN		
1000 g	2.5	5
1000-2000 g	3.0	6
2000-3000 g	3.5	8
3000 g to 6 mo old	3.5-4.0	8
PEDIATRIC		
18 mo	4.0	8
3 yr	4.5	8
5 yr	5.0	10
6 yr	5.5	10
8 yr	6.0	10
ADULT		
16 yr	7.0	10
Normal-sized woman	7.5-8.0	12
Normal-sized man	8.0-8.5	14
Large adult	9.0-10.0	16

Note: It is recommended to use a suction catheter with an outer diameter that is no more than half of the inner diameter of the endotracheal tube.
*ID, Inner diameter.

The practitioner can also easily compare the relative sizes of the tube and suction catheter at the bedside before suctioning. Suction catheters are sized by the French (Fr or F) scale of their OD. Endotracheal and tracheostomy tubes are sized by ID and OD in millimeters and often by ID in French. Review Table 11-1 if necessary. The following formula and example shows how to calculate the OD size of any suction catheter to find with which endotracheal or tracheostomy tube that size of suction catheter may be used. Because each French unit is about 0.33 mm, the OD in millimeters of a suction catheter can be found by multiplying the French size by 0.33. For example, calculate the OD of a 12 Fr suction catheter:

$$12 \text{ Fr} \times 0.33 = 3.96 \text{ (about 4.0) mm OD of the catheter}$$

Therefore this sized catheter could be used on an 8.0 mm ID endotracheal tube. See Fig. 12-3 for the relative sizes of this endotracheal tube and catheter.

There may also be some clinical use in knowing the ID of a suction catheter because it relates to the maximum particle size that can pass through it. The following formula can be used to interconvert from French to millimeters.

$$mm = \frac{Fr - 2}{4}$$

Example. What is the ID in millimeters of a 12 Fr suction catheter?

$$mm = \frac{12 - 2}{4}$$

$$mm = \frac{10}{4}$$

$$mm = 2.5 \text{ (See Fig. 12-3.)}$$

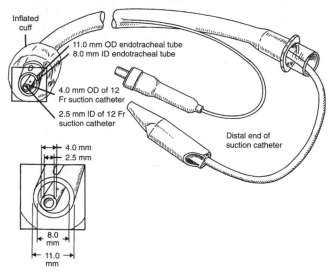

Fig. 12-3 Number 12 Fr suction catheter inside of 8.0-mm ID endotracheal tube. The OD of the catheter should be no more than one half of the ID of the tube so that the patient can still breathe around it.

a. Get the necessary catheter for an open airway suctioning procedure (Code: IIA1g) [Difficulty: An]

Open airway suctioning is used here to refer to the patient spontaneously breathing room air after being disconnected from the source of supplemental oxygen. This happens to the patient with a normal upper airway when the oxygen mask is removed for nasotracheal suctioning. It also happens when the patient with an endotracheal or tracheostomy tube has the aerosol T-piece (Briggs' adapter) or ventilator circuit removed for suctioning purposes.

These types of catheters have been in use for many years. There are two basic types, as shown in Fig. 12-4. Closing the thumb control, as shown in Fig. 12-5, allows the vacuum to be selectively applied to the secretions when desired. The tips of the catheters can vary greatly. There has been a considerable amount of effort spent trying to develop a catheter tip that most effectively removes secretions without damaging the tracheal mucosa. Fig. 12-6 shows some of the catheter tips that have been developed to minimize mucosal damage. Note that all feature at least one opening in the catheter that is back from the opening at the tip. Compare this with the single-end opening found on the oral suction catheter (see Fig. 12-2). The side openings are designed to prevent the vacuum from being applied to the tip when it makes contact with the mucosa.

Notice in Figs. 12-4 and 12-6 that most catheters are straight throughout their length. All of these catheters tend to enter the right mainstem bronchus during deep suctioning. This is because its angle off of the trachea is less

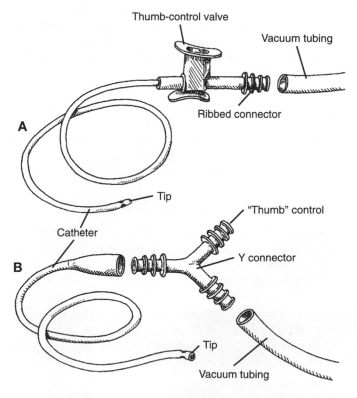

Fig. 12-4 Features of two types of suction catheters with angle-cut tips and side holes. **A,** Catheter has its own thumb control valve. **B,** Catheter must have a thumb control valve constructed from a Y connector.

acute compared with the angle of the left mainstem bronchus. Thus it is difficult, if not impossible, for any of these catheters to suction the left mainstem bronchus. The Coudé catheter has been designed with an angled tip to better enable it to be guided into the left (or right) mainstem bronchus. See the far right example in Fig. 12-6. When these catheters are used, the direction of the thumb control valve can help determine the angle of the bent tip.

Use of these traditional types of catheters during open airway suctioning always results in some level of hypoxemia. The use of a relatively new type of suction catheter may help to alleviate this problem. The insufflating suction catheter is designed to alternatively provide oxygen through the catheter or vacuum for suctioning. The thumb control end of the catheter is modified with two male-type tubing connectors and a way to switch the lumen of the catheter between them. The thumb control is set to direct the oxygen through the catheter and into the patient as the catheter is advanced. After the catheter has been deeply placed into the trachea for suctioning, the thumb control is switched from delivering oxygen to applying suction.

b. Get the necessary catheter for a closed airway suctioning procedure (Code: IIA1g) [Difficulty: An]

Closed airway suctioning is used here to refer to suctioning when the patient remains connected to the original source of oxygen. This may be done through a special aerosol T-piece or, more commonly, with the patient receiving mechanical ventilation. Spontaneously breathing patients are less likely to suffer hypoxemia with closed airway suctioning because they can continue to inhale the prescribed oxygen percentage.

In closed airway suctioning systems, a flexible, clear plastic sheath covers the catheter to maintain its sterility

(Fig. 12-7). The practitioner does not need gloves. When used for patients who need frequent suctioning, the self-contained systems have a financial advantage over the traditional catheter and gloves suctioning method because they can be reused. These closed-system suction catheters come with either the traditional straight tip or the Coudé tip for selective bronchial suctioning.

Another device to create a sealed system for endotracheal tube suctioning consists of an elbow adapter that has an inner plastic sleeve or diaphragm. As the traditional catheter is inserted into the opening on the elbow adapter, the sleeve or diaphragm conforms to the catheter so that there is no air leak (Fig. 12-8). This ensures that the ventilator delivered volumes and pressures are not lost through a leak.

c. Put the suctioning equipment together, make sure that it works properly, and identify any problems (Code: IIB1g) [Difficulty: An]

Refer to Fig. 12-4 for the attachment of an open airway suction catheter to the vacuum tubing. Fig. 12-7 shows the attachment of a closed airway suction catheter to the vacuum tubing. The other end of the vacuum tubing is attached to the vacuum regulator system.

With open airway suctioning, only a hand covered by a sterile glove can be allowed to touch the area of the catheter that enters the patient's trachea. The practitioner's other hand should also be gloved. A clean glove is acceptable because it does not touch the part of the catheter that will enter the patient's trachea.

While holding the body of the catheter, the thumb control valve, and vacuum connector with the sterile-gloved hand and the vacuum tubing with the clean-gloved hand, slip the vacuum tubing over the catheter's vacuum

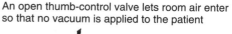

An open thumb-control valve lets room air enter so that no vacuum is applied to the patient

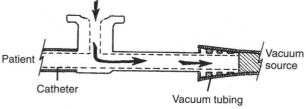

Fig. 12-5 Close-up of thumb control valve showing how room air is drawn into vacuum tubing when the valve is left open. Closing valve applies vacuum to catheter tip to suction secretions.

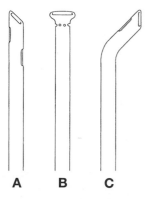

Fig. 12-6 Close-up of the ends of three different suction catheters. **A,** Shows a bevel cut of the tip with two offset side holes. **B,** Shows a ring tip with several side holes around it. **C,** Shows a Coudé (curved-tip) catheter, which may help in guiding it into either the left or right mainstem bronchus. (From Rarey KP, Youtsey JW: Respiratory patient care, Englewood Cliffs, NJ, 1981, Prentice-Hall. Used by permission.)

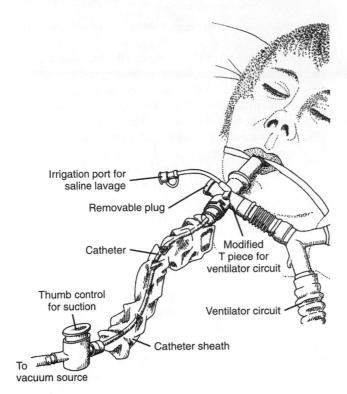

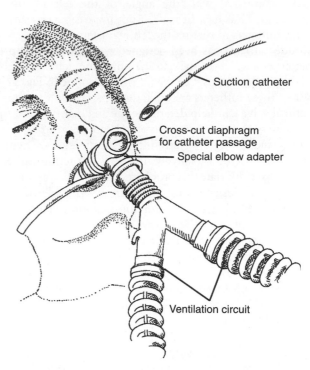

Fig. 12-7　Self-contained catheter and sheath suctioning system for closed-airway suctioning. (Based on the Kimberly-Clark/Ballard TRACH CARE® closed endotracheal suction device.)

Fig. 12-8　Features and placement of special elbow adapter for closed-airway suctioning without losing tidal volume or pressure during mechanical ventilation.

connector. The seal should be tight so that there is no vacuum leak. From now on, only the sterile-gloved hand may touch the part of the catheter that makes contact with the patient. The clean-gloved hand may touch only the thumb control valve and vacuum tubing. If the catheter is contaminated, it must be discarded.

The catheter can be tested for patency and vacuum at the tip by the three methods described earlier in the discussion on oropharyngeal suction devices. Note that only a *sterile* glove may be touched against the tip of the suction catheter to check for a vacuum.

The practitioner does not need gloves when a self-contained catheter is used for closed airway suctioning because the sheath covers the catheter to prevent contamination.

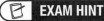　**EXAM HINT**

Remember that endotracheal suctioning is a sterile procedure. Contaminated gloves or catheter must be replaced with sterile equipment.

d. Fix any problems with the equipment (Code: IIB2g) [Difficulty: An]

The three common causes of an equipment failure and how to fix them are described in the earlier discussion on

oropharyngeal suction devices. Remember to completely withdraw the closed airway suctioning catheter from the endotracheal tube into the sheath, or it will act as a partial obstruction.

3. Specimen collectors

a. Get the necessary equipment (Code: IIA1g) [Difficulty: An]

A variety of specimen collectors (commonly called Lukens traps) exist. They are packaged as sterile so that there is no contamination of the sputum sample with nonpatient organisms. Figs. 12-9 through 12-12 show the key features and functions of several sputum sample collectors. The sputum sample is obtained through a suction catheter or bronchoscope.

The specimen jar has volume markings and screws into either a special lid used to suction the specimen or a regular lid for shipment to the laboratory. The special lids used in the systems featured in Figs. 12-9 and 12-10 must be connected to a sterile catheter. Fig. 12-11 shows a system with its own catheter. The vacuum source is provided to these specimen collectors by a length of vacuum tubing as in the previously described suction catheter systems. Fig. 12-12 shows a DeLee system sometimes used in the delivery room. The physician, nurse, or practitioner uses mouth suction to remove secretions from the newborn. In all of these examples, after the sample has been collected,

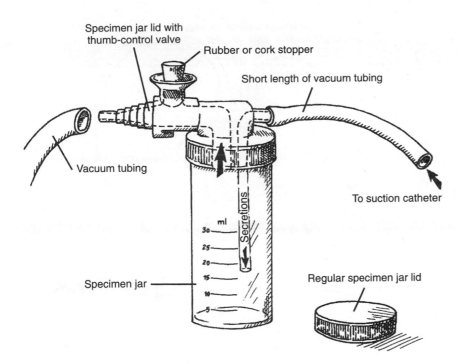

Specimen jar lid with
thumb-control valve

Rubber or cork stopper

Short length of vacuum tubing

Vacuum tubing

To suction catheter

Secretions

ml
30
25
20
15
10
5

Specimen jar

Regular specimen jar lid

Fig. 12-9   Features of sputum specimen collection system with thumb control valve.

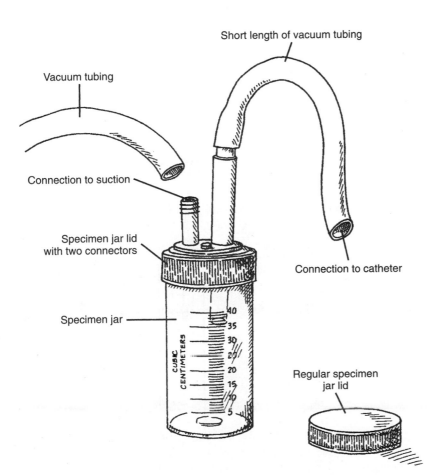

Short length of vacuum tubing

Vacuum tubing

Connection to suction

Specimen jar lid
with two connectors

Connection to catheter

Specimen jar

CUBIC CENTIMETERS

40
35
30
25
20
15
10
5

Regular specimen
jar lid

Fig. 12-10   Features of sputum specimen collection system without thumb control valve.

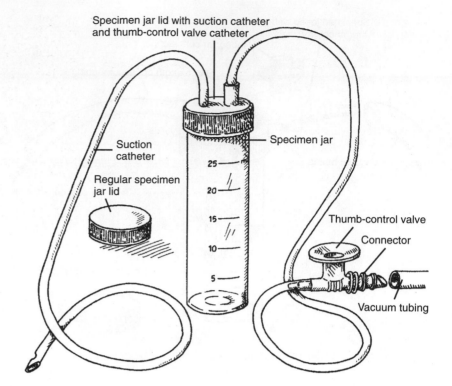

Fig. 12-11 Features of sputum specimen collection system with thumb control valve built into catheter.

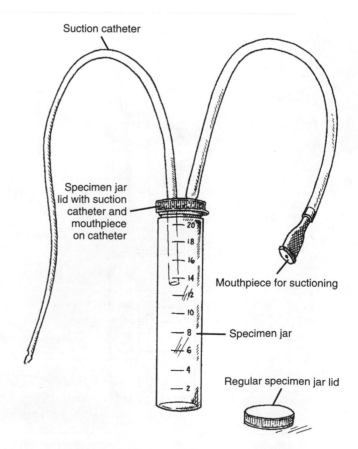

Fig. 12-12 Features of DeLee sputum specimen collection system with mouthpiece through which the practitioner can apply suction.

the special lid is unscrewed and replaced with the regular specimen jar lid.

b. Put the equipment together, make sure that it works properly, and identify any problems (Code: IIB1g) [Difficulty: An]

A properly working specimen collection system provides a vacuum to the tip of the suction catheter when the thumb control valve or mouthpiece is sealed and vacuum is applied. This is tested by dipping the catheter tip into a container of sterile water or saline solution. The liquid is drawn up the catheter and deposited in the specimen jar. (The water can be emptied out of the jar by simply unscrewing the jar and discarding it.)

c. Fix any problems with the equipment (Code: IIB2g) [Difficulty: An]

Failure to have a vacuum at the tip of the suction catheter may be caused by any of the previously mentioned possibilities. They can be checked and corrected by the methods listed earlier. There are two likely causes of an inability to suction secretions. One possible cause is that the jar is not screwed tightly into the special lid. This allows room air to be drawn in. Simply screw the lid in tightly. The second possible cause is that the secretion channel is plugged. Discard it and replace it with a new specimen collector.

MODULE B	Vacuum regulator systems

1. Get the necessary vacuum regulator system: vacuum pump, regulator, and collection bottle (Code: IIA1r) [Difficulty: An]

2. Put the equipment together, make sure that it works properly, and identify any problems (Code: IIB1r) [Difficulty: An]

The vacuum regulators come preassembled by the manufacturer. There are two basic types, which are described here. Components must be added to make them fully functional.

a. Portable vacuum systems

Portable units are designed to be moved with the patient. They may be mounted on a small platform (see Fig. 12-13) or mounted on a wheeled cart. The portable systems generally include an electrically powered vacuum pump with an on/off switch and a collection bottle. Some units have a control valve for adjusting the level of negative pressure. A negative pressure gauge is used to determine how much vacuum is being applied. A length of rubber vacuum tubing is used to pass the negative pressure from the pump to the collection bottle. Another length of vacuum tubing is used to pass the vacuum through to the

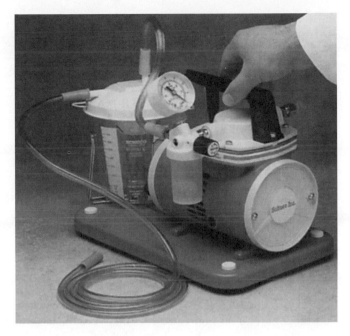

Fig. 12-13 Portable suction machine. Electrically powered motor, collection bottle and cap, and connecting tubing can be seen. (Courtesy Allied Health Care Products Inc, St Louis, MO.)

suction catheter. Portable systems are not as powerful as the central vacuum systems. They are not very effective at suctioning out large amounts of thick secretions.

In general, the following steps are needed to make the units operational:

1. Plug the vacuum pump into a working electrical outlet. Battery operated units should have fully charged batteries.
2. Place a clean, empty collection bottle into its holder on the cart. The bottle should be able to hold at least 500 mL of fluid.
3. Slip the rubber lid onto the open top of the collection bottle. Both vacuum tubing connectors on the lid must be patent.
4. Slip one end of a short length of vacuum tubing over the connector on the vacuum pump and the other end to one of the tubing connectors on the collection bottle lid.
5. Slip one end of a length of vacuum tubing over the other tubing connector on the collection bottle lid. The vacuum tubing should be no more than 3 feet long. The other end of the vacuum tubing is connected to the suction catheter when needed.
6. Turn on the unit and determine the negative pressure by:
   a. Pinching closed the long vacuum tubing
   b. Turning on the vacuum pump
   c. Observing the pressure on the negative pressure gauge

7. If the unit has a fixed vacuum level, the observed negative pressure should match that listed by the manufacturer.
8. If the unit has a variable vacuum level, adjust the vacuum control knob to the desired level.

b. Central vacuum systems

Central (wall) vacuum systems are usually available at each patient's bedside in all special care units. Each of the wall outlets is connected through a hospital-wide piping system to a large electrically powered vacuum pump. It is capable of generating a negative pressure far greater than what is needed in most patient care situations. A regulator is used to reduce the vacuum to the desired clinical level (see Fig. 12-14). Either a Quick Connect or Diameter Index Safety System (DISS) connector is used to attach the regulator to the central vacuum system.

Most regulators have a selector knob that allows the user to turn the vacuum off (Off setting) or switch between full vacuum (Full setting) and a regulated level of vacuum (Reg setting). The Full setting opens the unit to the maximum level of vacuum available from the central pump. The Reg setting allows the user to adjust the vacuum level through a wide range.

In general, the following steps are needed to make the units operational:

1. Connect the regulator into a working suction outlet.
2. Screw a clean, empty collection bottle onto its connector on the regulator. The bottle must be able to hold at least 500 mL of fluid.
3. Slip one end of a length of vacuum tubing over the tubing connector on the collection bottle. The vacuum tubing should be no more than 3 feet long. The other end of the vacuum tubing is connected to the suction catheter when needed.
4. Determine the negative pressure by:
   a. Pinching closed the vacuum tubing (see Fig. 12-15).
   b. Turning the selector knob to Reg.
   c. Observing the pressure on the negative pressure gauge

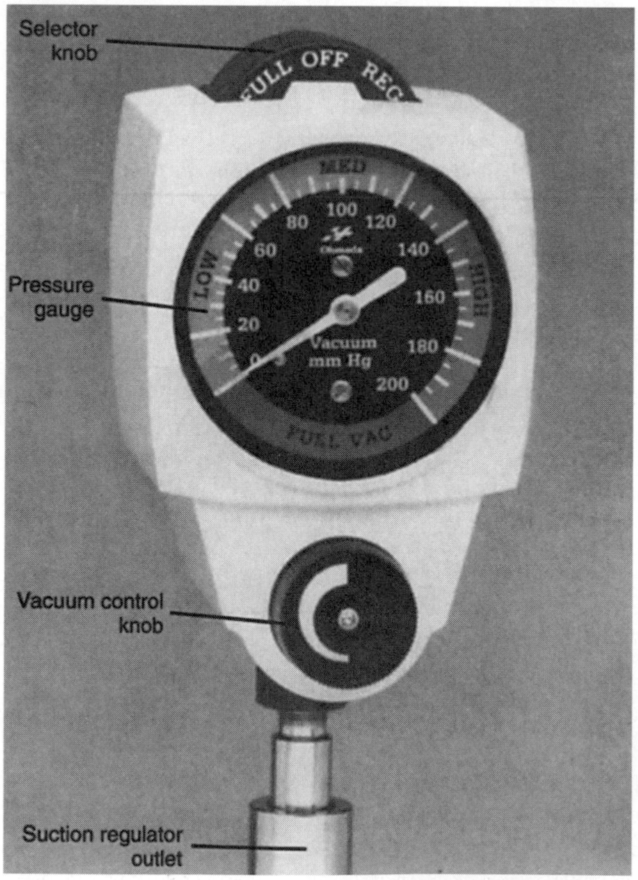

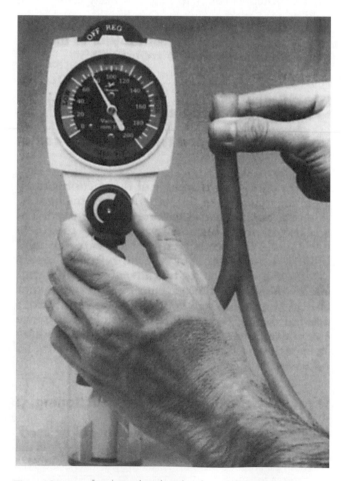

Fig. 12-14 Features of Ohmeda central vacuum regulator with three-position selector knob. (Courtesy Ohmeda, Madison, WI.)

Fig. 12-15 Setting the level of negative pressure on Ohmeda central vacuum regulator by pinching vacuum tubing and adjusting vacuum control knob. Vacuum pressure is seen on pressure gauge. (Courtesy Ohmeda, Madison, WI.)

5. Adjust the vacuum control knob to the desired level. If the secretions are too thick to be drawn up the suction catheter, the negative pressure must be increased.

3. Fix any problems with the equipment (Code: IIB2r) [Difficulty: An]

With a *portable* vacuum system, check the following when trying to determine the cause of a loss of vacuum:

a. The vacuum pump is plugged into a working electrical outlet.
b. The vacuum pump is turned on.
c. The vacuum control valve is set at the desired negative pressure.
d. The lid to the collection bottle is tightly sealed.
e. The vacuum tubing tightly connects the pump to the collection bottle and the collection bottle to the suction catheter.
f. There are no knots or obstructions in the vacuum tubing or catheter.
g. The collection bottle is not filled above its maximum level.

Correct any potential problems. Do not use a portable vacuum system that will not generate the negative pressure that it is supposed to.

With a *central* vacuum system, check the following when trying to determine the cause of a loss of vacuum:

a. The regulator is plugged into a working vacuum outlet.
b. The vacuum control valve is set at the desired negative pressure.
c. The collection bottle is tightly screwed onto the suction regulator outlet.
d. The vacuum tubing tightly connects the collection bottle to the suction catheter.
e. There are no knots or obstructions in the vacuum tubing or catheter.
f. The collection bottle is not filled above its maximum level.

Correct any potential problems. Do not use a central vacuum system outlet that will not generate the negative pressure that it should. Occasionally, there is less negative pressure than expected when the central vacuum system is being heavily used. There is no problem with the regulator or tubing and the vacuum pressure will increase when fewer people are using it.

MODULE C	Initiate suctioning procedures to remove tracheal and oral secretions (Code: IIIC6b) [Difficulty: An]

Tracheal or oral secretions must be actively removed by suctioning whenever the patient cannot clear them out and is at risk of obstructing the airway. Suctioning may be needed in patients who are unconscious and lack swallowing or coughing reflexes. Or the patient may be too weak to cough effectively to remove tracheal secretions. Often the physician writes a standing order to suction the patient on a regular basis or as needed. However, in many institutions there is a protocol to suction any patient who is at risk of obstructing his or her airway. For example, the comatose patient who vomits should have the mouth suctioned out even though there is no specific physician's order to do so.

Suctioning secretions from a patient's trachea, by any method, places the patient at risk. The following two factors must be understood, identified when they occur, and prevented or corrected.

1. Prevent hypoxemia during the suctioning procedure (Code: IIIB4c) [Difficulty: An]

Suctioning the trachea removes air (including oxygen), as well as secretions, from the lungs. Hypoxemia, however, can be minimized by hyperoxygenating the patient for 1 to 2 minutes before suctioning. It is generally recommended that the patient receive 100% oxygen, if possible. Infants younger than 6 months of age should be given a fractional concentration of inspired oxygen (F_IO_2) only 10% to 20% greater than their base level. This is because of the risk of retinopathy of prematurity (ROP), also known as retrolental fibroplasia.

Check the patient's arterial blood gas results or SpO_2 value to see whether the patient is hypoxic before beginning the procedure. SpO_2 values can also be monitored throughout the suctioning procedure to see how low the saturation drops and when the patient has been resaturated (>90%) after suctioning is performed. The patient's chart should also be checked for any history of cardiac problems. Sudden hypoxemia from suctioning can result in life-threatening dysrhythmias such as premature ventricular contractions (PVCs). Check the patient's pulse rate and rhythm before and after suctioning. If the patient is using a cardiac monitor, it should be watched for rate and rhythm changes that are related to the suctioning procedure. Tachycardia is frequently seen with hypoxemia. Check the blood pressure of any patient who has suctioning-related dysrhythmias. The patient's vital signs should return to normal when oxygenation is restored.

Any modern mechanical ventilator can be set to deliver 100% oxygen. The most current ventilators have a 100% oxygen button designed just for this purpose. Pushing it results in the patient receiving pure oxygen for 1 to 2 minutes (depending on the manufacturer). Several sigh breaths can also be delivered. A closed airway suction catheter can be used with the ventilator, as discussed earlier, to minimize hypoxemia.

A spontaneously breathing patient can have a non-rebreathing mask placed and set to deliver close to 100% oxygen. If a non-rebreathing mask is not available, turn up the oxygen flow or percentage on whatever appliance the patient is using. A spontaneously breathing patient with an endotracheal or tracheostomy tube can have 100% oxygen

BOX 12-1	Hazards and Complications of Endotracheal Suctioning

Cardiac arrest
Respiratory arrest
Hypoxemia
Cardiac dysrhythmias
Bronchospasm
Increased intracranial pressure
Hypertension
Hypotension
Apnea from interruption of mechanical ventilation
Pulmonary hemorrhage
Mechanical trauma to tracheal and bronchial mucosa
Infection to and/or from patient and respiratory care practitioner
Atelectasis

delivered through a Brigg's adapter/aerosol T-piece. A manual resuscitation bag can also be used to give the patient several sigh breaths.

All patients must be reoxygenated before another attempt at suctioning is made. Giving 100% oxygen after the suctioning episode helps the patient to reoxygenate faster. Giving several sigh breaths also helps reoxygenation to occur faster than normal tidal volume breathing does.

Vagus or vagal nerve stimulation. Vagal nerve endings are found in the hypopharynx and trachea. When they are mechanically stimulated by a suction catheter, any of the following may be seen:

a. The patient may have an induced bronchospasm.
b. The patient may become bradycardic.
c. The patient's blood pressure may drop because of the bradycardia.

Listen to the patient's breath sounds before and after suctioning to determine whether there is an increase in wheezing, which shows bronchospasm. Check the patient's heart rate and rhythm by palpation or cardiac monitor to determine whether he or she is becoming bradycardic. The blood pressure can also be measured to check for hypotension.

Further suctioning should be delayed, if possible, until the patient's wheezing and vital signs have returned to normal. It may be necessary to modify the suctioning procedure by not going as deeply and striking the carina, not twisting the catheter, or not suctioning for as long to reduce the risk of vagal stimulation. A local anesthetic such as lidocaine (Xylocaine) can be nebulized (with a physician's order) to reduce the local reaction to the catheter.

See Box 12-1 for hazards and complications of endotracheal suctioning. See Box 12-2 for contraindications and hazards and complications of nasotracheal suctioning.

BOX 12-2	Contraindications and Hazards and Complications of Nasotracheal Suctioning

Contraindications
  Absolute:
    Epiglottitis
    Laryngotracheobronchitis (croup)
  Relative:
    Blocked nasal passages
    Nasal bleeding
    Acute facial, neck, or head injury
    Bleeding disorder
    Upper respiratory tract infection
    Irritable airway
    Laryngospasm
Hazards and complications
  Cardiac arrest
  Respiratory arrest
  Hypoxemia
  Cardiac dysrhythmias
  Bronchospasm
  Increased intracranial pressure
  Hypertension
  Hypotension
  Pulmonary hemorrhage
  Infection to and/or from patient and respiratory therapist
  Atelectasis
  Pain
  Catheter misdirected into esophagus
  Gagging and/or vomiting
  Uncontrolled coughing
  Mechanical trauma: nasal turbinates, perforation of pharynx, nasal bleeding, bleeding of the tracheal and bronchial mucosa

---

EXAM HINT

Understand the importance of hyperoxygenating a patient before and after a suctioning procedure. Hypoxemia and vagal stimulation can result in unstable vital signs and bronchospasm. Be prepared to stop suctioning, give extra oxygen, or get help.

MODULE D	Respiratory care plan

1. **Participate in the development of the respiratory care plan [e.g. case management, development and application of protocols, disease management education] (Code: IC4) [Difficulty: An]**

Hearing coarse, intermittent expiratory sounds (rhonchi) indicates that there are secretions in the airway. Tracheal suctioning should clear these secretions and result in the return of normal breath sounds (or at least an improvement). Pneumonia and bronchitis result in chest

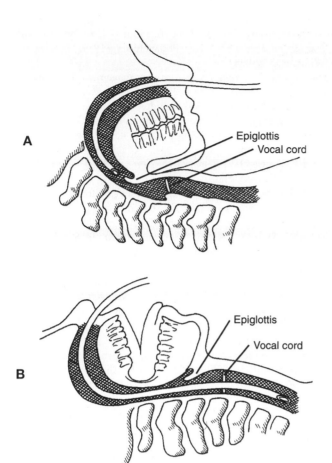

A

Epiglottis
Vocal cord

B

Epiglottis

Vocal cord

Fig. 12-16   Cross section through airway showing nasotracheal suctioning. **A,** With head in sniff position, catheter is advanced through nostril to level of vocal cords. **B,** During an inspiration, catheter is advanced into trachea. The patient will cough, and secretions can be suctioned out.

radiograph changes that show areas of infiltrate. Disease involvement of right or left lung (or both), individual lobes, and segments can be determined. As the patient's condition improves, the chest radiograph should show clearing of infiltrates.

2. Note the patient's subjective response to therapy (Code: IIIA1c) [Difficulty: An]

A conscious patient should be able to communicate with you about how he or she feels after suctioning of secretions. Hopefully, the feeling of dyspnea is improved.

3. Make a change in the size and type of suction catheter (Code: IIIC7b) [Difficulty: An]

As discussed earlier, the OD of the suction catheter should be no more than half the ID of the patient's endotracheal tube. If the secretions are easy to suction out, a smaller catheter may be used. The spontaneously

breathing patient is less likely to become hypoxic if the tube is less obstructed.

A catheter with a Coudé tip should be used if the catheter must be directed into one or the other mainstem bronchus (usually the left). Closed airway catheters such as those made by Ballard Medical Products offer two advantages over single-use catheters. First, they are more economical if the patient needs frequent suctioning. Second, a patient using a mechanical ventilator continues to be ventilated and oxygenated and have PEEP maintained during the suctioning episode. The newer catheters that offer intermittent or continuous insufflation of oxygen may reduce the hypoxemia that many patients experience during the suctioning procedure. However, they can be difficult to use and costly.

4. Observe changes in the patient's sputum production and consistency (Code: IIIA1c) [Difficulty: An]

The amount and consistency of sputum that a patient produces depends on the lung problem and whether it is worsening or improving. For example, if pneumonia or bronchitis is worsening, secretion production is increased. Also, if the patient is dehydrated the sputum contains less water than normal. The patient may complain that the secretions are "thicker" and harder to cough out. Airway suction may be needed to remove the secretions. As the patient's condition improves, there should be a return to normal sputum consistency and less should be produced. The patient should be able to cough it out effectively.

5. Change the level of vacuum used when suctioning (Code: IIIC7c) [Difficulty: An]

In general, the lowest possible vacuum level should be used that adequately removes secretions. Several authors have listed recommended maximum vacuum levels to be applied to adults, children, and neonates. However, the American Association for Respiratory Care (AARC) Clinical Practice Guidelines on suctioning state that there is a lack of experimental data to support these or any other written maximum pressures.

6. Instill an irrigating solution into the trachea (Code: IIIC7d) [Difficulty: An]

Sterile normal saline solution (0.9%) is widely accepted as useful to instill into the trachea to dilute and mobilize pulmonary secretions. It should be used whenever secretions are difficult to suction out. Also, because the secretions are easier to remove, the respiratory therapist can use a lower vacuum level. In adults, about 5 to 10 mL are instilled into the trachea and then suctioned out with any secretions. Less is used with children, but no universal guidelines are available. Neonates have been reportedly given a few drops to 0.33 mL.

7. Change the frequency of suctioning (Code: IIIC7a) [Difficulty: An]

Secretions obstruct the airways and should be removed if possible. Often this requires more than one suctioning episode. There is no harm in repeatedly suctioning the patient as long as he or she is reoxygenated between each session. Watch for any complications as listed in Boxes 12-1 and 12-2. Also, listen to the patient's breath sounds for rhonchi, or palpate the chest for secretions in between suctioning efforts. Stop suctioning when it is no longer needed.

8. Change the duration of the suctioning procedure (Code: IIIC7a) [Difficulty: An]

Suctioning generally takes between 5 and 10 seconds; the entire procedure should take between 10 and 15 seconds. Some patients may not be able to tolerate this. Be prepared to suction for a shorter period. Suction repeatedly rather than increase the suctioning time.

As listed in Boxes 12-1 and 12-2, stop the procedure if the patient becomes hypoxic or has tachycardia, bradycardia, dysrhythmias, hypotension, or bronchospasm. Bloody secretions may indicate mucosal damage and justify stopping the procedure. Hypoxemia, tachycardia, bradycardia, dysrhythmias, hypotension, bronchospasm, pneumothorax, or pulmonary hemorrhage that place the patient's life in danger indicate the cancellation of the suctioning order. Once the underlying problem has been corrected and safe suctioning can be performed, the order may be resumed.

 EXAM HINT

Past examinations have often tested understanding of the need to alter the suctioning procedure as discussed previously. Also be prepared to recommend changing the suctioning duration or frequency if the patient becomes hypoxemic or has a significant change in heart rate.

BIBLIOGRAPHY

AARC Clinical Practice Guideline: Endotracheal suctioning of mechanically ventilated adults and children with artificial airways, *Respir Care* 38:500, 1993.

AARC Clinical Practice Guideline: Nasotracheal suctioning, *Respir Care* 37:898, 1992.

Burton GG: Patient assessment procedures. In Barnes TA, editor: *Respiratory care practice*, St Louis, 1998, Mosby.

Caldwell SL, Sullivan KN: Suctioning protocol. In Burton GG, Hodgkin JE, editors: *Respiratory care*, ed 2, Philadelphia, 1984, Lippincott.

Eubanks DH, Bone RC: *Comprehensive respiratory care*, ed 2, St Louis, 1990, Mosby.

Guidelines for the prevention of nosocomial infections, *AARTimes*, 7(9):x, 1983.

Lewis RM: Airway Care, In Fink JB, Hunt GE, editors: *Clinical practice in respiratory care*, Philadelphia, 1999, Lippincott Williams & Wilkins.

Pettignano MM, Pettignano R: Airway management. In Barnhart SL, Czervinske MP, editors: *Perinatal and pediatric respiratory care*, Philadelphia, 1995, WB Saunders.

Plevak DJ, Ward JJ: Airway management. In Burton GG, Hodgkin JE, Ward JJ, editors: *Respiratory care*, ed 4, Philadelphia, 1997, Lippincott-Raven.

Rarey KP, Youtsey JW: *Respiratory patient care*. Englewood Cliffs, NJ, 1981, Prentice-Hall.

Roth P: Airway care. In Aloan CA, Hill TV, editors: *Respiratory care of the newborn and child*, ed 2, Philadelphia, 1997, Lippincott.

Scanlan C, Simmons K: Airway management. In Scanlan CL, Wilkins RL, Stoller JK, editors: *Egan's fundamentals of respiratory care*, ed 7, St Louis, 1999, Mosby.

Scott AA, Koff PB: Airway care and chest physiotherapy. In Koff PB, Eitzmann DV, Neu J, editors: *Neonatal and pediatric respiratory care*, ed 2, St Louis, 1993, Mosby.

Shapiro BA et al: *Clinical application of respiratory care*, ed 4, St Louis, 1991, Mosby.

Wilkins RL: Physical examination of the patient with cardiopulmonary disease. In Wilkins RL, Krider SJ, Sheldon RL, editors: *Clinical assessment in respiratory care*, ed 3, St Louis, 1995, Mosby.

Wilkins RL, Hodgkin, JE, Lopez B: *Lung sounds, a practical guide*, St Louis, 1988, Mosby.

Wojciechowski WV: Incentive spirometers, and secretion evacuation devices, and inspiratory muscle training devices. In Barnes TA, editor: *Core textbook of respiratory care practice*, ed 2, St Louis, 1994, Mosby.

SELF-STUDY QUESTIONS

1. Your patient is being mechanically ventilated with 60% oxygen and 8 cm of PEEP. Twice she has had her SpO_2 value and blood pressure fall when she was removed from the ventilator for suctioning. What should be recommended to prevent this from happening again?
   A. Switch to a smaller suction catheter.
   B. Switch to a larger suction catheter.
   C. Increase her PEEP to 10 cm water before and after the suctioning.
   D. Use a closed-system suction catheter.

2. It is difficult to remove the tracheal secretions from your adult patient when using 60 mm Hg of vacuum pressure. What should be done?
   A. Suction for 20 seconds.
   B. Suction more frequently.
   C. Increase the vacuum pressure to 80 mm Hg.
   D. Change from the central vacuum system to a portable one.

3. When selecting a catheter's OD for suctioning through an endotracheal tube, it is important that it be:
   A. No more than one fourth the ID of the tube
   B. No less than one half the ID of the tube
   C. No less than three fourths the ID of the tube
   D. No more than one half the ID of the tube

4. Your 40-year-old patient has pneumonia in her left lower lobe with a large amount of secretions. What would you recommend to be able to suction her better?
   A. Use the largest diameter suction catheter that is available.
   B. Use a suction catheter with a Coudé tip.
   C. Use the longest suction catheter that is available.
   D. Increase the length of time that you apply suction.

5. Your patient is receiving mechanical ventilation and has an 8.0 mm oral endotracheal tube in place. Over the course of the shift it is noticed that the patient has more tracheal secretions. What is the best course of action?
   A. Suction more often.
   B. Suction for longer periods.
   C. Change to a closed airway suction catheter.
   D. Administer nebulized atropine.

6. A conscious patient requires nasotracheal suctioning. During the suctioning procedure the patient's blood pressure drops to 100/60 mm Hg and heart rate drops from 110 to 60 beats per minute. What should be done?
   A. Change to a catheter with a larger diameter.
   B. Shorten the suctioning time.
   C. Insert an oropharyngeal airway before suctioning.
   D. Squirt 5 mL of saline down the suction catheter into the patient's trachea.

7. The respiratory therapist is called to set up a suctioning system for a new patient in the intensive care unit. To measure the vacuum pressure, what should be done?
   A. Check the manometer while occluding the catheter tip.
   B. Set the vacuum control to maximum.
   C. Close the thumb control valve on the catheter.
   D. Check the manometer while pinching off the connecting tubing.

8. A 16-year-old female patient is intubated with a 7.0-mm endotracheal tube and is receiving mechanical ventilation. After suctioning with a 14 Fr catheter it is noticed on the ECG monitor that the patient is bradycardic. What should be recommended?
   A. Administer 10 cm PEEP.
   B. Limit suctioning to twice a shift.
   C. Change to a 10 Fr catheter.
   D. Use a catheter with a Coudé tip.

9. An intubated patient with pneumonia must have a sputum sample sent to the laboratory for culture and sensitivity testing. What is the most appropriate way to get a sample?
   A. Place a Lukens trap between the suction catheter and the vacuum tubing.
   B. Suction the oropharynx with a sterile Yankauer suction catheter.
   C. Place a Lukens trap between the vacuum tubing and the collection bottle.
   D. Suction the patient and place the catheter inside the Lukens trap.

Answer Key

1. **D.** Rationale: A closed-system suction catheter allows the patient to be ventilated and keep the PEEP level while suctioning is being performed. This should help to prevent hypoxemia. Changing to a smaller or larger diameter open airway suction catheter will not significantly improve the patient's situation. When the patient is taken off of the ventilator and suctioned he or she will become hypoxemic. Additional PEEP will not prevent hypoxemia when the patient is taken off of the ventilator.

2. **C.** Rationale: Increasing the vacuum pressure from 60 to 80 mm Hg will result in the secretions being removed more quickly. The whole suctioning procedure is usually limited to 15 seconds. Suctioning for 20 seconds will remove more secretions but is also likely to cause hypoxemia. Suctioning more frequently will not prove effective if the suctioning level is too low at 60 mm Hg. A hospital's central vacuum system is more powerful than a portable one and will suction more effectively.

3. **D.** Rationale: It is commonly accepted practice to limit the size (OD) of a suction catheter to no more than one half the ID of the endotracheal or tracheostomy tube. This allows the patient to spontaneously breathe around the catheter during the procedure as shown in Fig. 12-3. See Table 12-1 for recommendations on tube size and suction catheter. A smaller catheter may be used but will not remove as many secretions with each suctioning effort. This may result in the need to suction more frequently. Too frequent suctioning can result in greater risk of trauma to the mucous membrane, hypoxemia, and vagal stimulation. A larger suction catheter prevents the patient from being able to breathe around it.

4. **B.** Rationale: A suction catheter with a Coudé tip may enable the catheter to be guided to either the left or right mainstem bronchus. A straight catheter has a tendency to go down the right mainstem bronchus of an adult. This is because it comes off of the trachea at the carina at a more acute angle than the left mainstem bronchus. (A newborn patient does not have a significant difference in the angle of the mainstem bronchi from the trachea.) As discussed in question 3, the diameter of the catheter should not be more the one half the ID of the endotracheal tube. Any adult-size suction catheter is long enough to suction adequately. Increasing the time of suctioning puts the patient at risk for hypoxemia.

5. **A.** Rationale: More frequent suctioning is called for if the patient has more secretions. Suctioning for longer periods of time puts the patient at risk for hypoxemia. There is no indication that a closed airway suction catheter is needed (hypoxemia or therapeutic PEEP) or will be more effective than a standard catheter. Nebulized atropine in a large enough dose decreases secretion production. However, a dose large enough to do this is also likely to cause tachycardia Atropine is rarely given to control secretions outside of the operating room. A physician's order is needed to give this medication.

6. **B.** Rationale: Because the patient is having an adverse reaction to the suctioning procedure, the suctioning time should be shortened. Changing to a catheter with a larger diameter increases the risk of trauma to the mucous membrane of the patient's nasal passage. Inserting an oropharyngeal airway before suctioning may stimulate the conscious patient's gag reflex. In addition, the airway may block the suction catheter from passing through the patient's oropharynx to the larynx and trachea. Squirting 5 mL of saline down the suction catheter into the patient's trachea will probably trigger coughing. This could worsen the patient's distress with the whole procedure.

7. **D.** Rationale: To seal the system and determine the set vacuum pressure, check the manometer while pinching off the

connecting tubing. The system is not sealed off if the therapist just occludes the catheter tip; the thumb control valve is still open. Setting the vacuum control to maximum without sealing off the system allows an air leak. Therefore the pressure cannot be measured. The system is not sealed off if the therapist just closes the thumb control valve on the catheter; the catheter tip opening is still open.

8. **C.** Rationale: Change to a 10 Fr catheter because the currently used 14 Fr catheter is too large for the endotracheal tube. See Table 12-1 for the catheter and tube combinations that should be used. A physician's order is needed to administer 10 cm PEEP. Also, there is no indication that the patient is having any difficulties other than bradycardia during the suctioning procedure. Suctioning should be done as often as needed and not limited to twice a shift. The patient experiences bradycardia whenever she is suctioned because the catheter is too large. There is no indication that a catheter with a Coudé tip is needed to guide the catheter down the left (or right) mainstem bronchus.

9. **A.** Rationale: The only way to get an uncontaminated sputum sample is to place a Lukens trap between the suction catheter and the vacuum tubing. This way the patient's secretions are collected within the Lukens trap after they have passed through the sterile suction catheter. Suctioning the patient's oropharynx with a sterile Yankauer suction catheter provides an oral sample—not a tracheal sample. It is likely that the patient's mouth contains additional microorganisms besides the ones causing the pneumonia. Placing a Lukens trap between the vacuum tubing and the collection bottle will provide a contaminated sample. This is because the vacuum tubing is not sterile like a suction catheter. The Lukens trap is designed to hold secretions and keep them from becoming contaminated. It is not designed to hold a suction catheter.

13 Intermittent Positive-Pressure Breathing

MODULE A	Initiate intermittent positive-pressure breathing (IPPB) therapy to achieve adequate spontaneous ventilation and oxygenation (Code: IIIB2a) [Difficulty: An]

 EXAM HINT

Past Written Registry Exams have averaged one question (1% of the exam) on IPPB. Usually the question deals with troubleshooting and correcting a problem with the treatment such as a leak, or adjusting the equipment settings to increase the tidal volume.

1. Indications

The following indications and guidelines are listed in the American Association for Respiratory Care (AARC) Clinical Practice Guideline on IPPB.

To treat atelectasis when other deep breathing methods are ineffective. Patients who are uncooperative, unconscious, or physically incapable of being coached in deep breathing and coughing techniques or in performing incentive spirometry may be helped by IPPB. The patient who cannot generate an inspiratory capacity (IC) of greater than 12 mL/kg, a vital capacity (VC) of greater than 15 mL/kg, or who has a postoperative IC less than 33% of the preoperative value can benefit from IPPB rather than incentive spirometry. An inspiratory pause at the end of the IPPB breath helps to better distribute the gas to open areas of atelectasis.

The AARC Guideline lists the following poor pulmonary function values as supporting the need for IPPB. This guideline suggests that the patient would have an ineffective cough: VC less than 70% of predicted or less than 10 mL/kg, forced expiratory volume in 1 second (FEV$_1$) less than 65% of predicted, or maximum voluntary ventilation (MVV) less than 50% of predicted.

To more effectively deliver aerosolized medications. If the patient cannot coordinate his or her breathing pattern to make use of a metered dose inhaler or hand-held nebulizer, IPPB may be used. Examples of when IPPB is preferable include any situation in which the patient is unconscious, uncooperative, or physically incapable. These patients are physically unable to make effective use of simpler methods of lung inflation (incentive spirometry) or to take an aerosolized medication (metered dose inhaler or hand-held nebulizer). Examples of these types of patients include the elderly, the chronically debilitated, patients with neuromuscular diseases, and patients with kyphoscoliosis. It may also be used to provide temporary support to home care patients.

To enhance the patient's cough effort and sputum clearance. The combination of aerosolized saline, with or without a bronchodilator or mucolytic, and deeper tidal volumes may help the patient to cough more productively. The practitioner must stop the treatment periodically to coach the patient's cough effort.

The following additional indications were listed in *Guidelines for the Use of Intermittent Positive Pressure Breathing (IPPB)*:

To treat impending ventilatory failure as seen by an increased arterial carbon dioxide pressure (PaCO$_2$). It may be possible to delay or avoid intubation and mechanical ventilation in the deteriorating chronic obstructive pulmonary disease (COPD) patient. The patient is able to relax and reduce the work of breathing (WOB) during a passive IPPB treatment. It may be necessary to give IPPB for 5 to 10 minutes as often as every one half to 1 hour. The treatment should also be given with the intention of helping the patient's cough and sputum clearance.

To help manage the patient with acute pulmonary edema. IPPB can help in the management by temporarily reducing the venous return to the heart. The IPPB procedure does not correct the underlying cardiac problem, which must be treated by other means.

To induce a sputum sample for culture and sensitivity or other diagnostic studies. Inducing a sputum sample by IPPB is indicated only if simpler methods have failed.

To deliver medications for special purposes when simpler methods do not work. IPPB should be used to deliver medication when simpler methods fail, for example, to deliver a local anesthetic such as lidocaine (Xylocaine) before a bronchoscopy procedure.

2. Contraindications

Untreated pneumothorax is listed by all authors and the AARC Guidelines as an absolute contraindication. An increased intrathoracic pressure converts a simple pneumothorax into a tension pneumothorax. The consequences can be fatal. Once a chest tube has been inserted into the pleural space and a pleural drainage system set up, IPPB can be administered. There may be an increase in the air leak, but it will not be life threatening.

The AARC Guideline lists the following as relative contraindications. Any patient with one of the following contraindications should be evaluated carefully before a decision about the clinical use of IPPB is made:

a. Active hemoptysis. Coughing up blood indicates

that a tear has occurred in the airway or lung tissues. The IPPB treatment should be stopped if there is a large amount of hemoptysis. Certainly massive hemoptysis (defined as greater than 600 mL of blood coughed out in a 16-hour period) contraindicates IPPB.

   b. Hemodynamic instability

   c. Intracranial pressure greater than 15 mm Hg

   d. Chest radiograph that shows a bleb

   e. Tracheoesophageal fistula

   f. Recent surgery on the esophagus, skull, face, or mouth

   g. Untreated, active tuberculosis (hazard to the practitioner)

   h. Nausea, air swallowing, or hiccups (singultation)

3. Hazards and precautions

The AARC guideline lists the following hazards and precautions for IPPB therapy:

   a. Pneumothorax

   b. Barotrauma

   c. Increased airway resistance from a bronchospastic reaction to the positive pressure or an adverse reaction to a medication. This can result in alveolar overdistention and air trapping.

   d. Hyperoxia when 100% oxygen is delivered to the patient. Some COPD patients who are hypercarbic and breathing on hypoxic drive may hypoventilate as a result.

   e. Secretions that may become impacted when the inhaled gas is not humidified adequately

   f. Nosocomial infection

   g. Decreased venous return (According to Realey, this is helpful in a patient with pulmonary edema.)

   h. Increased ventilation to perfusion mismatch. This may worsen any hypoxemia.

   i. Hyperventilation

   j. Psychologic dependence. This may be seen in the long-term home care patient who does not want to switch to another method of taking inhaled medications.

4. Initiation of therapy
a. Steps in the basic procedure

1. Check for a complete and proper order specifying the patient, oxygen percentage, frequency of treatment, medication, and any special considerations.

2. Gather the necessary equipment, medication, and so on.

3. Set up the equipment outside of the patient's room.

4. Introduce yourself, the department, and your purpose to the patient.

5. Confirm the patient's identity.

6. Have the patient sit up in bed or in a chair; an obese patient may stand.

7. Interview the patient.

8. Assess the patient's vital signs.

9. Assess the patient's breath sounds.

10. Prepare the IPPB unit for operation:

   a. If the unit is electrical, plug into a working outlet.

   b. If the unit is pneumatic, plug into either a compressed air or oxygen outlet as ordered.

   c. Set the following controls:

     1. Set sensitivity at -1 cm H_2O pressure.

     2. Set nebulizer to run on inspiration only.

     3. Adjust the flow as necessary.

     4. Set the peak pressure at about 10 to 15 cm H_2O.

   d. Test the nebulizer by turning on the machine.

   e. Cover the mouthpiece with a clean tissue to ensure that it cycles off at the preset pressure.

11. Instruct the patient to sip on the mouthpiece like a straw to turn the machine on. Have the patient relax and let the machine fill his or her lungs with air. The patient should hold his or her breath in for 2 to 3 seconds and exhale slowly.

b. Giving a passive treatment

Most authors describe the patient taking a passive treatment. In a passive treatment, the patient relaxes and lets the machine fill the lungs until the preset pressure is reached. As mentioned earlier, the patient is then told to hold in his or her breath before exhaling passively. This treatment is given with the intent of minimizing the patient's WOB. As slow a flow rate as possible is used so that any nebulized medication is deposited deeply into the small airways and lungs.

c. Giving an active treatment

Several authors advocate having the patient take an active treatment in which he or she interacts with the IPPB machine to get as deep a breath as possible.

Welch et al. have found that the patient's posttreatment IC is greatest when the practitioner: (1) uses as high a peak pressure as the patient can tolerate and (2) coaches the patient to inhale as deeply as possible with the IPPB machine. They and others believe that this is the best way to treat or prevent atelectasis.

5. Initial settings on the Bird Mark 7

The older version of the Mark 7 is used as the model respirator of the Bird series. The current Mark 8 has similar features. Other Bird units have slightly different controls and features. Refer to Fig. 13-1 for the following:

   a. Adjust the *air-mix* knob to the desired gas mix.

   b. Sensitivity should be set so that the patient has to generate about -1 cm H_2O pressure to cycle the unit on. Set the *sensitivity* control (on the left-hand side of the unit when facing it) to the reference number 15. This is at approximately the 2 o'clock position. Turning the control lever counterclock-

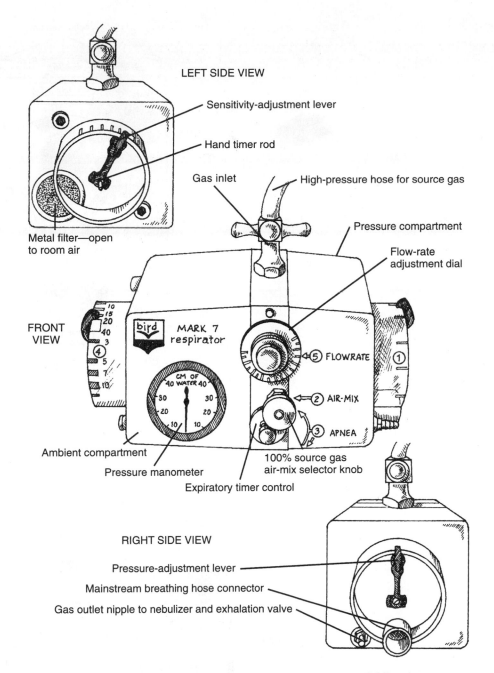

LEFT SIDE VIEW

Sensitivity-adjustment lever

Hand timer rod

Gas inlet

High-pressure hose for source gas

Pressure compartment

Flow-rate adjustment dial

Metal filter—open to room air

FRONT VIEW

bird MARK 7 respirator

⑤ FLOWRATE ①

② AIR-MIX

③ APNEA

Ambient compartment

Pressure manometer

Expiratory timer control

100% source gas air-mix selector knob

RIGHT SIDE VIEW

Pressure-adjustment lever

Mainstream breathing hose connector

Gas outlet nipple to nebulizer and exhalation valve

Fig. 13-1   Controls and features of the Bird Mark 7 IPPB unit.

wise makes the unit more sensitive. Push in the hand timer rod to note that the unit cycles on easily.

c. Flow should be set so that the patient feels comfortable with the inspiratory time. Set the *flow rate* knob so that the reference number 15 is at the 12 o'clock position; the *off* sign will be at the 8 o'clock position. Turning the *flow rate* knob counterclockwise increases the flow.

d. Peak pressure should be set at about 10 to 15 cm H_2O pressure. Set the *pressure* control (on the right-hand side of the unit when facing it) to the reference

number 15. This is at approximately the 10 o'clock position. Turning the control lever more clockwise increases the peak pressure. Hold a clean tissue against the patient's mouthpiece to see that the unit cycles off at the desired peak pressure.

6. Initial settings on the Bennett PR-II

The PR-II is used as the model respirator of the Bennett series. Other Bennett units have slightly different controls and features. Refer to Figs. 13-2 and 13-3 for the following:

a. Adjust the *air dilution* knob to the desired gas mix.

b. Sensitivity should be set so that the patient has to

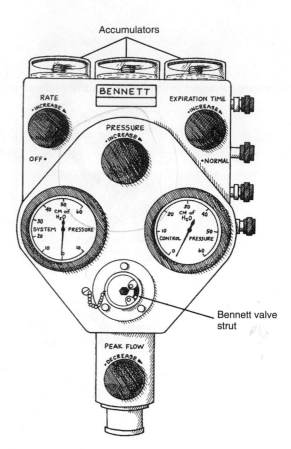

Fig. 13-2 Front controls and features of the Bennett PR-II IPPB unit.

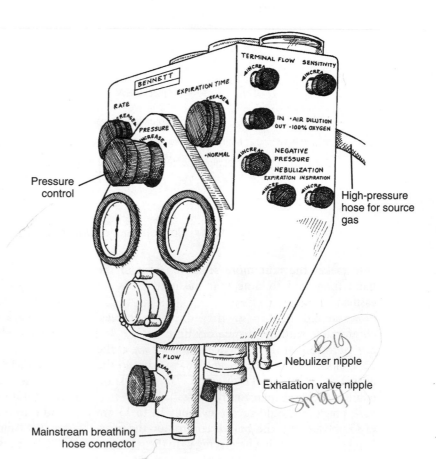

Fig. 13-3 Right side controls and features of the Bennett PR-II IPPB unit.

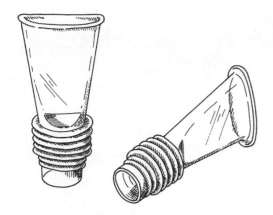

Fig. 13-4   Universal IPPB mouthpiece with a tapered 22- to 18-mm machine connector.

generate about -1 cm H_2O pressure to cycle the unit on. Turning the control lever counterclockwise makes the unit more sensitive. Push up on the Bennett valve strut to note that the unit cycles on easily.

c. Flow should be set so that the patient feels comfortable with the inspiratory time. The Bennett valve is designed to automatically open and close itself to allow the patient as much flow as desired. Set the *peak flow* control knob as counterclockwise as possible so that it is at the maximum setting. Turning the *peak flow* knob more clockwise will decrease the patient's peak flow.

d. Peak pressure should be set at about 10 to 15 cm H_2O pressure. Dial the *pressure* control clockwise until the *control pressure* gauge shows the desired peak pressure. Hold a clean tissue against the patient's mouthpiece to see that when the unit cycles off the *system pressure* gauge reads the same as the *control pressure* gauge.

e. Turn the *inspiration nebulization* control counterclockwise for medication to be nebulized only during an inspiration. Some practitioners believe that the *expiration nebulization* control should be turned on slightly so that the mouthpiece and circuit dead space is filled with medication before the next breath. Others are opposed to this because it wastes medication when the patient stops the treatment.

f. A small leak in the circuit, mouthpiece, or face mask can be overcome by adding some additional flow by turning on the *terminal flow* control. It is normally left off. Turn the control counterclockwise to add as much additional flow as necessary to overcome the leak.

Details on the design and control specifications for the various Bird and Bennett models can be found in the manufacturers' literature and books on respiratory therapy equipment.

MODULE B	Adjust IPPB therapy to achieve adequate spontaneous ventilation (Code: IIIB2a) [Difficulty: An]

1. Change the patient-machine interface (Code: IIIC1c) [Difficulty: An]

a. Mouthpiece

A conscious, cooperative patient can take a treatment with a mouthpiece. He or she must be instructed to place the mouthpiece between the teeth (or gums) and seal the lips around it so that there is no leak. Instruct the patient to sip gently on it to turn on the IPPB machine. As long as the lips are sealed and there are no other leaks, the positive-pressure breath will stop when the preset pressure is reached. Nose clips are often helpful to prevent a leak through the nose as the patient is learning how to take the treatment. The nose clips can be removed after the patient has learned how to seal the nasopharynx with the soft palate.

A variety of mouthpieces are available. All share the common features of a raised edge so that the teeth do not slip off and a 22-mm outer diameter (OD) connector end to insert into the IPPB circuit (Fig. 13-4).

b. Mouth seal (Bennett seal)

An unconscious, uncooperative, or aged patient who cannot seal his or her lips can be aided by placing a soft rubber seal around the mouthpiece. The practitioner gently holds the seal around the patient's lips to seal the airway so that the patient can trigger the breath and cycle the machine off (Fig. 13-5). Nose clips are also commonly needed.

c. Face mask

The face mask can be used if the mouth seal does not provide an airtight seal. This might be because of the patient's facial structure or lack of teeth. Mouth trauma, surgery, or lip sores are other reasons to use a face mask.

The mask should be clear and properly sized to fit comfortably over the patient's nose and mouth. The practitioner should be able to get a seal with a minimum amount of hand pressure (Fig. 13-6). The equipment connection opening in the mask has a 22-mm inner diameter (ID) so that it connects directly to the IPPB circuit. A 22-mm-OD male adapter and short length of aerosol tubing can be added for flexibility and patient comfort. The clear mask is important so that the practitioner can see whether the patient has vomited or has a large amount of secretions or saliva in his or her mouth. The mask should never be strapped to the patient's face so that the practitioner can attend to another patient.

This is the least effective patient attachment device if the therapeutic goal is to deliver an aerosolized medication. Much of the medication rains out on the patient's face or in the nasal passages if he or she is a nose breather.

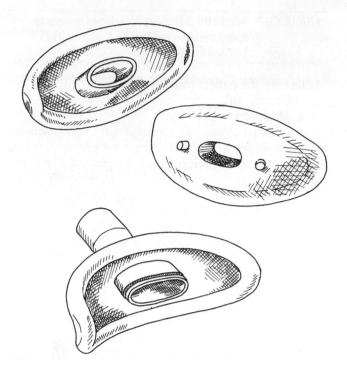

Fig. 13-5 *Top,* Bennett or mouth flange seal. *Bottom,* IPPB mouthpiece inserted into the seal.

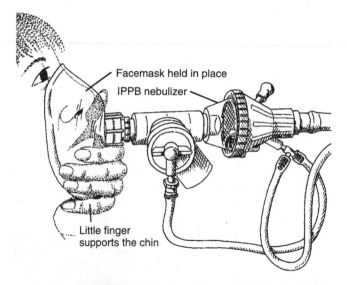

Fig. 13-6 Giving an IPPB treatment with the use of a face mask.

d. Tracheostomy/endotracheal tube (elbow) adapter

The elbow adapter is designed to connect the patient's tracheostomy or endotracheal tube to the IPPB circuit (or other respiratory care equipment). The IPPB end has a 22-mm-ID connector. The tracheostomy/endotracheal tube end has a 15-mm-ID connector (Fig. 13-7). If the patient has had the cuff deflated, it must be reinflated to seal the airway. An unsealed cuff results in an air leak, and the gas flow will not turn off.

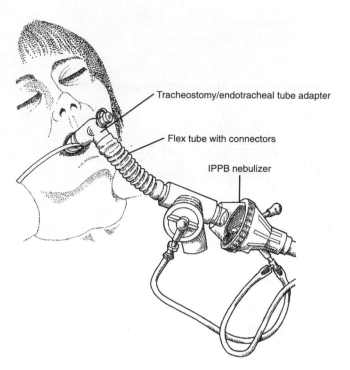

Fig. 13-7 Giving an IPPB treatment with the use of a tracheostomy/endotracheal tube adapter.

2. Adjust the sensitivity (Code: IIIC1a) [Difficulty: An]

The sensitivity of the IPPB unit refers to how much effort or work the patient must perform to turn the unit on for a breath. Commonly, the sensitivity is set so that the patient has to generate a negative pressure of only about -1 cm H_2O pressure to begin an inspiration. This can be seen by looking at the needle deflecting into the negative range on the pressure manometer. Ask the patient whether the machine can be easily turned on to get a breath. The IPPB unit should not be set at a level so sensitive that it self-cycles.

The sensitivity range on the Bird series is -0.01 to -5 cm H_2O. Turning the *sensitivity/starting effort* adjustment lever counterclockwise toward the smaller reference numbers makes the unit more sensitive. The sensitivity range on the Bennett series is -0.5 to -1 cm H_2O. Turning the *sensitivity* control counterclockwise makes the unit easier to turn on.

3. Adjust the fractional concentration of inspired oxygen (Code: IIIC1a) [Difficulty: An]

Compressed air or oxygen can power both the Bird and Bennett units. The patient's condition determines the oxygen percentage administered. The physician may include the oxygen percentage in the treatment order. Some departments have oxygen protocols in their treatment procedure. Generally, compressed air (21% oxygen) should be used whenever the patient does not need supplemental oxygen.

A patient with COPD who is retaining carbon dioxide and breathing on hypoxic drive should also be given room air via the IPPB unit. The patient may be allowed to keep wearing a nasal cannula with oxygen during the treatment so that the blood oxygen level is kept normal. The unavailability of piped-in compressed air should not be an excuse to give a patient a high oxygen percentage when it may be harmful. IPPB can be given through a gas-powered unit powered by a compressed air cylinder or an electrically powered unit.

Supplemental oxygen is given if either unit is powered by oxygen and the *air-mix/air dilution* knobs are set to dilute the source gas with room air. This is appropriate for patients who require supplemental oxygen and are not at risk of stopping their spontaneous ventilation. Most practitioners use this method of giving IPPB because piped oxygen is usually available in all patients' rooms.

Pure oxygen should be given to the patient who is severely hypoxemic. Examples include acute pulmonary edema, respiratory failure, and carbon monoxide poisoning. The *air-mix/air dilution* knobs must be set so that only the source gas (oxygen) is delivered to the patient.

For varying oxygen percentages on the Mark 7, note the following guidelines:

a. Pushing the *air-mix* knob into the center body results in pure source gas. This can be either air or oxygen.
b. Pulling the *air-mix* knob out of the center body results in a dilution of the source gas with room air. If oxygen is the source gas, the room air will dilute the delivered gas to between 60% and 90% (or more) oxygen.

For varying oxygen percentage on the PR-II, note the following guidelines:

a. Pulling the *air dilution* knob out of the body results in pure source gas. This can be either air or oxygen.
b. Pushing the *air dilution* knob into the body results in a dilution of the source gas with room air. If oxygen is the source gas, the room air will dilute the delivered gas to between 40% and 80% oxygen.
c. Turning on the *terminal flow* control results in the dilution of source gas with room air. This dilutes the final percentage if the source gas is oxygen.

4. Adjust the flow (Code: IIIC1a) [Difficulty: An]

The patient should initially feel comfortable with the flow rate and the inspiratory time. Ask the patient a simple question, such as, "Is the breath coming too fast or too slow?" He or she can give you a short answer or even a hand gesture in response. As the treatment progresses, the practitioner may be able to adjust the flow to modify the patient's breathing pattern to better achieve the therapeutic goal, for example:

a. Anxious patients may initially need a fast flow. As they are coached to relax and get used to the treatment, the practitioner should try to reduce the flow.
b. Slower flows result in medications being deposited deeper into the lungs. This is important if the patient is having a bronchodilator, mucolytic, or antibiotic nebulized.
c. Faster flows result in the deposition of medications in the upper airways. This is important if the patient is receiving racemic epinephrine for laryngeal edema or lidocaine for a local anesthetic of the upper airway before bronchoscopy.

Turning the *inspiratory time/flow rate* control counterclockwise increases the flow rate on the Bird series. Pulling the *air-mix* knob out from the center body increases the total flow by allowing room air to be entrained along with the source gas. Flow rate in the PR-II is determined by the patient's inspiratory effort and how open the Bennett valve is. Flow can be decreased somewhat by turning the *peak flow* control clockwise. Flow is not affected by the position of the *air dilution* knob.

5. Adjust the volume, pressure, or both (Code: IIIC1a) [Difficulty: An]

A review of the current respiratory care textbooks reveals that all authors agree that the basic goal of IPPB is to increase how deeply the patient inspires. Unfortunately, there is considerable difference about what inspiratory volume is being measured or by how much that breath should be increased for therapeutic goals to be achieved. The AARC has released the following on the subject:

a. The AARC Clinical Practice Guideline (1993) on IPPB: The tidal volume delivered during an IPPB-assisted breath should be at least 25% greater than the patient's spontaneous breaths.
b. The AARC Clinical Practice Guideline (1991) on incentive spirometry: IPPB is indicated to treat atelectasis rather than incentive spirometry if (a) the patient's IC is less than 33% of the preoperative value, or (b) the patient's VC is less than 10 mL/kg of ideal body weight.

If the therapeutic goal is to prevent or treat atelectasis, having the patient inspire a deeper than spontaneous tidal volume breath should help. It seems reasonable to follow the AARC guidelines both as indications and as clinical goals. They can be used as guidelines if an increased tidal volume is used as a substitute for the VC. Based on this assumption, an IPPB delivered tidal volume goal of at least 10 mL/kg of ideal body weight seems reasonable. Because all of the current IPPB units are pressure cycled, the only way to increase the inspired volume during a passive treatment is to increase the peak pressure. Coaching the patient during an active treatment results in a larger volume without the need for as great a peak pressure. Decrease the peak pressure if the patient complains of discomfort or cannot hold that much pressure without losing the lip seal.

6. Adjust expiratory retard (Code: IIIC1b) [Difficulty: An]

Expiratory retard is indicated in patients who have small airway disease and are air trapping on exhalation.

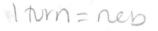

Over the course of an IPPB treatment, this can lead to an increased functional residual volume (FRC) with the increased risk of pulmonary barotrauma. Adding expiratory retard to the treatment has the same effect as pursed lips breathing. The increased back pressure on the smallest airways keeps them open longer so that the more distal air can be exhaled.

It is important to measure the exhaled volumes during the treatment and monitor the patient's response to know how much retard is needed. Too little retard results in some air trapping and an incompletely exhaled tidal volume. Too much retard results in an uncomfortably long expiratory time and an increased mean intrathoracic pressure. The proper amount of expiratory retard should result in the patient feeling comfortable with the breathing cycle and being able to completely exhale the tidal volume. Listening to the patient's breath sounds is also helpful. If wheezing is present, it can be minimized when the proper amount of retard is added. This is because the back pressure is properly adjusted to minimize the small airway collapse.

Bird makes a retard cap that fits over the exhalation valve port on their permanent circuit. The cap has a series of different size holes through which the exhaled gas can pass (Fig. 13-8). By rotating the cap progressively from the largest to the smallest opening and evaluating the patient at each setting, the proper size opening and amount of retard can be found.

Bennett makes a retard exhalation valve that can be substituted for the regular exhalation valve on their permanent circuit (Fig. 13-9). The valve consists of a spring attached to a nut and a diaphragm. As the nut is turned counterclockwise the spring pushes the diaphragm closer to the exhalation valve opening. This causes resistance to the exhalation of the tidal volume and a back pressure is created against the airways. If too much pressure is placed

against the exhalation valve opening, the patient will not be able to exhale back to atmospheric pressure. This should not be done without an order from the physician.

Be sure to ask the patient's opinion about the use of expiratory retard. The conscious, cooperative patient can tell you if he or she feels like more air is getting out by the use of the retard or if the lungs feel more full because too much retard is being used. Too much retard may also make the expiratory time uncomfortably long.

MODULE C   IPPB equipment

1. Get the proper IPPB circuit for the patient's treatment (Code: IIA1i1) [Difficulty: An]

The two most widely used IPPB machines are the Bird Mark 7/8 (or a variation on it found in the series) and the Bennett PR-II. Both are pneumatically powered and found in most hospitals. Each unit requires a circuit that is designed specifically for it. See Fig. 13-10 for a drawing of a permanent (reusable after cleaning) and disposable circuit for a Bird machine. See Fig. 13-11 for a drawing of a permanent (reusable after cleaning) and disposable circuit for a Bennett machine.

2. Put the IPPB circuit together, make sure that it works properly, and identify any problems (Code: IIB1i1) [Difficulty: R, Ap]

See Fig. 13-10 for the Bird setup and Fig. 13-11 for the Bennett setup.

a. General setup procedures
1. Check for plentiful source gas. Make sure that the oxygen or air tank has the proper regulator. Check the pressure in the gas cylinder.

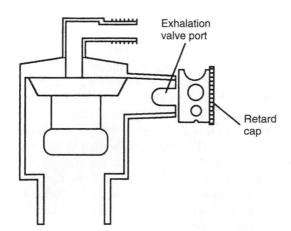

Fig. 13-8   Bird retard cap for providing adjustable expiratory resistance. (From McPherson SP: *Respiratory therapy equipment,* ed 5, St Louis, 1995, Mosby.)

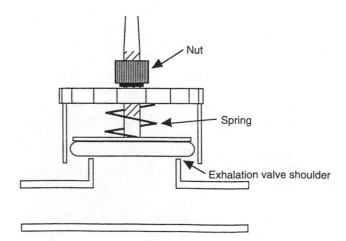

Fig. 13-9   Bennett retard exhalation valve for providing adjustable expiratory resistance. (From McPherson SP: *Respiratory therapy equipment,* ed 5, St Louis, 1995, Mosby.)

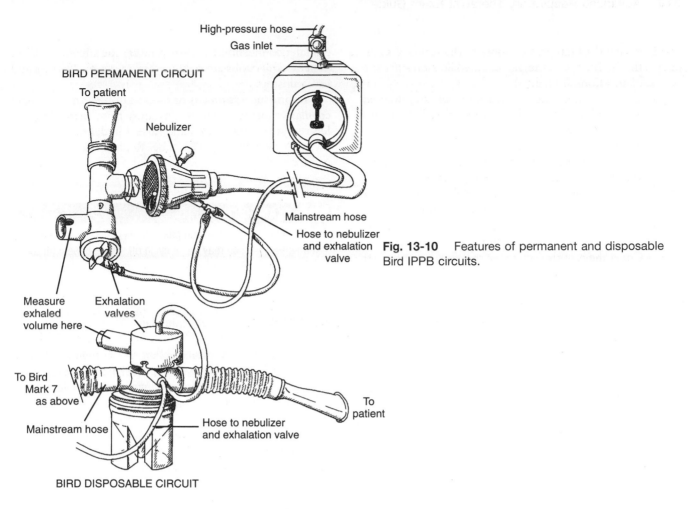

Fig. 13-10 Features of permanent and disposable Bird IPPB circuits.

BIRD PERMANENT CIRCUIT

High-pressure hose

Gas inlet

To patient

Nebulizer

Mainstream hose

Hose to nebulizer and exhalation valve

Measure exhaled volume here

Exhalation valves

To Bird Mark 7 as above

Mainstream hose

Hose to nebulizer and exhalation valve

To patient

BIRD DISPOSABLE CIRCUIT

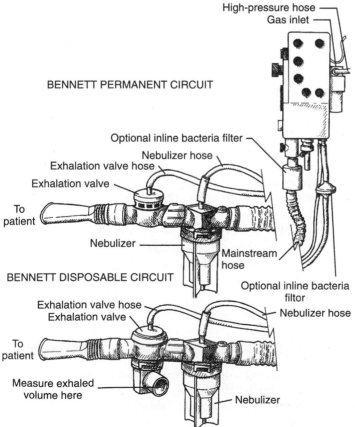

High-pressure hose

Gas inlet

BENNETT PERMANENT CIRCUIT

Optional inline bacteria filter

Nebulizer hose

Exhalation valve hose

Exhalation valve

To patient

Nebulizer

Mainstream hose

BENNETT DISPOSABLE CIRCUIT

Optional inline bacteria filtor

Exhalation valve hose

Exhalation valve

Nebulizer hose

To patient

Measure exhaled volume here

Nebulizer

Fig. 13-11 Features of permanent and disposable Bennett IPPB circuits.

2. Attach the high-pressure hose to the source gas and the IPPB unit at the gas inlet. Make sure that the connections are tight.

3. Bacteria filters are optional. They are inserted between the IPPB unit gas outlets and the mainstream and nebulizer hoses.

4. A cascade-type humidifier is optional. Some practitioners prefer to warm and humidify the mainstream gas before it reaches the patient.

5. Check to see that the IPPB circuit is put together properly and that all of the connections are tight.

6. Set the initial treatment parameters for sensitivity, flow, and peak pressure. Manually cycle the unit on. Cover the mouthpiece to see that the unit cycles off at the preset pressure.

7. Add any medication to the nebulizer. Check to see that the nebulizer is producing a mist.

b. Bird setup

1. One end of the mainstream (large bore) hose is connected to the mainstream breathing hose connector on the right side of the unit. The other end is connected to the nebulizer.

2. One end of the nebulizer (small bore) hose is connected to the small nipple on the right hand side of the unit. The other end is connected to a T-piece at the nebulizer.

3. A piece of small-bore hose is used to connect one limb of the T-piece and the exhalation valve. Gas flowing through this hose powers both the nebulizer and the exhalation valve.

c. Bennett setup

1. One end of the mainstream (large bore) hose is connected to the mainstream breathing hose connector on the underside of the unit. The other end is connected to the nebulizer.

2. One end of the nebulizer (medium bore) hose is connected to the larger of two nipples on the underside of the unit. The other end is connected to the nebulizer nipple.

3. One end of the exhalation (small bore) hose is connected to the smaller of two nipples on the underside of the unit. The other end is connected to the exhalation valve nipple.

3. Fix any problems with the equipment (Code: IIB2i1) [Difficulty: An]

Fixing a problem is only possible after the problem has been identified. The practitioner should be familiar with both permanent and disposable types of Bird and Bennett circuits. Leaks of any sort in the circuit prevent the unit from cycling off so that the patient can exhale. Tighten up any friction fit or screw-type connections to stop the leak. A leak at the source gas connection or high-pressure hose.

gas inlet connection results in a rather loud hissing sound. When connections are tightened properly, the hissing and leak will stop.

Debris such as mucus or blood can plug the nebulizer capillary tube and prevent any mist from being formed. Disassemble the nebulizer and rinse it under running water to try to clear the capillary tube. Replace the nebulizer if necessary.

🖢 EXAM HINT

There have been questions on past exams covering the reason(s) that an IPPB machine may fail to cycle off. Know to seal off an air leak around the patient's mouthpiece or within the circuit.

| MODULE D | Respiratory care plan |

1. Participate in the development of the respiratory care plan [e.g., case management, development and application of protocols, disease management education] (Code: IC4) [Difficulty: An]

Atelectasis is determined by characteristic chest radiograph findings and decreased or absent breath sounds over the affected area. Wheezing breath sounds is a finding indicating bronchospasm. Pulmonary edema has characteristic chest radiograph findings and cardiovascular indicators. Review discussion on these conditions and their findings in Chapters 1 and 5.

The patient should be fully cooperative to take full advantage of IPPB. It may be counterproductive to try to force an IPPB treatment on a combative or uncooperative patient. A patient who has a neuromuscular deficit may need assistance in holding the IPPB circuit or keeping a good mouth seal. A mouth seal or face mask treatment may have to be given. Be prepared to make a recommendation to have a patient use either incentive spirometry, positive end–expiratory pressure therapy, or IPPB for hyperinflation therapy. Also be prepared to make a recommendation for a patient to use either a metered dose inhaler, small volume nebulizer, or IPPB for the delivery of an aerosolized medication.

IPPB should be used only for hyperinflation therapy when less expensive options (such as incentive spirometry) are not practical. Bedside spirometry should confirm that IPPB is indicated and that the patient's IPPB breath is at least 25% greater than spontaneous breath. Breath sounds should be heard more clearly to the bases of the lungs. One of the goals of IPPB is to give the patient larger tidal volumes than normal. More secretions may be heard in the airways if the larger tidal volumes result in their mobilization. However, if the deeper breaths enable the patient to cough more effectively, more secretions should be coughed out. Wheezing should be diminished if a bronchodilator medication is nebulized to a patient with bronchospasm.

Ask about the patient's feelings toward the treatment and write them in the chart. Note any significant comments made by the patient. Note the patient's preferred flow and pressure or volume settings.

As previously mentioned, the general treatment length is 15 to 20 minutes. The patient may not be able to tolerate that length of time because of fatigue. This is often seen in aged or debilitated patients. Stop the treatment if the patient has a pulse change of 20 beats/min or more. It is most common to see the pulse increase because of a nebulized bronchodilator drug. A decreased venous return to the heart may be shown by an increased heart rate or drop in blood pressure.

The contraindications, hazards, and precautions to IPPB were discussed earlier. The treatment should be canceled if the patient has an untreated pneumothorax or massive hemoptysis. Other serious problems also justify the cancellation of the order.

BIBLIOGRAPHY

AARC Clinical Practice Guideline: Incentive spirometry, *Respir Care* 30:1402, 1991.

AARC Clinical Practice Guideline: Intermittent positive pressure ventilation, *Respir Care* 38:1189, 1993.

Branson RD, Hess DR, Chatburn RL, editors: *Respiratory care equipment*, ed 2, Philadelphia, 1999, Lippincott Williams & Wilkins.

Eubanks DH, Bone RC: *Comprehensive respiratory care*, ed 2, St Louis, 1990, Mosby.

Fink JB: Volume expansion therapy. In Burton GG, Hodgkin JE, Ward JJ, editors: *Respiratory care*, ed 4, Philadelphia, 1997, Lippincott.

Fink JB: Bronchial hygiene and lung expansion. In Fink JB, Hunt GE, editors: *Clinical practice in respiratory care*, Philadelphia, 1999, Lippincott Williams & Wilkins.

Fluck RJ Jr: Intermittent positive-pressure breathing devices and transport ventilators. In Barnes TA, editor: *Respiratory care practice*, ed 2, St Louis, 1994, Mosby.

McPherson SP: *Respiratory care equipment*, ed 5, St Louis, 1995, Mosby.

Miller WF: Intermittent positive pressure breathing (IPPB). In Kacmarek RM, Stoller JK, editors: *Current respiratory care*, Philadelphia, 1988, BC Decker.

Respiratory Care Committee of the American Thoracic Society: Guidelines for the use of intermittent positive pressure breathing (IPPB), *Respir Care* 25:365, 1980.

Scanlan CL, Wilkins RL, Stoller JK, editors: *Egan's fundamentals of respiratory care*, ed 7, St Louis, 1999, Mosby.

Shapiro BA et al: *Clinical application of respiratory care*, ed 4, St Louis, 1991, Mosby.

Wilkins RL, Scanlan CL: Lung expansion therapy. In Weizalis CP: Intermittent positive-pressure breathing. In Barnes TA, editor: *Respiratory care practice*, ed 2, St Louis, 1994, Mosby.

Welch MA et al: Methods of intermittent positive pressure breathing, Chest 78:463, 1980.

White GC: *Equipment theory for respiratory care*, ed 3, Albany, NY, 1999, Delmar.

SELF-STUDY QUESTIONS

1. In the emergency room, you are giving an IPPB treatment with metaproterenol sulfate (Alupent) to an asthmatic patient. During a break in the treatment, the patient complains that his lungs feel too full and he does not feel like all the IPPB volume is getting out. What would you recommend?
   A. Increase the flow.
   B. Add expiratory retard.
   C. Increase the system pressure.
   D. Change to 100% oxygen.

2. While giving an IPPB, a hissing sound is heard and the patient complains that the inspiratory time is too long. What is the most likely problem?
   A. The nebulizer hose is attached to the exhalation valve.
   B. The nebulizer medication jar is loose.
   C. The bacteria filter is missing.
   D. The inspiratory and expiratory hoses are reversed.

3. You are delivering an IPPB treatment to an elderly patient without teeth or dentures. He has difficulty keeping his lips tight around the mouthpiece and pressure fails to rise enough to cycle off the breath. What should be done?
   A. Switch the mouthpiece to a mask.
   B. Increase the inspiratory flow.
   C. Place nose clips on the patient.
   D. Change from IPPB to incentive spirometry.

4. You are about to give an asthmatic 16-year-old patient her second IPPB treatment with a bronchodilator medication. When checking the equipment you notice that it is set with a rather fast inspiratory flow. Her chart had a note that she was very anxious when first admitted. She seems calmer now. How would you start the treatment?
   A. Increase the pressure setting to deliver a larger breath.
   B. Keep the flow the same to deliver a larger breath.
   C. Make the machine as sensitive as possible to easily trigger it.
   D. Decrease the flow on the machine.

5. Your patient with atelectasis has a spontaneous tidal volume of 600 mL and weighs 82 kg (180 lb). Based on this information, what should his IPPB tidal volume be?
   A. 500 mL
   B. 600 mL
   C. 700 mL
   D. 900 mL

6. Atelectasis has been diagnosed by chest radiograph in a patient whom you are treating by IPPB. To evaluate the effectiveness of the treatment, which of the following would you evaluate?
   I. Repeat chest radiograph after the treatments have been given for 2 days
   II. Complete blood count
   III. Percussion note for the positions of the hemidiaphragms
   IV. Breath sounds
   V. MVV after the treatments have been given for 2 days
   A. I, III, IV
   B. I, II
   C. III, V
   D. III, IV, V

7. Your patient with COPD has been receiving IPPB treatments on a Bird Mark 7 for 5 days. Expiratory retard was added 4 days ago. Because the retard has not been evaluated since then, the physician asks you to do so. You proceeded to make the following adjustments in the retard cap settings and make the following observations:

Retard cap setting	Exhaled tidal volume (mL)	Wheezing	Patient's impression
1 (smallest)	850	None	Exhalation too long
2	825	Some in bases	Exhalation too long
3	800	Some in bases	Comfortable
4	700	All lobes	Lungs feel full

Based on this information, which retard cap setting would you recommend?
   A. 1
   B. 2
   C. 3
   D. 4

Answer Key

1. **B.** Rationale: Adding expiratory retard adds some back pressure to the patient's airways and allow for a more complete exhalation. Increasing inspiratory flow increases turbulence and increasing system pressure increases tidal volume. Neither of these will help the patient's problem of air trapping. There is no indication that the patient is hypoxic and needs 100% oxygen.

2. **B.** Rationale: A loose nebulizer medication jar would result in a hissing sound from the leaking air and a prolonged inspiratory time. If any of the hoses are misconnected, the IPPB machine will fail to function properly but the described problems will not be found. A missing bacteria filter does not cause any hissing sound or prolong the inspiratory time.

3. **A.** Rationale: The patient has a leak at the mouthpiece; correct it by switching to a face mask. Increasing the inspiratory flow will not correct the leak at the patient's mouth. Nose clips will not fix the patient's leak around the mouthpiece. There is no listed reason to switch the patient from IPPB to incentive spirometry.

4. **D.** Rationale: Because the patient is calmer now, it is best to reduce the flow from the IPPB machine. This allows the delivered tidal volume and medication to be more equally delivered to all areas of the lungs. There is no need at this time to deliver a larger tidal volume. The goal is to deliver medication effectively to the lungs. Machine sensitivity is not a problem at this time.

5. **D.** Rationale: The AARC Clinical Practice Guideline states that the an IPPB-assisted breath should be at least 25% greater than the patient's spontaneous tidal volume. This would result in an IPPB breath goal of at least 750 mL. Therefore the best answer is 900 mL.

6. **A.** Rationale: The chest radiograph should be repeated to determine if the lungs are more inflated in areas that earlier showed atelectasis. If atelectasis were decreased or gone, the patient's lung percussion note would reveal lowered hemidiaphragms indicating larger lung volumes. If atelectasis were decreased or absent, the patient's breath sounds would be normal in the former problem areas. There is no specific marker in the complete blood count for atelectasis or its correction. The MVV test is not specific for atelectasis.

7. **C.** Rationale: Expiratory retard cap setting 3 is best because the patient's tidal volume is adequate, wheezing is found only in the bases, and the patient is comfortable with the breath. The smaller settings (1 and 2) resulted in too long of an exhalation for patient comfort. With the largest setting (4) the patient's tidal volume decreased, wheezing was heard in all lobes, and the patient said that the lungs feel full.

14 Mechanical Ventilation of the Adult

A review of the most recent Written Registry Examinations has shown an average of 21 questions (21% of the examination) on mechanical ventilation of adult patients or questions that may apply to either adult, neonatal, or pediatric patients. Mechanical ventilation of the adult patient is the most heavily tested area on the examination. Also, several of the scenarios tested on the Clinical Simulation Examination deal with mechanical ventilation of the adult patient.

MODULE A	Review the patient's chart for the following data and recommend and perform the following diagnostic procedures

1. Work of breathing

a. Review the patient's chart for information on work of breathing (Code: IA1f4) [Difficulty: An]

Work of breathing (WOB) normally refers to how much energy the patient has to expend to inhale. Patients with stiff lungs and/or high airway resistance have an increased WOB. Exhalation is normally passive and requires no work. However, some patients with high airway resistance have to work to exhale. Look in the patient's chart for information on patient complaints of shortness of breath and easy tiring as signs of increased WOB.

A patient who has been intubated and placed on a modern mechanical ventilator with a microprocessor and graphics software can have WOB measured. See Fig. 14-1 for a pressure-volume loop tracing that shows a patient's WOB. WOB is minimized when the ventilator is set to minimize the negative pressure and inspiratory flow the patient has to generate.

b. Recommend that work of breathing be evaluated to get additional information (Code: IA2f) [Difficulty: An]

If the breathing of an intubated and ventilated patient appears to be unsynchronized with the ventilator, his or her WOB should be evaluated. Ask the conscious patient simple questions to try to determine what the problem is. If the ventilator is capable, program it to perform a pressure-volume loop of the patient's WOB. Be prepared to adjust parameters such as the machine's sensitivity and inspiratory flow to minimize the patient's workload.

2. Ventilator flow, volume, and pressure waveforms

a. Review the patient's chart for information on ventilator flow, volume, and pressure waveforms (Code: IA1f3) [Difficulty: An]

A patient who has been intubated and placed on a modern mechanical ventilator with a microprocessor and graphics software can have ventilator flow, volume, and pressure waveforms visualized on the monitor, stored in memory, or printed out. Look for this information and compare it with the patient's current situation.

b. Perform the procedure to measure ventilator flow, volume, and pressure waveforms (Code: IC1g) [Difficulty: An]

Follow the ventilator manufacturer's steps to direct the unit to create flow, volume, and pressure waveforms. The patient can be instructed, based on the breathing test, to either actively perform a breathing maneuver or lie passively as the ventilator delivers a breath.

c. Apply computer technology in the analysis of ventilator flow, volume, and pressure waveforms (Code: IIIA2c) [Difficulty: An]

d. Interpret ventilator flow, volume, and pressure waveforms (Code: IC2i) [Difficulty: An]

A number of flow, volume, and pressure waveforms have been included in this chapter for practice. In addition, review Figs. 4-1 and 4-11 for examples of pulmonary function test waveform tracings. The examples in this chapter include common clinical situations and have explanations to help with interpretation. For example, Fig. 14-2 demonstrates two ways that air trapping on exhalation can be identified as auto-positive end–expiratory pressure (PEEP).

EXAM HINT

Expect to see at least one examination question that either describes a waveform or shows a waveform that must be analyzed.

3. Airway resistance

a. Review the patient's chart for information on airway resistance (Code: IA1f4) [Difficulty: An]

Airway resistance may have been measured earlier in either the pulmonary function laboratory or on the ventilator. Compare any earlier values with new measurements. This is important for understanding the patient's

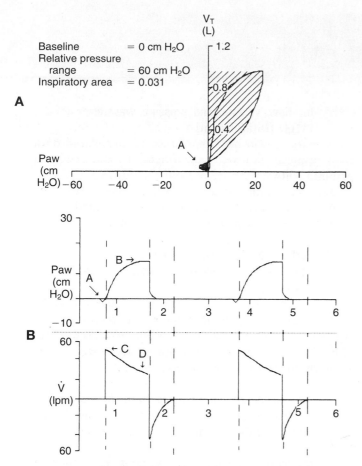

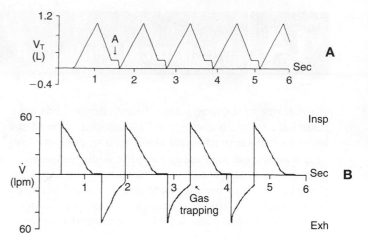

Fig. 14-1 Two graphic tracings of pressure support ventilation. **A,** Top graphic shows pressure-volume loop of a patient triggering a breath. *A,* Amount of work patient has to provide. Shaded area on right side indicates how much work was provided by ventilator. **B,** Bottom graphic shows pressure (P_{AW}) versus time and flow (V) versus time tracings. *A,* Where patient initiated a breath. *B,* Where ventilator cycled off when pressure support level of 15-cm water was reached. *C,* High peak flow at start of the breath. *D,* How flow rate decreases as pressure support level is reached. (Courtesy Mallinckrodt, Pleasanton, CA)

Fig. 14-2 Two graphic tracings of expiratory air trapping. **A,** Volume versus time. *A* shows that the exhaled tidal volume tracing does not reach the baseline. Inspiratory tidal volume is greater than expiratory tidal volume, indicating air trapping. **B,** Flow versus time. Inspiratory flow is the tracing above the horizontal baseline of zero flow. Expiratory flow is the tracing below the horizontal baseline. The patient's expiratory flow does not return to zero; this indicates air trapping. The higher the flow rate, the more air trapping there is. Air trapping leads to auto-PEEP. It can be minimized by increasing expiratory time, giving an erosolized bronchodilator to treat bronchospasm, or suctioning out any secretions. (Courtesy Mallinckrodt, Pleasanton, CA)

trends toward an improving or worsening pulmonary condition.

Airway resistance is measured in units of centimeters of water per liter per second at a standard flow rate of 0.5 L/sec (30 L/min). The normal spontaneously breathing adult's airway resistance (R_{AW}) is 0.6 to 2.4 cm water/L/sec; the normal 3 kg infant's R_{AW} is 30 cm H_2O/L/sec. Do not forget that this procedure is being performed on a patient with an intubated airway on a ventilator. The endotracheal tube adds to the patient's total R_{AW}. The smaller the tube the greater the resistance it offers to gas flowing through it. Altering inspiratory flow has an influence on the peak pressure measured for the calculation. As flow is lowered, gas turbulence is reduced and peak pressure is lowered.

Conversely, a higher flow creates more turbulence, and a higher peak pressure is seen.

b. Recommend the measurement of the patient's airway resistance (Code: IA2f) [Difficulty: An]

This calculation is important because it provides valuable information on the patient's pulmonary condition. The R_{AW} value indicates how difficult it is to move the tidal volume through the patient's airways and if aerosolized bronchodilating medications are effective.

It is reasonable to recommend an airway resistance measurement on any patient who has an increased airway resistance problem such as chronic obstructive pulmonary disease (COPD), asthma, bronchospasm, or wheezing breath sounds. It is also reasonable to measure airway resistance before and after a bronchodilator medication is given to determine if it had any benefit.

c. Determine the patient's airway resistance (Code: IC1a) [Difficulty: An]

Most of the microprocessor ventilators offer software for calculating all of these values. However, in other situations they must be calculated manually.

Procedure for calculating airway resistance

1. Cycle a tidal volume. The patient should be breathing passively; fighting the breath will result in an errone-

ously high peak pressure and assisting with the breath will result in an erroneously low peak pressure.

2. Note the peak airway pressure on the manometer.
3. Briefly prevent the tidal volume from being exhaled. No air should be moving. Note that the pressure manometer shows a peak pressure and then a static or plateau pressure that is stable as long as the tidal volume is held in the lungs. Record the plateau pressure.
4. Calculate the flow in liters per second by taking the flow in liters per minute and dividing it by 60 seconds.
5. Place the peak airway pressure, plateau pressure, and flow into the following formula and solve for airway resistance:

$$R_{AW} = \frac{\text{peak airway pressure} - \text{plateau pressure}}{\text{flow in L/sec}}$$

Example. A mechanically ventilated patient has a peak airway pressure of 30 cm water and plateau pressure of 20 cm water. The peak flow is set at 60 L/min.

Calculate peak flow in liters per second:

$$\frac{60 \text{ L/min}}{60 \text{ seconds}} = 1 \text{ L/sec}$$

Calculate airway resistance:

$$R_{AW} = \frac{\text{peak airway pressure} - \text{plateau pressure}}{\text{flow in L/sec}}$$

$$R_{AW} = \frac{30 \text{ cm H}_2\text{O} - 20 \text{ cm H}_2\text{O}}{1 \text{ L/sec}} = 10 \text{ cm H}_2\text{O/L/sec}$$

This value is greater than normal for a patient breathing spontaneously. However, remember that the patient's airway is intubated. This results in a smaller airway diameter and more resistance. Some practitioners use the calculated airway resistance as the basis for setting the pressure support ventilation (PSV) level (discussed later). An increased airway resistance may indicate bronchospasm or secretions in the airways. Delivering an aerosolized bronchodilator or suctioning should result in the resistance returning to the original level.

EXAM HINT

All past examinations have had questions that deal with identifying when the patient has an increased airway resistance and how it can be managed.

---

4. Lung compliance

a. Review the patient's chart for information on lung compliance (Code: IA1f4) [Difficulty: An]

This value may have been measured earlier in either the pulmonary function laboratory or on the ventilator. Compare any earlier values with new values. This is important for understanding the patient's

trends toward an improving or worsening pulmonary condition.

The compliance values indicate how easily the tidal volume can be delivered into the lungs. Static compliance (C_{st}) is the measurement of work required to overcome the elastic resistance to ventilation. It is a measurement of the compliance of the lungs and thorax (C_{LT}). Static compliance is measured in units of milliliters per centimeters of water pressure. The normal adult's static compliance is 100 mL/cm water; the normal 3-kg infant's static compliance is 5 mL/cm water.

Dynamic compliance (C_{dyn}), sometimes called *dynamic characteristic*, is the measurement of the combination of the patient's static compliance and airway resistance. As discussed previously, airway resistance is the pressure required to move a tidal volume through the airways. It is also known as *nonelastic resistance to ventilation*.

b. Recommend the measurement of the patient's lung compliance (Code: IA2f) [Difficulty: An]

It is reasonable to recommend that lung compliance be measured on any patient who has clinical evidence of a significant change in lung compliance. This may occur in conditions such as acute respiratory distress syndrome (ARDS), pneumonia, pulmonary edema, or pulmonary fibrosis. Compliance can be measured to document the worsening of the patient's condition as well as to determine if the compliance is improving with treatment.

c. Determine the patient's lung compliance (Code: IC1g) [Difficulty: An]

Most of the microprocessor ventilators offer software for calculating all of these values. However, in other situations they must be calculated manually.

1. Procedure for calculating the compliance factor.

Before the actual calculation of the patient's static and dynamic compliance can be performed, the static compliance of the breathing circuit should be determined. In most older ventilators some of the set tidal volume never reaches the patient because it is "lost" in the circuit. For highest accuracy in the calculation of static and dynamic compliance and the calculation of actual tidal and sigh volumes, this lost volume must be subtracted from the exhaled tidal volume. The phrase "compressed volume" is commonly used to describe this lost volume.

1. Remove the patient from the ventilator and manually ventilate him or her during this procedure.
2. Set the pressure limit as high as possible.
3. Block the breathing circuit at the patient connector.
4. Cycle a tidal volume.
5. Perform either of the following: (a) note the peak pressure developed in the circuit as the tidal volume stretches out the circuit; or (b) if the ventilator's peak

pressure hits the pressure limit, note the delivered tidal volume and the pressure limit.

Note: If the patient is on PEEP therapy, subtract the PEEP level from the measured peak pressure to find the true peak pressure.

6. The compliance factor is found by dividing the measured tidal volume by the peak pressure.

   Example. The patient has a set tidal volume of 600 mL. Using step 5b, the peak pressure is found to be 80 cm water, and the measured tidal volume is found to be 320 mL.

$$\text{Compliance factor} = \frac{320 \text{ mL}}{80 \text{ cm}} = 4 \text{ mL/cm water}$$

The compressed volume is found by multiplying the compliance factor by either the peak or plateau pressure. The compressed volume is then subtracted from the exhaled tidal volume to determine the patient's actual tidal volume.

⬅ EXAM HINT

Commonly examinations have had a question requiring the calculation of static and/or dynamic compliance. Be able to perform the following calculations.

---

2. Procedure for calculating static compliance.

1. Determine the compliance factor of the breathing circuit (as described previously).
2. Reattach the patient to the ventilator. Reset all controls to their ordered or preset positions.
3. Cycle a tidal volume. The patient should be breathing passively; fighting the breath will result in an erroneously high peak pressure and assisting with the breath will result in an erroneously low peak pressure.
4. Briefly prevent the tidal volume from being exhaled. No air should be moving. Note that the pressure manometer shows a peak pressure and then a static or plateau pressure that is stable as long as the tidal volume is held in the lungs. Note the *plateau pressure.*
5. Calculate the static compliance (C_{st}) using this formula:

$$C_{st} = \frac{\text{exhaled tidal volume} - \text{compressed volume}}{\text{plateau pressure} - \text{PEEP}}$$

in which compressed volume = compliance factor × plateau pressure.

3. Procedure for calculating dynamic compliance

1. Determine the compliance factor of the breathing circuit (as described previously).
2. Reattach the patient to the ventilator. Reset all controls to their ordered or preset positions.
3. Cycle a tidal volume. The patient should be breathing passively; fighting the breath will result in an erroneously high peak pressure and assisting with the breath will result in an erroneously low peak pressure.

4. Note the *peak pressure* on the manometer. If the pressure at the end of inspiration is less than peak pressure, the pressure at the end of inspiration should be used in the calculation.
5. Calculate the dynamic compliance (C_{dyn}) using this formula:

$$C_{dyn} = \frac{\text{exhaled tidal volume} - \text{compressed volume}}{\text{peak pressure} - \text{PEEP}}$$

in which compressed volume = compliance factor × peak pressure.

Example. Calculate the static and dynamic compliance on a ventilated patient *without PEEP therapy.*

The patient has an exhaled tidal volume of 600 mL. The peak pressure is 30 cm water and the static or plateau pressure is 20 cm water. The compliance factor has been determined to be 4 mL/cm water. The compressed volume at the plateau pressure is determined to be 80 mL (4 mL/cm compliance factor × 20 cm). The compressed volume at the peak pressure is determined to be 120 mL (4 mL/cm compliance factor × 30 cm).

$$C_{st} = \frac{600 \text{ mL} - 80 \text{ mL}}{20 \text{ cm} - 0}$$
$$= \frac{520 \text{ mL}}{20 \text{ cm}}$$
$$= 26 \text{ mL/cm water}$$

$$C_{dyn} = \frac{600 \text{ mL} - 120 \text{ mL}}{30 \text{ cm} - 0}$$
$$= \frac{480 \text{ mL}}{30 \text{ cm}}$$
$$= 16 \text{ mL/cm water}$$

Example. Calculate the static and dynamic compliance on a ventilated patient *with PEEP therapy.*

The same patient has an exhaled tidal volume of 600 mL. Because of refractory hypoxemia, 10 cm of PEEP therapy is started. The peak pressure is now 36 cm water, and the static or plateau pressure is now 25 cm water. The compliance factor has been determined to be 4 mL/cm water. The compressed volume at the plateau pressure is determined to be 60 mL [4 mL/cm compliance factor × 15 cm (25 cm − 10 cm PEEP)]. The compressed volume at the peak pressure is determined to be 104 mL [4 mL/cm compliance factor × 26 cm (36 cm − 10 cm PEEP)].

$$C_{st} = \frac{600 \text{ mL} - 60 \text{ mL}}{25 \text{ cm} - 10 \text{ cm}}$$
$$= \frac{540 \text{ mL}}{15 \text{ cm}}$$
$$= 36 \text{ mL/cm water}$$

$$C_{dyn} = \frac{600 \text{ mL} - 104 \text{ mL}}{36 \text{ cm} - 10 \text{ cm}}$$
$$= \frac{496 \text{ mL}}{26 \text{ cm}}$$
$$= 19 \text{ mL/cm water}$$

5. Interpret the patient's airway resistance, dynamic lung compliance, and static lung compliance values on the ventilator (Code: IB10d, IC2a, IC2i) [Difficulty: An]

Any increase in airway resistance and/or decrease in lung compliance creates an increase in the patient's WOB. Examples of conditions or situations in which there is an increased airway resistance include bronchospasm, secretions, mucosal edema, airway tumor, placement of a small endotracheal tube, and biting or kinking of the endotracheal tube. Lung compliance is decreased by pneumonia, pulmonary edema, ARDS, pulmonary fibrosis, atelectasis, consolidation, hemothorax, pleural effusion, air trapping, pneumomediastinum, and pneumothorax. Examples of chest wall and abdominal conditions that lower compliance include the various chest wall deformities, circumferential chest or abdominal burns, enlarged liver, pneumoperitoneum, peritonitis, abdominal bleeding, herniation, and advanced pregnancy. Correction of the problem should return the patient's ventilator pressure(s) to baseline and normalize the patient's WOB.

Six possible combinations of increasing or decreasing static and dynamic lung compliance exist. Each has its own possible causes and are covered in turn. The patient must be passive on the ventilator for the measured values to be accurate. Check two or three breaths for increased accuracy. Let the patient have a normal breath or two between each of the peak and plateau pressure measurement breaths.

a. Decreased dynamic compliance with stable static compliance

Decreased dynamic compliance with stable static compliance is noticed as an *increase* in the peak pressure with an unchanged plateau pressure (Fig. 14-3). It is caused by an increased airway resistance (bronchospasm, etc.). Correcting the underlying problem results in the peak pressure returning to the original level.

Note that the inspiratory resistance has doubled from the original 10 to 20 cm while the plateau pressure has not changed. This confirms that the problem originates in the airway or breathing circuit. The patient's lung compliance has not changed.

b. Increased dynamic compliance with stable static compliance

Increased dynamic compliance with stable static compliance is noticed as a *decrease* in the peak pressure with an unchanged plateau pressure (Fig. 14-4). This represents an improvement in the patient's airway resistance from the original condition. Secretions can be

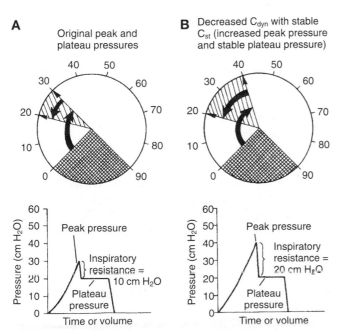

Fig. 14-3 Decreased dynamic compliance (C_{dyn}) with a stable static compliance (C_{st}). **A,** Original pressure manometer reading and pressure-volume curve. **B,** Altered pressure manometer reading and pressure-volume curve.

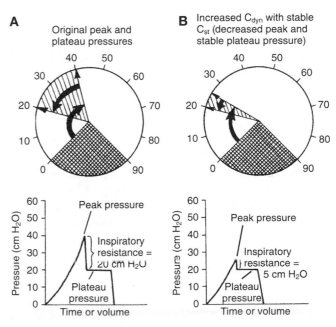

Fig. 14-4 Increased dynamic compliance (C_{dyn}) with a stable static compliance (C_{st}). **A,** Original pressure manometer reading and pressure-volume curve. **B,** Altered pressure manometer reading and pressure-volume curve.

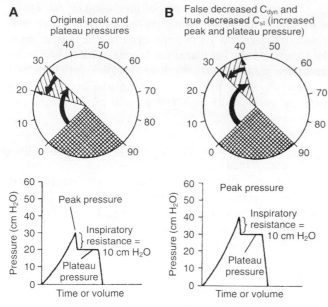

Fig. 14-5 False decreased dynamic compliance (C_{dyn}) with true decreased static compliance (C_{st}). **A,** Original pressure manometer reading and pressure-volume curve. **B,** Altered pressure manometer reading and pressure-volume curve.

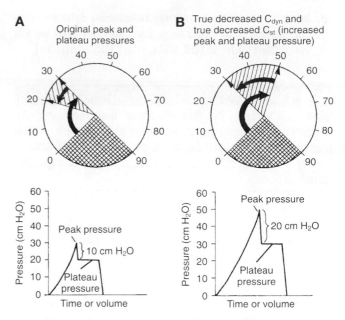

Fig. 14-6 True decreased dynamic compliance (C_{dyn}) with true decreased static compliance (C_{st}). **A,** Original pressure manometer reading and pressure-volume curve. **B,** Altered pressure manometer reading and pressure-volume curve.

diminished, mucous plugs cleared, bronchospasm corrected, and so on.

Note that the inspiratory resistance has decreased from the original level of 20 to just 5 cm. This confirms that the patient's airway resistance has decreased. The patient's lung compliance has not changed.

c. False decreased dynamic compliance with true decreased static compliance

False decreased dynamic compliance with true decreased static compliance is noticed as an *increase* in *both* the peak and plateau pressures (Fig. 14-5). This is seen when the patient's lung-thoracic compliance worsens. The plateau pressure is elevated and the static compliance is decreased.

As an artifact of the stiffer lungs, the peak pressure is also elevated, and the dynamic compliance is decreased. However, the difference between the peak and plateau pressures remains the same. This demonstrates that there is no real increase in the patient's airway resistance.

d. True decreased dynamic compliance with true decreased static compliance

True decreased dynamic compliance with true decreased static compliance is also noticed as an *increase* in *both* the peak and plateau pressures (Fig. 14-6). This is seen with the combination of a decreased lung compliance and an increased airway resistance. Causes of both of these problems were discussed earlier.

e. False increased dynamic compliance with true increased static compliance

False increased dynamic compliance with true increased static compliance is noticed as a *decrease* in *both* the peak and plateau pressures (Fig. 14-7). This is seen when the patient's lung-thoracic compliance improves. The plateau pressure decreases, and as an artifact, the peak pressure also decreases. Notice that the difference between the peak and plateau pressures remains the same. This indicates that the patient's airway resistance is unchanged.

f. True increased dynamic compliance with true increased static compliance

True increased dynamic compliance with true increased static compliance is also noticed as a *decrease* in *both* the peak and plateau pressures (Fig. 14-8). This is seen when both the patient's airway resistance and lung-thoracic compliance improve. Notice that the plateau pressure has decreased, thus indicating more compliant lungs. Also notice that the difference between the peak and plateau pressures has decreased. This demonstrates that the airway resistance has also decreased.

All six examples of increasing or decreasing static and/or dynamic lung compliance make use of a single tidal volume that is analyzed for peak and plateau pressures. Some practitioners advocate using several different tidal volumes (for example 8, 10, and 12 mL/kg of ideal body weight) when measuring dynamic and static pressures. The

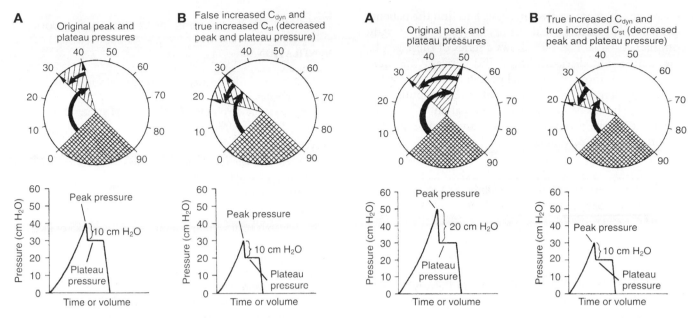

Fig. 14-7 False increased dynamic compliance (C_dyn) with true increased static compliance (C_st). **A,** Original pressure manometer reading and pressure-volume curve. **B,** Altered pressure manometer reading and pressure-volume curve.

Fig. 14-8 True increased dynamic compliance (C_dyn) with true increased static compliance (C_st). **A,** Original pressure manometer reading and pressure-volume curve. **B,** Altered pressure manometer reading and pressure-volume curve.

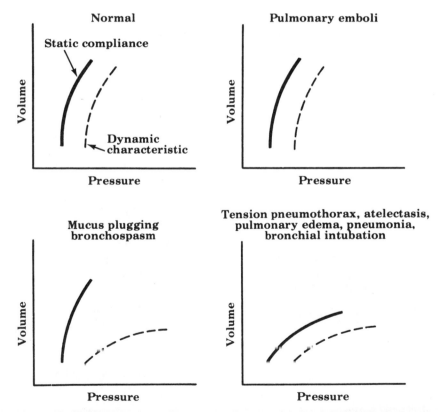

Fig. 14-9 Pressure-volume curves for normal airways and lungs, pulmonary embolism (no change in airway resistance or lung compliance), increased airway resistance, and decreased lung compliance. (From Pilbeam SP: *Mechanical ventilation: physiological and clinical applications,* St Louis, 1986, Multi-Media Publishing.)

measured values are plotted on a graph to find the patient's optimal tidal volume that results in the highest static compliance value. Fig. 14-9 shows a series of these graphs. The curves for diseased lungs and airways are quite different from those of a normal person or a patient with a pulmonary embolism. Because of this, a pulmonary embolism should be considered if the patient's condition deteriorates rapidly and there is no change in the dynamic or static compliance values.

MODULE B	Provide mechanical ventilation to adequately oxygenate and ventilate the patient

A number of physiologic criteria have been compiled to help the clinician determine when a patient is in respiratory or ventilatory failure (Box 14-1). Remember that the patient may not fail each and every criteria; however, the patient will often fail one or more criteria in each category.

1. Perform the following procedures to make sure that the patient is adequately oxygenated
   a. Minimize hypoxemia by positioning the patient properly (Code: IIIB4c) [Difficulty: An]
   This was discussed in Chapter 6.

   b. Administer oxygen, as needed, to prevent hypoxemia (Code: IIIB4c and IIIC3a) [Difficulty: An]
Oxygen administration and adjustment were discussed in Chapter 6. Briefly, the goal of oxygen administration is to keep the PaO_2 level of most patients between 60 and 90 torr and the SpO_2 level greater than 90%. Exceptions are the COPD patient who is breathing on hypoxic drive and the patient who is in a cardiac arrest situation. The following formula can be used to help guide the use of supplemental oxygen in most stable patients:

$$\text{Desired } F_IO_2 = \frac{\text{desired } PaO_2 \times \text{current } FiO_2}{\text{current } PaO_2}$$

Example. Your patient has a PaO_2 level of 55 mm Hg on 30% oxygen. The clinical goal is a PaO_2 level of 90 mm Hg. What oxygen percentage should the patient have?

$$\text{Desired } F_IO_2 = \frac{\text{desired } PaO_2 \times \text{current } FiO_2}{\text{current } PaO_2}$$
$$\text{Desired } F_IO_2 = \frac{90 \text{ mm Hg} \times 0.3}{55 \text{ mm Hg}}$$
$$\text{Desired } F_IO_2 = \frac{27}{55}$$
$$\text{Desired } F_IO_2 = 0.49 \text{ or } 49\% \text{ oxygen}$$

Those patients who have refractory hypoxemia (e.g., ARDS) will not respond with a normal increase in PaO_2 level as the oxygen percentage is increased. In the short

---

BOX 14-1	Indications for Ventilatory Support

VENTILATION
Apnea
$PaCO_2 \geq 55$ torr in a patient who is not ordinarily hypercapneic
Dead space: tidal volume (V_D/V_T ratio) of greater than 0.55-0.6 (55%-60%)

OXYGENATION
$PaO_2 <80$ torr on 50% oxygen or more
$P(A-a)O_2 <300-350$ torr on 100% oxygen
Intrapulmonary shunt >15%-20%

PULMONARY MECHANICS
Spontaneous tidal volume 3-4 mL/lb or 7-9 mL/kg of ideal body weight
Vital capacity <10-15 mL/kg
Maximum inspiratory pressured (MIP) < -20 to -25 cm water pressure
Forced expiratory volume in one second (FEV_1) <10 mL/kg
Respiratory rate <12 breaths/min or >35 breaths/min in an adult
Rapid, shallow breathing index (breaths/minute divided by tidal volume in liters) >105

MISCELLANEOUS
Unconscious patient
Unstable and unacceptable vital signs
Unstable cardiac rhythm caused by hypoxemia and/or acidosis
Worsening cardiopulmonary or other major organ system

---

term, use whatever oxygen percentage is needed to achieve the clinical goal. The risk of oxygen toxicity increases when the F_IO_2 is greater than 0.5 for periods of more than 48 hours. Always recheck the patient's arterial oxygen level after a change has been made in the F_IO_2.

Either of the following formulas can be used in the special situation of determining the flows of air and oxygen into a "bleed in" type of intermittent mandatory ventilation (IMV) or continuous positive airway pressure (CPAP) system to obtain an ordered F_IO_2. Either version can also be used for determining the gas flows, total flow, and oxygen/air ratio through an air entrainment (Venturi) mask.

The first formula follows:

$$(\text{L/min air} \times F_IO_2 \text{ of air}) + (\text{L/min } O_2 \times F_IO_2 \text{ pure } O_2) = \\ \text{total flow} \times \text{unknown } F_IO_2$$

The second formula follows:

$$F_1C_1 + F_2C_2 = F_TC_T$$

in which
F_1 = flow of first gas (oxygen)
C_1 = concentration of oxygen in the first gas (1.0 for pure oxygen)

F_2 = flow of second gas (air)

C_2 = concentration of oxygen in the second gas (0.21 for air)

F_T = total flow of both gases

C_T = concentration of oxygen in the mix of both gases

Use algebraic manipulation to solve for the unknown.

Example. Determine the oxygen percentage through a bleed in system that has an oxygen flow of 10 L/min and an airflow of 15 L/min. Determine the total flow through the system. Determine the ratio of oxygen to air.

$$(\text{L/min air} \times \text{FiO}_2 \text{ of air}) +$$
$$(\text{L/min O}_2 \times \text{FiO}_2 \text{ pure O}_2) = \text{total flow} \times \text{unknown F}_I\text{O}_2$$
$$(15 \times 0.21) + (10 \times 1.0) = (15 + 10) \times \text{unknown F}_I\text{O}_2$$
$$(3.15) + (10) = (25) \times \text{unknown F}_I\text{O}_2$$
$$13.15 = 25\, F_I\text{O}_2$$
$$(\text{Divide both sides by 25.})$$
$$0.526 \text{ or } 52.6\% = F_I\text{O}_2$$
$$\text{Total flow} = 15 + 10 = 25 \text{ L/min}$$
$$\text{Ratio} = \frac{10 \text{ L/min oxygen}}{15 \text{ L/min air}}$$

c. Adequately oxygenate the patient to prevent accidental hypoxemia before and after suctioning, changing the ventilator circuit, or performing other procedures in which the patient is disconnected from the ventilator (Code: IIIB4c) [Difficulty: An]

Ensuring adequate oxygenation when suctioning is discussed in Chapter 12. Briefly, remember to give the adult patient 100% oxygen for at least 30 seconds before suctioning. Perform the task as quickly and safely as possible to minimize time off the ventilator. Leave the patient on 100% oxygen for at least 1 minute after the procedure or until he or she returns to a stable condition as before the procedure. Children younger than 6 months of age can have the $F_I\text{O}_2$ increased by 10% for the procedure.

In an adult, it is acceptable to increase the inspired oxygen up to 100% before and after a procedure that requires disconnection from the ventilator. The goal is to prevent hypoxemia. The patient should be manually ventilated with a resuscitation bag if indicated. Always remember to return the patient to the original oxygen percentage when clinically indicated.

2. Initiate and adjust modes of ventilation (Code: IIIB2c) [Difficulty: An]

The following modes of ventilation are delivered through most types of electrically powered, volume-cycled ventilators such as the Servo 900 C, Nelcor Puritan-Bennett 7200, Drager Evita E4, and Bear 1000.

Control. Control (C) is the simplest method of providing ventilatory support and is used on an apneic patient. The ventilator is set with a mandatory respiratory rate and tidal volume. The machine is incapable of allowing any patient interaction. For example, the ventilator might be set to deliver a tidal volume of 700 mL at a rate of 14 times/min. Because of this limitation, it is rarely, if ever, used in modern medicine except when the patient must be kept sedated or pharmacologically paralyzed (Fig. 14-10, *A*, shows the pressure/time curve).

Assist/control. The assist/control (A/C) mode has a set backup respiratory rate but allows the patient to trigger additional machine-delivered breaths. A sensitivity control is adjusted to allow the patient to easily start a breath as needed. All tidal volumes are the same (Fig. 14-10, *B*, shows the pressure/time curve).

Intermittent mandatory ventilation. Intermittent mandatory ventilation (IMV) has a set backup respiratory rate and tidal volume that is delivered to the patient. In addition, in between the mandatory breaths, the patient can breathe spontaneously as frequently as desired. The patient can also take in as large a spontaneous tidal volume as needed. The sensitivity control is set so that the patient cannot trigger any extra ventilator tidal volumes. For example, the ventilator might be set to deliver a 700-mL tidal volume 8 times/min. Let us say that the patient breathes spontaneously 10 more times and has an average tidal volume of 400 mL. The total rate is counted at 18. The total minute volume is the combination of the machine's volume and the patient's volume (Fig. 14-10, *C*, shows the pressure/time curve).

Synchronous intermittent mandatory ventilation. Synchronous intermittent mandatory ventilation (SIMV) is similar to IMV except that the sensitivity control is functional. The patient can trigger a machine-delivered tidal volume during a preset time interval. The timing of the backup rate is such that the patient can get only as many ventilator breaths as are set. Spontaneous tidal volumes vary with the patient's efforts. The total respiratory rate and total minute volume would be calculated as discussed previously (Fig. 14-10, *D*, shows the pressure/time curve).

Pressure support ventilation. PSV is similar to intermittent positive-pressure ventilation (IPPB) in that when the patient initiates a ventilator breath, a preset pressure is delivered to the airway. The patient has the flexibility to determine the respiratory rate. The physician orders a PSV level that is enough to either overcome the patient's calculated airway resistance or to deliver a minimum tidal volume, depending on the clinical goal. The tidal volume will be stable if the patient passively takes the PSV breath, or it can be larger if the patient interacts actively with the pressure that is delivered (Figs. 14-1 and 14-10, *E*, show the pressure/time curve).

Pressure control ventilation. Pressure control ventilation (PCV) involves the delivery of tidal volume breaths that are pressure limited and time cycled. A set ventilator rate can be set and the patient can also trigger additional breaths. Because the pressure is limited, the tidal volumes may vary. This must be monitored closely in patients with frequently changing lung compliance and airway resistance. As the

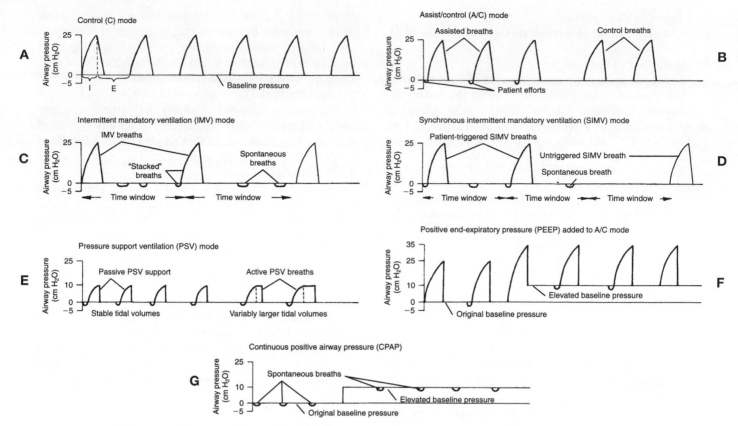

Fig. 14-10 Pressure versus time waveforms for various modes of mechanical ventilation. **A,** Control mode (C) shows no patient effort and consistent I:E ratios. **B,** Assist/control mode (A/C) shows that patient's initial effort triggers machine tidal volume breath. **C,** Intermittent mandatory ventilation mode (IMV) shows spontaneous tidal volume breaths occurring between predetermined machine tidal volume breaths. Note "stacked" breaths that happen when patient takes in a breath that is then supplemented by a machine breath. **D,** Synchronous intermittent mandatory ventilation mode (SIMV) shows that a patient effort within a time window results in delivery of machine tidal volume. Any other patient efforts within the time window result in a spontaneous tidal volume. If no patient efforts occur within the time window, machine tidal volume will be automatically delivered. **E,** Pressure support ventilation mode (PSV) shows how patient must initiate all breaths that are then supported to the predetermined airway pressure. Stable tidal volumes are seen if the patient inhales passively. Variably larger tidal volumes result if the patient inhales more actively. **F,** Positive end–expiratory pressure (PEEP) therapy can be added to A/C mode (as shown) or any other mode. The elevated baseline pressure prevents alveolar collapse. The sensitivity control must be set at -1 to -2 cm water so that the patient is able to trigger a breath without undue effort. **G,** Continuous positive airway pressure (CPAP) shows that the patient takes spontaneous tidal volumes while exhaling against an elevated baseline pressure.

inspiratory time is increased it can become longer than the expiratory time. This results in pressure control inverse ratio ventilation (PCIRV). Fig. 14-11 shows the volume, flow, and pressure tracings.

Positive end–expiratory pressure. Positive end–expiratory pressure (PEEP) is a residual pressure above atmospheric pressure maintained at the airway opening at the end of expiration. PEEP is administered through a mechanical ventilator and is not a mode by itself. Rather, it is used in conjunction with any of the previously mentioned modes.

PEEP is set to prevent the patient from exhaling back to ambient (atmospheric) pressure. The higher the level of PEEP, the more progressively the patient's functional residual capacity (FRC) is increased. The therapeutic goal of this is to increase the patient's arterial oxygen pressure (PaO_2). (Fig. 14-10, *F*, shows the pressure/time curve.)

Continuous positive airway pressure. Continuous positive airway pressure (CPAP) is a pressure above atmospheric maintained at the airway opening throughout the respiratory cycle during spontaneous breathing. CPAP is

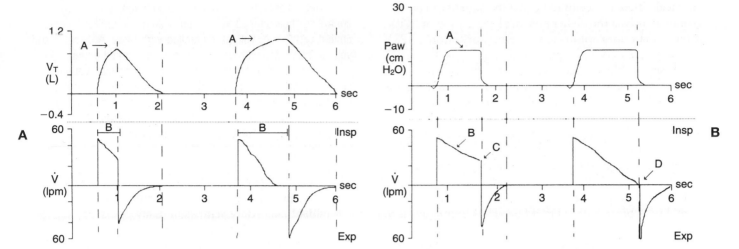

Fig. 14-11 Two sets of graphic tracings of pressure control ventilation. **A,** Two tracings show volume (V_T) versus time and flow ($\dot{V}$) versus time. *A* shows tidal volume; *B* shows inspiratory flow. Note how tidal volume increases as inspiratory time is increased. However, as shown in lower right tracing, as flow drops to zero no more volume is delivered. **B,** Two tracings show pressure versus time and flow versus time. *A* shows the pressure control level being reached with an inspiratory plateau or "square wave" appearance. *B* shows declining inspiratory flow. *C* shows final flow when inspiration is time cycled off and exhalation begins. This graphic can be used to help adjust a longer inspiratory time. If pressure control inverse ratio ventilation (PCIRV) were being optimally adjusted, the inspiration time could be increased until inspiratory flow reached zero (indicated by *D*). (Courtesy Mallinckrodt, Pleasanton, CA)

similar to PEEP in purpose and effect. It is different from the previously mentioned modes in that the patient does not receive any ventilator-delivered tidal volume breaths. The patient must be capable of providing all of the minute ventilation for carbon dioxide removal. CPAP can be delivered through some mechanical ventilators when the rate is turned off or through a free-standing system (Fig. 14-10, *G*, shows the pressure/time curve).

Airway pressure release ventilation. Currently only the Drager Evita and E4 ventilators offer the airway pressure release ventilation (APRV) mode (as well as other modes). They are microprocessor-controlled and include a monitor for patient data and graphics. The APRV mode has been used with success in ARDS patients who have not responded well to constant volume ventilation. APRV can be described simply as a mode in which the patient can breathe spontaneously at two different levels of CPAP. A difference from conventional CPAP is that the two levels are held for set periods of time. The ventilator options for this mode are quite simple. The practitioner sets the low pressure (P_{low}), high pressure (P_{high}), and times that the patient will be at those pressure levels. The low pressure is sometimes referred to as CPAP and high pressure as *release pressure*. The timing changes from low pressure to high pressure and back to low pressure effectively deliver a tidal volume. (See Fig. 14-12 for a pressure/time tracing.)

When comparing APRV with other modes of ventilation, there appear to be several similarities between it and

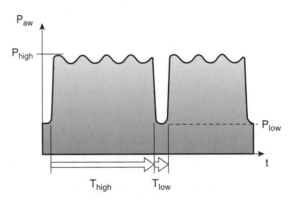

Fig. 14-12 Pressure versus time graphic of airway pressure support ventilation (APRV). The high pressure ensures a maximal, safe FRC and the low pressure maintains a normal FRC. The time spent at each pressure level is adjusted to meet the patient's needs and set a respiratory rate. Patient is able to breathe spontaneously at both pressure levels. When the high airway pressure is released (pressure release) the patient exhales a tidal volume to the low pressure level. (From Drager EVITA ventilator technical information.)

pressure control inverse ratio ventilation (PCIRV) with PEEP and bilevel ventilation. All have an elevated baseline pressure that allow the patient to breathe spontaneously. All have variable inspiratory times for the higher pressure level. None deliver a set tidal volume to the patient. The only real difference seems to be that the patient can breathe spontaneously at the higher pressure level only with APRV. If the patient does not make any respiratory efforts, APRV functions like PCV or bilevel ventilation.

A set of blood gases, vital signs, pulmonary artery catheter values, and so forth should be obtained on the current constant volume ventilator settings as a baseline before starting APRV. The following suggestions for initiating APRV are similar to those listed earlier for starting PCIRV:

1. Set the high pressure (release pressure) at the patient's optimal PEEP/CPAP level. Often this is in a range between the patient's static lung compliance pressure and peak pressure. See Fig. 14-32. The clinical goal is to safely maximize the patient's FRC.
2. Set the low pressure (CPAP) at the level of PEEP that was used on the constant volume ventilator. This is to maintain the patient's FRC. See point *A* of Fig. 14-32.
3. Set the inspired oxygen the same as before. Some may prefer to set it at 100%, as with PCIRV, until blood gas results show that it can be lowered.
4. Set the timing of the high pressure and low pressure values so that more time is spent at the high pressure than the low pressure. Often the low pressure time is limited to 1 to 1.5 seconds. Keep the same respiratory rate as before. Even if the patient is apneic, as the ventilator switches from high pressure to low pressure the patient exhales a tidal volume to blow off carbon dioxide.

Monitor the patient's ventilator delivered and spontaneous tidal volumes and rates. Check vital signs. Get an arterial blood gas (ABG) sample in about 15 minutes.

If the patient's initial blood gas results on APRV show hypoxemia, the following options are available: (1) increase the inspired oxygen percentage if it is not already at 100%, (2) increase the low pressure level, (3) increase the high pressure level, or (4) increase the time the patient is kept at the high pressure level. Reducing any or all of these options will decrease the patient's PaO_2 if it is too high.

If the blood gas results show hypoventilation, the following options are available: (1) increase the high pressure level, or (2) decrease the time at the high pressure level to increase the respiratory rate. Do the opposite to increase the $PaCO_2$ if the patient is being hyperventilated.

As with the previous ventilator modalities, the patient should be closely monitored and have an ABG drawn to evaluate every change.

EXAM HINT

The National Board of Respiratory Care (NBRC) examinations have used a variety of terms and phrases to describe modes or modifications of modes of ventilation, including the following.

Terms related to delivering a set tidal volume include volume ventilation; volume-cycled mechanical ventilation; volume-controlled ventilation; volume-preset ventilation; volume-controlled, flow limited ventilation; volume-controlled, pressure limited ventilation; volume controlled with SIMV, A/C, or C; and volume-controlled with continuous flow IMV circuit added.

Terms related to *not* delivering a set tidal volume include pressure-cycled ventilation; pressure control; pressure-controlled, pressure-limited, time cycled ventilation; pressure-controlled with constant inspiratory time; pressure-limited; and any previous term with inverse ratio ventilation.

---

3. **Begin and modify combinations of ventilatory techniques to adequately oxygenate the patient: synchronous intermittent mandatory ventilation (SIMV), pressure support ventilation (PSV), pressure control ventilation (PCV), and positive end-expiratory pressure (PEEP) (Code: IIIB4b) [Difficulty: An]**

The current generation of mechanical ventilators offers the physician and practitioner a number of options for how to best tailor ventilatory support to meet the patient's needs. The following should be considered when deciding what modes to use and combine.

a. **Increased work of breathing**

Patients who show increased WOB may have a very high airway resistance, as in status asthmaticus, or may have a very low lung-thoracic compliance, as in ARDS. Some practitioners believe that the C or A/C modes, when properly applied to a sedated patient, are best for these problems because the patient's breathing efforts are almost eliminated. Other practitioners believe that IMV or SIMV are physiologically superior modes of ventilation. More recently, PSV has been shown to be beneficial to patients with increased efforts at breathing from the high airway resistance caused by a small diameter endotracheal tube.

b. **Hypercapnia**

A patient may have hypercapnia (a high carbon dioxide level) because of sedation from a morphine or heroin overdose or may have COPD with worsening of the chronic hypercapnia. In either case, the patient becomes progressively more hypoxemic (unless given supplemental oxygen) as the carbon dioxide level rises. C or A/C modes are best for setting a minimum minute volume to determine the maximum carbon dioxide level. As the patient recovers, IMV/SIMV or PSV allow for the gradual reduction of ventilatory support. See Box 14-2 for indications of IMV/SIMV tolerance.

Mandatory minute ventilation (MMV) has also shown success at setting a minute volume that limits the rise in carbon dioxide as the patient is weaning. MMV is a relatively new variation on the IMV/SIMV mode. With MMV, the patient is assured of a preset minute volume regardless of his or her spontaneous breathing. It has been proposed as an effective way to ventilate and wean patients who can spontaneously breathe but who have an unreliable

---

BOX 14-2 Indications of Intermittent Mandatory Ventilation (IMV)/Synchronous Intermittent Mandatory Ventilation (SIMV) Tolerance

---

INDICATIONS THAT IMV/SIMV IS BEING WELL TOLERATED

Stable spontaneous respiratory rate
Stable heart rate
Stable spontaneous tidal volume
Stable vital capacity, MIP, and/or FEV_1
No use or stable use of accessory muscles of ventilation
Patient indicates he or she is comfortable
Stable blood gases

INDICATIONS THAT IMV/SIMV IS NOT BEING WELL TOLERATED

Increased spontaneous respiratory rate
Tachycardia or dysrhythmias such as premature ventricular contractions
A drop in the spontaneous tidal volume
A drop in the vital capacity, MIP, and/or FEV_1
Beginning or increased use of accessory muscles of ventilation
Patient complains of dyspnea
Deterioration of blood gases as seen by a falling PaO_2 or SpO_2 and a rapidly falling or rising $PaCO_2$

BOX 14-3 Patient Monitoring During Positive End-Expiratory Pressure (PEEP) or Continuous Positive Airway Pressure (CPAP) Therapy

---

GOOD TOLERANCE OF CPAP/PEEP THERAPY

Increased PaO_2
Increased static lung compliance
Stable cardiac output as shown by the following:
  Stable heart rate without rhythm disturbances
  Stable blood pressure
  The following, which can be measured only through a pulmonary artery/Swan-Ganz catheter:
    Stable or increased $P\bar{v}O_2$ (mixed venous oxygen)
    Stable cardiac output
    Decreased pulmonary vascular resistance
    Decreased intrapulmonary shunt

POOR TOLERANCE OF CPAP/PEEP THERAPY

Increased PaO_2 (This can be deceiving if this is the only information observed)
Decreased static lung compliance
Decreased cardiac output as shown by the following:
  Increased heart rate or rhythm disturbances
  Decreased blood pressure
  The following can be measured only through a pulmonary artery/Swan-Ganz catheter:
    Decreased $P\bar{v}O_2$ (mixed venous oxygen)
    Decreased cardiac output
    Increased pulmonary vascular resistance
    Increased intrapulmonary shunt

---

respiratory drive and unstable tidal volume. Examples include patients who have received narcotic, sedative, anesthetic, or neuromuscular blocking medications. Patient conditions for which MMV is indicated include encephalopathy and cerebral disorders such as stroke. In addition, MMV may be used during the recovery period of a neuromuscular disease. Ventilators that include the MMV mode are all controlled by a microprocessor and include the Bear 1000, Drager E4, and the Hamilton Veolar. The following parameters have been recommended for the initiation of MMV:

1. Set the ventilator tidal volume according to established guidelines (10 to 15 mL/kg of ideal body weight).
2. The spontaneous breaths may be taken through a demand valve or may be pressure supported.
3. Determine the minimum minute volume according to the patient's preexisting condition and the clinical goals:
   a. The patient who has been on IMV/SIMV should have the MMV set at 90% of the IMV delivered minute volume. For example, the patient has an IMV/SIMV rate of 5 breaths/min and tidal volume of 800 mL. Therefore the ventilator is delivering 4 L of minute volume (5 × 800 mL) and the MMV would be set at 3600 mL (90% of 4 liters).
   b. The patient who has been on A/C should have the mandatory minute volume set at 80% of the A/C delivered minute volume. For example, the patient has an A/C rate of 10 breaths/min and tidal volume of 1000 mL. Therefore the ventilator is delivering

10 L of minute volume (10 × 1000 mL) and the MMV would be set at 8 liters (80% of 10 L).
4. Set the inspired oxygen percent, inspiratory flow, and so forth as the patient's clinical condition requires.

Ideally MMV establishes a minimum safe volume of ventilation. If the patient inhales less than this volume, the ventilator delivers as many breaths as necessary at the preestablished tidal volume to make up the difference. Be aware that a patient breathing rapidly with a small tidal volume may move enough gas to exceed the minimum minute volume. Because of this risk, it is important to set a low tidal volume alarm and/or a high respiratory rate alarm to give warning. Do not let the programming of a MMV create a false sense of security with these patients.

c. Hypoxemia

If hypoxemia is secondary to a decreased FRC, as in ARDS or atelectasis, the treatment of choice for hypoxemia is CPAP on a freestanding system or PEEP on a conventional volume-cycled ventilator. If the problem is from an increased intrapulmonary shunt, the patient may need PEEP or CPAP as well as up to 100% oxygen. See Box 14-3 for patient monitoring during PEEP and CPAP. PCIRV and high frequency jet ventilation have been used with success in hypoxemic patients with a pulmonary air leak who have failed at conventional volume ventilation. All the following were discussed earlier as individual modes of ventilation. When a patient has more than one problem, more than one solution may be needed. The following are combinations of modes from which to choose:

d. Pressure control/pressure control inverse ratio ventilation, synchronous intermittent mandatory ventilation, and positive end-expiratory pressure

PCV or, if necessary, PCIRV have been used with success in patients with low compliance and a pulmonary air leak. By limiting the peak pressure, less air seems to leak out and the tissues are more likely to heal. Therapeutic PEEP is applied to increase the patient's FRC to correct hypoxemia. The SIMV feature is added to let the patient breathe spontaneously if desired and stay more synchronized with the ventilator. With lung healing, the PEEP level is decreased and the inspiratory time is shortened. SIMV with a constant tidal volume may be used during the weaning phase. Fig. 14-11 shows pressure and flow tracings during PCV.

e. Intermittent mandatory ventilation/synchronous intermittent mandatory ventilation with pressure support ventilation and positive end-expiratory pressure

IMV/SIMV is used to give the patient a controlled number of deep tidal volume breaths. The patient can breathe as often as desired in between the mandatory breaths. The patient's total minute volume can be determined by adding the combination of IMV/SIMV and pressure supported breaths. A maximum acceptable PaCO$_2$ can be established with the proper combination of IMV/SIMV breaths and pressure support level. A PS level of more than 10 cm water may be needed. In addition, the pressure support ensures that the airway resistance of the endotracheal tube is overcome. (See the airway resistance calculation earlier in the chapter.) PEEP therapy is applied to the level necessary to obtain a clinically safe PaO$_2$ at the lowest possible F$_I$O$_2$. Fig. 14-13, *A*, shows the pressure-time curve.

Patients who have both a ventilation and an oxygenation problem benefit from these modes of ventilation. They have the desire to breathe on their own but a very limited ability to do so. All three modes can be independently adjusted for more or less support as indicated by the patient's clinical condition and blood gas results.

f. Intermittent mandatory ventilation/synchronous intermittent mandatory ventilation with positive end-expiratory pressure

IMV/SIMV and PEEP therapy are applied as indicated. Pressure support is not needed if the patient is strong enough to overcome the airway resistance of the endotra-

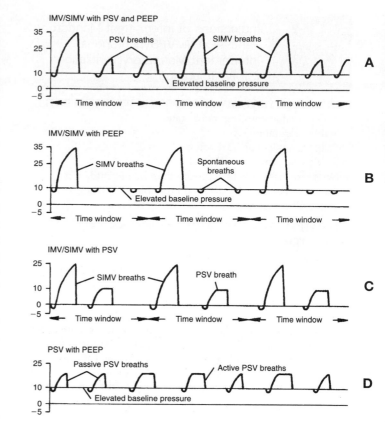

Fig. 14-13 Modification of combinations of IMV/SIMV, pressure support ventilation, and PEEP. **A,** IMV/SIMV with pressure support ventilation and PEEP. **B,** IMV/SIMV with PEEP. **C,** IMV/SIMV with pressure support ventilation. **D,** pressure support ventilation with PEEP. See text for descriptions of various combinations and their clinical application.

cheal tube and breathe with a clinically acceptable tidal volume. Fig. 14-13, *B,* shows the pressure-time curve.

g. Intermittent mandatory ventilation/synchronous intermittent mandatory ventilation with pressure support ventilation

IMV/SIMV and pressure support levels are increased or decreased based on the factors discussed earlier. This patient has the ability to provide some, but not all, of his or her own ventilation. The PaO$_2$ is clinically acceptable at an oxygen percentage probably no higher than 40%.

A fairly common clinical situation is seen in which the recovering patient does well on a gradually decreasing number of IMV/SIMV breaths until he or she can go no lower. The barrier seems to be the airway resistance of the endotracheal tube. (See the airway resistance calculation earlier in this chapter.) The addition of some pressure support overcomes that resistance so that the IMV/SIMV level can be further reduced. When the IMV/SIMV frequency is down to four or less, the patient is providing almost all of his or her minute volume. The greatest barrier to breathing is likely to be the resistance of the endotracheal tube. The decision can then be made to extubate the patient. Fig. 14-13, *C*, shows the pressure-time curve.

h. Pressure support ventilation with positive end–expiratory pressure

PSV and PEEP are applied as discussed earlier. This patient has the drive to breathe on his or her own; however, he or she has some limitation in the ability to overcome the resistance of the endotracheal tube or generate a consistently large enough tidal volume. (See the airway resistance calculation earlier in the chapter.) In addition, the patient has a significant oxygenation problem and needs some PEEP therapy. With recovery, both PS and PEEP can be reduced. They may be reduced individually or simultaneously as the patient's strength and/or oxygenation improve. Fig. 14-13, *D*, shows the pressure-time curve.

▣ EXAM HINT

There are usually two questions that require the therapist to evaluate a patient and make a change in the mode of ventilation. Frequently, one of the questions deals with identifying the need to increase the pressure support level to overcome the resistance of the endotracheal tube.

The following subjects are not specifically listed as testable on the Written Registry Examination. However, an analysis of the most recent examinations finds that there have been questions related to modifying the following ventilator settings.

Sensitivity. Sensitivity is the term used to describe the amount of work or effort the patient must perform to trigger the ventilator to deliver a tidal volume breath. Many ventilators require the patient to generate a *negative pressure* to trigger the unit. With these machines, the sensitivity is usually set at about −1 to −2 cm water pressure.

Several of the newer ventilators also have an option in which the patient generates an *inspiratory flow* to trigger a ventilator tidal volume breath. The Puritan-Bennett 7200 ventilator is an example of such a ventilator. The term "flow-by" is used to describe this sensitivity option on the ventilator. With a ventilator using flow sensitivity, the patient triggers a tidal volume when his/her inspiratory flow is about 2 L/min (33 mL/sec) less than the set baseline flow through the circuit.

Flow. Flow is adjusted to set the inspiratory time and inspiratory/expiratory (I:E) ratio to meet the patient's needs. Inspiratory flow should be great enough to meet the patient's needs and minimize WOB. Increase flow if the patient has signs of greater demand such as using accessory muscles of inspiration, lack of synchrony with the ventilator, or the pressure manometer deflects greatly

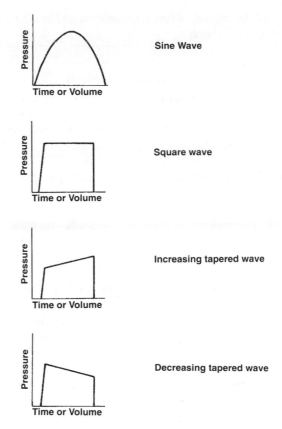

Fig. 14-14   Graphic tracings of typical inspiratory waveforms that are available on current mechanical ventilators.

below the baseline pressure or shows a low initial increase in inspiratory pressure.

In addition, most current generation ventilators offer more than one inspiratory flow pattern (Fig. 14-14). The sine wave is the most physiologically like a normal, spontaneous inspiration. The other wave forms can be compared with the sine wave to determine which one best meets the patient's needs. Ideally, the best flow pattern is one in which the patient's peak and mean airway pressures are lowest, exhalation is complete, breath sounds are improved bilaterally, heart rate and blood pressure are stable, and the patient feels most comfortable.

I:E ratio. The I:E ratio is adjusted to ensure that the patient can inhale in as physiologically appropriate a manner as possible and completely exhale the inspired tidal volume. Typically, the I:E ratio should be 1 to 2 or longer. Incomplete exhalation will cause air trapping and auto-PEEP (See Fig. 14-2).

▣ EXAM HINT

There are usually two questions related to modifying the inspiratory flow to meet the patient's need for a faster breath or modifying the I:E ratio. Remember that if the patient has auto-PEEP, the expiratory time must be increased to allow for a more complete exhalation.

Alarms. Alarm systems are different for each type of ventilator. Generally speaking, they are set with a safety margin of ±10% from the patient's normal ventilator settings. A variation of greater than 10% results in an audible or visual alarm condition. Most ventilators alarm if the I:E ratio is 1:1 or less.

Gas temperature. The goal for most patients is to minimize their humidity deficit by giving gas that is humidified and warmed to near body temperature. This can be accomplished by either a cascade- or wick-type humidifier or a heat-moisture exchanger (HME). It is common to see the gas warmed to 90° to 95° F (31° to 35° C). This decreases the patient's humidity deficit to a miniscule level and reduces the "rain out" of water vapor condensing in the ventilator circuit. A temperature probe should be placed in the inspiratory tubing as close to the patient as possible to monitor the inspired gas temperature.

4. Choose and adjust the tidal volume for mechanical ventilation

A spontaneously breathing 70-kg (154-lb) adult with normal lungs and metabolism needs a tidal volume at 7 to 9 mL/kg (3 to 4 mL/lb) of ideal body weight to adequately remove carbon dioxide. Splitting the differences, a spontaneous tidal volume of about 500 mL is considered normal. The Radford nomogram can be used for predicting normal spontaneous tidal volumes and rates based on body weights. It can be used to establish an initial tidal volume for most patients.

Most authors recommend a *set* ventilator tidal volume of *10 to 15 mL/kg* of ideal body weight. These are the values used by the NBRC in most patient situations. For example, the 70-kg (154-lb) adult with normal lungs needs a *set* mechanical ventilator tidal volume in the following range:

$$10 \text{ mL} \times 70 \text{ kg} = 700 \text{ mL}$$
$$15 \text{ mL} \times 70 \text{ kg} = 1050 \text{ mL}$$

This volume is higher than spontaneous for two reasons. First, some of the set volume is lost to the patient because of gas compression and tubing stretch/compliance (discussed previously). Second, some patients need larger-than-normal tidal volumes because their lungs are not functioning normally. Exceptions are patients with severe chronic restrictive lung disease, pneumonectomy patients, or patients with COPD. The tidal volume for these patients should be set at about 5 to 10 mL/kg of ideal body weight to avoid excessive ventilating pressure. In addition, giving a COPD patient a ventilator-delivered tidal volume in the normal range may result in blowing off too much carbon dioxide and causing a respiratory alkalosis.

It is common practice to get a set of ABG values after the patient is stable on the ventilator. The tidal volume can be adjusted within the range depending on whether the patient's arterial CO_2 pressure ($PaCO_2$) value is too high or low for the therapeutic goal. The most direct way to change alveolar ventilation is to modify the delivered tidal volume. If everything else remains the same, a larger tidal volume results in a lower $PaCO_2$ value. Conversely, while everything else remains the same, a smaller tidal volume results in a higher $PaCO_2$ value.

The following formula can be used to help predict what *tidal volume* produces a *desired PaCO₂* value:

$$[Vt - (VD_{anat} + VD_{mech})] \times f \times PaCO_2 = [Vt' - (VD_{anat} + VD_{mech})] \times f \times PaCO_2'$$

in which:

Vt = current tidal volume

Vd_{anat} = anatomic dead space. This is calculated at 1 mL/lb or 2.2 mL/kg of ideal body weight.

Vd_{mech} = added mechanical dead space

f = respiratory (ventilator) rate

$PaCO_2$ = actual patient $PaCO_2$ value

Vt' = *desired tidal volume*

$PaCO_2'$ = desired patient $PaCO_2$ value

Note that other, simpler formulas are available for calculating a change in minute volume or tidal volume. This one is presented because it takes into account more factors and can be used to calculate a change in tidal volume, rate, or mechanical dead space.

Example. The patient is a 70-kg (154-lb) man who is being ventilated on the control mode (he is apneic). His ventilator settings are a tidal volume of 1000 mL, rate of 12 times/min, fractional inspired oxygen concentration (F_IO_2) of 0.3, and no added mechanical dead space. His ABG values are an arterial oxygen pressure (PaO_2) of 90 torr, $PaCO_2$ of 30 torr, pH of 7.48, SaO_2 of 95%, and a base excess (BE) of 0. The clinical goal is to adjust the patient's tidal volume as needed to produce a $PaCO_2$ value of 40 torr. In summary:

Vt = 1000 mL current tidal volume

Vd_{anat} = 154 mL of anatomic dead space. This is calculated at 1 mL/lb or 2.2 mL/kg of ideal body weight.

Vd_{mech} = no added mechanical dead space

f = 12 times/min for the ventilator rate

$PaCO_2$ = 30 torr actual patient $PaCO_2$ value

Vt' = *desired tidal volume*

$PaCO_2'$ = 40 torr desired patient $PaCO_2$ value

Placing the data and goal into the formula results in the following:

$$[Vt - (VD_{anat} + VD_{mech})] \times f \times PaCO_2 = [Vt' - (VD_{anat} + VD_{mech})] \times f \times PaCO_2'$$
$$[1000 - (154 + 0)] \times 12 \times 30 = [Vt' - (154 + 0)] \times 12 \times 40$$

Simplifying produces the following:

$$[846] \times 12 \times 30 = [Vt' - 154] \times 480$$
$$304,560 = 480\ Vt' - 73,920$$
$$378,480 = 480\ Vt'$$
$$788\ mL = Vt'$$

The solution is to reduce the patient's tidal volume from 1000 to 788 mL.

 EXAM HINT

Every available NBRC examination has had several problems that require the test taker to determine an original ventilator tidal volume or a new tidal volume to correct for overventilating (low carbon dioxide level) or underventilating (high carbon dioxide level) a patient. Typically, start with a tidal volume of 10 mL/kg of body weight. Increase or decrease the tidal volume as needed from this starting point.

---

5. Choose and adjust the rate for mechanical ventilation

See Table 1-2 for a listing of the normal resting respiratory frequencies based on age. If the patient is apneic and has a normal temperature and an appropriately set tidal volume, the respiratory rates in the indicated ranges will produce a normal $PaCO_2$ level. This must be confirmed by ABG measurements. If the tidal volume cannot be changed, adjusting the respiratory rate will modify alveolar ventilation. A higher respiratory rate, while everything else remains the same, will result in a lower $PaCO_2$ level. Conversely, a lower respiratory rate, while everything else remains the same, will result in a higher $PaCO_2$ level.

As mentioned above, chronically hypercapneic patients must be ventilated with some caution. To give this type of patient a higher ventilator-delivered rate and larger tidal volume may result in blowing off too much carbon dioxide and cause a respiratory alkalosis. Adult patients with severe chronic restrictive lung disease or those who have had a pneumonectomy may need respiratory rates of 20 to 30 per minute or greater to meet their minute volume needs. This is because their delivered tidal volume must be smaller than normal because of their condition.

The same formula that was used to predict a tidal volume change can be used to help predict what *respiratory rate* will produce a desired $PaCO_2$ value:

$$[Vt - (VD_{anat} + VD_{mech})] \times f \times PaCO_2 =$$
$$[Vt - (VD_{anat} + VD_{mech})] \times f' \times PaCO_2'$$

Example. The patient is the same 70-kg (154-lb) man who is being ventilated on the control mode (he is apneic). His ventilator settings are a tidal volume of 1000 mL, rate of 12 times/min, fractional inspired oxygen concentration (F_IO_2) of 0.3, and no added mechanical dead space. His ABG values are an arterial oxygen pressure (PaO_2) of 90 torr, $PaCO_2$ of 30 torr, pH of 7.48, SaO_2 of 95%, and a base excess (BE) of 0. The clinical goal is to adjust the patient's rate as needed to produce a $PaCO_2$ value of 40 torr. In summary:

Vt = 1000 mL current tidal volume

Vd_{anat} = 154 mL of anatomic dead space. This is calculated at 1 mL/lb or 2.2 mL/kg of ideal body weight.

Vd_{mech} = no added mechanical dead space

f = 12 times/min for the ventilator rate

f' = *desired ventilator rate*

$PaCO_2$ = 30 torr actual patient $PaCO_2$ value

$PaCO_2'$ = 40 torr desired patient $PaCO_2$ value

Placing the data and goal into the formula results in the following:

$$[Vt - (VD_{anat} + VD_{mech})] \times f \times PaCO_2 =$$
$$[Vt - (VD_{anat} + VD_{mech})] \times f' \times PaCO_2'$$
$$[1000 - (154 + 0)] \times 12 \times 30 = [1000 - (154 + 0)] \times f' \times 40$$
$$[846] \times 12 \times 30 = [846] \times f' \times 40$$
$$304,560 = 33,840\ f'$$
$$9 = f'$$

The solution is to reduce the patient's respiratory rate from 12 to 9 breaths/min.

 EXAM HINT

Every available NBRC examination has had several problems that require the test taker to determine an original ventilator respiratory rate or a new respiratory rate to correct for overventilating (low carbon dioxide level) or underventilating (high carbon dioxide level) a patient. Typically start with a respiratory rate of 10 to 14 in an adult. Increase of decrease the rate needed from this starting point.

---

6. Choose and adjust the minute ventilation for mechanical ventilation

The subjects of minute ventilation and alveolar minute ventilation were covered in Chapter 4. Review the calculations as needed. Blood gases must always be evaluated for the $PaCO_2$ level to tell whether the patient's minute ventilation is adequate. A high carbon dioxide level indicates a need to increase the tidal volume, respiratory rate, or both. A low carbon dioxide level indicates a need to decrease the tidal volume, respiratory rate, or both. In both cases, the key to modifying the carbon dioxide level is to modify the alveolar ventilation. That is best accomplished by changing the tidal volume rather than the rate. The following formula can be used to calculate a change in the minute volume:

$$\dot{V}_E' = \frac{PaCO_2 \times \dot{V}_E}{PaCO_2'}$$

in which:

$\dot{V}_E'$ = *desired* minute volume

$\dot{V}_E$ = current minute volume

$PaCO_2$ = current carbon dioxide level

$PaCO_2'$ = *desired* carbon dioxide level

Example. The patient is the same 70-kg (154-lb) man who is being ventilated on the control mode (he is apneic). His ventilator settings are a tidal volume of 1000 mL, rate of 12 times/min, F_IO_2 of 0.3, and no added mechanical dead space. His ABG values are a PaO_2 of 90 torr, $PaCO_2$ of 30 torr, pH of 7.48, SaO_2 of 95%, and a BE of 0. The clinical goal is to adjust the patient's minute volume as needed to produce a $PaCO_2$ value of 40 torr. Placing the data and goal into the formula results in the following:

$$\dot{V}_E' = \frac{PaCO_2 \times V_E}{PaCO_2}$$
$$\dot{V}_E' = \frac{30 \times 12,000}{40}$$
$$\dot{V}_E' = \frac{360,000}{40}$$
$$\dot{V}_E' = 9,000 \text{ mL}$$

The goal can be accomplished by reducing the minute volume from 12,000 to 9,000 mL. As mentioned earlier, this is best done by reducing the tidal volume. Remember that the tidal volume must be kept at no less than 10 mL/kg of ideal body weight to avoid the development of atelectasis. The respiratory rate may be decreased, if necessary, to provide this reduced minute volume.

7. Begin and modify external negative-pressure ventilation

These ventilators have proven useful in patients with the following characteristics: (1) normal, intact upper airway, (2) ability to swallow, (3) normal airway resistance, (4) normal lung-thoracic compliance, and (5) ability to ventilate until respiratory muscle fatigue becomes too great.

Patients with the following disease conditions have been successfully ventilated by a negative-pressure ventilator: (1) neuromuscular defects such as poliomyelitis, postpolio syndrome, muscular dystrophy, and high spinal cord injury; (2) kyphoscoliosis with resulting restrictive lung disease; and (3) COPD during an acute worsening.

Negative-pressure ventilators work by creating a negative pressure either around the patient's whole body or over the anterior chest and abdomen. The negative pressure expands the thorax and a tidal volume is inhaled. If the patient needs supplemental oxygen, it must be given by nasal cannula or face mask. There are three basic types of external negative-pressure ventilators: Drinker body respirator, body wrap, and chest curaisse.

Drinker body respirator. With the Drinker body respirator (or "iron lung") and a smaller version (the Portalung), the patient must lie supine with the body inside the closed cylinder (Fig. 14-15). Only the head is exposed. The iron lung is the most powerful of the three types of negative-pressure ventilators and should be chosen to ventilate the more difficult hospitalized patients. The following steps are used to initiate ventilation:

1. Select a ventilator rate of about 5 to 10 breaths less than the patient's own. The rate can be varied between 14 and 24 per minute.
2. Gradually increase the negative pressure until the patient cannot speak during the inspiratory phase. A pressure of −7 to −15 cm water is enough for most patients. A maximum pressure of −35 cm water can be achieved. It is possible to create a positive pressure during exhalation, if needed, by closing a valve. This is usually limited to times when an assisted cough is called for.
3. Use a hand-held spirometer to measure the patient's tidal volume.
4. After a few minutes ask the patient, "Does the breath feel deep enough, too deep, or not enough? Do you have tingling fingers or feel dizzy (signs of hyperventilation)?"
5. Adjust the negativity and/or rate to meet the patient's needs.

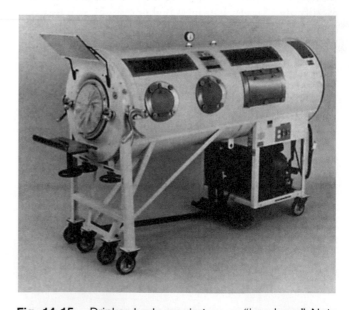

Fig. 14-15 Drinker body respiratory or "iron lung." Note the following features: Patient's head port is at left end and has foam rubber seal. Cylinder has two arm ports with seals, bed pan port, and two glass windows for viewing patient. Controls and motor for bellows are below cylinder at right end. Bellows covers right end of cylinder. Pressure gauge is located at top of cylinder. (From LifeCare, Boulder, CO.)

6. Draw an ABG sample after about 15 minutes. Speed is important because the unit must be opened to collect the sample.

In general, steps 2 through 6 should be used with the body wrap and chest curaisse units as well.

Body wrap. Body wrap devices are also called "pneumowraps," "raincoats," and "ponchos." All feature a wind-proof, water-permeable nylon parka. The patient slips into it and lies supine with only the head, hands, and feet exposed. Straps are used to tighten the parka at these sites to prevent air leaks. Ridged plastic anterior and posterior chest pieces are built into the parka (Fig. 14-16). Negative pressure draws the parka close to the skin and pulls the chest out for a breath to be inhaled. This is not as efficient as the iron lung and becomes even less so if the posterior chest piece is removed for better patient comfort. Despite the smaller tidal volume generated during passive breathing, these units are popular. Patients find that their portability and ease of entry and exit make them preferable to the iron lung for overnight or intermittent ventilatory assistance. It is recommended that the proper rate and negative-pressure settings be determined in the hospital and confirmed by an ABG analysis before the patient is sent home with the unit.

Chest curaisse. The chest curaisse is also known as the "chest shell" and "tortoise shell." It makes use of a vacuum pump similar to the body wrap device to control the negative pressure. The partial vacuum is applied to the patient by way of a hard plastic shell. It is fitted to cover the chest or preferably the chest and abdomen (Fig. 14-17). There should be a 2- to 3-inch gap between the shell and the patient's chest for maximum movement during inspiration.

The chest curaisse is the least efficient of all the negative-pressure ventilators because less of the patient's chest has vacuum applied to it. The patient shell can also cause skin abrasions if it is not carefully fitted to the patient's body contours. Again, it is recommended that the proper rate and negative-pressure settings be determined in the hospital and confirmed by an ABG analysis before the patient is sent home with the unit.

8. Begin and modify positive end–expiratory pressure therapy (Code: IIIB4a) [Difficulty: An]

PEEP is used as a means to increase a patient's FRC and thereby increase the PaO_2 level. PEEP is generally indicated in any bilateral, generalized pulmonary condition in which the FRC is decreased. Examples include generalized atelectasis, pulmonary edema, ARDS, and infant respiratory distress syndrome (RDS). All of these patients show a decreased lung compliance as measured by their static compliance (C_{st}). Specific indications for PEEP include:

a. Intrapulmonary shunt greater than 15%
b. Refractory hypoxemia ($PaO_2 < 60$ mm Hg despite an F_IO_2 of up to 0.8 to 1.0)
c. The patient has had an F_IO_2 of greater than 0.5 for 48 to 72 hours and shows no indication of a rapidly improving PaO_2. PEEP is added so that the F_IO_2 can be lowered to a safer level.

Before PEEP is begun, the patient should be carefully monitored to establish the baseline condition. The same parameters should be monitored after each change in the PEEP level to determine how the patient is tolerating it. The best or optimal level of PEEP is the level that results in the best delivery of oxygen to the tissues (not necessarily the arterial blood). Often, a secondary goal is to reduce the inspired oxygen to a safe level. The patient is at risk of oxygen toxicity if more than 50% oxygen is inhaled for more than 48 to 72 hours. See Box 14-3 for recommendations on what to monitor during the application of PEEP and how to evaluate the data.

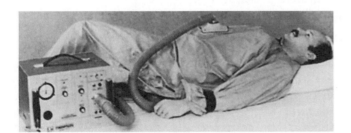

Fig. 14-16 Patient in body wrap external negative pressure ventilator (Pulmowrap). Note control box on left that contains vacuum motor. Hose connects vacuum motor to patient inside body wrap device. (From Hill NS: *Chest* 90:897, 1986.)

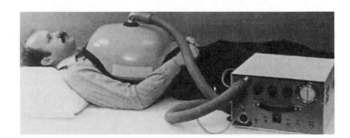

Fig. 14-17 Patient in chest curaisse (LifeCare). Note control box on right that contains vacuum motor. Hose connects vacuum motor to patient inside chest shell. (From Hill NS: *Chest* 90:897, 1986.)

The application of PEEP has risks. Clinically, these risks must be weighed against the potential benefit to the patient. In the profoundly hypoxic patient, PEEP can be lifesaving. Some clinicians use low levels of PEEP (up to 5 cm water) in patients with normal lungs or overly complaint lungs (emphysema) to maintain the baseline level of FRC. Hazards of PEEP include:

a. Pulmonary barotrauma: pneumothorax, tension pneumothorax, mediastinal emphysema, pulmonary interstitial emphysema (PIE) in the neonate, subcutaneous emphysema

b. Decreased venous return to the heart, causing a decreased cardiac output and tachycardia, decreased blood pressure, decreased tissue perfusion as measured by a decreased mixed venous oxygen ($P\bar{v}O_2$) level, decreased urine output

PEEP therapy is usually begun at initial levels of 2 to 5 cm water. After the patient's response is determined, 2 to 5 cm more PEEP may be applied. The patient is reevaluated. This process goes on until the best or optimal level of PEEP is determined. See Fig. 14-18 for a number of physiologic parameters that can be measured and evaluated.

There are different approaches to the application of PEEP to find the best level. One approach could be called minimum PEEP. It involves the application of PEEP to the minimum level that allows the inspired oxygen percentage to be lowered to a safer level. A clinical goal is to minimize the risk of oxygen toxicity. In this approach, PEEP is raised until the PaO_2 is greater than 60 torr or the SpO_2 is greater than 90% on 60% oxygen or less. Usually no more than 10 to 15 cm water of PEEP is needed.

Another approach could be called maximum or optimal PEEP. This approach has the clinical goal of reducing the patient's shunt fraction to less than 15%. Often this requires more pressure than the minimum PEEP approach. Because this higher pressure level is more likely to cause hemodynamic problems, the patient should have a pulmonary artery catheter inserted. With it, the patient's cardiac output, mixed venous oxygen level, pulmonary capillary wedge pressure, and pulmonary vascular resistance can be measured. In addition, the patient may need increased intravenous fluids, dopamine (Intropin), and digitalis (Digoxin) for cardiovascular support. The higher PEEP levels increase the risk of pulmonary barotrauma. Therefore the patient must be watched closely for signs of a pneumothorax.

As the patient begins to recover, the PEEP level may be reduced in steps of 2 to 5 cm water. Again, the patient is evaluated after every change in the PEEP level. If the patient's cardiovascular status is normal, the following are recommendations for how to decrease PEEP and oxygen levels:

a. Decrease PEEP first if the PaO_2 level is greater than 60 torr and the F_IO_2 is less than 0.5.

b. Decrease oxygen first if the PaO_2 level is greater than 60 torr and the is F_IO_2 greater than 0.5.

If the patient is showing an adverse reaction to the PEEP level such as decreased cardiac output or barotrauma, the PEEP level should be decreased before the oxygen percentage. Clinical judgment must be used to decide whether a high oxygen percentage or a high PEEP level is a greater danger to the patient. Minimize or remove the element that puts the patient at greater risk.

☞ EXAM HINT

Typically, there are three questions that deal with the clinical application and modification of PEEP. Know to increase PEEP if the patient is hypoxic, is receiving a high oxygen percentage, and is hemodynamically stable. Know to decrease PEEP if the patient is well oxygenated and receiving a moderate oxygen percentage, is not hemodynamically stable, or has a PEEP-related complication. A drop in the patient's cardiac output is a key indicator of excessive PEEP causing hemodynamic problems.

9. Begin and modify continuous positive airway pressure (Code: IIIB4a) [Difficulty: An]

CPAP has the same indications, hazards, and patient evaluation processes discussed earlier in PEEP therapy. One possible physiologic benefit of CPAP over PEEP is that there is less reduction in the venous return to the heart. This is because with CPAP the patient is breathing spontaneously. Therefore patients treated by CPAP may be able to tolerate higher pressure levels than those patients being ventilated with PEEP therapy.

CPAP is usually increased and decreased in steps of 2 to 5 cm water. As with PEEP, the patient is evaluated before CPAP is begun and again after every pressure change. See Box 14-3 for recommendations on what to monitor during the application of CPAP and how to evaluate the data.

Before a patient receives CPAP therapy, the practitioner and physician must be assured that the patient has the ability to breathe adequately to eliminate carbon dioxide. CPAP is contraindicated in an apneic patient or one who may become apneic. (This patient must be fully supported on the ventilator.) The patient must have an adequate respiratory rate, tidal volume, and minute volume. The heart rate and blood pressure should be stable. Maximum inspiratory pressure and vital capacity values may be acceptable or low. Blood gas analysis typically shows refractory hypoxemia but a normal or low $PaCO_2$ level. This shows that the patient would benefit from an elevated baseline pressure to increase the FRC but is quite capable of ventilating.

The patient must be carefully monitored for fatigue because the patient is providing all of the minute ventilation. Signs of fatigue include increasing respiratory

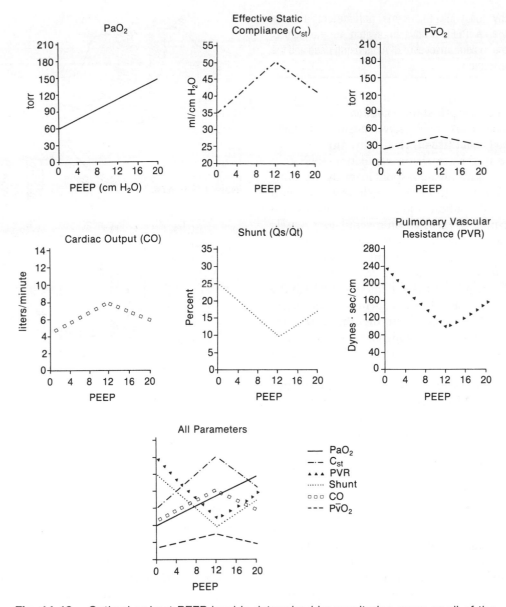

Fig. 14-18   Optimal or best PEEP level is determined by monitoring some or all of the following parameters: PaO$_2$, effective static compliance (C$_{st}$), pressure of mixed venous oxygen (P$\bar{v}$O$_2$), cardiac output (CO), shunt (Q̇s/Q̇t), and pulmonary vascular resistance (PVR). Ideally, as functional residual capacity (FRC) is increased by PEEP, lung compliance is improved and ventilation and perfusion are better matched. Cardiac output should remain stable. It can be measured by use of pulmonary artery (Swan-Ganz) catheter or indirectly followed by monitoring patient's heart rate and blood pressure. As can be seen, the optimal PEEP is found at 12 cm water pressure. Excessive PEEP is seen by the resulting drop in static compliance and cardiac output.

rate, decreasing tidal volume or vital capacity, decreasing maximum inspiratory pressure, and tachycardia. Blood gas measurement may show a stable or decreasing PaO$_2$ value. A rising PaCO$_2$ level is a definite sign of fatigue. The patient may complain of dyspnea. The practitioner may notice the patient is working harder than normal to breathe, as shown by the increased use of the accessory muscles of ventilation and heavy perspiration. When these signs occur, CPAP therapy should be discontinued and mechanical ventilation instituted in a mode that best fits the patient's needs.

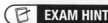 **EXAM HINT**

Know that CPAP can be used and increased if the patient's carbon dioxide level is normal and hypoxemia is present. Increase or decrease CPAP by following the same parameters used to evaluate a change in PEEP. Know to switch to mechanical ventilation when the maximum level of CPAP is being used and the patient is still hypoxemic.

10. Noninvasive positive pressure ventilation

a. Begin nasal/mask noninvasive positive pressure ventilation (Code: IIIB4a) [Difficulty: An]

Noninvasive positive pressure ventilation (NPPV) is indicated in stable, unintubated, spontaneously breathing patients who present with any of the following clinical situations: elevated carbon dioxide level, hypoxemia despite supplemental oxygen, chronic ventilatory muscle dysfunction, or sleep apnea from upper airway obstruction. Most of the time, these patients are ventilated with the aid of a nasal mask similar to that used to deliver mask CPAP. A full face mask is needed if the patient leaks through the mouth with a nasal mask. If the patient is critically ill, unstable, must be intubated to secure the airway for secretion removal, and/or needs a high level of therapeutic PEEP to maintain the FRC, he or she should be placed on a standard volume-cycled ventilator.

Often, patients receiving NPPV are ventilated with two different levels of positive pressure. This is referred to as *bilevel ventilation*. The baseline pressure is greater than zero (CPAP or PEEP) and the peak pressure is set to deliver a desired tidal volume (similar to pressure support ventilation). Both levels can be independently adjusted. If only the baseline pressure is elevated, the patient is receiving CPAP. If only the peak pressure is elevated, the patient is receiving pressure support ventilation. Respironics has developed two devices for bilevel ventilation that can be used in the hospital or home for noninvasive mask ventilation. They are the BiPAP S-D and newer BiPAP S/T-D Ventilatory Support System. Supplemental oxygen is not available through the machines; however, it can be added though a side port on the nasal mask to meet clinical goals.

The patient must have a properly fitting nasal or face mask to receive noninvasive ventilation. These ventilation masks are similar to CPAP masks and are referred to as such. CPAP masks come in different sizes for children older than 3 years of age and adults. Nasal masks are designed to cover only the nose. They allow the patient to eat, drink, speak, and use the mouth as a second airway for breathing in case there is a malfunction of the CPAP system. The mouth also acts as a pressure relief route if the CPAP pressure should become too great. Pressures of up to 10 to 15 cm water can usually be maintained (Fig. 14-19). Usually the mask is made of a transparent plastic. Face masks are designed to cover the nose and mouth. They are similar in design to the masks used during bag-mask ventilation and also made of a transparent plastic. The face mask must be used if the patient has persistent mouth

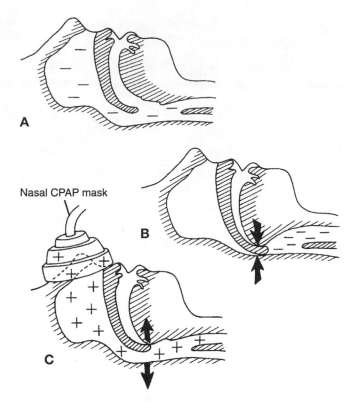

Fig. 14-19 Effect of nasal continuous positive airway pressure (CPAP) mask. **A,** Normal upper airway remains patent during sleep. **B,** Abnormal upper airway of patient with obstructive apnea collapses on inspiration during sleep. **C,** Pressure from nasal CPAP mask keeps abnormal upper airway patent during sleep. (Modified from Scanlan CL. In Scanlan CL, Spearman CB, Sheldon RL, editors: *Egan's fundamentals of respiratory care,* ed 5, St Louis, 1990, Mosby.)

breathing and cannot use a nose mask. With a good seal, pressures of greater than 15 cm water can be maintained.

Both types of CPAP mask have a soft, very compliant seal to closely fit the contours of the face. Straps are needed to hold the mask in place. (Fig. 14-20.) Too large a mask will not seal and will allow gas to leak and pressure to drop. The patient may show increased snoring or airway obstruction with periods of apnea. A mask that is too small or misfitting can cause an uneven distribution of pressure on the face. This can lead to abrasions or pressure sores and ulcers on the face.

The BiPAP S/T-D system can be used for bilevel ventilation or in the CPAP mode. It makes use of a relatively simple smooth interior circuit and does not have a humidifier, alarm system, or the other attachments seen in a volume-cycled ventilator. A bacteria filter should be inserted between the BiPAP unit and the patient circuit. If a humidifier is desired, it must be a cascade- or wick-type of humidifier. An HME cannot be used because it creates too much resistance.

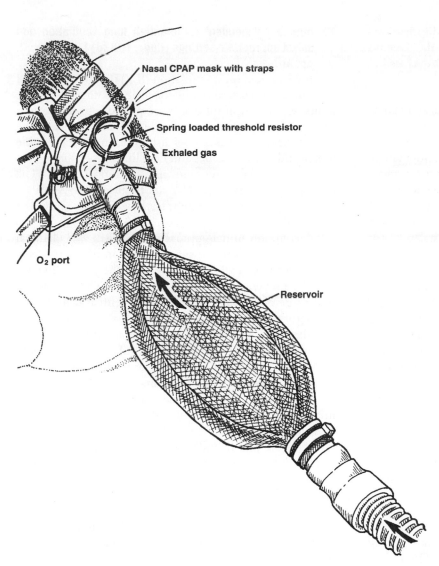

Nasal CPAP mask with straps

Spring loaded threshold resistor

Exhaled gas

O₂ port

Reservoir

Fig. 14-20 Nasal CPAP mask in place on adult patient. Note straps to hold mask in place to create a seal around the patient's nose. If patient needs supplemental oxygen, small bore tubing can be connected to the oxygen port.

b. Modify nasal/mask noninvasive ventilation (Code: IIIB4a) [Difficulty: An]

The bilevel settings must be determined at the bedside by asking for the patient's subjective opinion, listening to breath sounds, checking vital signs, and evaluating ABG values. If supplemental oxygen is needed it can be added at a port on the patient's mask, at the humidifier, or at the outlet from the BiPAP unit. Up to 15 L/min can be added without affecting the performance of the BiPAP system. It is not possible to know the delivered oxygen percentage until after the bilevel ventilation settings are determined. The oxygen flow should be then be gradually increased while the patient's SpO_2 value rises to the desired saturation level.

Only the function of the BiPAP S/T-D system is reviewed because it is newer and has more features. The operator can choose among the following five modes of operation:

1. Expiratory positive airway pressure (EPAP) from 2 to 20 cm water. This is functionally similar to CPAP.

2. Inspiratory positive airway pressure (IPAP) from 2 to 25 cm water. This is functionally similar to setting the peak pressure on a pressure-cycled ventilator. The patient must trigger each IPAP assisted breath.

3. Spontaneous (S) functions like the pressure support mode in which the patient must initiate each assisted breath. The therapist can set IPAP and EPAP levels. This delivers bilevel ventilation.

4. Spontaneous/timed (S/T) delivers between 6 and 30 ventilator breaths per minute when the patient's respiratory rate drops below the set number. Otherwise, it functions like the spontaneous mode and delivers bilevel ventilation.

5. Times (T) varies the percent of each cycle in IPAP from 10% to 90%. This allows the therapist to set an I:E ratio. All of the first four functions are maintained, except that the patient cannot trigger an IPAP breath.

With the BiPAP units, the difference between IPAP and EPAP is called pressure boost and delivers the tidal volume. It is important to remember that the delivered tidal volume varies depending on changes in the patient's airway resistance and lung-thoracic compliance as well as the machine settings.

11. Initiate high frequency ventilation and select appropriate settings (Code: IIIB2b) [Difficulty: R, Ap, An]

High frequency ventilation (HFV) is needed whenever the patient's condition calls for a higher respiratory rate or smaller tidal volume than usually delivered on a conventional volume-cycled ventilator. A high frequency ventilator can deliver a respiratory rate far higher than the limit of 150/min set by the Food and Drug Administration (FDA) on all conventional adult and neonatal/pediatric ventilators.

The FDA has approved HFV for use on adults during bronchoscopy and laryngoscopy procedures and when a patient with a bronchopleural fistula cannot be managed on a conventional ventilator. Although patients with ARDS have not been officially approved for HFV, the procedure has been employed when a patient is hypoxic despite maximum settings on a conventional ventilator. (Box 15-8 lists clinical uses for HFV with infants and children.)

Currently there are three different ways to deliver HFV. The first involves the use of a conventional ventilator set at a rate of up to the FDA maximum of 150/minute. This method is called high frequency positive pressure ventilation (HFPPV). With it, the set tidal volume is decreased to something less than standard (less than 10 mL/kg). The second involves the use of a high frequency jet ventilation (HFJV) and a special endotracheal tube with a standard lumen and an additional small diameter air entrainment lumen. (See Fig. 14-23.) The HFJV unit is connected to the air entrainment lumen. Gas from the HFJV unit entrains other gas through the main lumen to create the patient's tidal volume. HFJV units can deliver a small tidal volume several hundred times per minute. The third method involves a high frequency oscillation (HFO) ventilator. HFO makes use of a conventional endotracheal tube (as does HFPPV). However, the delivered tidal volume is the smallest and the respiratory rate can be the fastest of all three methods. Table 15-2 has a comparison of all three methods. The equipment used for HFJV and HFO are described later in this chapter. Table 14-1 lists considerations for the initial settings and adjustment of HFV delivered to infants and adults by either a jet ventilator or oscillator ventilator.

Current clinical experience is recommended with any HFV method. Although adults patients have been successfully treated with HFV, there is far greater use of these techniques with infants and children. Therefore Chapter 15 has further discussion.

12. Initiate independent (differential) lung ventilation and select appropriate settings (Code: IIIB2d) [Difficulty: R, Ap, An]

Independent lung ventilation (ILV) involves the use of a separate mechanical ventilator for each lung. A double lumen endotracheal tube must be placed into the patient to allow this procedure. (See Figs. 11-23 and 11-24 and the related discussion.) Box 14-4 lists indications for double lumen endotracheal tubes and ILV. In all cases, the patient has one normal lung and one abnormal lung. The overriding concerns with ILV are to adequately ventilate the patient through the normal lung and to allow the injured lung to heal.

A common initial approach is to select two identical ventilators that allow for synchronization of the patient's respiratory rate. The Servo 900C and the Drager Evita 1 and Evita 4 ventilators are suited for this. They allow one unit to be designated the "primary" ventilator to set the respiratory rate for it and the "secondary" unit. Each unit can then also have the same mode and I:E ratio. This synchronized independent lung ventilation method still allows for the independent setting of tidal volume, oxygen percentage, and PEEP for each lung.

For example, an 80 kg adult male normally receives an initial tidal volume of about 800 mL (10 mL × 80 kg). If both lungs functioned normally, each would receive 400 mL. However, with unilateral lung disease, the bad lung receives little tidal volume and the normal lung receives too much and becomes overdistended. It is therefore important to set the initial tidal volume to the good lung at *half* the normal volume for both lungs. Using this patient example, the normal lung's initial tidal volume should be set at 400 mL (5 mL × 80 kg). To avoid changing too many parameters at once, the same oxygen percentage and PEEP level are kept as originally set. The abnormal lung is ventilated based on its pathologic condition or may be left unventilated.

After 15 minutes, check the patient's ABG values. Depending on the results, adjust the ventilator settings for the good lung as would typically be done to remove carbon dioxide and maintain oxygenation. The ventilator settings for the diseased lung must be carefully adjusted to allow healing and prevent complications such as atelectasis and pneumonia.

When the patient has a bronchopulmonary fistula, the air leak through the bad lung can be so great that a high frequency ventilator must be used rather than a conventional ventilator.

In this situation there can be no synchronization of rate or any other parameters. The good lung conventionally is ventilated to maintain the patient's blood gas values. The high frequency ventilator is set to provide some support with a small tidal volume and low ventilating

TABLE 14-1   High-Frequency Ventilation Operational Considerations

	Infant jets	Adult jets	Infant oscillators	Adult oscillators
Initial recommended frequency	7 Hz (IMV background rate of 2)	5 Hz	15 Hz	3-5 Hz
Initial tidal volume parameters	Jet drive pressure to produce 90% of CMV peak pressure; I time 0.02 sec	Jet drive pressure of 25-35 psi; I:E = 1:2-1:1	Amplitude to create chest vibration visually; I:E = 1:1	Amplitude to create chest vibration visually; I:E = 1:2-1:1
To change effective V_A	Alter drive pressure*; alter inspiratory time†; alter frequency‡	Alter drive pressure*; alter inspiratory time†; alter frequency‡	Alter pressure amplitudes*; alter inspiratory time†; alter frequency‡	Alter pressure amplitudes*; alter inspiratory time†; alter frequency‡
To change mean P_{AW} (for $\dot{V}/\dot{Q}$ effects on PaO_2)	Alter applied PEEP; alter inspiratory time†	Alter applied PEEP (if available); alter inspiratory time†	Alter bias flow pressures; alter inspiratory time†	Alter bias flow pressures; alter inspiratory time†

CMV, Continuous mandatory ventilation; *I*, inspiratory; *I:E*, inspiratory/expiratory; *IMV*, intermittent mandatory ventilation; *PaO$_2$*, arterial oxygen pressure; *P$_{AW}$*, airway pressure; *PEEP*, positive end-expiratory pressure; *V$_A$*, alveolar ventilation; *$\dot{V}/\dot{Q}$*, ventilation-perfusion.

*↑ Pressure = ↑ tidal volume = ↑V_A.

†↑ Inspiratory time = ↑ tidal volume = ↑V_A *unless* air trapping develops, in which case tidal volume may ↓.

‡Frequency response may be variable—↑ frequency may increase total ventilation *but* ↑ frequency can ↓ tidal volume through shorter inspiratory time and pulse attenuation through narrow endotracheal tubes.

(From MacIntyre NR: High-frequency ventilation. In MacIntyre NR, Branson RD: *Mechanical Ventilation*, Philadelphia, 2001, WB Saunders.)

BOX 14-4	Indication for Double-Lumen Endotracheal Tubes and Independent Lung Ventilation

Thoracic surgery
  Pneumonectomy
  Some lobectomies
  Thoracic aortic surgery
  Thoracoscopy
  Some esophageal surgery
Selective airway protection
  Secretions (tuberculosis, bronchiectasis, or abscess)
  Whole-lung lavage
  Massive hemoptysis
Bronchopleural fistula
Unilateral lung disease
  Unilateral parenchymal injury
    Aspiration
    Pulmonary contusion
    Pneumonia
    Massive pulmonary embolism
    Reperfusion edema
    Asymmetrical ARDS
    Asymmetrical pulmonary edema
  Atelectasis
Unilateral airflow obstruction
  Single-lung transplant for chronic airflow obstruction
  Unilateral bronchospasm
Severe bilateral lung disease
  ARDS
  Aspiration
  Pneumonia

From Tuxen D: Independent Lung Ventilation. In Tobin MJ, editor: *Principles and Practice of Mechanical Ventilation*, New York, 1994, McGraw-Hill, pp 571-588.

pressures. The clinical goal is to prevent excessive lung pressure so that the lung tear heals.

The patient can be converted back to breathing through one conventional ventilator when normal functioning returns to the injured lung. This can be done when the peak pressure, plateau pressure, and mean airway pressure for both lungs are about the same. When these values match, or are close, they indicate similar lung compliance and airway resistance values. The first step in converting from ILV to conventional ventilation involves combining the proximal ends of the double lumen endotracheal tube with a Y adapter. By doing this, one ventilator can deliver tidal volume breaths to each lung. It is suggested that the PC mode be used so that excessive pressure is not applied to the healing lung. Set the peak pressure at or just below the previous peak pressure used with the healing lung. Set the PEEP level at the previous pressure used with the healing lung. Check the patient's ABG values after 15 minutes. Be prepared to adjust the conventional ventilator as needed to get the desired blood gas values. Watch for problems with the healing

lung and be prepared to go back to independent lung ventilation if necessary. When it appears certain that the patient is tolerating conventional ventilation, the double lumen endotracheal tube should be removed and replaced with an appropriate single lumen tube. This allows for better suctioning and results in less airway resistance through the tube. Wean and extubate the patient when appropriate.

MODULE C	Mechanical ventilation equipment

Note: The literature produced by the manufacturers and the descriptions used in many standard texts break down the various ventilators into more categories than used by the NBRC. To avoid confusion, this text uses the NBRC's more simplified terminology. A *pneumatically powered ventilator* is defined here as a ventilator powered by compressed gas and without any electrically powered control systems (electrically powered alarm systems may or may not be added). An *electrically powered ventilator* is defined here as a ventilator that is either electrically powered or controlled. Most volume-cycled ventilators fall into this category. *Microprocessor ventilators* are electrically powered, but controlled by one or more microprocessors (computers). Many of the most current volume-cycled ventilators have microprocessors to control their functions. *Fluidic ventilators* typically make use of electrical circuits with flip-flops to respond to changes in gas flow and pressure through the system. Fluidic ventilators are powered by compressed gas. *Noninvasive positive pressure ventilators* are designed for home use or short-term hospital use and are electrically powered and controlled. They have fewer controls and alarms than hospital-based critical care ventilators. A nasal or full face mask, rather than an endotracheal tube, is used to attach the ventilator to the patient.

1. Pneumatically powered ventilators
a. Get the necessary equipment for the procedure (Code: IIA1e1) [Difficulty: An]

The only commonly used pneumatically powered ventilators are the Bird series and the Bennett PR 2. A control or backup rate can be set on these units in case the patient is apneic. All other controls and functions are the same as discussed in Chapter 13. The following equipment and procedures are necessary:

1. Bennett PR 2 or Bird ventilator with an air/oxygen blender and hoses
2. Bennett or Bird breathing circuit
3. Bacteria filters
4. Proper humidification system: either a passover- or cascade-type humidifier or an HME, (discussed later). Put sterile, distilled water in the passover- or cascade-type humidifier.

5. One or two water traps for condensation from the circuit

6. Add an alarm system(s) such as a low-volume bellows spirometer or a low-pressure/disconnection alarm

7. If a low-volume bellows spirometer alarm is used, a length of large-bore tubing is needed to connect the exhalation valve to the bellows

b. Put the equipment together, make sure that it works properly, and identify any problems (Code: IIB1e1) [Difficulty: An]

Refer to Figs. 13-10 and 13-11 in Chapter 13 for the IPPB circuits. The ventilator and circuits are similar to those used in IPPB therapy with the following exceptions:

1. Set the ordered oxygen percentage on the blender; set the Bird *air-mix* and Bennett *air dilution* selection controls to pure source gas from the blender. Analyze the F_IO_2 through a port in the inspiratory limb of the circuit.

2. If a passover or cascade humidifier is used, a short length of large-bore tubing is connected between the outlet of the mainstream in-line bacteria filter and the inlet of the humidifier. The inspiratory limb of the circuit is connected to the outlet of the humidifier. If an HME is used, it is added between the circuit and the tracheostomy/endotracheal tube adapter (Fig. 14-21).

3. A tracheostomy/endotracheal tube adapter is always used to connect the circuit to the patient (Fig. 14-21).

4. Add at least one disconnection alarm to the circuit. It could be a low-volume bellows spirometer alarm (e.g., on the Puritan-Bennett MA-1 ventilator) on the expiratory limb or a low-pressure or disconnection alarm added into the inspiratory limb of the circuit with a Briggs adapter/T-piece.

5. Water traps are placed in the lowest part of the inspiratory and expiratory limbs of the circuit to hold any condensed water vapor.

Fig. 14-22 shows a complete circuit to a volume-cycled ventilator. It is essentially the same circuit as used on a pressure-cycled ventilator.

c. Fix any problems with the equipment (Code: IIB2e1) [Difficulty: An]

Both of these types of ventilators send gas through the circuit during an inspiration and do not cycle off until the preset pressure is reached. Test the tightness of the circuit, backup rate, and delivered tidal volume by placing a test lung on the patient connection of the circuit. Set the controls to deliver the prescribed order. Be prepared to make final adjustments once either unit has been placed on the patient. The patient's airway resistance and lung compliance greatly affect the functioning of both units.

Troubleshooting problems with these units were

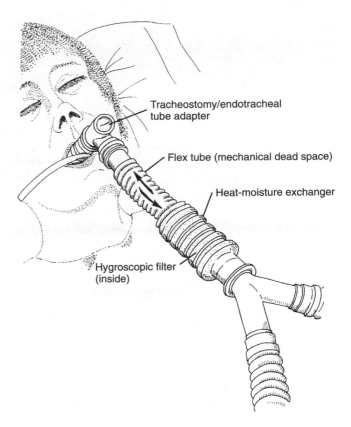

Fig. 14-21 Heat-moisture exchanger (HME) inserted into patient's breathing circuit. Any extra tubing placed between Y of circuit and endotracheal tube acts as mechanical dead space.

discussed in Chapter 13. Make sure that all connections are tight; there are more now with the addition of the humidification system and expiratory limb to the spirometer.

A defective exhalation valve or one in which the small-bore tubing has popped off sends gas through the circuit and not to the patient. If a bellows spirometer is being used, you will notice that it fills during inspiration instead of during expiration as normal.

2. Electrically powered ventilators
a. Get the necessary equipment for the procedure (Code: IIA1e1) [Difficulty: An]

The majority of mechanical ventilators are electrically powered or controlled. They primarily function as volume-cycled units, meaning that a preset volume is delivered from the ventilator with each breath regardless of the patient's condition. Each ventilator is unique in its abilities, modes, and so forth. It is beyond the scope of this book to discuss each and every volume-cycled ventilator. They are presented in a generic manner. The learner should become familiar with the function of the Servo 900 C and other widely used machines.

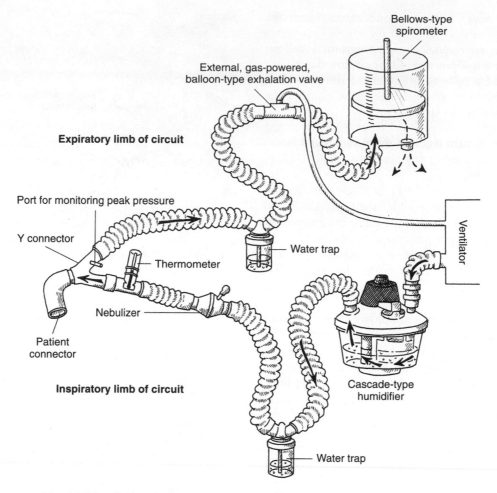

Fig. 14-22 Patient breathing circuit for continuous mechanical ventilation.

b. Put the equipment together, make sure that it works properly, and identify and fix any problems (Code: IIB1e1) [Difficulty: An]

c. Fix any problems with the equipment (Code: IIB2e1) [Difficulty: An]

Each ventilator must be learned for its specifics. Generally speaking, the following steps should be taken to ensure that the ventilator is functioning properly:

1. Select the proper ventilator for the physician's orders and patient's needs.
2. Attach the circuit properly and make sure that all connections are tight (see Fig. 14-22).
3. Select the appropriate humidification device: a passover-type, cascade-type, or HME. Put sterile, distilled water in the passover or cascade unit.
4. Preset all of the physician-ordered parameters and any other settings that are needed to make the ventilator fully functional.
5. Place a test lung on the circuit at the patient connection.
6. Make sure that the ventilator delivers the preset rate, volume, oxygen percentage, I:E ratio, and so forth.

A low volume can be caused by a leak; check all connections, and tighten them as needed. The volume can be measured directly as it leaves the ventilator and at the exhalation valve to help determine the source of the wrong volume. If the unit shows a volume entering the exhalation valve and spirometer instead of the test lung during inspiration, the exhalation valve is broken. All alarms must be working properly. Batteries must be replaced when discharged.

3. Microprocessor ventilators
a. Get the necessary equipment for the procedure (Code: IIA1e1) [Difficulty: An]

The microprocessor ventilators (e.g., Nelcor Puritan-Bennett 7200, Bear 1000, Drager Evita 4) are the most advanced generation of mechanical ventilators. They are electrically powered but controlled by one or more microprocessors (computers). They offer all commonly found modes of ventilation. In addition, many of these machines offer computer software for measuring bedside spirometry for weaning, WOB, and other parameters that give the clinician much valuable information. Airway resistance and static and dynamic lung compliance can be automatically calculated. Flow, volume, and pressure tracings are graphically displayed on the computer screen. Auto-PEEP can be documented and measured. These units offer the greatest amount of patient data and clinical flexibility of all currently available ventilators. The most challenging patients can probably be best cared for on one of these machines.

    b. Put the equipment together, make sure that it works properly, and identify and any problems (Code: IIB1e1) [Difficulty: An]

    c. Fix any problems with the equipment (Code: IIB2e1) [Difficulty: An]

All of the previous general discussion on electrically powered ventilators applies to the microprocessor ventilators as well. An additional advantage to these units is that they self-diagnose most problems and display the problem for you. If a microprocessor should fail, the unit should be removed from the patient. The biomedical department or manufacturer has to replace the computer chip.

4. Fluidic ventilators
    a. Get the necessary equipment for the procedure (Code: IIA1e1) [Difficulty: An]

Examples of commonly available fluidic ventilators include the Sechrist IV-100B and Bio-Med MVP-10. Both are neonatal/pediatric units. The Monaghan 225 is an example of an adult fluidic ventilator.

    b. Put the equipment together, make sure that it works properly, and identify any problems (Code: IIB1e1) [Difficulty: An]

Make sure that high pressure gas hoses between the unit and wall outlets are tightly connected to prevent leaks. The patient circuit and humidification system must be properly installed and operating.

    c. Fix any problems with the equipment (Code: IIB2e1) [Difficulty: An]

Typically, fluidic ventilators are pneumatically powered and have fluidic controls. Make sure that the oxygen and air sources are up to the required pressure (usually 50 psig). Fluidic controls are very sensitive to any obstruction and to changes of other settings. Make sure that gas inlet and outlet filters are kept clear of obstructions.

5. Noninvasive positive pressure ventilators
    a. Get the necessary equipment for the procedure (Code: IIA1e3) [Difficulty: An]

NPPV ventilators are intended for adult patients who are capable of breathing spontaneously for a limited period of time. The unit is typically used for a short period of time with a patient who is having breathing difficulty but does not require intubation and full ventilatory support. Current ventilators include the Respironics BiPAP S/T-D,

Nellcor Puritan-Bennett KnightStar 320, and Healthdyne Quantum PSV.

    b. Put the equipment together, make sure that it works properly, and identify any problems (Code: IIB1e3) [Difficulty: An]

    c. Fix any problems with the equipment (Code: IIB2e3) [Difficulty: An]

Follow the manufacturer's guidelines for putting the circuit on the unit and adding a cascade- or passover-type humidifier. Also, a properly sized nasal or full-face mask is needed to attach the circuit to the patient. Check carefully for any leakage between the mask and patient's face.

6. High frequency ventilators
    a. High frequency jet ventilators (HFJV)
        1. Get the necessary equipment for the procedure (Code: IIA1e2) [Difficulty: R, Ap, An]

Examples of freestanding jet ventilators include the Instrument Development Corporation Model VS600, Bunnell Life Pulse, and APT 1010. Bear Medical Systems developed the BEAR Jet, which must be used with a volume-cycled ventilator that is placed in the CPAP or IMV mode during use of the jet.

In addition, a special endotracheal tube must be placed into the patient before HFJV can be initiated. Ideally, the patient must be intubated with a HiLo Jet tube from Mallinckrodt (Fig. 14-23) or the similar APT Ultracheal tube. These tubes are designed with a catheter through which the jetted gas is sent to the main lumen. Based on the physical principles that govern jets, additional gas is entrained through the main lumen. This entrained gas should be humidified if the jet gas is dry. All exhaled gas passes out through this main lumen. If the jet ventilator is used with a conventional volume-cycled ventilator, the exhaled tidal volume can be measured through the ventilator's spirometry system. The ventilator's alarm systems can also be used and IMV breaths and PEEP can be added if needed. If the patient is too unstable to be extubated and reintubated, a special endotracheal tube adapter can be added (Fig. 14-24). Jet gas enters through the cannula and additional inspiratory and all expiratory gas go through the main lumen of the adapter.

        2. Put the equipment together, make sure that it works properly, and identify any problems (Code: IIB1e2) [Difficulty: R, Ap, An]
        3. Fix any problems with the equipment (Code: IIB2e2) [Difficulty: R, Ap, An]

Fig. 14-25 shows a schematic drawing of a HFJV. Although the currently available ventilators have basic differences in how they are designed, they share these common features:
1. 50 psig source gas(es) of oxygen or oxygen and air are needed to generate a driving pressure.

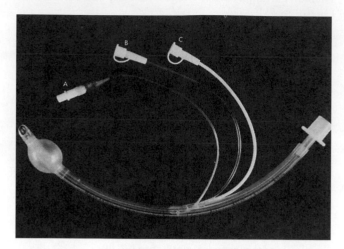

Fig. 14-23 A HiLo Jet endotracheal tube from Mallinckrodt. This special purpose endotracheal tube features four lumens. *A,* Pilot line to the cuff. *B,* Jet catheter used for delivering small bursts of tidal volume gas from a high frequency jet ventilator (HFJV). It opens within the endotracheal tube above the cuff. *C,* Catheter for measuring proximal airway pressure within endotracheal tube near its tip. The main lumen of the endotracheal tube is used for suctioning and adding entrained, humidified gas from a conventional volume-cycled ventilator. (From McPherson SR: *Respiratory therapy equipment,* ed 4, St Louis, 1990, Mosby.)

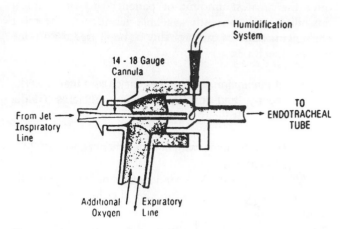

Fig. 14-24 Schematic drawing of tracheostomy/endotracheal tube adapter that has been modified for use with high frequency jet ventilator (HFJV). Jet injector cannula has been added to tracheostomy/endotracheal tube adapter. A needle has been pushed through endotracheal tube adapter to drip saline into it for humidity. This system would be used if patient could not be intubated with HiLo Jet endotracheal tube. (From Carlon GC et al: *Crit Care Med* 9:45, 1981.)

2. A patient circuit specifically suited to the jet ventilator.
3. A drive pressure control lets the operator set the peak pressure of the jet.
4. An inspiratory time control sets the I:E ratio.
5. Rate can be varied within the limits set by the unit.
6. The inspired oxygen percentage can be dialed either on the unit itself or on an external air-oxygen blender before going into the unit.
7. Humidification must be provided by either a dedicated cascade system or one joined to a volume-cycled ventilator. The BEAR Jet does not have a humidification system of its own. It is used with a conventional volume ventilator and the entrained gas is humidified through the cascade-type humidifier on it.

As with any ventilator, make sure that all connections are tight. Leaks are a particular problem because of the high pressures leaving the unit and the small tidal volumes that are delivered.

b. High frequency oscillator ventilators (HFOV)

1. Get the necessary equipment for the procedure (Code: IIA1e2) [Difficulty: R, Ap, An]

The Percussionaire VDR 4 is the only high frequency oscillation (HFO) ventilator (HFOV) available exclusively for adults. The unit is able to deliver conventional, large tidal volumes as well as very small oscillated tidal volumes.

The SensorMedics 3100A High-Frequency Oscillatory Ventilator is FDA approved for neonatal patients. However, it has been used successfully with smaller adult patients. Both units require a special circuit made just for it.

2. Put the equipment together, make sure that it works properly, and identify any problems (Code: IIB1e2) [Difficulty: R, Ap, An]

3. Fix any problems with the equipment (Code: IIB2e2) [Difficulty: R, Ap, An]

Experience with the equipment is recommended to assemble the circuit as needed. The SensorMedics 3100A circuit is designed to combine two separate flows of gas for the patient's tidal volume. As with any circuit, make sure that all connections are tight. The SensorMedics 3100A ventilator is controlled by a microprocessor that can help to diagnose any problems with the equipment.

7. Continuous mechanical ventilation (CMV) breathing circuits

a. Get the necessary equipment for the procedure (Code: IIA1i1) [Difficulty: An]

Either a permanent or a disposable circuit may be selected based on the type of ventilator on which it must be placed. A circuit with an external exhalation valve must be used with older ventilators such as the Bennett

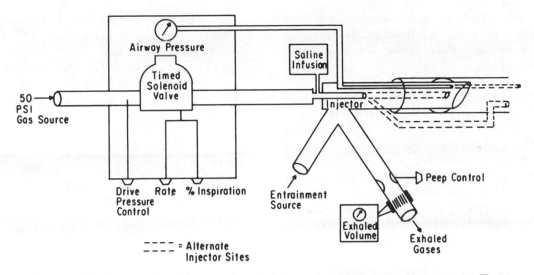

Fig. 14-25 Schematic diagram of a high-frequency jet ventilator concept. (From MacIntyre NR: *Jet ventilation in the adult with breathing rates up to 150 BPM,* Riverside, CA, 1985, Bear Medical Systems.)

MA-1 and Bear 1 and 2. The Nelcor Puritan-Bennett 7200, BEAR 1000, Servo 900 C, and other newer ventilators feature internal exhalation valves and do not need a circuit. If the patient must receive aerosolized medications, the circuit should either include a nebulizer or be able to accept one. If not included, the nebulizer or metered dose inhaler adapter must be added into the inspiratory limb of the circuit.

Also consider if it is better to use an unheated or heated circuit. Usually the circuit is unheated. With these, a cascade-type humidifier or HME is used to warm and humidify the inspired gas. However, some practitioners prefer to use a heated circuit in the care of neonates. These circuits either have heated wires loosely running through the lumen of the tubing or have a wire embedded within the tubing itself. A heated-wire circuit offers finer control over the temperature of the inspired gas and minimizes condensation. Follow the manufacturer's guidelines to make sure that the system can adequately humidify the minute volume that is being used.

b. Put the equipment together, make sure that it works properly, and identify any problems (Code: IIB1i1) [Difficulty: An]

Assemble the circuit with the features needed to manage the patient. Common, but not universal, features of the inspiratory limb of the circuit include a water trap, a humidification system, a nebulizer, a thermometer or temperature probe, a pressure monitoring port, and an oxygen monitoring port. Common, but not universal, features of the expiratory limb of the circuit include an exhalation valve and a water trap.

The heated-wire circuits must be used only with the humidifier that they are specifically designed to work with. The humidifier has a thermostat that regulates warming the humidifier water and heated wires to the same temperature. Never cover a heated-wire circuit with a patient's sheets or blanket or any other material. Do not rest the circuit on anything such as the bed rail, patient's body, or medical equipment. These circuits should always be supported on a boom arm or tube-tree.

All circuits use a Y-connector to tie the inspiratory and expiratory limbs together and attach the circuit to the patient. See Fig. 14-22 for a generic ventilator circuit. Make sure that the water level is properly maintained in the humidifier.

c. Fix any problems with the continuous ventilation circuit (Code: IIB2i1) [Difficulty: An]

Check the circuit and connections for leaks if the volume returned from the patient is less than what was set or delivered. The set volume should be measured with a hand held spirometer as it exits the ventilator, at connection points through the circuit, and at the exhalation valve and/or ventilator spirometer. The volume control or ventilator spirometer may be out of calibration. If the unit shows a volume entering the spirometer instead of the test lung during inspiration, the exhalation valve is broken. Replace a circuit with a leak or defective exhalation valve that cannot be fixed.

d. Change the patient's ventilator circuit as needed (Code: IIIC8a) [Difficulty: An]

A circuit must be replaced if it is damaged in a way that

prevents the patient from being ventilated. This is most commonly seen in circuits with external exhalation valves. If the valve is damaged and will not close, the circuit should be replaced.

Routine circuit changes are done for infection control purposes. A circuit that is not clean in appearance (mucus or blood contamination) should be changed. The American Association for Respiratory Care (AARC) clinical practice guideline on ventilator circuit changes includes the following recommendations:

1. The circuit should be changed every 24 hours if a nebulizer is used for humidification.
2. The circuit may be used for up to 5 days if a cascade- or wick-type humidifier is used for humidification.
3. If a HME is used, it should be changed every 24 hours.

8. Ventilator breathing circuits: PEEP valve assembly

a. Get the necessary equipment for the procedure (Code: IIA1i2) [Difficulty: An]

There are a variety of PEEP systems that can be added to a ventilator or CPAP circuit. Consult an equipment book for the details of their operation. A number of newer ventilators such as the Servo 900 C and Nelcor Puritan-Bennett 7200 have internal exhalation valves and PEEP-generating venturi systems. There is nothing to assemble at the bedside. Failure to generate PEEP indicates that the exhalation valve or PEEP-generating venturi system has failed in some manner.

Most older ventilators (Bennett MA-1 and Bear 1 and 2) use a balloon-like exhalation valve. There is a direct relationship between the volume of gas that is kept in the balloon, the pressure and resistance that it creates, and the PEEP level that is generated.

b. Put the equipment together, make sure that it works properly, and identify any problems (Code: IIB1i2) [Difficulty: An]

The key thing to check with any PEEP-generating system is that the proper level of PEEP is generated and maintained. Once the ordered PEEP level is set, it should be seen as stable on the pressure manometer throughout the respiratory cycle. Sensitivity should be set at no more than −1 to −2 cm water. That way, the PEEP level is maintained at close to the ordered level even during an assisted breath. For example, PEEP is set at 10 cm, and the sensitivity is set at −1 cm. When the patient triggers a breath, it will occur at 9 cm PEEP.

c. Fix any problems with the equipment (Code: IIB2i2) [Difficulty: An]

Malfunctioning internal exhalation valves or PEEP generation venturi systems cannot be easily repaired at the bedside. The ventilator must be replaced. Balloon-type exhalation valves are prone to the following two problems:

1. The small-bore tube carrying gas from the ventilator to

the balloon valve is pulled off. Reconnect the tubing to either the ventilator nipple connection or exhalation valve nipple connection.
2. The balloon is torn, and the gas leaks out. This can be confirmed by disassembling the exhalation valve assembly. Replace the balloon and reassemble the exhalation valve.

EXAM HINT

Both of these problems are exhibited when the inspiratory tidal volume flows past the patient and directly into the exhaled tidal volume spirometer. Little or no airway pressure is generated. The patient is poorly ventilated, if at all. This problem must be corrected immediately while the patient is manually ventilated.

---

9. CPAP systems: breathing circuits

a. Get the necessary equipment for the procedure (Code: IIA1i2) [Difficulty: An]

Most current generation ventilators have a built-in CPAP mode. No additional circuitry is needed. After switching to the CPAP mode, set the desired level by adjusting the PEEP/CPAP dial and watching the reading on the pressure manometer.

There are several manufacturers of CPAP systems for home use in the treatment of obstructive sleep apnea patients. These CPAP systems typically include an air pump to generate flow to the patient, CPAP generating device, circuit designed to work with the system, patient mask(s), and alarm system.

Free-standing CPAP breathing circuits used in hospitals vary considerably. No manufacturer has developed a system that dominates the marketplace. Most commonly, each respiratory care department develops its own breathing circuit to meet its own needs.

b. Put the equipment together, make sure that it works properly, and identify any problems (Code: IIB1i2) [Difficulty: An]

Fig. 14-26 shows the typical components used in a CPAP breathing circuit. The components include:

1. Air/oxygen blender
2. Pediatric or adult flowmeter on the blender
3. Cascade-type humidifier
4. Inspiratory circuit of large-bore or aerosol tubing with the following additions: water trap, one-way valve, and thermometer
5. Y-connector to connect the inspiratory and expiratory limbs of the circuit
6. Patient connector (elbow adapter) to endotracheal or tracheostomy tube, CPAP prongs, or CPAP mask
7. Expiratory circuit of large-bore or aerosol tubing with the following additions: water trap, high pressure pop-off valve (not shown), pressure manometer for measuring the CPAP level, low-pressure or disconnec-

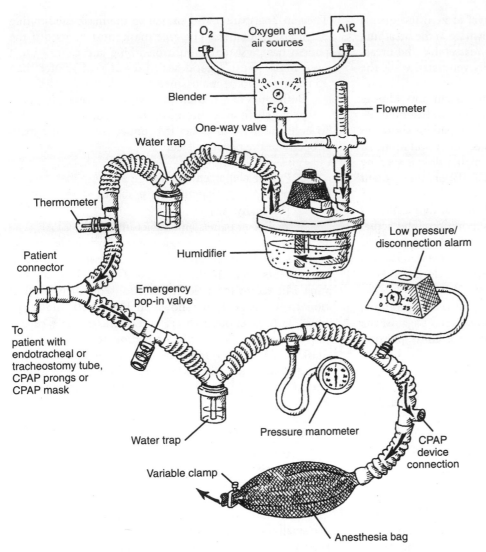

Fig. 14-26 Patient breathing circuit for continuous positive airway pressure (CPAP).

tion audible alarm, anesthesia bag as a reservoir, variable resistance clamp on the tail of the anesthesia bag, Brigg's adapters/T-pieces for connecting the various features, emergency pop-in valve in case gas flow is stopped, and CPAP device.

The CPAP level is adjusted by means of a variety of devices collectively called *threshold resistors,* which include the following:

1. A column of water with a length of expiratory tubing inserted the needed depth below the surface.
2. A vertically mounted ball bearing. It creates a resistance as gas flows up past it. These ball bearing resistors come in weights of 2.5, 5, and 10 cm water.
3. A spring-loaded resistor that is adjusted to apply the desired CPAP level against the airway.
4. A free-standing venturi PEEP system. Gas from the venturi jet creates backpressure against the escaping patient tidal volume.

Air exits through each of these devices when it is working properly. All CPAP systems must be adjusted by checking the pressure level on the manometer. Set the

low-pressure or disconnection audible alarm to sound at a few centimeters below the CPAP level. For example, if 10 cm CPAP is ordered, set the alarm to sound if the pressure drops below 8 cm of CPAP.

c. Fix any problems with the equipment (Code: IIB2i2) [Difficulty: An]

Flow through the CPAP breathing circuit must be sufficient to meet the patient's needs. Adjust the flowmeter setting and clamp on the anesthesia bag so that it is somewhat inflated with excess air escaping out past the clamp. With all of the devices, gas escapes through the path of least resistance. All or some may escape through the anesthesia bag, the CPAP device, or both. The bag should collapse somewhat during the patient's inspiration and expand somewhat during the expiration. The CPAP level should not drop more than 1 or 2 cm from the baseline during an inspiration.

Make sure that the water level is properly maintained in the humidifier. Fill it with sterile, distilled water as often as necessary.

A sudden drop in the CPAP level to zero indicates a disconnection at the patient or somewhere in the breathing circuit. Check all connections and reassemble the break. The patient may need to be manually ventilated while the problem is corrected.

If the CPAP level drops more than 2 cm water during an inspiration, the flow is inadequate and should be increased. Flow is also inadequate if the patient shows an increased use of accessory muscles of respiration or complains of increased WOB. Too high a flow is seen by an inadvertently high level of CPAP or the patient complaining of difficulty exhaling.

Water column systems must be frequently monitored because of water loss caused by evaporation. The actual CPAP level is progressively less than desired as the water is gradually lost. This system must regularly have water added to it or have the expiratory tubing inserted deeper to keep the desired CPAP level.

The ball bearing resistor system must be mounted vertically for gravity to keep the desired weight against the circuit. If it falls over and is horizontal, the CPAP pressure will be lost.

10. CPAP systems: masks

a. Get the necessary equipment for the procedure (Code: IIA1a3) [Difficulty: An]

A CPAP mask and breathing circuit are primarily used for patients who have obstructive sleep apnea. CPAP, by means of the mask, forces the soft tissues open to the point that the airway is never obstructed (see Fig. 14-19). The patient is now able to sleep normally and remain oxygenated. The patient should have the CPAP mask, breathing circuit, and proper CPAP level determined by a sleep study in the hospital. The patient can use the system at home once it is set up properly and he or she has been trained in its use.

In recent years, a CPAP mask has been used with a noninvasive mechanical ventilator to temporarily assist the breathing of a patient with respiratory distress. The hope is to support the patient's breathing long enough to treat the underlying problem(s). If successful, the patient does not need to be intubated. These patients require careful assessment and monitoring.

CPAP masks come in different sizes for children older than 3 years of age and adults. There are two different types of masks. Nose masks are designed to cover only the nose. They allow the patient to speak and offer the mouth as a second airway for breathing in case there is a malfunction of the CPAP system. The mouth also acts as a pressure relief route if the CPAP pressure should become too great. Pressures of up to 15 cm water can usually be maintained in an adult. Pressures of up to 10 cm water can usually be maintained in a child.

Face masks are designed to cover the nose and mouth. They are transparent and similar to the mask used during bag-mask ventilation. The face mask must be used if the patient has persistent mouth breathing and cannot use a nose mask. With a good seal, pressures of greater than 15 cm water can be maintained.

Both types of CPAP mask have a soft, very compliant seal to closely fit the contours of the face. Straps are needed to hold the mask in place. It is imperative that the mask properly fit the patient's face.

b. Put the equipment together, make sure that it works properly, and identify any problems (Code: IIB1a3) [Difficulty: An]

Several companies manufacture mask CPAP systems for home care. These are relatively simple circuits and do not have a humidification system or the other attachments seen in the hospital. Check the manufacturer's literature for specific directions on their application to the patient. As shown in Fig. 14-20, the straps must be tight enough to seal the mask to the face but not so tight as to cut off circulation to the skin. Any mask CPAP system must be able to generate enough flow to meet the patient's minute volume and peak flow needs. The CPAP level must be stable throughout the breathing cycle.

c. Fix any problems with the equipment (Code: IIB2a3) [Difficulty: An]

Too large a mask does not seal and allows gas to leak out. This is seen as a decreased CPAP pressure on the manometer. The patient may show increased snoring or airway obstruction with periods of apnea. A mask that is too small or misfitting can cause an uneven distribution of pressure on the face. This can lead to abrasions or pressure sores and ulcers on the face.

A sudden drop in the CPAP level to zero indicates a disconnection at the patient or somewhere in the breathing circuit. Check all connections and reassemble the break. If the CPAP level drops more than 2 cm water during an inspiration, the flow is inadequate and should be increased. Flow is also inadequate if the patient shows an increased use of accessory muscles of respiration or complains of increased WOB. Too high a flow is seen by an inadvertently high level of CPAP or by the patient complaining difficulty exhaling.

EXAM HINT

There are usually two questions that relate to troubleshooting equipment problems. Expect a question that involves a leak with the loss of delivered tidal volume. If the source of the leak is a loose CPAP or NPPV mask, it must be adjusted or replaced. Also be prepared to troubleshoot problems with a leak in the circuit tubing or the exhalation valve.

11. Humidifiers: passover and cascade type

a. Get the necessary equipment for the procedure (Code: IIA1b) [Difficulty: An]

A cascade-type humidifier is indicated in these situations:

1. The patient has thick or copious secretions. An increase in the amount or thickness of secretions or a change from white to yellow or green justifies the switch to a cascade-type humidifier.
2. The patient will probably require mechanical ventilation for more than 96 hours.
3. The patient cannot have mechanical dead space added to the breathing circuit. If the patient's (especially a child's) tidal volume is smaller than the HME's dead space, it should not be used. IMV systems typically are set up without mechanical dead space, so an HME should not be used.
4. An HME should not be used for a patient receiving very large tidal volumes. This is because the filter's ability to hold moisture is exceeded and the patient will breathe in some dry air. Check the manufacturer's literature for the maximum recommended tidal volume.
5. If the patient has a large air leak, as seen with a deflated cuff or bronchopleural fistula, an HME should not be used. With a large air leak, more air is inspired than expired and the exchanger will not be able to fully humidify the inspired tidal volume.

b. Put the equipment together, make sure that it works properly, and identify any problems (Code: IIB1b) [Difficulty: An]

The general discussion of this equipment was presented in Chapter 7. See Fig. 14-22 and Fig. 14-26 for setups in ventilator and CPAP breathing circuits. Both types are capable of providing 100% relative humidity. Passover-type systems are preferred with neonates.

The humidifier's temperature is usually maintained between 31 and 35° C. Normally, the temperature should never be greater than 37° C at the patient's airway. An exception to this rule is the hypothermic patient. Inhaled gas that is warmed a few degrees above normal body temperature speeds the rewarming process.

Typically, a temperature probe is added into the inspiratory limb of the circuit near the Y. If a heated-wire circuit is being used with an infant, the temperature probe should be outside of the incubator and away from a radiant warmer's direct heat. The humidifier should provide at least 30 mg/L of water vapor.

Make sure that the water level is kept in the recommended range to properly humidify the gas. Avoid being sprayed with any circuit water during disconnections from the patient. It is considered contaminated and should be disposed of like any other contaminated fluid from the patient.

An AARC Clinical Practice Guideline recommends that a cascade- or wick-type of humidifier and patient circuit be changed at least every 5 days for infection control purposes. The guideline also recommends that a nebulizer used for humidification purposes and the patient circuit be changed every 24 hours for infection control purposes.

c. Fix any problems with the equipment (Code: IIB2b) [Difficulty: An]

A loose connection at the humidifier (or anywhere else in the circuit) results in a loss of volume and/or pressure to the patient. Check the entire circuit. When the leak is fixed the volume and pressure are restored. The humidifier should warm to the desired temperature. Do not use a humidifier that does not warm properly.

12. Humidifiers: heat and moisture exchangers

a. Get the necessary equipment for the procedure (Code: IIA1b) [Difficulty: An]

HMEs are designed to be warmed by the patient's exhaled breath and absorb the water vapor from the gas. The next inspired volume is then warmed and humidified by evaporation. The key element in the exchanger is a hygroscopic filter medium. Under ideal conditions, the units can achieve up to 70 to 90% body humidity. They should minimally provide 30 mg/L of water at 30° C. The general discussion of this equipment was presented in Chapter 7. See Fig. 14-21 for a setup in a ventilator breathing circuit.

An HME is indicated in the following situations:

1. The patient has few, if any, secretions.
2. The patient will probably be weaned from the ventilator within 96 hours.
3. The patient is being transported on mechanical ventilation.

An HME is contraindicated in the following situations:

1. The patient has thick, bloody, or large amounts of secretions.
2. The patient has a large air leak such that the exhaled volume is less than 70% of the inhaled tidal volume. This results in a relatively dry hygroscopic filter. (Patients with uncuffed or torn cuffs on their endotracheal tubes or large bronchopleurocutaneous fistulas have large tidal volume leaks.)
3. The patient's temperature is less than 32° C.
4. The patient's spontaneous minute volume is greater than 10 L/min
5. Always remove the HME when delivering nebulized medications through the circuit.

Consider the following when selecting an HME:

1. Select a unit with the smallest possible dead space volume. Watch for an increase in the patient's $PaCO_2$ if the HME adds too much dead space or the patient's tidal volume is too small.

2. Pick the unit that provides the greatest percentage of body humidity. Do not use one that cannot meet the above minimal standards.
3. If the patient had a known pulmonary infection, select an HME that is also a bacteria filter.
4. Should the unit be disposable or reusable? Staffing, infection control, and equipment processing considerations make a difference in choosing which unit to use.

b. Put the equipment together, make sure that it works properly, and identify any problems (Code: IIB1b) [Difficulty: An]

Most of these units are preassembled by the manufacturer. There is nothing to add. It may be necessary to attach a length of large-bore or aerosol tubing or an elbow adapter to make the unit fit onto the Y or endotracheal tube. All come with standard 15- or 22-mm connector ends. Air should flow easily through them with little resistance (see Fig. 14-21).

An AARC Clinical Practice Guideline states that HMEs can be used for up to 4 days if the patient does not have a major secretion problem. Each individual HME can be used for at least 24 hours unless it is obviously fouled. The whole patient circuit should be changed at least every 5 days for infection control purposes.

c. Fix any problems with the equipment (Code: IIB2b) [Difficulty: An]

Any disconnections can be easily noticed and reconnected. Replace any unit that has a mucous plug or other debris obstructing the channel. This might be demonstrated by the patient's peak airway pressure suddenly rising. Typically, HME units are replaced every 24 hours.

> **EXAM HINT**
>
> When secretions are coughed into an HME, it becomes obstructed. This is seen as a rapid increase in the peak pressure during an inspiration. Remove the obstructed HME. Either replace it or change to a cascade-type humidifier.

---

13. H-valve assembly for intermittent mandatory ventilation (IMV)

a. Get the necessary equipment for the procedure (Code: IIA1i3) [Difficulty: R, Ap]

Hudson RCI is a manufacturer of an H-valve and related components depicted in Fig. 14-27, which is an example of a closed- or positive-pressure type of IMV system. The same H-valve can be added into the ventilator circuit as shown in Fig. 14-28, which is an example of an

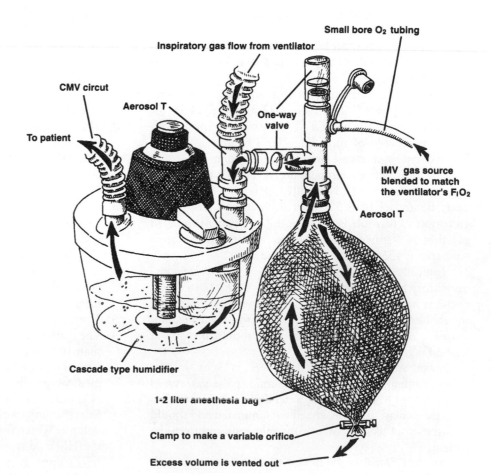

Fig. 14-27 Detail of a closed- or positive-pressure IMV system.

CMV circut
To patient
Aerosol T
Inspiratory gas flow from ventilator
Small bore O₂ tubing
One-way valve
IMV gas source blended to match the ventilator's FᵢO₂
Aerosol T
Cascade type humidifier
1-2 liter anesthesia bag
Clamp to make a variable orifice
Excess volume is vented out

open- or ambient-pressure IMV system. These IMV systems have been added to older ventilators such as the Bennett MA-1.

b. Put the equipment together, make sure that it works properly, and identify any problems (Code: IIB1i3) [Difficulty: R, Ap]

Closed- or positive-pressure IMV system. See Fig. 14-27 for the typical set-up of the Hudson RCI closed- or positive-pressure IMV system. Gases from both the ventilator and IMV system flow through the cascade-type humidifier. IMV flow must be great enough to keep the bag inflated so that the excess gas flows through the humidifier to the patient or is vented out past the partially clamped orifice on the anesthesia bag. IMV flow should never be so great that the pressure manometer on the ventilator shows a constant positive pressure (unless therapeutic PEEP is being applied).

Open- or ambient-pressure IMV system. See Fig. 14-28 for the typical set-up of an open- or ambient-pressure IMV system. A 100 to 200 mL length of aerosol tubing is added for a reservoir instead of the anesthesia bag. The IMV gas is humidified by either a heated, large volume nebulizer (as shown) or a second cascade humidifier. Gas from the ventilator flows through the original cascade humidifier.

Both IMV system configurations must have a thermometer placed into the inspiratory limb of the circuit near the patient to ensure that the desired temperature is maintained. Make sure in both configurations that the oxygen percentage is the same through both the IMV system and the ventilator. Ventilator alarms for low exhaled volume and/or patient disconnection must be functional.

c. Fix any problems with the equipment (Code: IIB1i3) [Difficulty: R, Ap]

Closed- or positive-pressure IMV system. Placing the one-way valve backwards prevents any flow from passing through to the patient. If the flow through the IMV system is too great, the bag will overfill and pressure will build up

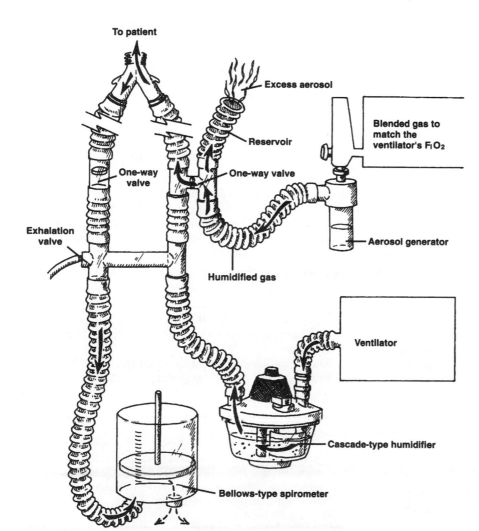

Fig. 14-28   Detail of an open- or ambient-pressure IMV system.

To patient

Excess aerosol

Reservoir

One-way valve

One-way valve

Blended gas to match the ventilator's F$_I$O$_2$

Exhalation valve

Aerosol generator

Humidified gas

Ventilator

Cascade-type humidifier

Bellows-type spirometer

in the circuit. The patient may complain of difficulty exhaling and a positive pressure will be seen on the manometer. The flow to the IMV system must be decreased.

The opposite problem is inadequate flow through the IMV system. This is seen as the reservoir bag collapsing on inspiration, the patient complaining of not getting enough air, or the pressure gauge registering a negative pressure on inspiration. Obviously, the flow to the system must be increased.

Open- or ambient-pressure IMV system. Flow through the nebulizer must be great enough that excess mist can be seen escaping from the reservoir during a patient's spontaneous inspiration. Increase the flow if mist is not seen. Placing the one-way valve backwards prevents any added flow from passing through to the patient; placing the valve in the reversed position results in the IMV breath being vented out into room air. Placing the valve properly allows gas to pass through to the patient as intended.

14. Perform volume, flow, and pressure calibration on a ventilator for quality control (Code: IIB3b) [Question difficulty: R, Ap]

Follow the manufacturer's guidelines for quality control procedures on a mechanical ventilator. The microprocessor ventilators usually have a software package that performs self-diagnostic tests on the unit. Obviously, the ventilator should deliver the volume, flow, and pressure that is set on the controls. Do not use a unit that fails a quality control check.

MODULE D	Evaluate and monitor the patient's response to mechanical ventilation

1. Observe the patient's subjective response to being mechanically ventilated (Code: IIIA1c) [Difficulty: An]

Because a patient with an intubated airway cannot speak, it is necessary to communicate by asking simple questions that can be answered in a *yes* nod or *no* shake of the head. Other methods of communication are a pad of paper and pencil or picture boards.

It is not possible to predict how a patient will react to the initiation of mechanical ventilation or its prolonged need. Some patient's react with relief and relax when the WOB is reduced. Others may become angry at the limitations imposed on them. Still others may become depressed. The issue of a patient's emotional reaction to illness is discussed in detail in Chapter 1.

2. Measure the patient's lung compliance and airway resistance (Code: IC1a and IC1g) [Difficulty: An]

These measurements and their interpretation are presented earlier in this chapter.

3. Interpret the ventilator flow, volume, and pressure waveforms (Code: IC2i) [Difficulty: An]

Review and interpret the various waveforms presented in the chapter and the flow-volume loops in Chapter 4.

4. Measure the tidal volume (Code: IIIA1h) [Difficulty: An]

The patient's exhaled tidal volume is usually measured and recorded in his or her chart. Many of the newer ventilators also display an inhaled and exhaled tidal volume. If possible, compare the two volumes. If they do not match closely, check for a leak or other reason for the difference. The patient on an IMV, SIMV, or PSV mode should have both the machine delivered and spontaneous tidal volumes measured and recorded.

The weaning patient must have his or her spontaneous tidal volume measured along with the vital capacity. They and other parameters are used to judge weanability (discussed later; see Box 14-5 for more information).

BOX 14-5	Indications That the Patient Can Probably Be Weaned From the Ventilator

OXYGENATION

$PaO_2 \geq 80$ torr or $SpO_2 > 90\%$ on 50% oxygen or less
$P(A-a)O_2 < 300-350$ torr on 100% oxygen
Intrapulmonary shunt of less than 15%

VENTILATION

$PaCO_2 < 55$ torr in a patient who is not ordinarily hypercapneic
Dead space/tidal volume ($V_D:V_T$) ratio <0.55-0.6 (55%-60%)
Rapid, shallow breathing index (breaths/minute divided by tidal volume in liters) <105

PULMONARY MECHANICS

Spontaneous tidal volume of 3-4 mL/lb or 7-9 mL/kg of ideal body weight
Vital capacity of at least 10-15 mL/kg
Maximum inspiratory pressure (MIP) > -20 to -25 cm water pressure
Forced expiratory volume in one second (FEV_1) >10 mL/kg
Respiratory rate of 12-35/min (adult)

MISCELLANEOUS

Conscious and cooperative patient who wants to breathe spontaneously
Stable and acceptable normal blood pressure and temperature
Stable cardiac rhythm; heart rate should not increase by more than 15% to 20%
Corrected underlying problem that led to ventilatory support
Normal fluid balance and electrolyte values
Proper nutritional status

5. Measure the respiratory rate (Code: IIIA1h) [Difficulty: An]

Count and record the machine-delivered respiratory rate. If the patient is on an IMV, SIMV, or PSV, count and record both the machine and spontaneous rates. The weaning patient should have his or her spontaneous rate counted and recorded.

6. Measure the inspiratory/expiratory ratio (Code: IIIA1h) [Difficulty: An]

The I:E ratio should be calculated and recorded. Some newer ventilators display it. Others show inspiratory time and expiratory time. The I:E ratio can then be calculated as shown in Table 14-2.

7. Measure airway pressures (Code: IIIA1h) [Difficulty: An]

a. Peak pressure (or P_{peak}): The peak pressure reached during the delivery of a tidal volume is the pressure required to push the gas through the circuit, endotracheal tube, and the patient's airways, and to expand the lungs. The sigh volume requires a greater pressure because it is a larger volume. These pressures should be recorded regularly whenever the patient and machine are checked. The importance of peak pressure in calculating dynamic compliance was discussed earlier in the chapter.

b. Plateau pressure (or P_{plat}): The plateau pressure is found when the tidal volume has been delivered to the lungs and is temporarily held within them. The importance of plateau pressure in calculating static compliance was discussed earlier in the chapter.

c. Baseline pressure: The baseline pressure is the pressure measured at the end of exhalation. Normally it is seen as zero on the ventilator's pressure manometer. (Remember that in this case zero is actually local barometric pressure.) If the patient has therapeutic PEEP or CPAP, the baseline pressure will be greater than zero.

8. Monitor mean airway pressure (Code: IIIA1h) [Difficulty: An]

Mean airway pressure (P_{AW}) is the average pressure over an entire breathing cycle. Most of the newer ventilators display a mean airway pressure. This pressure results from changes in the patient's peak and baseline pressures plus the I:E ratio.

9. Test the ventilator alarm systems and adjust them as needed (Code: IIIA1h) [Difficulty: An]

All alarm systems must function properly. Test all audible and visual alarms. The practitioner should be familiar with the most widely used adult and infant ventilators and their alarm systems. It is common practice to set most alarms at $\pm10\%$ from the set value. For example:

1. The tidal volume is 1000 mL. Set the low-volume alarm at 900 mL and the high-volume alarm at 1100 mL.
2. The minute volume is 10,000 mL. Set the high-volume alarm at 11,000 mL and the low- volume alarm at 9000 mL.
3. The oxygen percentage is set at 40%. Set the high-percentage alarm at 45% and the low-percentage alarm at 35%.
4. The low-pressure or disconnection alarm is set to sound if the ventilator-delivered pressure is about 5 cm water below the peak pressure. For example, if the peak pressure has been about the 40 cm water, the low-pressure or disconnection alarm should be set at 35 cm water. If a leak or disconnection occurs, the alarm sounds when the peak pressure does not reach 35 cm water. If the patient is on a CPAP system, the

TABLE 14-2 Time Variables in Mechanical Ventilation

Term	Symbol	Formula for calculation
Frequency (rate)	f	Count breaths/min or $\dfrac{60}{t_I + t_E}$
Cycle time	$t_I + t_E$	Add $t_I + t_E$ or $\dfrac{60}{f}$
Inspiratory time	t_I (I)	$t_I = \dfrac{60}{f} - t_E$ or $t_I = \%t_I \times (t_I + t_E)$
Expiratory time	t_E (E)	$t_E = \dfrac{60}{f} - t_I$
Inspiratory/expiratory ratio	$I:E$ or t_I/t_E	$I:E = \dfrac{t_I}{t_E}$, usually numerator
Percent inspiratory time	$\%t_I$	$\%t_I = \dfrac{t_I}{t_I + t_E} \times 100$

From Scanlan CL: Physics and physiology or ventilatory support. In Scanlan CL, Spearman CB, Sheldon RL, editors: *Egan's fundamentals of respiratory care*, ed 5, St Louis, 1990, Mosby.

low-pressure or disconnection alarm should be set to sound if the pressure drops about 2 to 3 cm water below the set level. For example, if the patient is on 10 cm water CPAP, the alarm should be set at 8 cm water.

Many types of alarms have a timer that can be set to delay when the alarm sounds. If the alarm is on a ventilator, the delay should be set for about 3 to 5 seconds longer than the cycling time. For example, if the patient has a back-up rate of 10 times/min, the cycling time between mandatory breaths is 6 seconds. Set the timer to delay the alarm sounding for about 10 seconds. If the patient is disconnected from the ventilator and the peak pressure does not reach 35 cm water, the alarm will sound in 10 seconds. If the patient is on a CPAP system, the timer may be set for no delay or a short delay. Adjust all the alarms to fit the clinical setting and the patient's condition. Some may need tighter limits, and others may need wider limits than those just discussed.

10. Monitor the cuff pressure to the patient's endotracheal or tracheostomy tube (Code: IIIA1j) [Difficulty: An]

This was presented in Chapter 11. Review it if necessary.

11. Auscultate the patient's chest and interpret the breath sounds (Code: IB4a) [Difficulty: An]

This was presented in Chapter 1. Review it if necessary.

MODULE E	Recommend and/or make modifications in therapeutic procedures based on the patient's response

1. Change the type of mechanical ventilator (Code: IIIC8a) [Difficulty: An]

Selecting the type of mechanical ventilator is discussed earlier in this chapter. Briefly, a pressure-cycled unit can be used with a patient without cardiopulmonary disease. Most patients with conditions that cause abnormal airway resistance or lung compliance should be placed on electrically powered volume-cycled units. The microprocessor ventilators offer more ventilating options and monitoring of clinical information. They are best for the most critical patients. Noninvasive ventilation and negative-pressure ventilation are used with patients who do not need intubation and have some ability to breathe for themselves.

Be prepared to change from one type of ventilator to another as the patient's condition warrants. A ventilator that is malfunctioning should be replaced with one that is capable of providing the same level of ventilatory support.

2. Change the ventilator breathing circuit (Code: IIIC8a) [Difficulty: An]

Changing circuits was discussed earlier in this chapter.

Briefly, change a circuit that has a leak or is contaminated. Routine changes are done for infection control purposes.

3. Change the oxygen percentage (Code: IIIB4c and IIIC3a) [Difficulty: An]

As discussed earlier, the goal of oxygen administration is to keep the PaO_2 level of most patients between 60 and 90 torr and the SpO_2 level greater than 90%. Exceptions are the patient who is breathing on hypoxic drive and the patient who is in a cardiac arrest situation. The COPD patient who has a chronically low PaO_2 level and chronically high $PaCO_2$ level may be allowed to have a PaO_2 value as low as 50 to 55 torr and an SpO_2 value as low as 85%. The patient who is extremely hypoxic must be given up to 100% oxygen. Those patients who have refractory hypoxemia (e.g., ARDS) do not respond with a normal increase in the PaO_2 level as the oxygen percentage is increased.

4. Change the mode of ventilation (Code: IIIB2c) [Difficulty: An]

Changing the mode of ventilation was discussed earlier in this chapter. Be prepared to change the mode as the patient's condition varies.

📋 EXAM HINT

There is usually one question that requires changing the mode of ventilation, depending on the patient's condition. This could involve a patient who can breathe spontaneously being changed from the A/C mode to the SIMV mode, or it could involve a patient receiving volume-cycled ventilation being changed to pressure-cycled ventilation because of a very high plateau pressure.

---

5. Change the mechanical dead space (Code: IIIC8c) [Difficulty: An]

Mechanical dead space is added to increase the patient's $PaCO_2$ level. This is done by having the patient rebreathe gas from his or her anatomic dead space. This high CO_2 gas is then inhaled back to the alveolar level and increases the patient's $PaCO_2$ level. The more dead space tubing there is, the more carbon dioxide is retained. It is important to realize that this same rebreathed volume of gas is lower in oxygen because of its diffusion into the patient's pulmonary circulation. If a large amount of mechanical dead space is added, it will be necessary to increase the F_IO_2 to keep the ordered level. Measure the oxygen percentage between the dead space and the endotracheal or tracheostomy tube adapter.

Mechanical dead space is used only in the C and A/C modes. It should not be used in IMV/SIMV, pressure support, or CPAP modes. Typically, a length of large-bore or aerosol tubing is added into the breathing circuit between the Y and the patient's endotracheal or tracheostomy tube (see Fig. 14-22). The following formula can be used to predict what amount of *mechanical dead space* (Vd_{mech}') produces a desired $PaCO_2$ level:

$$[(Vt - Vd_{anat}) - Vd_{mech}] \times f \times PaCO_2 = [(Vt - Vd_{anat}) - Vd_{mech}'] \times f \times PaCO_2'$$

In which:

V_T = current tidal volume

V_{Danat} = anatomic dead space. This is calculated at 1 mL/lb or 2.2 mL/kg of ideal body weight.

V_{Dmech} = current mechanical dead space

f = ventilator rate

$PaCO_2$ = actual patient $PaCO_2$ value

V_{Dmech}' = *desired mechanical dead space*

$PaCO_2'$ = desired patient $PaCO_2$ value

Example. Your patient is a 70-kg (154-lb) male who is being ventilated on the Control mode (he is apneic). His ventilator settings are tidal volume of 1000 mL, rate of 12/min, F_IO_2 of 0.3, no added mechanical dead space. His ABGs are PaO_2 of 90 torr, $PaCO_2$ of 30 torr, pH of 7.48, SaO_2 of 95%, BE 0. The clinical goal is to adjust the patient's mechanical dead space as needed to produce a $PaCO_2$ of 40 torr. In summary:

V_T = 1000 mL current tidal volume

V_{Danat} = 154 mL anatomic dead space. This is calculated at 1 mL/lb or 2.2 mL/kg of ideal body weight.

V_{Dmech} = no added mechanical dead space

f = 12 for ventilator rate

$PaCO_2$ = 30 torr actual patient $PaCO_2$ value

V_{Dmech}' = *desired amount of mechanical dead space*

$PaCO_2'$ = 40 torr desired patient $PaCO_2$ value

Placing the data and goal into the formula results in the following equation:

$$[(V_T - V_{Danat}) - V_{Dmech}] \times f \times PaCO_2 = [(V_T - V_{Danat}) - V_{Dmech}'] \times f \times PaCO_2'$$
$$[(1000 - 154) - 0] \times 12 \times 30 = [(1000 - 154) - V_{Dmech}'] \times 12 \times 40$$

Simplifying produces the following equation:

$$[846] \times 12 \times 30 = [846 - V_{Dmech}'] \times 480$$
$$304,560 = (846 \times 480) - (V_{Dmech}' \times 480)$$
$$304,560 = 406,080 - 480\, V_{Dmech}'$$
$$-101,520 = -480\, V_{Dmech}'$$
$$211.5 \text{ mL} = V_{Dmech}'$$

The solution is to increase the patient's mechanical dead space from zero to 212 mL.

 EXAM HINT

There is usually one question that deals with recommending the addition of mechanical deadspace when ABG results show that the patient is being hyperventilated.

6. **Change the level of noninvasive positive pressure ventilation (Code: IIIB4a) [Difficulty: An]**

NPPV was discussed earlier in this chapter. Briefly, if the patient's tidal volume must be increased, the level of positive pressure must be increased. Lowering the level of positive pressure decreases the tidal volume. Blood gases and vital signs should always be monitored after any change is made.

7. **Initiate and change combinations of ventilatory techniques to adequately oxygenate the patient (Code: IIIB4b) [Difficulty: An]**

Change the tidal volume and sigh volume. The specific tidal volume to select was discussed earlier in this section. Conditions in which the tidal volume should be increased include atelectasis, consolidation, and when the present tidal volume is at the small end of the normal range and the patient has an elevated carbon dioxide level or low oxygen level. The NBRC has used the upper level for a set tidal volume in an adult as 15 mL/kg of ideal body weight.

Conditions in which the tidal volume should be decreased include air trapping, hyperinflated lungs as seen on the chest radiograph by wide intercostal margins or flattened hemidiaphragms, and when the present tidal volume is at the large end of the normal range and the patient has a decreased carbon dioxide level. The NBRC has used the lower level for a set tidal volume in an adult as 10 mL/kg of ideal body weight.

An additional consideration is whether or not to give the patient a sigh breath. People normally sigh every few minutes. A sigh is a volume larger than the normal tidal volume. It serves the purpose of opening up atelectatic alveoli and reorienting the surfactant in the alveoli so that they are stable.

Most patients being ventilated in the A/C mode receive a ventilator sigh volume just as they do a tidal volume. A sigh volume is typically 1.5 to 2 times the tidal volume if the tidal volume is in the low to middle range of normal. If the patient has atelectasis or consolidation, a larger sigh volume may be indicated. The patient may not need a sigh volume at all if the set tidal volume is at the 15 mL/kg upper limit. A sigh volume may be contraindicated in a patient with bullous emphysema, a pneumothorax, or cardiac status that is sensitive to high peak pressures. The patient who is air trapping the tidal volume should have a smaller (or possibly no) sigh volume. Compare the inspired and expired volumes to ensure that there is no air trapping. Most current ventilators allow the clinician to tailor the sigh frequency to best meet the patient's clinical needs. The sigh frequency should be increased in patients with atelectasis or consolidation. The sigh frequency may need to be decreased or eliminated in patients who are air trapping the tidal or sigh volume. Sighs are usually not given when the patient is on the IMV/SIMV mode.

☞ EXAM HINT

Expect to see at least one question about setting or adjusting the tidal volume and one question about setting or adjusting the sigh volume.

Change the respiratory rate. Respiratory rate was discussed earlier in this chapter. Increase the backup rate on the ventilator if the patient has an elevated carbon dioxide level and the tidal volume is at the high end of the normal range. Decrease the backup rate on the ventilator if the patient has a decreased carbon dioxide level and the tidal volume is at the low end of the normal range.

Change the PEEP or CPAP level. PEEP therapy was discussed earlier in this chapter. Remember that therapeutic PEEP is indicated in situations in which the patient has bilaterally small lungs with a reduced FRC. This results in hypoxemia. The proper level of PEEP restores the FRC and improves oxygenation. Watch for side affects of barotrauma or decreased cardiac output from too much pressure. The patient should be carefully monitored with blood gas analysis and vital sign checks before starting PEEP and after each change.

CPAP therapy was discussed earlier. Briefly, all of these considerations for PEEP apply to CPAP except that the patient must be able to breathe adequately to maintain a normal carbon dioxide level.

Change the inspiratory plateau level. Inspiratory plateau (also known as inflation hold) is a technique in which the patient is temporarily prevented from exhaling the ventilator-delivered tidal volume. See Fig. 14-29 for the pressure/time waveform. Inspiratory plateau is added therapeutically to improve the distribution of the tidal volume. Patients with ARDS and pulmonary edema can benefit from it. Oxygenation should improve in direct proportion to the duration of the inspiratory plateau. The duration of inspiratory plateau is measured in different ways, depending on the ventilator. For example, the Bear 1000 and Nelcor Puritan-Bennett 7200 can have it added in steps of 0.1 second up to several seconds total. The Servo 900 C can have it added as a variable percentage of the total duration of the breathing cycle. It is important to reduce the inspiratory plateau as the patient's ventilation and lung compliance improve. Patients' with normal ventilation and compliance should not receive any inspiratory plateau.

Notice that the use of an inspiratory plateau increases the inspiratory phase of the breathing cycle. This results in a shorter expiratory time if the rate is kept the same. Or, the rate must be reduced to keep the same I:E ratio. Again, as discussed earlier, make sure that the tidal volume is completely exhaled. The patient's condition should be monitored closely to determine if the level of inspiratory plateau is appropriate.

Nontherapeutic inspiratory plateau is added temporarily to determine the plateau pressure on the ventilator. This is considered to be the pressure needed to deliver the tidal volume. With this information, the patient's effective static

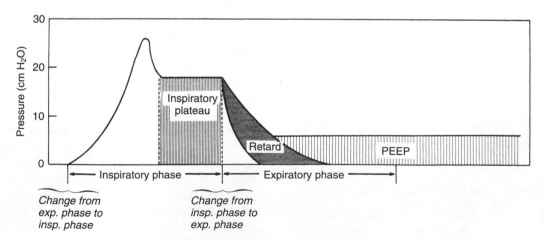

Fig. 14-29 Pressure-time waveform showing how exhalation can be modified. Inspiratory plateau (inflation hold) is seen when the tidal volume is held within the lungs for a period of time. With expiratory retard, the gas is more slowly exhaled than during a passive breath. These two modifications of exhalation may or may not be combined with PEEP. (From Kirby RR, Smith RA, Desautels DA. In Burton GG, Hodgkin JE, editors: *Respiratory care: a guide to clinical practice,* ed 2, Philadelphia, 1984, Lippincott.)

compliance can be calculated. Its calculation and interpretation were discussed earlier in this chapter. An inspiratory plateau of 0.5 to 1.0 second is usually long enough to find the plateau pressure. Remember to turn off the inspiratory plateau afterward.

Change the expiratory retard level. Expiratory retard was first discussed in Chapter 13. It is indicated in any patient who is air trapping and not exhaling completely. It functions like pursed-lip breathing in the spontaneously breathing patient. The back pressure prevents the collapse of the smallest airways (see Fig. 14-29 for the pressure/time waveform). Expiratory retard may be indicated in a patient with asthma, emphysema, or bronchitis. It is important with these types of patients to measure the inspiratory and expiratory tidal volume. Air trapping is confirmed by the expiratory volume being less than the inspiratory volume. When listening to the patient's breath sounds, there is no pause at the end of exhalation before the next inspiration is started. In extreme cases, the pressure manometer does not return to the baseline level. These patients should be checked for the presence and level of auto-PEEP. The proper level of expiratory retard is determined by trial and error. The following parameters should be monitored to find the proper amount:

a. The inspiratory and expiratory tidal volumes should be the same.
b. The patient's breath sounds should reveal wheezing to be absent or minimal and a silent pause at the end of exhalation before the next tidal volume is delivered.
c. There should be no auto-PEEP.
d. The patient should subjectively feel that he or she has exhaled completely before the next breath is given.

It is important to monitor the patient frequently when expiratory retard is being used. As the patient is treated with bronchodilating medications, the bronchospasm should diminish. Expiratory retard should not be needed when the airway resistance has returned to normal.

 EXAM HINT

There is usually one question that deals with the indications for or application of either inspiratory plateau or inflation hold.

Change the pressure support level. When the pressure support level is adjusted to deliver a tidal volume, it is called PSV_{max} (for maximum pressure support ventilation). The clinical guidelines for PSV_{max} follow:

1. Use enough pressure to deliver a tidal volume of 10 to 12 mL/kg of ideal body weight.
2. The patient should not have to assist the ventilator at a rate greater than 20 times/min to achieve acceptable ABG values.

PSV_{max} has been used in patients who have had acute respiratory failure that is resolving. Usually these patients have been maintained on the A/C mode for several days to minimize their WOB while undergoing treatment for their condition. It is believed that PSV_{max} is ideal for reconditioning their diaphragm and other respiratory muscles. Reconditioning occurs when the assist or "trigger" pressure for the breath is kept at low as possible (−1 to −2 cm water pressure) and the tidal volume large. This pattern results in a low respiratory muscle work load. As the patient continues to improve, the PSV level is reduced. The patient's tidal volume is stable if the patient passively takes in the PSV supported breath. The tidal volume can be larger if the patient interacts actively with the pressure that is delivered. See Fig. 14-1 for a pressure and flow versus time curves and Fig. 14-10, *E*, for a pressure/time curve.

The pressure support level has also been used as a way to overcome the airway resistance caused by the patient's endotracheal tube. (See the example calculated earlier in this chapter.) It is believed that too small an endotracheal tube prevents some patients from successfully weaning by the IMV/SIMV mode. The addition of enough pressure support to overcome the additional WOB caused by the tube enables the patient to wean successfully and the airway to be extubated.

The pressure support level is reduced, as tolerated, when the patient's lung-thoracic compliance or airway resistance improves. As both return toward normal, the only barrier to extubation is the resistance offered by the endotracheal tube. Some practitioners advocate extubation when the PSV level is 10 cm water or less. This is probably the pressure level needed to overcome the tube's resistance. Therefore the patient should tolerate extubation without any increase in the WOB.

 EXAM HINT

Expect to seen one question that requires an increase in the pressure support level if the patient is working too hard when inhaling through a small endotracheal tube or if the SIMV rate is quite low.

Change the pressure control ventilation level. PCV involves the delivery of tidal volume breathes that are pressure limited and time cycled. It has been advocated for patients with bilateral low compliance conditions such as is seen with ARDS. The pressure control (PC) level is set as low as possible to achieve an adequate tidal volume for gas exchange. It is important to monitor the exhaled volume continuously because the tidal volume decreases if the patient's lung compliance or airway resistance worsens. If either or both improve, the tidal volume increases. The patient with a pulmonary air leak loses variable amounts of tidal volume out of the chest tube depending on the same changes in compliance and resistance. It is important to evaluate an ABG sample with a change in the PC level or tidal volume.

The PCV mode is well tolerated by many patients because of the freedom they have to set the rate, inspiratory flow through the demand valve, and minute volume. PCV may also be combined with SIMV and PSV as the clinical situation indicates. The following are some suggestions for initial PC settings:

a. Set the level of PEEP at the same level used on the constant volume ventilator. This maintains the patient's FRC.
b. Set the PC level at the patient's static lung compliance pressure. Be prepared to increase this pressure. The clinical goal is to give a tidal volume close to that delivered previously.
c. Set the rate the same as before.
d. Set the inspired oxygen the same as before. Some may prefer to set it at 100% until blood gas results show that it can be lowered.
e. Set the inspiratory time under PC so that the I:E ratio is the same as before.

Check the patient's vital signs for tolerance and get an ABG sample in about 15 minutes. If the airway resistance or lung compliance worsens, the PC level must be increased to maintain or increase the tidal volume. Obviously, as the patient's airway resistance and lung compliance improve (or pulmonary air leak decreases) the PC level must be decreased to maintain the desired tidal volume.

Make a change in inverse ratio ventilation. Inverse ratio ventilation (IRV) has been used with success in adults with ARDS who do not respond to PCV. Increased inspiratory time and decreased expiratory time should be used in any condition in which the patient has a small time constant of ventilation. (Time constant of ventilation (Tc) = $C_{LT} \times R_{AW}$) This is seen clinically as a normal airway resistance but a low lung-thoracic compliance. Examples of conditions in which this is seen include ARDS, pulmonary edema, pneumonia, or an enlarged abdomen. Increasing the inspiratory time to create an inverse I:E ratio keeps the lungs inflated longer to provide more time for oxygen to diffuse. In addition, it keeps the alveoli open longer to help prevent atelectasis and maintain the FRC.

Typically, patients being considered for IRV are already being ventilated in the PC mode. Therefore the merging of the two modes is called pressure control inverse ratio ventilation (PCIRV). The following have been recommended as initial PCIRV settings:

a. If the patient is being switched from volume-cycled ventilation to PCIRV, set the PC level at the patient's static lung compliance pressure. However, if the patient was already on PCV at a higher pressure, keep this higher pressure.
b. Set the oxygen at 100%.
c. Keep the current respiratory rate.

d. Keep the I:E ratio at 1:1 for now.
e. PEEP should be removed if it is currently at less than 8 cm water. Cut the PEEP level in half if it is currently at more than 8 cm water. As the I:E ratio is made inverse, air-trapping increases the patient's FRC.

Draw a set of ABGs after 15 minutes on PCIRV and check the patient's vital signs. Monitor the exhaled tidal volume for a decrease. If the ventilator gives a real-time graph of pressure, volume, and flow these should be monitored for air-trapping (auto-PEEP). See Fig. 14-2 for an auto-PEEP flow/time tracing.

If the initial set of blood gases on PCIRV does not show adequate oxygenation, the inspiratory time should be increased. The inspiratory time must be progressively increased and expiratory time decreased if the patient's lung compliance worsens. It is also possible to alternate a 2 to 3 cm water increase in the PC level with small increases in the inspiratory time. Blood gases must be analyzed with each increase in inspiratory time, decrease in expiratory time, or increase in PC. Once an acceptable PaO_2 is established it is usually not necessary to make further increases in the inspiratory time if the patient's pulmonary condition does not worsen. Look for an increase in $PaCO_2$ or end-tidal CO_2 as a sign of inadequate tidal volume. It may be necessary to increase the PC level or decrease the inspiratory time to increase the tidal volume. Also monitor the patient's vital signs and cardiac output, if possible, to look for a decrease in cardiac output. PCIRV ratios as inverse as 3:1 or 4:1 have been reported. When this happens, the pressure-volume curve takes on a characteristic "square wave" shape as shown in Fig. 14-11, *B*.

It is very important to return the I:E ratio toward normal as the patient's lung compliance improves. This is done by gradually decreasing the inspiratory time and/or increasing the expiratory time. The patient's blood gas result should be evaluated with each step to be sure that oxygenation is maintained at a safe level.

Monitor the mean airway pressure to determine the patient's response to respiratory care. Mean airway pressure (P_{aw} or MAP) is the average pressure over an entire breathing cycle. A number of current neonatal and adult ventilators are able to calculate the value (Fig. 14-30). Mean airway pressure is influenced by the patient's lung-thoracic compliance (C_{LT}), airway resistance (R_{AW}), and ventilator settings. If a volume-cycled ventilator is being used, a decrease in compliance or an increase in resistance results in an increase in the mean airway pressure. This is because it takes more pressure to deliver the tidal volume; a higher peak pressure is seen. Conversely, if the patient's compliance increases or the resistance decreases, the P_{aw} decreases. It is important to further evaluate the patient when a change in P_{aw} is noticed. This is because the new pressure, by itself, does not clarify whether there has been a change in compliance, resistance, or both. Any treatments that improve lung compliance and reduce airway resistance

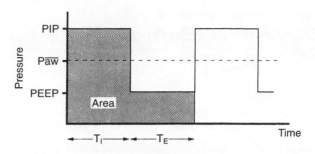

Fig. 14-30 Pressure/time tracing showing mean airway pressure (P_{aw}). *PIP* is peak inspiratory pressure, *PEEP* is positive end–expiratory pressure, T_I is inspiratory time, T_E is expiratory time. (From Chatburn RL: *Respir Care* 36:569, 1991.)

are shown by a reduced mean airway pressure. It is important to calculate both dynamic and static compliance (discussed earlier) when trying to determine how the patient's condition has changed.

In general, an increase in mean airway pressure increases the patient's oxygenation. This is because the alveoli are kept open longer, allowing more time for diffusion and preventing alveolar collapse. (Fig. 15-9 shows how several ventilator adjustments can change the mean airway pressure.) If alveolar ventilation is improved, the $PaCO_2$ may also be reduced. If the mean airway pressure is too high there is an increased risk of pulmonary barotrauma and decreased cardiac output. This is especially true if PEEP is increased to raise the $P_{\overline{aw}}$. Watch the patient closely whenever a ventilator change is made that increases the $P_{\overline{aw}}$. A sudden deterioration in cardiopulmonary function may be caused by a pneumothorax. A reduction in urine output, an increased heart rate, and decreased blood pressure are often seen when the cardiac output is reduced. The mean airway pressure should be reduced if any of these situations is seen. To prevent these complications, it is necessary to reduce the mean airway pressure whenever the patient's pulmonary condition improves. As the compliance increases toward normal it is not necessary to use as high a mean airway pressure to maintain acceptable blood gases.

Recommend the use of sedatives or muscle relaxants (paralyzing agents) as needed. An adult who is attempting to inhale or exhale out of sequence with the ventilator is said to be "bucking" or "fighting" the ventilator. This problem is most commonly seen in the Control and A/C modes. If the asynchrony between the patient's efforts and the ventilator is too great, there is an increased risk of hypoxemia, air trapping, and pneumothorax. Carefully evaluate the patient to determine if he or she is breathing rapidly because of pain, anxiety, or improper adjustment of the ventilator. Make sure that the inspiratory flow, respiratory rate, pressure limit, and so forth are correctly set for the patient's condition. Sedation or paralysis should be considered only after all other causes of asynchrony have

been ruled out. It is important to consider the following patient conditions before making a medication choice for controlling the patient's breathing efforts:

1. Is the patient in pain? If so, an opiate analgesic such as morphine sulfate is commonly given intravenously for fast onset. Morphine has the additional effects of reducing anxiety and inducing sleep. Because, like all opiates, it is a central nervous system depressant, make sure that the ventilator alarm systems are functioning properly in case the patient becomes disconnected.

2. Is the patient agitated? Asynchrony with the ventilator for no known reason can often be attributed to anxiety or fear. The benzodiazepines are the drug of choice for treatment of agitation. They include diazepam (Valium) and midazolam (Versed). When given intravenously they produce a sedating effect within minutes.

3. Does the patient need to be paralyzed? If it is necessary to cause total muscular relaxation along with apnea, a skeletal muscle paralyzing agent should be used. Usually a short-term, depolarizing neuromuscular blocker such as succinylcholine (Anectine) is used during a difficult intubation. A single intravenous dose paralyzes a combative patient for about 10 minutes. For paralysis during mechanical ventilation, one of the following long-term, nondepolarizing neuromuscular blocking agents is commonly used: pancuronium (Pavulon), atracurium (Tracrium), and vecuronium (Norcuron). These are all given intravenously and cause paralysis lasting 2 to 4 hours.

Remember that these paralyzing agents have no effect on the patient's ability to feel pain or to be afraid of what is happening. Pain medications, such as morphine, must be given as necessary. A sedating agent, such as Valium, is always given to counteract the emotional stress of being awake but unable to move.

 EXAM HINT

Expect to see one question requiring the therapist to recommend a medication for sedating an agitated patient receiving mechanical ventilation.

Wean the patient from the ventilator. Indications that the patient will tolerate weaning should include some, if not all, of the criteria listed in Box 14-5. It is not necessary that the patient pass each and every criteria. However, the more the patient can attain, the more likely he or she is to successfully wean. Individual physicians and practitioners may favor some of these conditions over others and may include other factors not listed.

There are patients who will not wean successfully even though objective criteria indicated that they should. Conversely, some patients can wean successfully even when objective criteria indicate that the patient will not succeed. The key point to keep in mind is that each patient must be evaluated individually. Look at the objective criteria, as well as how the patient actually performs during weaning.

Each of the five methods presented here has its advocates and a body of clinical evidence to show that it is a valid weaning technique. The practitioner must evaluate the patient before recommending any particular weaning method. The patient must also be evaluated during the weaning trial to determine if the method chosen is meeting his or her needs. The practitioner must be prepared to discontinue weaning if the patient is failing and be ready to try another weaning approach to help ensure success.

Ventilator discontinuance. Ventilator discontinuance is widely used with patients who have been ventilated for a short period and are now fully prepared to breathe on their own (Fig. 14-31, *A*). When the patient is stable, awake, and alert and meets the criteria listed in Box 14-5, he or she can be prepared for weaning. The patient should be instructed about the weaning, suctioned, and put in Fowler's or semi-Fowler's position if possible. The ventilator circuit is disconnected, and an aerosol and oxygen mix is breathed in through a T-piece (Brigg's adapter). The oxygen percentage should be the same as originally inspired or up to 10% higher, depending on the patient's PaO_2 level on the ventilator.

Ventilator discontinuance and weaning begin at the same moment. The patient goes from having the ventilator provide 100% of the minute volume needs to providing none of it. The patient should be watched continuously because he or she is now breathing totally independently. Vital signs and respiratory mechanics should be measured every 5 to 10 minutes throughout the procedure. If the patient deteriorates, ventilator therapy is reestablished. After a rest period, intermittent ventilator discontinuance or another mode of weaning might be tried. If the patient is stable, an ABG sample should be taken after about 20 minutes. Alternatively, pulse oximetry and end-tidal carbon dioxide can be monitored. If the blood gas results are acceptable and the patient appears stable, the weaning is continued or the patient can be extubated. Approximately 75% of patients who tolerate this procedure can be extubated.

Intermittent ventilator discontinuance. This method is used after the previously mentioned method proves less than successful. The patient is started on a schedule of intermittent weaning periods and rest periods on the ventilator (Fig. 14-31, *B*). The method shown has a cycle of lengthening weaning periods and shortening rest periods. This goes on until the patient is weaning for an extended period, as discussed earlier. Another method involves a cycle of set rest periods (commonly 0.5 to 1 hour) and lengthening weaning periods as the patient becomes stronger. Again, blood gas values should be monitored after about 20 minutes of weaning. The weaning period can be extended as long as the patient is stable or until extubated.

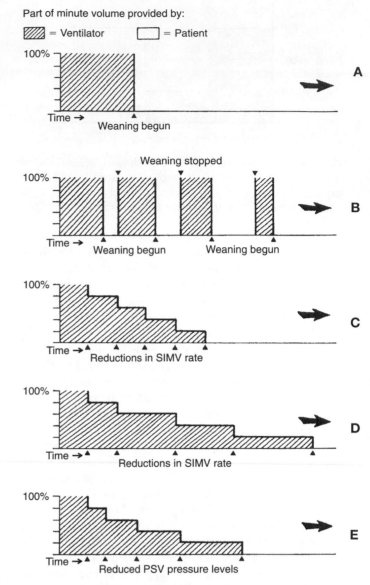

Fig. 14-31 A-E, Options for weaning a patient from mechanical ventilator. *PSV,* Pressure support ventilation; *SIMV,* synchronous intermittent mandatory ventilation.

Regular steps in SIMV weaning. As discussed earlier, IMV/SIMV was originally developed as a ventilating mode and has since become a widely-used weaning mode. It allows the patient a more gradual transition toward totally providing all of the WOB. SIMV seems to work especially well in weaning patients who have been ventilator dependent for an extended period. By gradually taking over more of the WOB, the patient reconditions respiratory muscles that may have atrophied through lack of use. The patient is also gaining self-confidence that complete weaning will occur. An additional benefit is that all ventilator alarm systems are functional and the patient does not need to be directly watched as closely as in the two previously mentioned weaning methods.

This particular SIMV weaning pattern can be applied to a patient who is stable and making rapid progress (Fig. 14-31, *C*). The weaning pattern might involve the

IMV rate being reduced in increments of about 2 per minute on a set time schedule. About 20 minutes after reducing the SIMV rate, blood gas values should be monitored. The patient's respiratory mechanics are monitored closely. It is important to calculate the patient's spontaneous minute volume (rate × tidal volume). It should be approximately the same volume as was subtracted from the ventilator-delivered minute volume. The process continues as long as the patient tolerates each decrease in the SIMV rate. The stable, strong patient can be rather quickly weaned down to an SIMV rate of 2 to 4 times/min. The decision is often made at this point to either use a T-piece, as discussed earlier, or to extubate the airway.

Irregular steps in SIMV weaning. This method is applied when the regular SIMV method is unsuccessful. Often, the patient starts out on a cycle of regular reductions in the SIMV rate. This goes on until a point is reached at which the patient has a setback and cannot tolerate any further reductions in the SIMV rate. The rate may be kept at that level for an extended period until the patient is ready for a further decrease (Fig. 14-31, *D*). Further drops in the IMV rate proceed as the patient tolerates them. No attempt is made to set up a regular pattern of reducing the rate.

It may be necessary to increase the rate to higher previous levels if the patient has a serious setback. One possible cause that may prevent the SIMV rate from dropping is the resistance to breathing through the demand-valve and breathing circuit. A trial on a T-piece (which offers no resistance) may prove to be the final step in weaning. If the patient fails this, the reason is probably the resistance caused by the endotracheal tube. The pressure support weaning method should then be tried on the patient.

Weaning by pressure support ventilation. The PSV mode is available on most modern electrically powered and microprocessor ventilators. It can be used as the newest weaning method (Fig. 14-31, *E*). When used as a weaning method, the pressure support level is gradually reduced. Decreasing pressure support steps of 2 to 5 cm water are commonly made. The patient has to gradually increase the WOB to inspire a tidal volume. Blood gas values and respiratory mechanics should be evaluated after each drop in the pressure support level. A modest pressure support level of 2 to 5 cm water is maintained to overcome any resistance of the endotracheal tube. If the patient does well during an extended trial of minimal pressure support, extubation is performed unless the endotracheal tube is needed for other reasons.

The criteria listed in Box 14-5 can be used in evaluating any patient being weaned by any of these methods. General signs that the patient is not tolerating weaning include anxiety, agitation, a large increase or decrease in the respiratory rate, angina, tachycardia, an increase in premature ventricular contractions or other serious dysrhythmias, bradycardia, hypertension, hypotension, cyanosis, hypoxemia, and hypercarbia with acidemia. The patient probably will not exhibit all of these signs. Some tend to be seen together because they relate to the patient's WOB. Others appear to give conflicting signals of success or failure. It is the practitioner's responsibility to evaluate the patient's condition to determine whether weaning should be continued or ventilatory support resumed.

Make a recommendation to extubate the patient. Extubation can usually be safely accomplished when the patient has met the criteria listed in Box 14-5, has demonstrated the ability to breathe effectively for a clinically significant period of time as measured by the listed criteria, has acceptable blood gas results, is alert enough to protect his or her airway, and can effectively cough out any secretions. It may be found that some patients need the endotracheal tube even though they no longer need ventilatory support. The tube provides a suctioning route if the patient is unable to cough out large amounts of secretions. The tube also protects the airway from the risk of aspiration in a comatose patient who may vomit.

| MODULE F | Respiratory care plan |

1. Participate in the development of the respiratory care plan [e.g., case management, development and application of protocols] (Code: IC4) [Difficulty: An]

Be prepared to make recommendations on changing ventilator parameters based on the patient's pathological condition, blood gas values, chest radiograph findings, breath sounds, and vital signs. Common recommendations follow.

EXAM HINT

Past Written Registry Examinations have had questions about the management of patients with the specific conditions such as increased intracranial pressure (ICP), COPD, congestive heart failure, ARDS, and pneumothorax. In addition, the Clinical Simulation Examination has at least one adult scenario on each of the following: a patient with COPD, a patient with trauma, a patient with cardiovascular disease, and a patient with neuromuscular or neurologic diseases. The management of these patients is briefly discussed in the following text.

Increased intracranial pressure. Intracranial pressure (ICP) is the pressure within the cranium (skull) and is normally less than 10 mm Hg. It is measured by a catheter placed into the subarachnoid space, subdural space, or ventricular space. The most common cause of an increased ICP is an acute head injury in which the brain is shaken. Other causes of increased ICP include craniotomy for brain tumor resection and stroke (cerebral vascular accident [CVA]). Any significant increase in the pressure within the skull will further injure the brain. Clinical experience has shown that when the ICP exceeds 20 mm Hg, the patient's outcome significantly worsens.

The A/C mode is usually selected with constant volume ventilation so that the patient is assured of a set minute volume if apnea occurs. It has been demonstrated that hyperventilating the patient to a $PaCO_2$ between 25 and 30 torr lowers the increased ICP. This is the result of the lowered carbon dioxide pressure causing cerebral vasoconstriction. Because the cerebral blood flow is decreased by hyperventilation, it is important to maintain the patient's PaO_2 in the 90 to 110 torr range.

Chronic obstructive lung disease (COPD). Patients with COPD are usually well known because of previous hospitalizations for acute exacerbations related to problems such as a lung infection or heart failure. When the patient must be ventilated, it is important to maintain baseline "normal" blood gas values. This usually means accepting moderate hypoxemia and hypercarbia with a compensated respiratory acidosis. Ventilating the patient to provide textbook normal ABGs must be avoided. This is because the COPD patient cannot maintain this level of breathing efficiency when ready to come off of the ventilator.

The A/C or SIMV mode may be used with either a constant volume set or PC used to set the tidal volume. A COPD patient must have the ventilator adjusted, including the addition of mechanical dead space, to maintain the patient's normally elevated $PaCO_2$ level. A PaO_2 of 60 to 70 torr is usually adequate. Keep the plateau pressure (alveolar pressure) less than 30 cm water to avoid overdistension of the patient's compliant lungs and resulting volutrauma.

If the patient has air trapping and auto-PEEP, a small amount of therapeutic PEEP may be added to help the patient exhale and trigger the ventilator. Increase the therapeutic PEEP in 1 cm water steps until the patient is synchronized with the ventilator. Many COPD patients need 5 cm water of PEEP or more. When the condition that caused the sudden deterioration is corrected, the patient should be weaned off of the ventilator as soon as possible to prevent atrophy of the ventilatory muscles.

Congestive heart failure (CHF). Patients with CHF usually also have a pulmonary edema problem. This results in hypoxemia and low lung compliance. Mechanical ventilation with the A/C or SIMV mode with constant volume ventilation is needed to reduce the patient's WOB, deliver supplemental oxygen, and add therapeutic PEEP. Usually a pulmonary artery catheter is placed to measure pulmonary artery pressure (PAP), pulmonary capillary wedge pressure (PCWP), and cardiac output (CO). If the PEEP level is increased and the patient's cardiac output decreases, the PEEP should be reduced to its previous level. The patient must be given a diuretic such as furosemide (Lasix) to increase urine output. The patient's heart function is improved by giving digitalis (Lanoxin). Closely follow the patient's cardiovascular values to monitor improvement following the administration of a diuretic and digitalis. Reduce the PEEP and inspired oxygen as the pulmonary edema problem is corrected.

Acute respiratory distress syndrome (ARDS). ARDS is caused by a variety of pulmonary and circulatory conditions that result in nonhomogenous damage to alveolar capillary membranes throughout the lungs. This results in noncardiac pulmonary edema with decreased pulmonary compliance and hypoxemia. Like the patient with CHF, the patient with ARDS needs mechanical ventilation to reduce the WOB, provide supplemental oxygen, and provide therapeutic PEEP. A pulmonary artery catheter is also needed to follow the patient's cardiovascular status. Also shunt ($\dot{Q}s$) studies may be performed.

Unlike the patient with CHF, the patient with ARDS does not respond as favorably to diuretic and digitalis medications. The continued problem of low compliance and resulting high ventilating pressures has been linked to volutrauma. Recent research as lead to the following lung protective strategies.

Small tidal volume ventilation.

Initially, most ARDS patients are started on the A/C or SIMV mode with constant volume ventilation. Unfortunately, many severe ARDS patients cannot be managed in this manner. The stiff lungs result in a very high plateau pressure and risk of pulmonary volutrauma. Recent studies have shown that the plateau pressure found in the alveoli (Pplat) must be kept ≤35 cm water to avoid this serious complication. To lower a dangerously high alveolar pressure, the tidal volume must be reduced. Many clinicians recommend that the patient be switched from constant volume ventilation to PCV to do this. Resent evidence has shown a higher survival rate in ARDS patients when the tidal volume was lowered from 12 mL/kg to 6 mL/kg of ideal body weight.

If the initial set of blood gases on PC with a small tidal volume do not show adequate oxygenation, the inspiratory time must be increased. Some ARDS patients need an increased inspiratory time such that the I:E ratio is inverse. This results in PCIRV. The advantages of PCIRV over conventional volume ventilation are the lowered peak airway pressure and the longer inspiratory time. The lowered peak pressure is thought to reduce the risk of volutrauma. The longer inspiratory time allows alveoli with long time constants of ventilation to fill and areas of atelectasis to reopen.

Permissive hypercapnia.

The small tidal volumes used with PCIRV can result in failure to blow off carbon dioxide to a normal level. There are times when this must be clinically accepted. Permissive hypercapnia involves allowing a $PaCO_2$ of ≥50 torr up to 100 to 150 torr. It is very important to prevent the carbon dioxide level from rising too rapidly because it causes cerebral vasodilation and increases the patient's ICP. To minimize this risk, the $PaCO_2$ should not be allowed to rise faster than 10 torr/hour to a maximum of 80 torr. If the $PaCO_2$ must be allowed to rise to >80 torr, the rate of increase must be slower than 10 torr/hour.

The high $PaCO_2$ also results in a respiratory acidosis. Keep the patient's arterial pH at ≥7.25 to avoid problems related to the acidosis. It may be necessary to administer intravenous bicarbonate to correct the respiratory acidosis. When the patient recovers, the $PaCO_2$ can be gradually lowered. If permissive hypercapnia was used for less than 24 hours, the $PaCO_2$ can probably be lowered by 10 to 20 torr/hr. If permissive hypercapnia was used for more than 24 hours or bicarbonate was given to buffer the pH, the $PaCO_2$ must be lowered more slowly. It is important to monitor the patient's arterial pH throughout this process to prevent too rapid an increase.

Lung inflection points.

An optimal PEEP study is justified to find the PEEP level needed correct the low lung compliance, severe hypoxemia, and large shunt problems these patients have. If possible, the lungs low and high inflection points should be determined. They relate to the lung compliance points at FRC and near total lung capacity. (Review Fig. 14-18 if needed.) A modern microprocessor ventilator with graphics software and a monitor should be employed to evaluate the these conditions. Set the unit to display a pressure/volume loop as shown in Fig. 14-32. Point *A* on the figure shows the low inflection point. This identifies the pressure needed to open up alveoli and establish the patient's FRC. When the therapeutic PEEP level is set at or above the lungs' low inflection point, they will be most effectively ventilated. This PEEP will likely need to be maintained for several days until the patient begins to recover. Point *B* on the figure shows the high inflection point. This identifies the highest lung volume and highest lung pressure that should be allowed. Further pressure does not greatly increase tidal volume and can result in volutrauma to any overstretched alveoli. Many clinicians use the high inflection point as the maximum pressure allowed with PCV to deliver a tidal volume.

Auto-PEEP recognition.

Auto-PEEP is end–expiratory pressure in the lungs that cannot be seen on the ventilator's pressure manometer. (The terms *inadvertent PEEP* or *intrinsic PEEP* are also used). Auto-PEEP is caused by air trapping because of an inadequate expiratory time. It becomes more likely when the inspiratory time is increased or the expiratory time is decreased, or in patients with long time constants of ventilation. Simply put, the next breath is delivered before the patient has exhaled completely. This problem is frequently seen in a patient with status asthmaticus or COPD because of early small airway closure. In patients with ARDS receiving PCIRV, the long inspiratory times used increase the risk of expiratory air trapping. Auto-PEEP is more likely to be found when the I:E ratio becomes 2:1 or greater.

The level of auto-PEEP can be determined in different

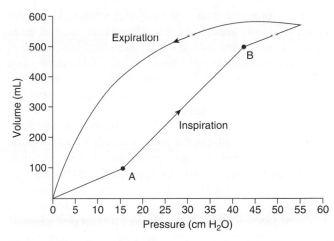

Fig. 14-32 Pressure-volume loop showing lower and upper inflection points in an ARDS patient. *A*, Shows lower inflection point indicating opening pressure of alveoli. This is minimum PEEP level needed to maintain patient's FRC. *B*, Shows upper inflection point indicating that lungs are being overstretched. This should be upper limit of peak airway pressure to avoid overdistension and volutrauma. Flattening of pressure-volume loop to right of point *B* shows that little volume is delivered despite increased pressure.

ways depending on the type of ventilator being used. It can be measured on the pressure manometer of most ventilators, such as the Servo 900 B. The trapped expiratory gas can also be seen on the graphic display of microprocessor ventilators such as the BEAR 1000, Nellcor Puritan Bennett 7200, Hamilton Veolar, and Drager Evita 4. The following procedure can be followed for determining the presence or level of auto-PEEP:

1. Note the delivery of a tidal volume.
2. Watch the pressure gauge as it drops to zero (or the level of therapeutic PEEP) at the end of exhalation. Make sure that the patient is exhaling passively to get an accurate reading.
3. Reduce the rate control to delay the next breath.
4. Occlude the expiratory tubing (or push the expiratory-hold button on the Servo 900 C or add inflation hold on other ventilators) to prevent any further exhalation for about 3 to 5 seconds.
5. If the pressure gauge is being monitored, note any pressure rise above the baseline pressure. Or, if the ventilator has a graphics monitor, noting the failure of the exhaled tidal volume or expiratory flow to return to baseline confirms the presence and amount of auto-PEEP (see Fig. 14-2).
6. Listen to the patient's breath sounds during a standard breath and during the prolonged exhalation. It is likely that during the standard breath the expiratory sounds will be heard until the inspiratory sounds begin. During the prolonged exhalation the expiratory sounds continue for a

longer time and then end with silence. This silent pause time indicates that there is no more expiratory airflow.

It is important to add any auto-PEEP to the amount of therapeutic PEEP the patient has. This should be recorded as the total PEEP. For example, the patient has 5 cm of therapeutic PEEP and 2 cm of auto-PEEP for 7 cm of total PEEP. It may be felt that the total PEEP level places the patient at risk for volutrauma or decreased venous return and lowered cardiac output. The amount of auto-PEEP can be reduced by decreasing the inspiratory time, increasing the expiratory time, or decreasing the tidal volume. Lack of auto-PEEP can be confirmed by this procedure. If the auto-PEEP cannot be eliminated, therapeutic PEEP can be added to match it. By raising the baseline pressure, the patient can more easily trigger an assisted or SIMV breath. It is especially important to decrease the auto-PEEP and therapeutic PEEP levels as the patient's lung compliance improves and airway resistance returns to normal.

With ARDS, as the lungs become more compliant, the PCIRV inspiratory time must be reduced toward normal to prevent the pressure from compressing the heart. Full exhalation of the tidal volume must be assured. This is not usually a problem because the stiff lungs rapidly recoil to the resting level (FRC).

Pneumothorax.

Recognize the signs of a pneumothorax on a mechanically ventilated patient (suddenly rising peak and plateau pressures, hypoxemia, mediastinal shift to the side opposite the pneumothorax, hyperresonant percussion note over the pneumothorax, and asymmetrical chest movement on inspiration) and be prepared to recommend the insertion of a pleural chest tube or to treat a tension pneumothorax (discussed later in this chapter and in Chapter 17). Common causes of the pneumothorax include lung puncture during the insertion of a CVP line via the subclavian vein, overinflated lungs from too large a tidal volume on the ventilator, punctured lung from a sharp broken rib, and thoracentesis.

Remember to get an ABG after every ventilator change that could result in a different PaO_2 (pulse oximetry or transcutaneous oxygen may be substituted) or $PaCO_2$ (end-tidal CO_2 or transcutaneous carbon dioxide may be substituted). Mixed venous blood gas values should also be obtained when possible.

Physical responses to mechanical ventilation, as measured by the vital signs, can vary considerably. A patient who is anxious, angry, or in pain will have an increase in the vital signs. A patient who is relaxed has reduced WOB, and whose blood gas values are now normal will have a return to normal vital signs. Watch carefully for the patient whose drop in blood pressure coincides with a tachycardia. This patient may be having decreased venous return to the heart from an increased intrathoracic pressure.

Because an intubated patient cannot speak, it is necessary to communicate by asking simple questions that can be answered in a *yes* nod or *no* shake of the head. Other methods of communication are a pad of paper and pencil or picture boards. It is not possible to predict how a patient will react to the initiation of mechanical ventilation or its prolonged need. Some patients react with relief and relax when the WOB is reduced. Others may become angry at the limitations imposed on them or become depressed.

2. Treat a tension pneumothorax (Code: IIID2) [Difficulty: R, Ap, An]

A chest radiograph and physical examination of the patient will reveal if air (or fluid) is abnormally found around the lung(s) or heart. If a patient has a tension pneumothorax, a pleural chest tube must be inserted on the affected side to remove the air and relieve the pressure within the chest. In an emergency, a large-gauge needle may be placed between the second and third ribs (second intercostal space) in the midclavicular line. These and related subjects are discussed in detail in Chapter 17. A nontension pneumothorax of greater than 10% is often also treated by inserting a pleural chest tube. In addition, a pleural chest tube is placed to remove blood or other fluid from the pleural space.

A pneumomediastinum, pneumopericardium, or pneumoperitoneum that puts the patient at risk must also be treated. A chest tube is then inserted into the area where the abnormal air is found. The same chest tube would also remove any abnormal collection of fluid. A pericardial chest tube is usually placed behind the heart to remove any blood that may leak out after open heart surgery.

3. Measure the volume of air lost through a patient's pleural chest tube (Code: IIIC8b) [Difficulty: Ap, An]

If the patient is being ventilated on a constant volume ventilator, the amount of air that is lost through the pleural chest tube can be calculated. This is done by subtracting the measured exhaled volume from the measured inhaled volume (the set tidal volume). The following equation demonstrates:

Inspired tidal volume = 500 mL
Exhaled tidal volume = − 400 mL

100 mL of tidal volume is lost
through the pleural chest tube

It is not always possible to measure a consistent tidal volume when PCV or a similar mode is used. In a case like this it is possible to make only a qualitative judgment on pleural air leak. In other words, if air is seen to bubble out through the pleural drainage system, an air leak is present. When the air stops bubbling, the pleural tear has healed. See Chapter 17 for a complete discussion on pleural drainage systems.

EXAM HINT

There is usually one question that deals with recognizing that a patient is losing tidal volume through a pleural chest tube.

BIBLIOGRAPHY

AARC Clinical Practice Guideline: Humidification during mechanical ventilation, *Respir Care* 37:887, 1992.

AARC Clinical Practice Guideline: Patient-ventilator system checks, *Respir Care* 37:882, 1992.

AARC Clinical Practice Guideline: Endotracheal suctioning of mechanically ventilated adults and children with artificial airways, *Respir Care* 38:500, 1993.

AARC Clinical Practice Guideline: Ventilator circuit changes, *Respir Care* 39:797, 1994.

AARC Clinical Practice Guideline: Long-term invasive mechanical ventilation in the home, *Respir Care* 40:1313, 1995.

AARC Clinical Practice Guideline: Removal of the endotracheal tube, *Respir Care* 44:85, 1999.

AARC Clinical Practice Guideline: Selection of device, administration of bronchodilator, and evaluation of response to therapy in mechanically ventilated patients, *Respir Care* 44:105, 1999.

Aloan CA, Hill TV, editors: *Respiratory care of the newborn and child*, ed 2, Philadelphia, 1997, Lippincott-Raven.

American Association for Respiratory Care: Consensus statement on the essentials of mechanical ventilation, *Respir Care* 37:1000, 1992.

Banner MJ, Lampotang S: Clinical use of inspiratory and expiratory waveforms. In Kacmarek RM, Stoller JK, editors: *Current respiratory care*, Philadelphia, 1988, BC Decker.

Barnes TA (ed): Core *Textbook of respiratory care practice*, ed 2, St Louis, 1994, Mosby.

Barnhart SL and Czervinske MP: *Perinatal and pediatric respiratory care*, Philadelphia, 1995, WB Saunders.

Bone RC: Pressure-volume measurements in detection of bronchospasm and mucous plugging in acute respiratory failure, *Respir Care* 21(7):620, 1976.

Bone RC: Monitoring ventilatory mechanics in acute respiratory failure, *Respir Care* 28:5, 1983.

Boysen PG, McGough E: Pressure-control and pressure-support ventilation: flow patterns, inspiratory time, and gas distribution, *Respir Care* 33(2):620, 1988.

Branson RD et al: Altering flowrate during maximum pressure support ventilation (PSV$_{max}$): effects on cardiorespiratory function, *Respir Care* 35:1056, 1990.

Branson RD, Chatburn RL: Technical description and classification of modes of ventilator operation, *Respir Care* 37:1026, 1992.

Branson RD, Hess DR, Chatburn RL, editors: *Respiratory care equipment*, ed 2, Philadelphia, 1999, Lippincott Williams & Wilkins.

Branson RD, Hurst JM: Laboratory evaluation of moisture output of seven airway heat and moisture exchangers, *Respir Care* 32:741, 1987.

Burton GC, Hodgkin JE, Ward JJ, editors: *Respiratory care: a guide to clinical practice*, ed 4, Philadelphia, 1997, Lippincott-Raven.

Cairo JM, Pilbeam SP: *Mosby's respiratory care equipment*, ed 6, St Louis, 1999, Mosby.

Chang DW: *Clinical application of mechanical ventilation*, ed 2, Albany, NY, 2001, Delmar.

Chatburn RL: A new system for understanding mechanical ventilation, *Respir Care* 36:1123, 1991.

Chatburn RL: Classification of mechanical ventilators, *Respir Care* 37:1009, 1992.

Corbridge T, Hall JB: Status asthmaticus in the adult: assessment, drug therapy, and mechanical ventilation, *Respir Manage* 21(5):119-126.

Dantzker DR, MacIntyre NR, Bakow ED, editors: *Comprehensive respiratory care*, Philadelphia, 1995, WB Saunders.

Drinker PA, McKhann CF III: The iron lung: first practical means of respiratory support, *JAMA* 256:1476, 1986.

Felix WR, MacDonnell KF, Jacobs L: Resuscitation from drowning in cold water, *N Engl J Med*, 304(14):843, 1981.

Fink JB, Hunt GE, editors: *Clinical practice in respiratory care*, Philadelphia, 1999, Lippincott- Raven.

Flasch M: Negative-pressure ventilatory support in the home, *Respir Ther* 16:21, 1986.

Greer K: Hypothermia: a quiet killer, *Adv Respir Ther*, Jan 15, 1990.

Guidelines for invasive applications with BiPAP systems, Respironics: Monroeville, Penn.

Gurevitch MJ: Selection of the inspiratory/expiratory ratio. In Kacmarek RM, Stoller JK, editors: *Current respiratory care*, Philadelphia, 1988, BC Decker.

Hess DR, Kacmarek RM: *Essentials of mechanical ventilation*. New York, 1996, McGraw-Hill.

Hess DR, McCurdy S, Simmons M: Compression volume in adult ventilator circuits: a comparison of five disposable circuits and a nondisposable circuit, *Respir Care* 36:1113, 1991.

Hill NS: Clinical application of body ventilators, *Chest* 90:897, 1986.

Hill NS et al: Efficacy of nocturnal nasal ventilation in patients with restrictive thoracic disease, *Am Rev Respir Dis* 145:365, 1992.

Hirsch C, Kacmarek RM, Stanek K: Work of breathing during CPAP and PSV imposed by the new generation mechanical ventilators: a lung model study, *Respir Care* 36:815, 1991.

Kacmarek RM: The role of pressure support ventilation in reducing work of breathing, *Respir Care* 33:99, 1988.

Kacmarek RM et al: Determination of ventilatory reserve in mechanically ventilated patients: A comparison of techniques, *Respir Care* 36:1085, 1991.

Kacmarek RM, Hess D: Pressure-controlled inverse-ratio ventilation: panacea or auto-PEEP? *Respir Care* 35:945, 1990.

Kirby RR: Modes of mechanical ventilation. In Kacmarek RM, Stoller JK, editors: *Current respiratory care*, Philadelphia, 1988, BC Decker.

MacIntyre NR: Pressure support ventilation: potential clinical application, Winter 1986, pp 1-7, Mead Johnson Pharmaceutical Division.

MacIntyre NR: Pressure support: inspiratory assist. In Kacmarek RM, Stoller JK, editors: *Current respiratory care*, Philadelphia, 1988, BC Decker.

MacIntyre NR: Weaning from mechanical ventilatory support: volume-assisting intermittent breaths versus pressure-supporting every breath, *Respir Care* 33:121, 1988.

MacIntyre NR, Branson, RD: *Mechanical ventilation*. Philadelphia, 2001, WB Saunders.

Martz KV, Joiner JW, Rodger MS: *Management of the patient-ventilator system: a team approach*, ed 2, St Louis, 1984, Mosby.

Pennock BE et al: Pressure support ventilation with a simplified ventilatory support system administered with a nasal mask in patients with respiratory failure, *Chest* 100:1371, 1991.

Pilbeam SP: *Mechanical ventilation: physiological and clinical applications*, ed 3, St Louis, 1998, Mosby.

Product literature on the suggested protocol for initiation of the BiPAP S/T or BiPAP S/T-D Ventilatory Support System, Respironics, Monroeville, Pennsylvania.

Quan SF, Parides GC, Knoper SR: Mandatory minute volume (MVV) ventilation: an overview, *Respir Care* 35:898, 1990.

Scanlan CL, Wilkins RL, Stoller JK, editors: *Egan's fundamentals of respiratory care*, ed 7, St Louis, 1999, Mosby.

Schinco MA, Formosa VA, Santora TA: Ventilatory management of a bronchopleural fistula following thoracic surgery, *Respir Care* 43:1064, 1998.

Shapiro BA et al, editors: *Clinical application of respiratory care*, ed 4, St Louis, 1991, Mosby.

Shelledy DC, Mikles SP: Newer modes of mechanical ventilation. I. Pressure support. *Respir Manage* pp 14-20, July/Aug 1988.

Shelledy DC, Mikles SP: Newer modes of mechanical ventilation. II. Mandatory minute volume ventilation, *Respir Manage* pp 21-28, July/Aug 1988.

Stoller JK: Establishing clinical unweanability, *Respir Care* 36: 186, 1991.

Strumpf DA et al: An evaluation of the Respironics BiPAP Bi-Level CPAP device for delivery of assisted ventilation, *Respir Care* 35:415, 1990.

The Acute Respiratory Distress Syndrome Network: Ventilation with lower tidal volumes as compared with traditional tidal volumes for acute lung injury and the acute respiratory distress syndrome. May 2000. http://www.nejm.org/content/brower/1.asp

Tobin MJ: Monitoring of pressure, flow, and volume during mechanical ventilation, *Respir Care* 37:1081, 1992.

Tobin MJ, Lodato RF: PEEP, auto-PEEP, and waterfalls, *Chest* 96:449, 1989.

Waldhorn RE: Nocturnal nasal intermittent positive pressure ventilation with bi-level positive airway pressure (BiPAP) in respiratory failure, *Chest* 101:516, 1992.

Whitaker K: *Comprehensive perinatal & pediatric respiratory care*, ed 2, Albany, NY, 1997, Delmar.

White GC: *Equipment theory for respiratory care*, ed 3, Albany, NY, 1999, Delmar.

Wright J, Gong H: "Auto-PEEP": Incidence, magnitude, and contributing factors, *Heart Lung* 19:352, 1990.

SELF-STUDY QUESTIONS

1. PCIRV is indicated in the following condition:
   A. Asthma
   B. Chronic bronchitis
   C. Pulmonary contusion
   D. ARDS

2. Mean airway pressure is defined as:
   A. P_{peak} minus the plateau pressure
   B. P_{peak} divided by inspiratory time
   C. The average pressure throughout the breathing cycle
   D. Tidal volume divided by peak pressure

3. Clinical factors causing decreased lung compliance include:
   I. Pulmonary edema
   II. Pulmonary fibrosis
   III. Emphysema
   IV. ARDS
   A. I and II only
   B. II and III only
   C. I, II, and IV only
   D. I, II, III, and IV

4. MMV ventilation is:
   I. Similar to A/C ventilation
   II. Indicated when weaning a patient with an unstable respiratory drive
   III. Designed to make sure that at least a minimum minute volume is delivered
   IV. A substitute for CPAP
   A. II and III only
   B. I only
   C. III only
   D. I and IV only

5. The Food and Drug Administration has approved high frequency ventilation for management of all of the following situations *except*:
   A. Laryngoscopy
   B. Near drowning
   C. Bronchopleural fistula
   D. Bronchoscopy

6. Weaning should be terminated when:
   I. The patient's rapid, shallow breathing index is 120.
   II. Cardiac dysrhythmias occur.
   III. The patient's $PaCO_2$ is 60 torr.
   IV. The patient's PaO_2 is 70 torr on 40% oxygen.
   A. I and III only
   B. II and IV only
   C. II, III, and IV only
   D. I, II, and III only

7. If a patient has just returned from surgery for a left pneumonectomy, the ventilator-delivered tidal volume should be:
   A. Less than normal based on ideal body weight
   B. The same as normal based on ideal body weight
   C. Larger than normal based on ideal body weight
   D. The same volume as delivered before surgery

8. The "iron lung" negative-pressure ventilator is indicated for all the following types of patients *except*:
   A. ARDS
   B. Neuromuscular defects
   C. Kyphoscoliosis
   D. COPD in acute failure

9. The parameters found with an ideal optimal PEEP study are:
    I. Pulmonary compliance improves
    II. PaO_2 rises
    III. Percent shunt decreases
    IV. Pulmonary vascular resistance increases
    V. Pulmonary vascular resistance decreases
    VI. Blood pressure falls and heart rate increases
    A. II, IV, and VI only
    B. I, II, III, and V only
    C. II, III, V, and VI only
    D. I, II, III, and IV only

10. What would be a patient's static compliance (C_{st}) if the corrected tidal volume is 600 mL, the ventilator's peak pressure is 65 cm water, the plateau pressure is 48 cm water, and there is 12 cm water of PEEP?
    A. 9 mL/cm water
    B. 11 mL/cm water
    C. 13 mL/cm water
    D. 17 mL/cm water

Use the following information for questions 11 and 12: Your ventilated patient has an exhaled tidal volume of 700 mL. Because of refractory hypoxemia, 6 cm of PEEP therapy is started. The peak pressure is 35 cm water and the static or plateau pressure is 25 cm water. The compliance factor has been determined to be 4 mL/cm water.

11. Calculate the static compliance (C_{st}) for this patient.
    A. 19 mL/cm water
    B. 24 mL/cm water
    C. 28 mL/cm water
    D. 32 mL/cm water

12. Calculate the dynamic compliance (C_{dyn}) for this patient.
    A. 16 mL/cm water
    B. 19 mL/cm water
    C. 24 mL/cm water
    D. 32 mL/cm water

13. When preparing for an HFJV with an APT 1010 unit it is necessary to have all of the following *except:*
    A. Spirometer to measure tidal volume
    B. Jet injector line
    C. High-pressure oxygen source
    D. Humidifier

14. Over the course of an 8-hour shift, the respiratory therapist notices that a patient receiving constant volume ventilation has had an increase in the peak pressure from 25 to 40 cm water. What could have caused this change?
    I. Airway resistance decreased
    II. Lung compliance increased
    III. Airway resistance increased
    IV. Lung compliance decreased
    A. III only
    B. IV only
    C. III and IV only
    D. I and II only

15. A 45-year-old patient has developed ARDS. The physician asks the respiratory therapist for the best ventilator adjustment to reduce the patient's intrapulmonary shunting. The therapist should recommend:
    A. Increasing the inspiratory time.
    B. Increasing the sigh volume.
    C. Decreasing the respiratory rate.
    D. Increasing the PEEP.

16. A trauma patient has a pleural chest tube to the left lung. A Nellcor Puritan Bennett 7200 ventilator is delivering an inspiratory tidal volume of 800 mL. The expiratory tidal volume is shown to be 600 mL. What could best explain the volume difference?
    A. Air leak through the chest tube
    B. Deflated endotracheal tube cuff
    C. Miscalibrated spirometers
    D. Bronchospasm and auto-PEEP

17. In a patient with ARDS, the indication to switch from volume-cycled ventilation to pressure-cycled ventilation is:
    A. Peak pressure of 35 cm water or greater.
    B. Lung compliance less than 35 mL/cm water.
    C. Plateau pressure of 35 cm water or greater.
    D. Peak pressure and plateau pressure total 35 cm water.

18. A 70-kg (154-lb) patient suffering from a stroke is being mechanically ventilated in the A/C mode with the following settings:

Minute ventilation	8.4 L
I:E ratio	1:2
F_IO_2	0.35
Rate	12
Mechanical dead space	150 mL

His ABG results are as follows:

pH	7.30
$PaCO_2$	51 torr
HCO_3-	24 mEq/L
PaO_2	107 torr

On the basis of this information, it would be most appropriate to recommend:
    A. Decreasing the F_IO_2
    B. Decreasing the minute ventilation
    C. Increasing the respiratory rate
    D. Decreasing the mechanical dead space

19. The chest radiograph of a patient receiving mechanical ventilation reveals atelectasis in both bases. In addition, the patient's breath sounds are diminished bilaterally and she has a low grade fever. Which of the following ventilator adjustments should the respiratory therapist recommend?
    A. Increasing the flow rate
    B. Lengthening the expiratory time
    C. Increasing the ventilator frequency
    D. Increasing the ventilator sigh volume

20. When permissive hypercapnia is being used to help manage a patient with ARDS, the following should be remembered:
    I. Bicarbonate may be given to increase the pH if needed.
    II. The carbon dioxide level is allowed to rise in a controlled manner.
    III. The pH should be kept between 7.45 and 7.35.
    IV. The pH should be kept greater than 7.25.
    V. The $PaCO_2$ should be kept between 40 and 50 torr.
    A. I, II, and IV only
    B. III and V only
    C. II and IV only
    D. II and V only

21. Your patient has the desire to breathe spontaneously and has a tidal volume that is 4 mL/kg of ideal body weight. Because

of facial trauma from an automobile accident, she has an endotracheal tube that is smaller than the ideal size. She also suffered lung contusions in the crash. Her PaO_2 is 63 torr on 55% oxygen. What ventilator mode(s) would you recommend for her?

A. A/C with flow-by for triggering the ventilator.
B. Low level pressure support ventilation with PEEP.
C. SIMV with low level pressure support and PEEP.
D. SIMV with high level pressure support (PSV_{max}).

22. An apneic 60-kg (132-lb) patient is being ventilated with the PC mode. Her ventilator settings are:

tidal volume	700 mL
rate	10/min
oxygen	60%
mechanical dead space	100 mL

Her ABG shows:

PaO_2	66 torr
$PaCO_2$	55 torr
pH	7.32
Base excess	0

Considering this information, all of the following individual ventilator adjustments would improve her ABG values *except*:

A. Increase the respiratory rate to 14/min.
B. Increase the tidal volume to 800 mL.
C. Change to an SIMV mode with a rate of 10/min.
D. Remove the mechanical dead space.

23. Indications that the patient is tolerating SIMV include all of the following *except*:

A. The respiratory rate is increased.
B. The heart rate is stable.
C. The blood gas results are stable.
D. Accessory muscles of ventilation are not being used.

24. Your 55-kg (120-lb) female patient is being ventilated with an SIMV rate of 10, tidal volume of 600 mL, 10 cm water of therapeutic PEEP, and 35% inspired oxygen. She has an 8.0 mm ID tracheostomy tube. Her spontaneous tidal volume is 350 mL and rate is 10/min. The most recent ABG shows PaO_2 95, $PaCO_2$ 42, and pH 7.40. What would you recommend?

A. Reduce the SIMV rate to 3
B. Reduce the PEEP to 7 cm water
C. Increase the SIMV rate to 12
D. Add 10 cm of pressure support

25. Five adult patients are being weaned from mechanical ventilation. Their bedside spirometry values are shown below.

	f	$\dot{V}E$ (L)	Vt (mL)	FEV_1 (mL/kg)	MIP (cm water)
Patient 1	7	2.45	350	5	−35
Patient 2	12	5.4	450	10	−30
Patient 3	15	8.25	550	15	−20
Patient 4	37	11.1	300	13	−15
Patient 5	40	17.0	425	7	−15

Which of the following patients may be ready for extubation?

A. Patients 1 and 2
B. Patients 1 and 4
C. Patients 2 and 3
D. Patients 3 and 5

26. The measurements below are obtained on a patient while he is being mechanically ventilated:

	6 PM	8 PM
Total respiratory rate	14	14
PEEP (cm water)	8	8
P plateau (cm water)	15	15
P peak (cm water)	30	45
Compliance (mL/cm water)	40	40

In this situation, the most appropriate action would be to:

A. Increase therapeutic PEEP.
B. Administer a bronchodilating agent.
C. Administer a diuretic agent.
D. Administer a paralyzing agent.

27. When working with a patient who recently had a bowel resection and is receiving a paralyzing medication to prevent fighting against the ventilator, it is important to:

A. Give the patient caffeine as a central nervous system stimulant.
B. Give the patient a sedative medication for pain.
C. Give the patient a narcotic medication for pain.
D. Talk quietly because the patient is probably sleeping.

28. If your ventilator-dependant patient has a large amount of thick tracheal secretions, it is best to:

A. Use a cascade-type humidifier warmed to body temperature.
B. Use a HME for his or her humidity needs.
C. Use no humidification system so that the secretions will dry out to some extent.
D. Either B or C is acceptable.

29. All of the following are needed to assemble a free-standing CPAP system *except*:

A. An exhaled volume spirometer
B. A low pressure or disconnect alarm
C. Water traps in the inspiratory and expiratory tubing
D. A device to create the CPAP pressure

30. A patient with a closed head injury and increased ICP is being mechanically ventilated in the A/C mode with an F_IO_2 of 0.3, a rate of 12, and a tidal volume of 700 mL. Her ABG results are shown below:

pH	7.44
$PaCO_2$	35 torr
PaO_2	295 torr

The physician orders a $PaCO_2$ of 25 torr for the patient. What should the respiratory therapist change on the ventilator to accomplish this?

A. Add 100 mL of mechanical dead space
B. Increase the tidal volume by 100 mL
C. Change to the PC mode
D. Decrease the ventilator rate to 10/min

31. Expiratory retard is indicated in the ventilator management of a patient with:

A. Pulmonary edema
B. Bronchospasm and air trapping
C. Pleural effusion
D. Pneumothorax

32. If the gas flow is inadequate to a closed- or positive-pressure IMV system all of the following will be seen *except*:

A. The anesthesia bag will be overinflated.
B. The pressure gauge will show a negative pressure during inspiration.
C. The anesthesia bag will be underinflated.
D. The patient's WOB will be increased.

33. An 80-kg (176-lb) male patient with bilateral pneumonia is being ventilated in the PC mode. The following data are available:

	8 AM	**12 PM**
Set respiratory rate	12/min	12/min
Total respiratory rate	16/min	26/min
Exhaled tidal volume	800 mL	600 mL
Inspiratory pressure	28 cm water	28 cm water

What is the most appropriate thing to do at this time?
A. Sedate the patient
B. Increase the set respiratory rate
C. Add 5 cm PEEP
D. Increase the inspiratory pressure

34. A 17-year-old female patient has been admitted with status asthmaticus and placed on a Drager Evita 4 ventilator. The physician wants to know if she has any auto-PEEP. Which ventilator waveform would be best for determining if the patient has any auto-PEEP?
A. Maximum voluntary ventilation tracing
B. Flow/volume loop
C. Flow/time
D. Pressure/time

Answer Key

1. **D.** Rationale: ARDS results in stiff lungs that are at risk of volutrauma if too large a tidal volume is forced into them. PCIRV is used with these patients because the peak pressure is limited to a safe level. The long inspiratory time used with PCIRV helps to oxygenate the patient. Asthma and chronic bronchitis are noted for high airway resistance, not stiffness of the lungs. These patients need a long expiratory time for complete exhalation. PCIRV would likely cause more air trapping because of the long inspiratory time and short expiratory time. A pulmonary contusion is a lung bruise from trauma. It is neither helped or hindered by PCIRV.

2. **C.** Rationale: Mean airway pressure is the average pressure throughout the breathing cycle. It is found by determining a series of inspiratory pressure and expiratory pressure points during short time intervals through a patient's breath cycle. See Fig. 14-30 for an example. P_{peak} minus the plateau pressure gives a general indication of airway resistance. P_{peak} divided by inspiratory time is used as a respiratory care calculation. Tidal volume divided by peak pressure is used to calculate dynamic compliance. See question 12 for an example.

3. **C.** Rationale: Pulmonary edema, pulmonary fibrosis, and ARDS are all conditions in which the lungs become stiff. This results in decreased lung compliance and increased WOB. Emphysema is caused by the loss of connective tissue within the lungs and results in increased lung compliance. As a result, the lungs are overinflated.

4. **A.** Rationale: MMV ventilation is used to provide a secure minimum minute volume to unstable patients. Often, these patients have an unstable respiratory drive because of a stroke or brain injury. MMV is a variation on SIMV; it does not allow the patient to trigger each breath like the A/C mode does. MMV is not like CPAP because MMV delivers mandatory tidal volume breaths.

5. **B.** Rationale: Near-drowning patients are traditionally ventilated with the A/C or SIMV mode with a constant volume. HFV has been shown effective in ventilating patients with airway procedures such as laryngoscopy and bronchoscopy. HFO has been shown effective in patients with a bronchopleural fistula because the small tidal volumes and low driving pressures do not force gas out through the lung tear. This allows the tissues to heal.

6. **D.** Rationale: Review the indications for ventilatory support in Box 14-1. These indications include a rapid, shallow breathing index of >105, $PaCO_2$ of >55 torr, and cardiac dysrhythmias. The patient is not dangerously hypoxic with a PaO_2 of 70 torr.

7. **A.** Rationale: Because the patient's left lung has been removed, he or she should have a delivered tidal volume that is about half of normal for two lungs. Giving a normal or larger than normal tidal volume for two lungs is likely to overdistend the patient's one remaining lung.

8. **A.** Rationale: ARDS is characterized by very stiff lungs. A negative-pressure ventilator is unable to generate enough pressure to adequately ventilate any patient with low lung compliance. Also, an iron lung does not offer any modes other than Control and cannot add PEEP. The other three conditions (neuromuscular defects, kyphoscoliosis, and COPD in acute failure) are not as challenging to ventilate. These patients are not intubated and only require assisted ventilation for a short period of time. Negative-pressure ventilation has been used with these patients successfully.

9. **B.** Rationale: Review Box 14-3 and Fig. 14-18 for information on the evaluation of an optimal PEEP study. As PEEP establishes the patient's FRC the pulmonary compliance should improve. Ventilation better matches perfusion so that shunt will decrease and PaO_2 will rise. In addition, the patient's pulmonary vascular resistance (PVR) decreases as the lungs are properly ventilated and bloodflow through them is normalized. If too much PEEP is applied, the lungs will be overstretched. This causes the PVR to increase and cardiac output to drop as venous return to the lungs and heart is decreased. As a result, the patient's blood pressure falls and heart rate increases.

10. **D.** Rationale:

$$C_{st} = \frac{\text{exhaled tidal volume} - \text{compressed volume}}{\text{plateau pressure} - \text{PEEP}}$$

In this situation use the corrected tidal volume because the compressed volume has already been subtracted from the exhaled tidal volume. The following equation results:

$$C_{st} = \frac{600 \text{ mL}}{48 - 12}$$
$$= \frac{600 \text{ mL}}{36}$$
$$C_{st} = 17 \text{ mL/cm water}$$

11. **D.** Rationale: Static compliance (C_{st}) is calculated as follows:

$$C_{st} = \frac{\text{exhaled tidal volume} - \text{compressed volume}}{\text{plateau pressure} - \text{PEEP}}$$

compressed volume =
compliance factor × plateau pressure (4 mL/cm water × 25 cm water) = 100 mL

$$C_{st} = \frac{700 \text{ mL} - 100 \text{ mL}}{25 - 6}$$
$$= \frac{600 \text{ mL}}{19}$$
$$C_{st} = 32 \text{ mL/cm water}$$

12. **B.** Rationale: Dynamic compliance (C_{dyn}) is calculated as follows:

$$C_{dyn} = \frac{\text{exhaled tidal volume} - \text{compressed volume}}{\text{peak pressure} - \text{PEEP}}$$

compressed volume =
compliance factor × peak pressure (4 mL/cm water × 35 cm water) = 140 mL

$$C_{dyn} = \frac{700 \text{ mL} - 140 \text{ mL}}{35 - 6}$$
$$= \frac{560 \text{ mL}}{29}$$
$$C_{st} = 19 \text{ mL/cm water}$$

13. **A.** Rationale: HFJV involves the delivery of very small tidal volume breaths at a very high rate. It is impractical to try to measure these very small tidal volumes. The other three listed items plus a high-pressure air source, suitable patient circuit, and the ventilator itself are needed for HFJV.

14. **C.** Rationale: An increased airway resistance (caused by bronchospasm or airway secretions) causes the peak pressure to increase. A decrease in lung compliance (caused by pulmonary edema, pneumonia, or pleural effusion) causes the plateau pressure to increase. This, in turn, drives up the peak pressure. Without having both the peak and plateau pressures, there is no way to know more specifically what has caused the peak pressure to rise. If either the lung compliance had increased or the airway resistance had decreased, the peak pressure would have decreased.

15. **D.** Rationale: Therapeutic PEEP increases a patient's FRC. This increased lung volume enables better ventilation and perfusion matching. As a result, intrapulmonary shunting past underventilated alveoli is reduced. Increasing inspiratory time and sigh volume improves alveolar filling and may help to increase oxygenation. However, they do not increase FRC and, therefore, do not reduce shunting.

16. **A.** Rationale: A 200 mL air leak through the pleural chest tube would explain the difference in delivered and returned tidal volumes. If the patient had a deflated endotracheal tube cuff, the delivered tidal volume would be decreased. The selected ventilator is microprocessor driven and has the ability to monitor itself. There would have been a warning of a system failure such as miscalibrated spirometers. There is no indication that the patient has asthma or any condition causing bronchospasm. This ventilator has the ability to monitor auto-PEEP and none is indicated.

17. **C.** Rationale: Recent research has shown that alveolar overstretching and damage can occur when the plateau pressure is 35 cm water or greater. Therefore the patient should be switched from volume-cycled ventilation to pressure-cycled ventilation (pressure control) with a peak pressure of no higher than 35 cm water. A high peak pressure may be caused by high airway resistance or lung stiffness. Lung compliance is calculated from tidal volume divided by plateau pressure. There is no direct connection between calculated lung compliance and alveolar overstretching. Both peak pressure and plateau pressure should be monitored. However, the combination has no direct connection to alveolar overstretching.

18. **D.** Rationale: Interpretation of the patient's ABG results indicate hypercarbia and resulting respiratory acidosis. The best solution to the problem is to remove the 150 mL of mechanical dead space. There is no urgent need to decrease the patient's 35% oxygen because this is not a toxic amount. Decreasing the patient's minute volume further raises the carbon dioxide level and lowers the pH. Although increasing the respiratory rate would help to blow off some carbon dioxide, the best solution is to remove the dead space. After another set of ABG's are drawn and analyzed, the rate can be increased if still needed to blow off CO_2.

19. **D.** Rationale: Atelectasis is best treated by giving the patient a larger sigh volume. This should help to open up alveoli that have collapsed or are prone to collapsing. Changing flow rate, expiratory time, and ventilator frequency have no impact on lung volume.

20. **A.** Rationale: Permissive hypercapnia involves the gradual increasing of a patient's carbon dioxide level such that the pH does not become overly acidotic. It may be necessary to give the patient intravenous bicarbonate to keep the pH greater than 7.25. During permissive hypercapnia, the patient's $PaCO_2$ can rise well above 50 torr and the pH will probably fall below the normal range of 7.35.

21. **C.** Rationale: SIMV allows the patient to breath spontaneously when she wants to while still receiving support from the ventilator. A low level of pressure support should help to reduce her added WOB from the small endotracheal tube. Therapeutic PEEP is justified because of her PaO_2 measurement of only 63 torr on 55% oxygen. The A/C mode does not allow her to take any totally spontaneous tidal volume breaths. In addition, she would benefit from some therapeutic PEEP. A high level of pressure support (PSV_{max}) does not offer her the "safety net" of support offered by SIMV at this stage of her recovery. Some therapeutic PEEP is needed.

22. **C.** Rationale: Interpretation of the patient's ABG values shows an increased carbon dioxide level with resulting respiratory acidosis. An SIMV rate of 10/min does not increase the patient's baseline minute volume from the PC rate of 10. Because the patient is apneic, she will not be adding to the minute volume total. The patient's minute volume will be increased by both a higher respiratory rate and a larger tidal volume. Removing the mechanical dead space will prevent the patient from rebreathing her own carbon dioxide. All three of these options result in a lower $PaCO_2$ and correction of the low pH.

23. **A.** Rationale: Review Box 14-2 for indications of SIMV tolerance/intolerance if needed. An increased respiratory rate (usually accompanied by a falling tidal volume) indicates that the patient is fatigued and needs more ventilator support. Review the rapid, shallow breathing index calculation shown in Box 14-1 if needed. Stable vital signs and blood gas values indicate good tolerance of the WOB. Lack of accessory muscle use indicates that the diaphragm is strong enough to ventilate the patient.

24. **B.** Rationale: ABG results show adequate oxygenation. Therefore the PEEP level can be safely reduced from 10 to 7 cm water. A drop in SIMV rate from 10 to 3 is too large. A smaller rate drop from 10 to about 6 is more reasonable at this stage in the patient's recovery. ABG results show adequate ventilation. There is no need to increase the SIMV rate at this time. There is no indication that the patient has an increased airway resistance problem that would justify the addition of pressure support. Her tracheostomy tube is the appropriate size and her spontaneous rate and tidal volume are adequate.

25. **C.** Rationale: Review Box 14-5 for indications of the ability to wean. Only patients 2 and 3 have all parameters within the normal ranges listed. Patient 1 has a low respiratory rate, tidal volume, and forced expiratory volume in one second (FEV_1). Patient 4 has a fast respiratory rate, low tidal volume, and low MIP. Patient 5 has a fast respiratory rate, low FEV_1, and low MIP.

26. **B.** Rationale: The only patient parameter that has changed significantly is the increase in P peak from 30 to 45 cm water. This can be caused only by an increase in airway resistance. Although several things can cause this (bronchospasm, secretions, biting or kinking of the endotracheal tube), the only option that fits is giving a bronchodilating agent. Increasing PEEP has no effect on airway resistance. A diuretic agent (such as Lasix) would help to eliminate pulmonary edema and lower a patient's plateau pressure (P plateau). However, this value is unchanged, so no worsening is indicated. A paralyzing agent will not affect any of the recorded patient values.

27. **C.** Rationale: Even though the patient is paralyzed and cannot request a medication for pain relief, the patient can feel the surgical pain. Paralyzing medications do not block touch (pain) or the other senses. A narcotic medication (morphine) is justified for pain relief. Caffeine does not have a role in the care of a patient who has been pharmacologically paralyzed. A sedative medication may be given to relieve any anxiety the patient may have but it would not affect the patient's pain. Unfortunately, there is no easy way to tell when the paralyzed patient is awake or sleeping. Regardless, it is important to talk normally to the patient so that he or she knows what medical care is being given.

28. **A.** Rationale: An AARC Clinical Practice Guideline recommends the use of a cascade-type humidifier warmed to body temperature to help liquify thick secretions. A HME should be used only if the patient has few secretions. The secretions should not be allowed to dry out. If they did it would be very difficult to remove them by suctioning.

29. **A.** Rationale: A spirometer is not needed because the patient's tidal volumes cannot be accurately measured while on the CPAP system. If a spirometer were incorporated into the CPAP system, it would register continuous flow rather than patient volumes. An alarm system is needed for patient safety and water traps are used to keep the tubing clear. A pressure-generating device must be added to set and maintain the CPAP level.

30. **B.** Rationale: Increasing the tidal volume from 700 to 800 mL will decrease the patient's $PaCO_2$ toward the goal. Another ABG sample should be taken in 15 minutes to see if the ordered $PaCO_2$ of 25 torr has been achieved. Adding 100 mL of mechanical dead space will raise, rather than lower, the patient's carbon dioxide level. Changing to the PC mode with the same settings will maintain the same minute volume and same $PaCO_2$ as present. Decreasing the ventilator rate from 12 to 10/min results in a higher, rather than lower, carbon dioxide level.

31. **B.** Rationale: Expiratory retard acts like pursed lips breathing in a patient with bronchospasm to put backpressure on the small airways. This results in a more complete exhalation. None of the other conditions is helped by expiratory retard. It is possible that the pneumothorax would be worsened by the added pressure, causing more air to leak through the torn lung tissue.

32. **A.** Rationale: Review Fig. 14-27 for the closed- or positive-pressure IMV system. If flow is not adequate to the reservoir bag, it will be underinflated, not overinflated. When the patient inspires, there will be a negative pressure shown on the pressure gauge. This negative pressure confirms that the patient is having to work harder than normal to inhale.

33. **D.** Rationale: The drop in patient tidal volume is significant. Probably the patient's lung compliance has worsened. The patient has increased his respiratory rate to make up for the lost minute volume. The best solution is to increase the pressure control inspiratory pressure to produce the previous tidal volume of 800 mL. Sedating the patient will result in a dramatic drop in minute volume with resulting hypercarbia and hypoxia. Increasing the set respiratory rate will deliver a higher minute volume and relieve the patient of some of the burden of triggering the ventilator. However, it will not correct the main problem—a decreased tidal volume. Without blood gas results to document hypoxia, there is no indication to add PEEP.

34. **C.** Rationale: The flow/time tracing enables any auto-PEEP to be detected. See Fig. 14-2 for the graphic. The maximum voluntary ventilation tracing is done in the pulmonary function laboratory to evaluate a patient's overall breathing ability. It is not useful for detecting auto-PEEP. A flow/volume loop can be done on many microprocessor ventilators and is helpful in evaluating flow at the end of exhalation. However, the flow/time tracing is the best detector of auto-PEEP. A pressure/time tracing (see Fig. 14-1, *B*, top graphic) is not helpful in detecting auto-PEEP.

MODULE A	Perform continuous positive airway pressure and continuous mechanical ventilation to achieved adequate artificial ventilation and/or recommend modifications in ventilatory support based on the patient's response

Analysis of the most recent versions of the Written Registry Examination reveals an average of two questions (2% of the test) that deal with the application of continuous positive airway pressure (CPAP) or mechanical ventilation to the neonate. The National Board of Respiratory Care (NBRC) tests much more heavily on the application of these techniques with adult patients. Of the 10 scenarios presented in the Clinical Simulation Examination, expect one neonatal and one pediatric patient. CPAP and/or mechanical ventilation may be involved in both situations.

1. Initiate and adjust continuous positive airway pressure (CPAP) breathing (Code: IIIB4a) [Difficulty: An]

a. Physiologic effects

CPAP and positive end-expiratory pressure (PEEP) increase the patient's functional residual capacity (FRC). In neonates, the most common cause of a decreased FRC is infant respiratory distress syndrome (RDS). This condition is caused by the lack of surfactant in the lungs of the premature neonate. The neonate with RDS has relatively airless lungs that are prone to atelectasis. This results in hypoxemia. In addition, each tidal volume breath requires a greater than normal inspiratory effort (see Fig. 15-1). The restoration of FRC in the neonate increases its PaO_2, decreases the percentage of shunt, narrows the alveolar to arterial difference in oxygen, and reduces its work of tidal volume breathing. CPAP must be used with caution in neonates with persistent pulmonary hypertension (PPHN) of the newborn. An excessive amount of pressure in the alveoli compresses the capillary bed. This decreases pulmonary blood flow, which in turn increases blood flow through the patent ductus arteriosus and worsens the problem.

b. Indications, contraindications, and hazards

CPAP is indicated for any condition that results in an unacceptably low PaO_2 secondary to a decreased FRC. Some neonates respond so well to CPAP that mechanical ventilation is not needed. In addition, CPAP has been used to keep open the airways of infants with tracheal malacia or other conditions in which the airways collapse abnormally.

In general, contraindications include any CPAP-related condition that results in a worsening of the patient's original status. Some neonates cannot tolerate CPAP and progressively hypoventilate as the pressure level is increased. Clinical judgment is needed to decide how high the $PaCO_2$ should be allowed to rise before discontinuing the CPAP and beginning mechanical ventilation. In general, the $PaCO_2$ should not be greater than 50 torr as long as the pH is at least 7.25. An absolute contraindication is apnea resulting in hypoxemia and hypotension. These infants should be mechanically ventilated. Box 15-1 gives a complete listing of indications, contraindications, and hazards.

c. Initiation

> **EXAM HINT**
>
> Questions on the Written Registry Examination typically ask about the indications to start CPAP, the initial CPAP setting, CPAP adjustment, and when to switch from CPAP to mechanical ventilation.

Before starting CPAP, a set of baseline arterial blood gases should be taken. Transcutaneous oxygen monitoring or pulse oximetry may be substituted in some clinical situations if oxygenation is the only parameter that must be measured. The neonate's vital signs should also be recorded. Assemble the CPAP circuit and pressure device. The decision must be made whether to apply the CPAP above the epiglottis (Figs. 15-2 and 15-3) or to intubate the infant and apply the CPAP within the trachea. Nasal CPAP (NCPAP) or nasopharyngeal tube CPAP (NP-CPAP) are both widely used to apply pressure from above the epiglottis. The neonate or infant must have an endotracheal tube placed to apply CPAP within the trachea. Among the factors to be considered are the neonate's gestational age and weight, the amount of secretions that need to be suctioned, the pulmonary problem, and the likelihood of mechanical ventilation eventually becoming necessary. More mature and larger infants with few secretions and relatively stable pulmonary conditions will most likely have CPAP applied above the epiglottis by nasal prongs or nasopharyngeal tube. In contrast, less mature and smaller infants (less than 1000 to 1200 g) who need suctioning and have relatively unstable pulmonary conditions will probably be intubated. Mechanical ventilation can then be easily started if needed.

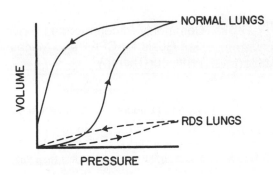

Fig. 15-1 Pressure-volume curves for normal neonate and for one with infant respiratory distress syndrome (RDS). Normal neonate's lungs inhale a relatively large tidal volume at low pressure. Note how when the same pressure is placed against the lungs of infant with RDS the tidal volume is much smaller. To get a normal tidal volume the RDS infant must generate a much greater negative pressure. (From Carlo WA, Martin RJ: *Pediatr Clin North Am* 33:221, 1986.)

CPAP is usually started at about 4 to 5 cm water pressure whether the pressure is applied above or below the epiglottis. The inspired oxygen percentage is usually kept at the previously set level. It is important to make only one change at a time so that each adjustment in care can be evaluated for its own effect. For example, if you simultaneously increased the oxygen percentage by 10% and started 5 cm water of CPAP, it would not be known whether the increase in PaO_2 was from the additional oxygen, the CPAP, or both. Usually the long-term inspired oxygen is limited to 40% to 50% because of concern of the possibility of pulmonary oxygen toxicity.

d. Adjustment and weaning

Blood gases and vital signs must be evaluated at the starting CPAP level. The heart rate, blood pressure, and respiratory rate should be stable or improved. Blood gases should be measured in about 10 minutes. See Table 15-1 for the recommended blood gas limits. In general, the PaO_2 should be kept between 60 and 70 torr, $PaCO_2$ less than 50 to 55 torr, and pH at least 7.25. If the PaO_2 is too low and the patient's vital signs are acceptable, the CPAP may be increased in a step of 2 cm water. The vital signs and blood gases should then be reevaluated. If necessary, the process of adding CPAP and reassessing the patient can be continued. It is rare to find that more than 10 cm water CPAP is necessary. The maximum CPAP level in a neonate is generally held to be 12 cm water; the maximum CPAP level in an infant is generally held to be 15 cm water.

Mechanical ventilation is usually indicated if more than these maximum CPAP pressures are needed to correct hypoxemia. Depending on the patient, even levels less than these maximum CPAP pressures may not be well tolerated. The infant may become exhausted from exhaling against the back pressure of the CPAP system. That is seen

INDICATIONS
Infant respiratory distress syndrome (RDS)
Atelectasis
Pulmonary edema
Apnea of prematurity
Tracheal malacia
Recent extubation
Transient tachypnea of the newborn
Physical examination shows some, if not all, of the following:
  Respiratory rate 30-40% greater than normal
  Substernal and suprasternal retractions
  Nasal flaring
  Expiratory grunting
  Cyanosis
  Chest radiograph shows atelectasis or pulmonary edema
Arterial blood gases showing:
  PaO_2 less than 50 torr on 60% or more oxygen
  Adequate ventilation with a $PaCO_2$ less than 50 torr and pH greater than 7.25
Weaning from mechanical ventilation when the intermittent mandatory ventilation (IMV) rate is about 4-12/min, the pulmonary condition is improved, blood gases show acceptable $PaCO_2$, and there is acceptable PaO_2 on PEEP. The CPAP level is set to match the level of PEEP used on the ventilator.

CONTRAINDICATIONS
Prolonged apnea leading to hypoxemia and hypotension (begin mechanical ventilation)
Untreated pneumothorax or other evidence of a pulmonary gas leak
Unstable cardiovascular status such as bradycardia and hypotension
Inadequate ventilation with a $PaCO_2$ greater than 50 torr and pH less than 7.25
Unilateral pulmonary problem: untreated congenital diaphragmatic hernia
Nasal CPAP should not be used on a patient with cleft palate, choanal atresia, or tracheoesophageal fistula

HAZARDS
Persistent pulmonary hypertension of the newborn (PPHN)
Increased intracranial pressure that can cause intraventricular hemorrhage
Decreased cardiac output
CPAP may be ineffective if the neonate weighs less than 1000-1200 grams

clinically as decreased chest movement from the smaller tidal volume. The $PaCO_2$ will probably increase. It may be necessary to place the infant on mechanical ventilation to decrease the work of breathing and then add PEEP to maintain the FRC. When nasal prongs or a nasopharyngeal tube are used, CPAP pressures of greater than 8 cm water may cause the infant's mouth to open. This results in the

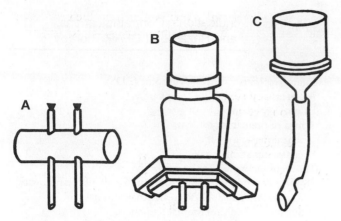

Fig. 15-2 Nasal CPAP devices for infants. **A,** Jackson-Reese tubes. **B,** Argyle nasal cannula (prongs). **C,** Endotracheal tube cut shorter for nasopharyngeal insertion (NP tube). (From Blodgett D: *Manual of pediatric respiratory care procedures,* Philadelphia, 1982, JB Lippincott.)

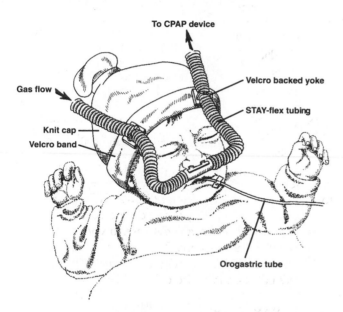

Fig. 15-3 An assembly for supporting nasal CPAP prongs in an infant. (Modified from advertisement of Stayflex tubing system from Ackrad.) (From Sills JR: *Respiratory care registry guide,* ed 1, St Louis, 1994, Mosby.)

loss of CPAP. A crying infant also opens its mouth and loses the CPAP. In either case, the CPAP pressure gauge drops to zero or fluctuates below the set pressure.

As the patient improves, it is necessary to reduce the CPAP level so as not to cause pulmonary barotrauma. The pressure level can be reduced in steps of about 2 cm water. The vital signs and blood gases should be reassessed after each step. The apparatus is usually removed when the CPAP level is down to 2 to 4 cm water. The infant is then placed into an oxyhood at the same oxygen percentage as before or 5% to 15% higher. If the infant has an

TABLE 15-1	Commonly Recommended Blood Gas Goals for CPAP and Mechanical Ventilator Therapy	
	Age of neonate	
	Less than 72 hours	**Greater than 72 hours**
PaO$_2$ (torr)	60-70	50-70
PtcO$_2$ (torr)	Greater than 50,* less than 90*	Greater than 40,* less than 90*
SpO$_2$	92-96%	92-96%
PaCO$_2$ (torr)	35-45†	45-55
PtcCO$_2$ (torr)	May be used after correlation with PaCO$_2$ as discussed in Chapter 3.	
pH	7.25-7.45	7.25-7.45

*PtcO$_2$ values may be used after they have been shown to correlate within 15% of the PaO$_2$ from an arterial blood gas.
†With CPAP, this value may be increased to 50 to 55 torr as long as the pH is at least 7.25.
NOTE: Keep the PaO$_2$ no greater than 80 torr in the premature neonate to reduce the risk of retinopathy of prematurity.

endotracheal tube that is needed for suctioning or a secure airway, the pressure is usually left at 2 to 4 cm water. After extubation, the infant is placed into an oxyhood as before.

If the infant was breathing more than 50% oxygen while on the CPAP, it may be more important to lower the oxygen before decreasing the CPAP level. The following guidelines may prove helpful when deciding whether to first lower the oxygen percentage or the CPAP level:

a. If the patient has been breathing more than 50% oxygen for more than 48 hours and has stable vital signs without any pulmonary barotrauma, decrease the oxygen first. Lower the inspired oxygen in 5% to 15% steps and check the oxygenation level after each reduction. Attempt to get the oxygen down to 40%, if possible. Then decrease the CPAP level.

b. If the patient is breathing 50% oxygen or less and has unstable vital signs or pulmonary barotrauma, decrease the CPAP first. After the CPAP is reduced (or removed entirely) and the patient is stable, reduce the inspired oxygen percentage.

2. Mechanical ventilation

a. Change the type of ventilator to be used on the patient (Code: IIIC8b) [Difficulty: An]

Most neonatal patients requiring life support receive time-triggered, pressure-limited, time-cycled mechanical ventilation (TPTV). These ventilators are pneumatically powered with electrical controls and alarm systems. They are used in the IMV mode and feature a continuous flow of gas. They are pressure limited to prevent an excessive peak airway pressure and can have therapeutic PEEP added. Furthermore, they are capable of reaching the Food and Drug Administration (FDA) limited rate of 150 breaths/

min. The majority of neonatal and small pediatric patients can be effectively ventilated on these types of units.

High frequency ventilation (HFVF) with a small tidal volume has been approved by the FDA for use in the rescue of neonates with RDS and a bronchopulmonary fistula or pulmonary interstitial emphysema (PIE) who fail under conventional TPTV ventilation. HFV has also been used in the short-term support of neonates with a congenital diaphragmatic hernia until corrective surgery can be performed.

A volume-cycled ventilator can be used on an infant who weighs more than 10 kg (22 lb). Any conventional volume-cycled ventilator can be used if it can be set to deliver a tidal volume as small as 50 mL. Volume-oriented ventilation can also be performed with a neonatal TPTV-type ventilator if the patient is apneic. This technique is discussed later.

When selecting a ventilator it is important to choose one that offers the features needed to ventilate the patient. For example, if real-time graphics are needed to evaluate the patient's response to a ventilator adjustment, the proper unit will be needed. Any selected ventilator must be able to meet the typical tidal volume goal for a neonatal or small pediatric patient of 6 to 8 mL/kg. A patient receiving HFV for an FDA-approved pulmonary problem has a smaller tidal volume goal.

b. Initiate and adjust different combinations of assist/control (A/C), intermittent mandatory ventilation (IMV), synchronous intermittent mandatory ventilation (SIMV), and therapeutic PEEP (Code: IIIB2c and IIIB4b) [Difficulty: An]

With traditional neonatal TPTV, a set tidal volume is not ordered and cannot be measured. With volume-cycled ventilation of a pediatric patient, the tidal volume is ordered just as it is with an adult patient. Typically the therapist is expected to set the following ventilator controls based on a protocol or the patient's condition and response to the ventilator: sensitivity, flow, I:E ratio, alarms, and humidified gas temperature.

1. Sensitivity

There is no sensitivity control on traditional continuous flow TPTV-type neonatal ventilators. The IMV mode is used with these units. Some of the newer ventilators have the ability to sense a neonate's respiratory effort and trigger a machine delivered breath. The BEAR Cub does this with an add-on feature that senses a change in flow when the neonate inspires. The Drager Babylog 8000 has this flow-sensing feature built into the unit. The Sechrist IV-200 uses two electrocardiogram leads on the neonate's chest to sense a change in electrical impedance (skin resistance) as a sign of respiratory effort. A child on a volume-cycled ventilator should have the sensitivity set at about −1 to −2 cm water pressure. No matter which method the ventilator

uses to sense the patient's respiratory effort, the neonate or child should not have to work very hard to trigger a machine tidal volume.

2. Flow

Flow is adjusted to set the inspiratory time and I:E ratio and/or to meet the patient's needs.

3. I:E Ratio

The I:E ratio is adjusted to ensure that the patient can inhale in as physiologically appropriate a manner as possible and can completely exhale the inspired tidal volume. A ventilator with real-time graphics can reveal the presence of auto-PEEP (incomplete exhalation).

4. Alarms

Alarm systems are different for each type of ventilator. Generally speaking, they are set with a safety margin of ±10% from the patient's normal ventilator settings. A variation of greater than 10% results in an audible or visual alarm condition.

5. Humidified gas temperature

The goal for most patients is to minimize their humidity deficit by giving gas that is humidified and warmed to near body temperature. It is common to have the gas warmed to 90° to 95°F/35°C. It should be measured in the inspiratory limb of the circuit as close to the patient as possible.

A review of the literature dealing with neonatal critical care shows that there are few universally accepted strategies for the use and modification of CPAP/PEEP and mechanical ventilation. What is presented here is an attempt to describe what are widely accepted approaches to neonatal TPTV and related therapy. The approach used in this discussion focuses on adjusting the ventilator and treating a neonate based on its pathologic problem.

3. Indications for mechanical ventilation

All authors agree that apnea is an absolute indication for mechanical ventilation. A general indication is any condition that causes respiratory failure. This is usually documented by unacceptable arterial blood gases. Box 15-2 lists indications for mechanical ventilation.

MATH REVIEW

TIME CONSTANTS OF VENTILATION

Note: This concept has not been directly tested by the NBRC. It is hoped that understanding the concept of time constants as used here and in the later text will help the reader understand lung pathology and why certain ventilator adjustments are made.

It is important in any patient requiring mechanical ventilation to consider both the patient's lung-thoracic compliance and

BOX 15-2 Common Indications for the Initiation of Mechanical Ventilation

RESPIRATORY FAILURE
PaO₂ less than 50 torr despite maximal CPAP therapy (10-12 cm water) and 60% or more inspired oxygen
PaCO₂ greater than 60 torr and pH less than 7.25

NEUROLOGIC
Complete apnea
Apneic periods leading to hypoxemia and bradycardia
Intracranial hemorrhage
Drug depression

PULMONARY CONDITIONS
Infant respiratory distress syndrome (RDS)
Diffuse pneumonia
Pulmonary edema
Meconium aspiration
Diaphragmatic hernia

PROPHYLACTIC USE
Cyanotic congenital cardiac defect
Persistent pulmonary hypertension of the newborn (PPHN)
Postoperatively after major thoracic or abdominal surgery

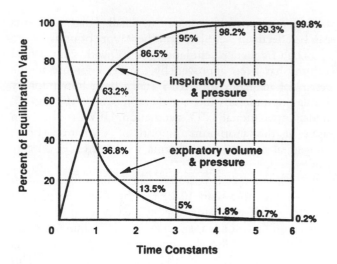

Fig. 15-4 Graphic presentation of the percentage of inspiratory and expiratory volume and pressure in comparison with time constants of ventilation. (From Chatburn RL: *Respir Care* 36:569, 1991.)

airway resistance when setting inspiratory and expiratory times. This is especially important in neonates because, in comparison with adults, they are less compliant and have greater resistance. In addition, neonates are usually ventilated at faster rates. As a review, the respective lung-thoracic compliances (C_{LT}) and airway resistances (R_{AW}) of normal adults and infants are shown here:

Adult lung-thoracic compliance: 100 mL/cm water pressure (0.1 L/cm water pressure)
Neonatal lung-thoracic compliance: 5 mL/cm water pressure (.005 L/cm water pressure; about 20 times stiffer than an adult)
Adult airway resistance: 2 cm water/L/sec
Neonatal airway resistance: 20 to 40 cm water/L/sec (about 10 to 20 times more resistance to airflow than an adult)

The placement of an endotracheal tube to facilitate mechanical ventilation will results in a total pulmonary resistance ranging from 50 to 150 cm water/L/sec. The time constant of ventilation (T_c or time constant of the respiratory system T_{RS}) is calculated as the product of compliance and resistance:

Time constant in seconds = compliance (L/cm water) × resistance (cm water/L/sec)

For example, using these values for a spontaneously breathing normal neonate, its time constant is calculated as:

T_c = compliance (.005 L/cm water) × resistance (30 cm water/L/sec)
= .005 × 30 seconds
= .15 seconds

Although technically impractical to measure the time constant of ventilation at the bedside, the concept is important

because it relates to two important clinical considerations during mechanical ventilation. First, it relates to the pressure that develops at the alveolar level as the tidal volume is delivered. For each time constant, progressively more of the peak inspiratory pressure (PIP) is applied within the alveoli (see Fig. 15-4). As can be seen, at three time constants 95% of the PIP is applied to the alveoli. At five time constants, virtually the entire PIP is applied at the alveolar level. Second, the time constant relates to how rapidly the lung recoils to baseline (FRC) during an exhalation. As shown in Fig. 15-4, it will takes three time constants to exhale 95% and five time constants to completely exhale.

The clinical significance of this relates directly to the pulmonary condition of the patient. Infants with stiff lungs and normal resistance, as found in RDS, have a short time constant. Alveolar pressure quickly increases to match the peak inspiratory pressure. The lungs then rapidly recoil during exhalation so that there is little chance of air trapping. Infants with normal compliance and increased resistance, as found in meconium aspiration, have a long time constant. It takes a relatively long time for the alveolar pressure to reach the PIP. Also, a relatively long time is needed for the exhalation to be complete. Because of this, these infants are at risk for air trapping and auto-PEEP.

4. Initiation and adjustments based on the patient's condition
a. Patients with normal cardiopulmonary function
Patients with normal cardiopulmonary function may need mechanical ventilation because of apnea from anesthesia, paralysis, or a neurologic condition. The initial TPTV ventilator parameters for this type of patient are listed in Box 15-3. Once mechanical ventilation is established, it is important to evaluate the patient's blood

BOX 15-3	Common Mechanical Ventilator Parameters for Neonates With Normal Lungs

Delivered tidal volume: 6-8 mL/kg (This may be estimated by calculation if the neonate is apneic and the pressure limit is not reached until the end of the inspiratory time.)

Pressure limit (peak inspiratory pressure or PIP): 10-20 cm water

Frequency: 10-20/min

I:E ratio: 1:2 to 1:10

Inspiratory time (T_I): at least 0.4 seconds

Expiratory time (T_E): at least 0.5 seconds

PEEP: none unless 2-4 cm water is added to replace "epiglottal PEEP"

Inspiratory flow: sufficient to see the chest move and hear bilateral breath sounds during the inspiration. 5-8 L/min commonly used; or start with at least twice the infant's estimated minute volume (respiratory rate × estimated tidal volume of 7 mL/kg). Check the blood gases for the $PaCO_2$.

Oxygen percentage: 40%

---

gases, vital signs, breath sounds, and any other pertinent clinical information before changing any ventilator parameters.

As the patient recovers and begins to breathe spontaneously, it will probably be necessary to reduce the ventilator-delivered minute volume. This encourages the child to breathe more because the final goal is to completely wean and extubate the patient. The most accepted way to reduce the ventilator-delivered minute volume is to reduce the ventilator rate. A reduction of about 10% is a good starting place but must be tailored to meet the patient's needs. The tidal volume is maintained as originally set. Obtain a set of blood gases in 10 to 20 minutes (or follow the transcutaneous or pulse oximetry values) and check the patient's vital signs to see how well the adjustment is tolerated.

If the blood gases show an elevated $PaCO_2$, the ventilator-delivered minute volume must be raised. This can be done by increasing either the alveolar ventilation or respiratory rate. Alveolar ventilation can be increased by either increasing the inspiratory flow or pressure limit (if it has been reached) to increase the tidal volume. The ventilator rate may be increased if the flow and pressure limit cannot be increased. An increase of about 10% is a good starting place but must be tailored to meet the patient's needs. As before, blood gases and vital signs should be monitored after every change to see if the increase is well tolerated and accomplishing what was intended.

If the blood gases show that the $PaCO_2$ is lower than desired, the ventilator-delivered minute volume must be decreased. The first parameter to adjust is usually the rate. Try decreasing the rate by about 10% and check another set

of blood gas values. If other parameters need to be reduced, try decreasing the inspiratory flow or inspiratory time about 10% to decrease the tidal volume. Again, check the blood gas values after every adjustment.

If the blood gases show that the PaO_2 is higher or lower than necessary, the oxygen percentage must be adjusted. An increase or decrease of about 5% is a good starting place but must be adjusted as needed. If the patient does not respond to the increased oxygen as expected, the patient should be reevaluated. It may be necessary to reclassify him or her into one of the following categories.

MATH REVIEW

CALCULATION OF ESTIMATED TIDAL VOLUME DURING TPTV MECHANICAL VENTILATION

The NBRC examination content outline does not specifically list estimated tidal volume calculations. However, the information may be useful in understanding concepts presented later in the text.

If the neonatal patient receiving TPTV is apneic and neither assisting nor fighting against the ventilator-delivered breath, it is possible to calculate an approximate tidal volume. This is referred to as volume-oriented ventilation by some authors. The following formula is used:

$$\text{Calculated tidal volume} = (T_I \times \dot{V}) - V_c$$

In which:

T_I = inspiratory time (It is important that either the pressure limit is not reached or the pressure limit is reached at the same time inspiratory time is completed. If the pressure limit is reached before the inspiratory time limit is reached, part of the inspiratory time is spent as an inflation hold and no additional tidal volume is delivered.)

$\dot{V}$ = inspiratory flow rate on the ventilator in mL/sec

V_c = volume compressed in the circuit and ventilator (This is found by multiplying the peak inspiratory pressure by the manufacturer's stated compliance factors for the circuit and ventilator.)

For example, estimate the delivered tidal volume for an apneic 5 kg infant. The ventilator parameters are: inspiratory flow 5.5 l/min, frequency of 20/min, I:E ratio of 1:3, inspiratory time of 0.75 seconds, and expiratory time of 2.25 seconds. Peak inspiratory pressure (PIP) is 15 cm water. The internal compliance of the ventilator is 0.4 mL/cm water and the circuit compliance factor is 1.6 mL/cm water.

$$\text{Calculated tidal volume} = (T_I \times \dot{V}) - V_c$$

In which:

T_I = .75 seconds

$\dot{V}$ = 5.5 L/min. This is converted to mL/sec by dividing the flow in L/min by 60 seconds. So 5.5 L/min = .092 L/sec or 92 mL/sec

V_c = 0.4 + 1.6 mL/cm water = 2 mL/cm water = 2 mL/cm water × 15 cm water PIP = 30 mL

Therefore:

$$\text{Calculated tidal volume} = (0.75 \text{ sec.} \times 92 \text{ mL/sec}) - 30 \text{ mL}$$
$$= (69 \text{ mL}) - 30 \text{ mL}$$
$$= 39 \text{ mL}.$$

This is within the ideal tidal volume range of 30 to 40 mL (based on 5 kg weight × 6 to 8 mL/kg).

It must be emphasized that this is only a calculated tidal volume. Leaks in the system, a decrease in the patient's compliance, or an increase in the patient's resistance decreases the true tidal volume. Conversely, an increase in the patient's compliance or a decrease in the patient's resistance increases the true tidal volume. Also, if the pressure limit is reached before the inspiratory time is completed, less volume than expected will be delivered. This is because part of the inspiratory time is spent as an inflation hold and no additional tidal volume is delivered (see Fig. 15-5). Finally, the infant must be completely passive during the delivery of the breath.

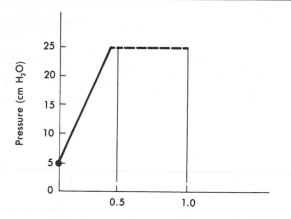

Fig. 15-5 Pressure-time curve seen with pressure limit set at 25 cm water and inspiratory time being increased from 0.5 to 1 second. Pressure limit is reached when inspiratory time is about 0.5 second. As inspiratory time is increased to 1 second (or greater), the pressure limit is held at 25 cm water resulting in a "square wave" pressure curve. (From Betis P, Thompson JE. In Koff PB, Eitzman DV, Neu J: *Neonatal and pediatric respiratory care,* St Louis, 1988, Mosby.)

b. Patients with decreased lung compliance and normal airway resistance such as Infant Respiratory Distress Syndrome (RDS)

Although RDS is the most common cause of decreased lung compliance and normal airway resistance, it is seen in other lung conditions including pneumonia and pulmonary edema (see Fig. 15-6). The greatest challenge presented in the care of these infants is to oxygenate them without causing oxygen toxicity or pulmonary barotrauma. Common recommendations for the initial ventilator settings are listed in Box 15-4. As discussed earlier, blood gases, vital signs, and so forth must be monitored after the infant is placed on the ventilator. Any further adjustments can then be determined and evaluated by another set of blood gases and vital signs.

BOX 15-4   Common Mechanical Ventilator Parameters for Neonates With Low Compliance and Normal Resistance

Delivered tidal volume: 6-8 mL/kg
Pressure limit: 20-25 cm water (This may need to be increased up to 35-40 cm water.)
Frequency: 30-60/min (This may need to be raised up to 150/min.)
I:E ratio: 1:2 (This may eventually need to be altered to an inverse I:E ratio.)
Inspiratory time (T_I): between 0.4 and 0.7 seconds (This may need to be increased.)
Expiratory time (T_E): at least 0.5 seconds (This may need to be decreased.)
PEEP: 2-4 cm water initially (This may need to be increased up to 8-10 cm water.)
Inspiratory flow: sufficient to see the chest move and hear bilateral breath sounds during the inspiration. 5-8 L/min commonly used. As a general rule, the faster the rate is, the higher the flow must be to deliver an adequate tidal volume. Check the blood gases for the $PaCO_2$.
Oxygen percentage: 40% (This may need to be increased to keep the SpO_2 greater than 92%.)

Fig. 15-6 Comparison of the lung volumes and capacities of a 6-year-old child, normal infant, and an infant with IRDS. Note relatively high compliance and low resistance of a normal child compared with an infant, and infant with RDS compared with normal infant. (From Chatburn RL, Lough MD. In Lough MD, Doershuk CF, Stern RC, editors: *Pediatric respiratory therapy,* ed 3, St Louis, 1985, Mosby.)

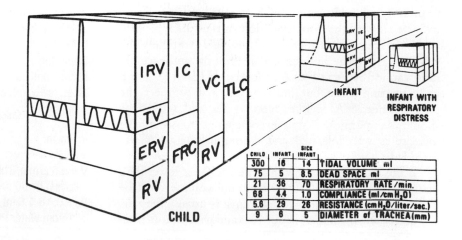

CHILD	INFANT	SICK INFANT	
300	16	14	TIDAL VOLUME ml
75	5	8.5	DEAD SPACE ml
21	36	70	RESPIRATORY RATE /min.
68	4.4	1.0	COMPLIANCE (ml/cm H₂O)
5.6	29	28	RESISTANCE (cm H₂O/liter/sec.)
9	8	5	DIAMETER of TRACHEA (mm)

The issue of time constants of ventilation help to better understand the various options available for adjusting the ventilator. As presented earlier, the time constant of ventilation (T_c or time constant of the respiratory system T_{RS}) is calculated as the product of compliance and resistance. For example, using the following values for a mechanically ventilated neonate with RDS, its time constant is calculated as:

T_c = compliance (.001 L/cm water because the lungs are less compliant) × resistance (100 cm water/L/sec because the infant is intubated) Simplify as follows:

= .001 × 100 second

= .1 seconds (Compare this with a T_c of .15 for a normal, spontaneously breathing neonate.)

Neonates with RDS have a relatively short time constant; therefore the tidal volume and ventilating pressure are delivered rather quickly to the lungs. However, because the lungs are so stiff, there is usually no problem with the tidal volume being fully exhaled as long as five time constants are allowed. An expiratory time of at least 0.5 seconds is usually set initially. The various options available for increasing oxygenation are discussed on the following pages.

1. Administer oxygen, as needed, on the ventilator to prevent hypoxemia (Code: IIIC3a) [Difficulty: An]

Up to 100% oxygen can be given to the neonate in the short term. Hypoxemia cannot be tolerated and supplemental oxygen is usually the best way to correct it. See Chapter 14 for equations that can be used to predict the oxygen percentage change needed to correct the patient's hypoxemia. Although hypoxemia cannot be tolerated, there are several limiting factors. First, it is commonly held that giving more than 50% oxygen for more than 48 to 72 hours increases the risk of pulmonary oxygen toxicity. Second, if more than 80% oxygen is given, some poorly ventilated alveoli will have all of the oxygen absorbed from them, leading to denitrogenation absorption atelectasis. Third, keep the neonate's PaO_2 below 80 torr to minimize the risk of retinopathy of prematurity (ROM). Fourth, if the hypoxemia is caused by a decreased FRC because of the lack of surfactant and small lung volumes, increasing the oxygen will not markedly increase the PaO_2. Other solutions, such as those discussed later, must be used.

2. Increased inspiratory flow

Increasing the flow increases the tidal volume until the pressure limit is reached. Increasing the tidal volume should result in an increased PaO_2 and is likely to reduce the $PaCO_2$. If the pressure limit is reached, the delivered tidal volume is held in the lungs for the duration of the inspiratory time. This acts as an inflation hold and should also increase the PaO_2. The mean airway pressure is raised

by increasing the flow. (See Fig. 15-7 for the pressure waveforms seen during low-flow and high-flow conditions.) Under high-flow conditions the pressure waveform takes on a characteristic square shape (square wave) because the pressure limit is reached. This pattern of ventilation is currently widely used with these types of patients.

3. Increased inspiratory time leading to inverse ratio ventilation

As with increasing the flow, increasing the inspiratory time increases the tidal volume until the pressure limit is reached. If the pressure limit is reached, any increased inspiratory time acts as inflation hold. This also raises the mean airway pressure and should result in an increased PaO_2. (See Fig. 15-5 for the pressure waveform change as the inspiratory time is increased.)

Some authors have advocated an increased inspiratory time as an important way to improve oxygenation. This has led to the use of inverse I:E ratios of up to 3:1 (.33) or 4:1 (.25) to produce an adequate PaO_2. The inspiratory time

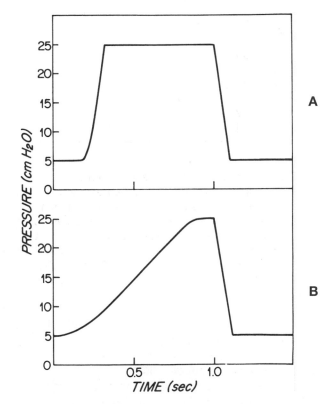

Fig. 15-7 Comparison of pressure-time curves showing influence of inspiratory flow when the pressure limit is set at 25 cm water pressure. **A,** Curve at high flow rate. Pressure limit is reached very early in the inspiratory time with resulting "square wave" flow pattern. **B,** Curve at low flow rate. Pressure limit is not reached until inspiratory time is almost 1 second. (From Chatburn RL, Lough MD. In Lough MD, Doershuk CF, Stern RC, editors: *Pediatric respiratory therapy,* ed 3, St Louis, 1985, Mosby.)

should be increased in small time increments and followed in 10 to 20 minutes with a blood gas to determine if the desired improvement in oxygenation was achieved. Inspiratory time is increased only as long as necessary to result in a satisfactory PaO_2. Great care must be taken to adjust expiratory time, respiratory rate, or both when a prolonged inspiratory time is used. Obviously, expiratory time must be reduced to keep the same rate as the inspiratory time is increased, or the rate must be reduced as the inspiratory time is increased if the expiratory time cannot be reduced. Care must be taken to ensure that the tidal volume is fully exhaled to avoid auto-PEEP.

As the neonate's lung compliance improves, the inspiratory time must be decreased for two reasons. First, the alveolar pressure is more readily transmitted throughout the lungs and may decrease venous return to the heart. That results in a decreased cardiac output. Second, the more normal lungs are more prone to barotrauma or volutrauma. The inspiratory time should be decreased in small time increments and followed with a set of blood gases to be sure that the neonate is not hypoxemic.

4. Increased positive end-expiratory pressure (PEEP)

Increased PEEP has the greatest effect on improving the patient's FRC and is probably the most effective at increasing the PaO_2. As discussed in regard to CPAP therapy, the pressure is usually started out at 4 to 5 cm water. A blood gas is then checked and, if necessary, PEEP is added in 2 to 3 cm water increments. Commonly, between 4 and 7 cm are needed; it is rare for more than 10 cm of PEEP to be needed. Another blood gas should be checked for PaO_2 after every addition of pressure. PEEP has the greatest impact on raising the mean airway pressure of all the options presented here. Excessive PEEP may cause a decreased venous return to the heart and decreased cardiac output. It also may cause barotrauma resulting in PIE, pneumothorax, or pneumomediastinum. Care must be taken to carefully evaluate the patient after each increase in PEEP. Watch for a sudden deterioration in the patient's condition as a sign of a pulmonary air leak. As the patient's PaO_2 improves, the PEEP level should be reduced in steps of about 2 to 3 cm water. As always, recheck the blood gases with each adjustment.

5. Increased pressure limit

To deliver a larger tidal volume, it may become necessary to increase the pressure limit when it is reached by the peak inspiratory pressure. It may also be necessary to raise the pressure limit to restore the original tidal volume after the addition of PEEP. This is because the original tidal volume is reduced when PEEP is added and the peak inspiratory pressure reaches the pressure limit. This is shown in Fig. 15-8. To restore the original tidal volume the pressure limit (and peak inspiratory pressure) must be increased by the same amount as the added PEEP. It is

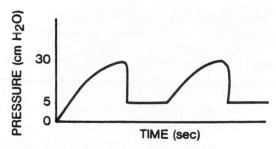

Fig. 15-8 Pressure-time curve showing effect of addition of PEEP on tidal volume. Initially, tidal volume is delivered by pressure difference of 30 cm water (difference between 0 and 30 cm water pressure). With addition of 5 cm water PEEP, pressure difference is reduced to 25 cm water (difference between 5 and 30 cm water pressure). This results in less tidal volume being delivered. (From Burgess WR, Chernik V: *Respiratory therapy in newborn infants and children,* ed 2, New York, 1986, Thieme.)

important to remember that as PEEP is reduced, the pressure limit must also be reduced by the same amount. This maintains the original tidal volume.

6. Increased respiratory rate

Increasing the ventilator respiratory rate increases the minute volume and probably raises the PaO_2 and lowers the $PaCO_2$. Patients with stiff lungs and short time constants of ventilation often respond well to an increased respiratory rate. To that end, some authors advocate using a rate of up to 150/min on a conventional time-triggered, pressure-limited, time-cycled mechanical ventilator, if necessary. (It should be noted that the FDA has set the upper rate limit of 150/min on these units.) A rate of greater than 150/min is termed high frequency ventilation (HFV) and requires a special ventilator. This procedure and the needed equipment are discussed later.

7. Instillation of exogenous surfactant

In 1991 the FDA approved the use of exogenous surfactant that can be directly instilled into the lungs of RDS neonates. Exosurf Neonatal (a synthetic product), Survanta (a bovine lung extract), and Curosurf (a pig lung extract) have been successfully used clinically. These drugs have proven very beneficial to premature neonates with inadequate natural surfactant. After the drug is administered, the patient's lung compliance improves dramatically. Usually, the drug allows rapid reductions in the ventilator-delivered oxygen percentage, rate, pressure limit, and PEEP.

Each of the options discussed in this section has its advocates; however, it seems logical that the best possible care would come from the proper application of each option when it is best suited to the patient's condition. To that end, Chatburn, Waldemar, and Lough (1983) have developed a rather comprehensive approach to the adjustment of the various ventilator parameters to optimize the care of the RDS infant. They use the initial and subsequent blood gas results to direct the various ventilator changes that have been discussed. Because of the complexity of the logic in the algorithm, it is recommended that their articles, listed in the references, be read to fully appreciate its use.

c. Patients with increased airway resistance and normal lung compliance such as meconium aspiration syndrome (MAS)

Although meconium aspiration is a commonly seen cause of increased airway resistance, it is also seen in infants with excessive airway secretions or bronchospasm. These neonates usually have normal lung compliance and their clinical problem is getting enough air into and out of the lungs. The meconium or other obstruction causes uneven airflow and results in hypoxemia, air trapping, auto-PEEP, and an increased risk of barotrauma or volutrauma. Because of these issues, there are two key clinical goals. The first is to minimize turbulence during inspiration by reducing the inspiratory flow rate as much as possible. The second is to give a long enough expiratory time to prevent air trapping. Common recommendations for the ventilator settings are listed in Box 15-5. As discussed earlier, blood gases, vital signs, and so forth must be monitored after the infant is placed on the ventilator. Listen to the breath sounds to detect the end of exhalation and a pause before the start of the next inspiration. This is to ensure that the exhalation has been complete and there is no air trapping that would lead to auto-PEEP. Any further adjustments can then be determined and evaluated by another set of blood gases and vital signs.

Look again at the issue of time constants of ventilation to better understand the various options for adjusting the ventilator. Using the following values for a mechanically ventilated neonate with meconium aspiration, its time constant is calculated as follows:

T_c = Compliance (.005 L/cm water) × resistance (150 cm water/ L/second because the infant is intubated and has an obstructive problem) Simplify as follows:

= .005 × 150 second

= .75 second (Compare this with a T_c of 0.15 for a normal, spontaneously breathing neonate and a T_c of 0.1 for a ventilated infant with RDS.)

This relatively long time constant means that the tidal volume and peak inspiratory pressure are rather slowly delivered to the alveoli. There is little chance of causing barotrauma or volutrauma from high ventilating pressures, however, it takes a fairly long inspiratory time to deliver an adequate tidal volume. Care must be taken to provide enough expiratory time for the tidal volume to be exhaled completely. Briefly then, the challenge is to deliver an adequate tidal volume to maintain acceptable blood gases at a rate slow enough to prevent air trapping on exhalation.

BOX 15-5	Common Mechanical Ventilator Parameters for Neonates With Increased Airway Resistance and Normal Lung Compliance

Delivered tidal volume: 6-8 mL/kg

Pressure limit: less than 20 cm water

Frequency: 20-40/min

I:E ratio: 1:3 to 1:10

Inspiratory time (T_I): between 0.4 and 0.7 seconds (This may need to be increased.)

Expiratory time (T_E): at least 0.5 seconds (This may need to be increased.)

PEEP: 2-4 cm water if needed

Inspiratory flow: sufficient to see the chest move and hear bilateral breath sounds during the inspiration. 5-8 L/min commonly used.

Oxygen percentage: 40% (This may need to be increased to keep the SpO_2 greater than 92%.)

In general, the inspiratory flow and rate are kept low, inspiratory and expiratory times are kept relatively long, and the I:E ratio should favor a long time for complete exhalation. Furthermore, it is important to frequently suction the airway to remove meconium or secretions. Postural drainage and percussion are also provided to mobilize the secretions so that they can be suctioned out. Usually these procedures and the natural breakdown of meconium result in reduced airway resistance within a few days. Ventilatory support can then be lessened.

d. Patients with persistent pulmonary hypertension (PPHN) of the newborn

PPHN is also referred to as persistent pulmonary hypertension (PPH), persistent fetal circulation (PFC), or persistence of the fetal circulation. Infants with PPHN present clinically with an elevated pulmonary artery pressure and a right-to-left shunt through a patent ductus arteriosus and/or the foramen ovale. Because of this, their oxygenation fluctuates greatly. The problem may be seen right after birth or up to 24 hours later. PPHN seems to result from fetal hypoxemia and acidosis. These, in turn, are caused by or associated with maternal drug addiction, infection, preeclampsia, abruptio placenta, postterm gestation, oligohydramnios, and meconium staining or aspiration. The following four tests are done to help confirm the diagnosis:

1. Hyperoxia test: This is the first test and is done after an arterial blood gas has shown a low PaO_2. The test involves having the patient inspire 100% oxygen for about 10 minutes and obtaining a second arterial blood gas. If the PaO_2 does not improve to more than 50 torr, a fixed right-to-left shunt is proven. The shunt may be from PPHN or a cyanotic heart

defect. If the PaO_2 does go over 100 torr, the neonate probably has parenchymal lung disease and should be treated accordingly.

2. Preductal and postductal arterial blood sampling: Simultaneously draw and then analyze (1) a blood gas sample from the right radial or brachial artery to check the preductal PaO_2, and (2) a blood gas sample from the left brachial, left radial, either femoral artery, or the umbilical artery catheter to check the postductal PaO_2. Compare the results. A drop in saturation from preductal to postductal blood of greater than 10% or a drop in PaO_2 of greater than 15 to 20 torr indicates shunting. For example, a preductal PaO_2 of 70 torr and a postductal PaO_2 of 45 torr indicates significant shunting. This same test may be performed noninvasively with either transcutaneous oxygen monitoring or pulse oximetry monitoring. The $PtcO_2$ monitors should be placed over the right upper chest for preductal blood and left upper chest, abdomen, or either thigh for postductal blood. Pulse oximetry monitors should be placed on the right hand for preductal blood and left hand or either foot for postductal blood. Again, a greater than 15 to 20 torr drop in preductal to postductal $PtcO_2$ or a greater than 10% drop in saturation in preductal to postductal SpO_2 confirms a significant shunt.

   It is important to note that if the neonate has a shunt through the foramen ovale instead of the ductus arteriosus, this test will be negative. The preductal and postductal oxygen levels will be the same. Shunting through the foramen ovale is seen in as many as 50% of PPHN babies.

3. Hyperoxia-hyperventilation test: The infant is manually ventilated with 100% oxygen at a rate and pressure adequate to significantly reduce the carbon dioxide level. When this "critical $PaCO_2$" (usually between 20 and 30 torr) is reached, the pulmonary artery pressure drops, the lungs are better perfused, and the PaO_2 improves. Although the patient's color will likely change from cyanotic to pink and the $PtcO_2$ and SpO_2 values will improve, the test is confirmed by a postductal PaO_2 of greater than 80 torr. The critical $PaCO_2$ value, ventilation rate, and manometer pressure on the manual ventilator should be recorded. These values can be used later to set the mechanical ventilator parameters.

4. Echocardiography: This procedure can be used to identify an intracardiac shunt through the foramen ovale or evidence of increased right ventricular pressure as a sign of pulmonary hypertension.

Any infant who shows signs of PPHN, such as positive results to any of these tests or the need for more than 70% oxygen to prevent hypoxemia, should be considered for hyperventilation therapy. The goal is to reduce pulmonary artery hypertension and thus reduce shunting and improve the PaO_2. This is accomplished by hyperventilating the patient to his or her critical $PaCO_2$. Box 15-6 lists common ventilator parameters used to treat persistent pulmonary hypertension. Once the proper ventilator settings are found and the blood gas goals are met, the patient is maintained at this level for 1 or more days. It is often necessary to pharmacologically paralyze the infant with pancuronium bromide (Pavulon) or a similar drug to ensure that the patient's breathing is synchronized with the ventilator. This is especially important when high ventilator rates are needed. After about 24 hours, the ventilator is adjusted to increase the $PaCO_2$ by 1 to 2 torr. If the peak inspiratory pressure is greater than 45 cm water it should be reduced first. A blood gas is drawn to see if the PaO_2 is stable and if the $PaCO_2$ increased the desired small amount. If this first reduction in support is tolerated, it may be slowly followed by further reductions. Each step back from hyperventilation should be small so that the $PaCO_2$ increases only by 1 to 2 mm Hg each time.

As this happens, the patient should be supported in every other way. The medication tolazoline (Priscoline) is a pulmonary vasodilator that has proven to be successful in about one of six neonates with PPHN. Watch for signs of pulmonary barotrauma or bronchopulmonary dysplasia

---

BOX 15-6　Common Mechanical Ventilator Parameters to Treat a Neonate With Persistent Pulmonary Hypertension

Delivered tidal volume: 6-8 mL/kg initially. 8-10 mL/kg may be needed to hyperventilate the neonate

Pressure limit: 20-25 cm water. Use as little pressure as possible but be prepared to raise up to 35 cm water to deliver an adequate tidal volume

Frequency: 60-100/min may be needed to decrease the $PaCO_2$ to the critical level of probably between 20 and 30 mm Hg. A rate of up to 150/min has been used.

I:E ratio: 1:2 (This depends on the respiratory rate needed to decrease the carbon dioxide level.)

Inspiratory time (T_I): Between 0.4 and 0.7 seconds (This must be decreased at higher respiratory rates.)

Expiratory time (T_E): at least 0.5 seconds (This must be decreased at higher respiratory rates.)

PEEP: none if possible to lower the mean airway pressure and prevent crushing of the pulmonary capillary bed. 2-4 cm water may be used if needed.

Inspiratory flow: sufficient to see the chest move and hear bilateral breath sounds during the inspiration. 5-8 L/min commonly used initially. Flow must be increased at higher respiratory rates.

Oxygen percentage: up to 70%-100% to keep the postductal PaO_2 greater than 55 torr and ideally between 115 and 120 torr.

from the high peak pressures and oxygen percentages required with these patients.

1. Modify special gases: inhaled nitric oxide (Code: IIIC4) [Difficulty: Ap, An]

At the time of this writing, inhaled nitric oxide (iNO) gas is being used as a pulmonary artery vasodilator in limited clinical trials approved by the FDA. These early investigations indicate clinical improvement when a small amount of nitric oxide is inhaled by a neonate with PPHN or RDS. It is important to keep the concentration of iNO to a therapeutic dose of less than 2 parts per million (ppm). This is because nitric oxide combines with oxygen to form nitrogen dioxide (NO_2). A level of nitrogen dioxide greater than 10 ppm can cause cell damage, hemorrhage, and pulmonary edema leading to death.

Patients who receive iNO are usually receiving mechanical ventilation. In addition, special iNO measurement and delivery systems are needed and levels of inspired oxygen, nitric oxide, and nitrogen dioxide must be measured. Because of the experimental nature of iNO at this time, there are no standard procedures that are widely adopted. If the FDA fully approves iNO, the NBRC will likely test its clinical use.

e. Patients with bronchopulmonary dysplasia (BPD)

The neonate who develops BPD is usually born prematurely with a low birth weight. He or she is a survivor of RDS but has suffered serious lung damage in the process. It is controversial whether high peak pressures, high mean airway pressures, high inspired oxygen percentages, or a combination of these factors is the main cause of BPD. It is important to try to minimize all of them so that new lung tissues can grow to replace lung tissue that has been damaged. It is important to try to wean these infants as quickly as possible to avoid further ventilator-induced damage. If acceptable blood gases can be maintained with a ventilator rate of less than 15/min, the infant may be extubated. Nasal CPAP may be used to help maintain the PaO_2. See Box 15-7 for the commonly recommended ventilator settings for a BPD patient.

A number of medications are used to help optimize the patient's pulmonary function. Methylxanthines such as aminophylline or caffeine are beneficial as respiratory stimulants. There is further evidence that they help to strengthen the diaphragm and decrease muscle fatigue. The diuretic furosemide (Lasix) has been widely reported to improve lung compliance and airway resistance by decreasing any pulmonary edema fluid. Remember that patients receiving furosemide must be given a potassium-chloride supplement to replace what is lost through the kidneys. Some authors have reported the use of corticosteroids to be helpful in weaning because of increased pulmonary compliance. This possible advantage must be balanced against the known problems associated with the prolonged use of the medication. Finally, a dietary supplement of vitamin E may increase lung healing. Hopefully the use of surfactant replacement therapy early in the treatment of the RDS neonate will reduce the incidence of BPD.

BOX 15-7   Common Mechanical Ventilator Parameters for Neonates With Bronchopulmonary Dysplasia

Delivered tidal volume: 6-8 mL/kg

Pressure limit: as low as possible and not to exceed 25 cm water

Frequency: as low as possible to maintain the $PaCO_2$ between 35 and 45 torr. Some authors report accepting a $PaCO_2$ as high as 55 to 65 torr to minimize the need to increase peak and mean pressures.

I:E ratio: 1:2 to 1:10

Inspiratory time (T_I): between 0.3 and 0.7 seconds

Expiratory time (T_E): at least 0.5 seconds to allow for a complete exhalation

PEEP: no more than 2-4 cm water

Inspiratory flow: sufficient to see the chest move and hear bilateral breath sounds during the inspiration. 5-8 L/min commonly used initially.

Oxygen percentage: as low as possible to keep the PaO_2 between 55 and 65 torr. Some authors report accepting a PaO_2 as low as 35 torr to minimize the need to increase peak and mean pressures. It must be noted that a PaO_2 below 55 torr increases the risk of pulmonary hypertension.

---

5. Monitor the mean airway pressure to evaluate the patient's response to respiratory care (Code: IIIA1h) [Difficulty: An]

Mean airway pressure ($P\overline{aw}$) is the average pressure over an entire breathing cycle. A number of current neonatal and adult ventilators are able to calculate the value. $P\overline{aw}$ is influenced by both the patient's lung thoracic compliance (C_{LT}) and airway resistance (R_{AW}). If the ventilator settings are unchanged, a decrease in compliance or an increase in resistance will result in an increase in the mean airway pressure. This is because in a neonatal ventilator, the pressure limit is reached earlier and held for the duration of the inspiratory time. Conversely, if the patient's compliance increases or the resistance decreases, the $P\overline{aw}$ will decrease. It is important to further evaluate the patient when a change in $P\overline{aw}$ is noticed. This is because the new pressure by itself does not show you whether there has been a change in compliance, resistance, or both. Any treatments that improve lung compliance and reduce airway resistance are shown by a reduced mean airway pressure.

In general, an increase in mean airway pressure increases the patient's oxygenation. This is because the alveoli are kept open longer, allowing more time for diffusion and preventing alveolar collapse. If alveolar ventilation is improved, the $PaCO_2$ will also be reduced. There is clinical evidence that a mean airway pressure of 12 or more cm water pressure is associated with an increased risk of pulmonary barotrauma and decreased cardiac output. This is especially true if PEEP is increased to raise the $\overline{Paw}$. Watch the patient closely whenever a ventilator change is made that increases the $\overline{Paw}$. A sudden deterioration in cardiopulmonary function may be caused by a pneumothorax. A reduction in urine output, an increased heart rate, and decreased blood pressure are often seen when the cardiac output is reduced. The mean airway pressure should be reduced if either of these situations is seen. To prevent these complications, it is necessary to reduce the mean airway pressure whenever the patient's compliance improves.

Usually the mean airway pressure is the result of the patient's lung compliance, airway resistance, and the various ventilator settings. The initial mean airway pressure should be considered along with the ventilator settings when interpreting the first set of arterial blood gases. Based on the blood gas results, ventilator adjustments may be needed. Note the $\overline{Paw}$ at each adjustment.

A number of ventilator control adjustments influence the patient's mean airway pressure. (See Fig. 15-9 for several examples of airway pressure tracings based on ventilator control changes.) If the patient's compliance and resistance are stable, the $\overline{Paw}$ will be *increased* by the following: (1) an increased inspiratory flow, (2) an increased pressure limit (assuming the pressure limit has been previously reached), (3) an increase in PEEP, (4) an increased inspiratory time (assuming no change in ventilator rate and a decreased expiratory time), and (5) a decreased expiratory time (assuming an increased ventilator rate). These ventilator adjustments should result in an increased PaO_2 and possibly a decreased $PaCO_2$. Measure blood gases to be sure of the patient's response.

If the patient's compliance and resistance are stable, the $\overline{Paw}$ will be *decreased* by the following: (1) a decreased inspiratory flow, (2) a decreased pressure limit (assuming the pressure limit has been previously reached), (3) a decrease in PEEP, (4) a decreased inspiratory time (assuming no change in ventilator rate and an increased expiratory time), and (5) an increased expiratory time (assuming a decreased ventilator rate). These ventilator adjustments may result in a decreased PaO_2 and possibly an increased $PaCO_2$. Measure blood gases to be sure of the patient's response.

It should be noted that of all the various controls that have an influence on the mean airway pressure, PEEP has the greatest impact. There is usually a one-for-one relationship between the addition or removal of PEEP and the resulting $\overline{Paw}$. For example, the $\overline{Paw}$ is 10 cm water when 5 cm water of PEEP is added. The resulting $\overline{Paw}$ is seen to become 15 cm water. If 2 cm of PEEP is removed the $\overline{Paw}$ will drop to 13 cm water.

6. Initiate high-frequency ventilation (HFV) and select appropriate settings (Code: IIIB2b) [Difficulty: R, Ap, An]

HFV involves the use of a ventilator respiratory rate that is much greater than commonly needed. The Food and Drug Administration defines HFV as a rate of more than 150/min. Because of this FDA definition of HFV, conventional neonatal TPTV ventilators are not considered high frequency ventilators. Several manufacturers have developed ventilators capable of rates significantly greater than 150/min. One of these must be used when HFV is indicated. The FDA has also set some guidelines for the appropriate use of HFV. See Box 15-8 for the clinical indications for HFV.

Despite the FDA guidelines, many respiratory thera-

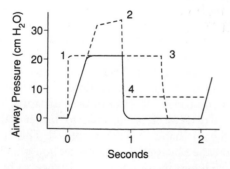

Fig. 15-9 Pressure-time tracings showing four different ventilator settings that can be used to increase mean airway pressure. *1,* Inspiratory flow is increased. *2,* Pressure limit is increased. *3,* Inspiratory time is increased. This also changes the I:E ratio by reducing expiratory time if rate is kept the same. *4,* PEEP is added. (From Harris TR. In Goldsmith JP, Karotkin EH, editors: *Assisted ventilation of the neonate,* Philadelphia, 1981, WB Saunders.)

BOX 15-8	Common Clinical Indications for the Use of High Frequency Ventilation in Infants and Children

Severe hypoxemia and hypercarbia unresponsive to
  conventional ventilation techniques:
    Infant respiratory distress syndrome (RDS)
    Acute respiratory distress syndrome (ARDS)
    Pneumonia
    Aspiration syndromes
    Pulmonary hemorrhage
Conventional ventilation with a persistent pulmonary air leak:
    Pneumothorax
    Bronchopleural fistula
    Pulmonary interstitial emphysema (PIE)
    Pneumomediastinum
    Pneumoperitoneum
Persistent pulmonary hypertension of the newborn (PPHN)
Pulmonary hypoplasia
Bronchoscopy, laryngoscopy, or tracheal surgery

pists consider a rate of greater than 40/min on a neonatal patient to be HFV. When a conventional TPTV ventilator is used to deliver a respiratory rate of up to 150/min, the term high frequency positive pressure ventilation (HFPPV) is used. Experience has shown that many RDS infants can be successfully managed with conventional TPTV ventilator set to deliver a small tidal volume at a rate between 40 and 150/min. However, when these methods fail, true HFV is needed.

Ventilator manufacturers have developed two different technologies for delivering FDA-defined HFV. The first is called high frequency jet ventilation (HFJV). With HFJV, small jets of gas are directed down the patient's endotracheal tube. These gas jets entrain additional gas into the tube. The two combined volumes of gas make up the patient's tidal volume. The patient exhales passively because of normal lung recoil. The second method is called high frequency oscillation (HFO) or high frequency oscillatory ventilation (HFOV). With HFO, a pumping device (piston, diaphragm, or sound speaker) actively pushes a small tidal volume into the patient from a continuous flow of gas (called bias flow) passing through the circuit and by the endotracheal tube. HFO technology can deliver very high rates because the patient actively exhales the delivered tidal volume. This active exhalation is created by the back stroke of the pumping device that pulls the tidal volume out of the patient's airways and lungs. See Table 15-2 for a comparison of HFV methods and characteristics.

Initial HFV settings depend on the patient's diagnosis, clinical situation, current conventional ventilator settings and the type of high frequency ventilator to be used. Generally speaking, the initial HFV settings include a tidal volume large enough to see chest movement and a continuation of the patient's original mean airway pressure, PEEP level, and oxygen percentage. The I:E ratio should be set at 1:2 and the high frequency rate should be between 10 and 15 Hertz (Hz) depending on the infant's body weight. (A Hz is defined as 1 respiratory cycle/sec; 60 respiratory cycles/min. For example, a rate of 600/min is 10/sec or 10 Hz.) After the patient is stabilized on HFV,

arterial blood gases should be drawn and analyzed, vital signs assessed, and a chest radiograph obtained. In a patient without a pulmonary air leak, a chest radiograph finding of lung expansion to T8 to T9 on the right hemidiaphragm, without intercostal bulging, is believed to show the best lung volume. Once established, the HFV rate is seldom changed. Adjustments in tidal volume are made by increasing or decreasing what is referred to as either drive pressure (with HFJV) or amplitude (with HFO). Increasing drive pressure/amplitude increases the tidal volume and decreases the carbon dioxide level. The patient's oxygenation should also improve as the mean airway pressure is increased. Decreasing drive pressure/amplitude decreases the tidal volume and increases the carbon dioxide level. If the patient's oxygenation should decrease too much, additional therapeutic PEEP may be needed. See Fig. 15-10 for a protocol on initiation and adjustment of HFO. Fig. 15-11 shows a protocol for weaning from HFO.

7. Test the ventilator alarm systems and adjust them as needed (Code: IIIA1h) [Difficulty: An]

All alarm systems must function properly, so test all audible and visual alarms. The respiratory therapist should be familiar with the most widely used neonatal ventilators and those that can be used with pediatric as well as adult patients. It is common practice to set most ventilator alarms at ±10% from the set value.

If the patient is on a CPAP system, the low-pressure or disconnection alarm should be set to alarm if the pressure drops about 2 cm water below the set level. For example, if the patient is on 8 cm water CPAP, the alarm setting should be set at 6 cm water.

Many types of alarm systems have a timer that can be set to delay when the alarm sounds. For example, if the neonatal patient has a ventilator rate of 30/min, the cycling time between mandatory breaths is 2 seconds. The delay should be set so that the alarm sounds in 1 to 2 seconds after a mandatory breath fails to be delivered. If the patient is on a CPAP system, the timer may be set for no delay or a short delay after the CPAP pressure drops below the set

TABLE 15-2	High-Frequency Ventilation		
	HFPPV	**HFJV**	**HFO**
Rate	60-150/min	<600/min	<1200/min
V_T	3-5 mL/kg	2-5 mL/kg	1-3 mL/kg
I/E ratio	1:3-1:2	1:3-1:2	1:3-1:2
Technical application	Conventional ventilator	Special ventilator	Special ventilator
F_1O_2	0.21-1.0	0.21-1.0	0.21-1.0
PEEP	0-20	0-20	0-20
Expiration	Passive	Passive	Active
Gas movement	Bulk flow	Bulk flow	Diffusion

HFJV, High frequency jet ventilation; *HFO,* high frequency oscillation; *HFPPV,* high frequency positive pressure ventilation.

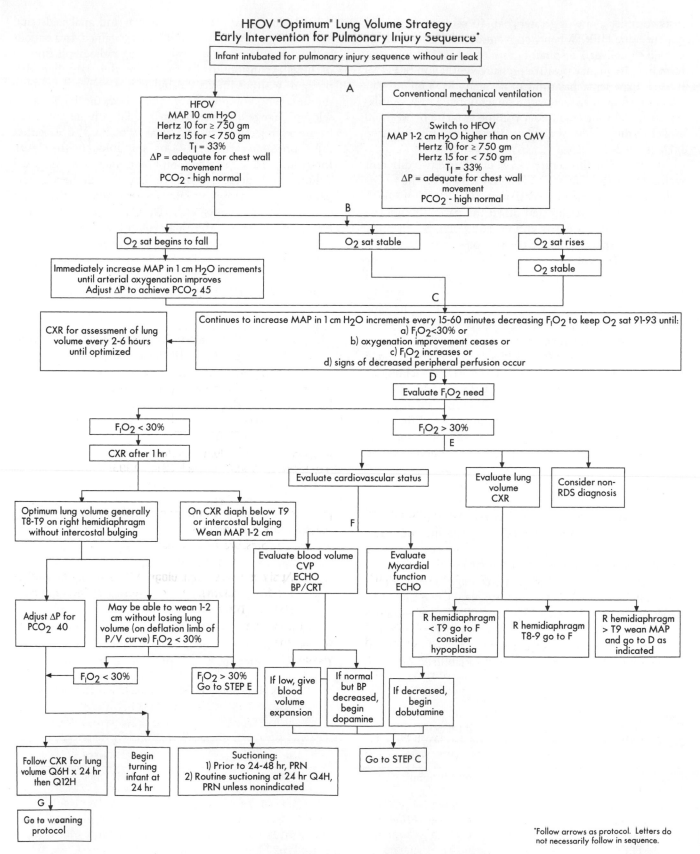

Fig. 15-10 Optimum lung volume HFOV strategy flow chart. (From Minton S, Gerstmann D, Stoddard R: *Cardiopul Rev,* Yorba Linda, Calif, 1995, Sensormedics Corp. PN 770118-001.)

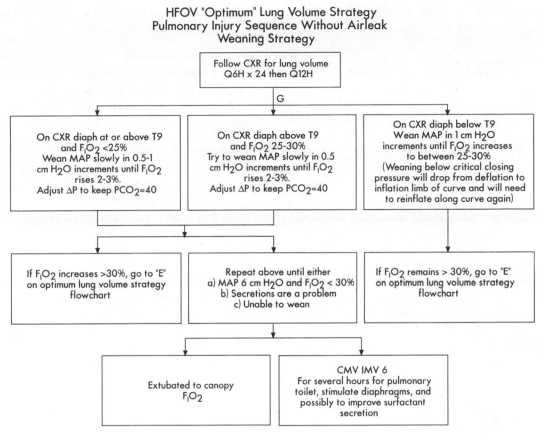

HFOV "Optimum" Lung Volume Strategy
Pulmonary Injury Sequence Without Airleak
Weaning Strategy

Fig. 15-11   HFOV flow cart for weaning from optimum lung volume strategy. (From Minton S, Gerstmann D, Stoddard R: *Cardiopul Rev,* Yorba Linda, Calif, 1995, Sensormedics Corp. PN 770118-001.)

value. Always adjust all alarm systems to fit the clinical situation and the patient's condition.

8. Ventilator flow, volume, and pressure waveforms

a. Review existing information in the patient's chart (Code: IA1f3) [Difficulty: An]

A patient who has been intubated and placed on a modern mechanical ventilator with a microprocessor and graphics software can have ventilator flow, volume, and pressure waveforms visualized on the monitor. Some units allow the information to be stored in memory or printed out. Look for this information and compare it with the patient's current situation.

b. Perform the procedure to measure ventilator flow, volume, and pressure waveforms (Code: IC1g) [Difficulty: An]

Because not every ventilator can provide waveform information, the correct unit must be selected for the patient. The Drager Babylog 8000 has the monitor and graphics software built into the unit. Other neonatal ventilators, such as the VIP Bird, can be upgraded to provide graphic information. Some ventilators, such as the Hamilton Galileo, can be used with any size patient and provide waveform information. Follow the ventilator manufacturer's guidelines to direct the unit to create flow, volume, or pressure waveforms.

c. Apply computer technology in the analysis of ventilator flow, volume, and pressure waveforms (Code: IIIA2c) [Difficulty: An]

Follow the ventilator manufacturer's guidelines to direct the unit to create flow, volume, or pressure waveforms.

d. Interpret ventilator flow, volume, and pressure waveforms (Code: IC2i and IIIA1e) [Difficulty: An]

Ventilator flow, volume, and pressure waveforms offer much clinically useful information. For example, expiratory flow can be monitored to look for air trapping and auto-PEEP. As discussed earlier, this is a concern if the neonate has obstructive airway disease or if a high respiratory rate is being used. Volume can be monitored as an indicator of improving or worsening lung compliance. Pressure can also be monitored as it relates to improving or worsening lung compliance. Less pressure is needed to deliver the desired tidal volume if the patient's lung compliance is improving. Conversely, more pressure is needed to deliver the desired tidal volume if the patient's lung compliance is worsening.

MODULE B   Mechanical ventilation equipment

1. Ventilators

As discussed in Chapter 14, the literature produced by the manufacturers and the descriptions used in many standard texts break the various ventilators into more categories than used by the NBRC. To avoid confusion, this text uses the NBRC's more simplified terminology. A pneumatically powered ventilator is defined here as powered by compressed gas. It may be electrically controlled with electrical alarm systems. Fluidic ventilators are defined here as being pneumatically powered and partially or completely controlled by fluidic methods. Fluidic controls make use of compressed gas for cycling and other ventilator functions. Both of these types of neonatal ventilators use compressed air and oxygen that go to an air-oxygen mixer (blender) to determine the inspired oxygen. The gas then goes to a flow meter where the continuous flow per minute through the ventilator circuit is set. Depending on the ventilator, either compressed air or oxygen are used to drive the other control functions in fluidic ventilators.

An electrically powered ventilator is defined here as being electrically powered and controlled. Compressed air and oxygen go to a blender where the inspired oxygen is set. A microprocessor ventilator is defined here as being controlled by a microprocessor; it may be pneumatically or electrically powered. All of these types of ventilators are limited to the 150 breaths/min maximum rate set by the FDA. A high frequency ventilator is capable of delivering a respiratory rate of more than 150/min.

a. Pneumatic ventilators
1. Obtain the equipment necessary for the procedure (Code: IIA1e1) [Difficulty: An]

It is beyond the scope of this text to discuss in detail the functions of pneumatic ventilators and the following types of ventilators. Refer to the manufacturer's literature for specific information. Examples of neonatal pneumatic ventilators include the Babybird, BEAR BP200, BEAR Cub, and Healthdyne 105. They are used to deliver conventional TPTV mechanical ventilation to the majority of neonatal and pediatric patients. The Bio-Med Devices MVP-10 is an example of a pediatric transport ventilator.

2. Put the equipment together, make sure that it works properly, and identify any problems (Code: IIB1e1) [Difficulty: An]
3. Fix any problems with the equipment (Code: IIB2e1) [Difficulty: An]

Make sure that the air and oxygen high pressure hoses are screwed tightly into the air-oxygen blender. A gas leak is heard as a whistling or hissing sound. If either gas source is cut off to the blender its alarm will sound.

b. Fluidic ventilators
1. Obtain the equipment necessary for the procedure (Code: IIA1e1) [Difficulty: An]

The Sechrist IV-100B and IV-200 ventilators are pneumatically powered and electrically and fluidically controlled.

2. Put the equipment together, make sure that it works properly, and identify any problems (Code: IIB1e1) [Difficulty: An]
3. Fix any problems with the equipment (Code: IIB2e1) [Difficulty: An]

Fluidic ventilators are prone to the same kind of problems with leaking high pressure air and oxygen hoses as pneumatic ventilators. In addition, they are very sensitive to obstructions. Make sure that all inlet filters are intact and free of debris.

c. Electric ventilators
1. Obtain the equipment necessary for the procedure (Code: IIA1e1) [Difficulty: An]

At the time of this writing, there are no exclusively neonatal units that fit the earlier definition of an electric ventilator; however, some adult ventilators such as the Servo 900C, Nellcor Puritan Bennett 7200, and Drager Evita 2 Dura can deliver tidal volumes small enough for a pediatric patient.

2. Put the equipment together, make sure that it works properly, and identify any problems (Code: IIB1e1) [Difficulty: An]
3. Fix any problems with the equipment (Code: IIB2e1) [Difficulty: An]

Make sure that the electrical power source is secure. Do not use a unit that does not power up or operate properly.

d. Microprocessor ventilator
1. Obtain the equipment necessary for the procedure (Code: IIA1e1) [Difficulty: An]

The LifeCare PLV-102 and Nelcor Puritan Bennett Companion 2801 are microprocessor controlled and electrically powered. They are home care ventilators that can deliver tidal volumes small enough for pediatric patients (50 mL).

2. Put the equipment together, make sure that it works properly, and identify any problems (Code: IIB1e1) [Difficulty: An]

Both the LifeCare PLV-102 and the Nelcor Puritan Bennett Companion 2801 must have a stable electrical supply. They also must have an oxygen source for adding to the tidal volume if more than room air is required by the patient. An oxygen analyzer should also be put inline to monitor the oxygen percentage because it varies with a changing respiratory rate or tidal volume.

3. Fix any problems with the equipment (Code: IIB2e1) [Difficulty: An]

The Infrasonics Infant Star series, Drager Babylog 8000, and VIP Bird Infant/Pediatric Ventilator are electrically and pneumatically powered and controlled by a microprocessor. Some of the current generation of primarily adult ventilators are capable of delivering tidal volumes and rates appropriate for infants. Examples include the Nelcor Puritan Bennett 7200 and BEAR 1000 ventilators. Microprocessor ventilators typically come with self-diagnostic software. If a problem is detected the unit will display it on the monitor. There is little to repair with these units at the bedside. Occasionally a computer chip must be replaced in the department.

e. High frequency ventilators
1. Obtain the necessary equipment for the procedure (Code: IIA1e2) [Difficulty: R, Ap, An]

The Bunnell Life Pulse High Frequency Ventilator provides HFJV. The SensorMedics 3100A High-Frequency Oscillatory Ventilator and Infrasonics Infant Star 950 Ventilator are examples of HFO ventilators.

2. Put the equipment together, make sure that it works properly, and identify any problems (Code: IIB1e2) [Difficulty: R, Ap, An]

Hands-on experience with these ventilators is recommended. The following are needed for proper assembly of a HFJV: (1) a pressurized oxygen source, (2) a pressurized air source, (3) an air-oxygen proportioner (blender), (4) a pressure regulator for controlling the patient's peak pressure, (5) an injector line to add the jet volume to the endotracheal tube, and (6) an intravenous infusion pump to supply a steady drip of water to the jet ventilator injector line for nebulization.

An HFO ventilator needs the following basic accessories for assembly: (1) a pressurized oxygen source, (2) a pressurized air source, (3) an air-oxygen proportioner (blender), and (4) a passover or cascade humidifier.

3. Fix any problems with the equipment (Code: IIB2e2) [Difficulty: R, Ap, An]

Make sure that gas sources are stable, all tubing connections are tight, and humidification systems are functioning properly. Because the patient's tidal volume is very small, it cannot be accurately measured. Any leaks will result in an undetectable loss of delivered tidal volume.

2. Ventilator breathing circuits
a. Obtain the necessary equipment for the procedure (Code: IIA1i1) [Difficulty: An]

Conventional neonatal ventilators use a circuit that has all of the standard features of an adult circuit as discussed in Chapter 14. A special circuit made of noncompliant tubing is needed with the SensorMedics 3100A ventilator. In addition, to complete an HFJV circuit, a Hi-Lo Jet endotracheal tube or special endotracheal tube adapter is needed to deliver the jetted gas and add the entrained gas for the tidal volume. These are shown in Chapter 14.

b. Put the equipment together, make sure that it works properly, and identify any problems (Code: IIB1i1) [Difficulty: An]

c. Fix any problems with the equipment (Code: IIB2i1) [Difficulty: An]

Conventional neonatal ventilator circuits are basically the same as adult circuits with an inspiratory limb and an expiratory limb. Water traps are usually added. An obvious difference is the smaller diameter so that there is less compressible volume. Some are smooth bore to minimize gas turbulence and some have a heated wire running through them to keep a constant temperature and eliminate condensation. It is important that a heated-wire circuit be used only with the servo-controlled humidifier for which it is designed. Mixing circuits and humidifiers can lead to either overheating or under heating problems. Furthermore, do not cover a heated-wire circuit with a blanket. The circuit should not be allowed to touch the patient to avoid burns. If the patient is inside an incubator, the circuit's temperature probe must be kept outside.

An added feature is a third small-bore tubing for measuring the proximal airway pressure. The tube runs from the patient Y to the proximal airway pressure nipple on the ventilator. Make sure that all the connections are tight to prevent gas leaks.

d. Change the patient's ventilator circuit (Code: IIIC8a) [Difficulty: An]

Commonly, disposable single patient use corrugated plastic circuits are used. They are inexpensive and meet the needs of most patients. Condensation is drained out into water traps that are placed at low points in the natural draping of the inspiratory and expiratory limbs of the circuit. If excessive moisture is a problem or if the gas temperature must be maintained within a narrow range, a heated-wire circuit may be used. These types of circuits are built with a heated wire either loosely threaded through the lumen or coiled within the tubing itself. They are integrated with the humidification system and a servo unit for automatic temperature regulation. As expected, these circuits are considerably more expensive than the disposable types and may be sterilized and reused between patients.

Another possible concern with disposable, corrugated circuits is their relatively high internal resistance and compressible volume. The corrugations lead to gas turbulence that increases as the flow is raised. When the tubing is warmed it becomes more stretchable. This results in more tidal volume lost to the circuit instead of being delivered to the patient. When high flow rates and ventilating pressures are needed, as in HFV, a smooth bore and low compressible volume circuit is used instead of the standard disposable type.

3. Continuous positive airway pressure (CPAP) devices
a. Obtain the necessary equipment for the procedure (Code: IIA1a3) [Difficulty: An]

Nasal CPAP devices are widely used with neonates who are born prematurely and have RDS. Their immature lungs lack sufficient surfactant and need the CPAP pressure to keep the alveoli open. Often, nasal CPAP meets the patient's needs so that endotracheal intubation and mechanical ventilation can be avoided. Nasal CPAP works with neonates because they are obligate nose breathers.

Nasal CPAP is associated with the hazards of gastric distension and reflux aspiration. These occur when the airway pressure forces air into the stomach. A gastric tube is usually inserted to vent the air out. There are two different devices for administering nasal CPAP. A nasopharyngeal tube is actually an endotracheal tube that has been cut shorter (see Fig. 15-2, C). Select a tube that is the largest that can be easily inserted into the patient. Nasal prongs come in short and long versions (see Fig. 15-2, A and B); both types involve prongs that fit into both nostrils. The prongs come in different diameters so that the proper size can be found to fit the internal diameter of the infant's nares.

b. Put the equipment together, make sure that it works properly, and identify any problems (Code: IIB1a3) [Difficulty: An]

Follow the manufacturer's instructions for assembly of the CPAP device and CPAP circuit. See Figs. 15-2 and 15-3 as well as the illustration of the CPAP circuit in Chapter 14 (Fig. 14-26) for general assembly guidance.

c. Fix any problems with the equipment (Code: IIB2a3) [Difficulty: An]

A sudden drop in the CPAP level to zero indicates a disconnection at the patient or somewhere in the breathing circuit. Check all connections and reassemble the break. The patient may need to be manually ventilated while the problem is corrected.

If the CPAP level drops more than 2 cm of water pressure during an inspiration, the flow is inadequate and should be increased. Flow is also inadequate if the patient shows an increased use of accessory muscles of respiration or appears to have an increased work of breathing. Too high a flow is seen by an inadvertently high level of CPAP or the appearance that the patient is having a difficult time exhaling. A common problem with small diameter tubes like these is mucous plugging. A plugged tube may result in

a backup of gas and can increase CPAP; however, depending on the CPAP system, there may be no change in pressure. Careful patient monitoring is important. Watch for a decrease in a drop in oxygenation, an increase in the respiratory rate, or retractions as signs of airway obstruction. Suction to clear out the mucous plug or remove the tube and place a new one.

4. Continuous positive airway pressure (CPAP) circuit
a. Obtain the necessary equipment for the procedure (Code: IIA1a3) [Difficulty: An]

The general discussion and an illustration related to CPAP systems was presented in Chapter 14. Freestanding neonatal systems are similar to those used with adults. All currently available neonatal ventilators offer a CPAP mode. This allows the practitioner to easily switch the intubated neonate from IMV to CPAP without the need to set up new equipment.

b. Put the equipment together, make sure that it works properly, and identify any problems with it (Code: IIB1a3) [Difficulty: An]

c. Fix any problems with the equipment (Code: IIB2a3) [Difficulty: An]

The previous discussion about putting together and fixing problems with the CPAP device applies to the CPAP circuit.

> **EXAM HINT**
>
> A sudden drop in CPAP level indicates a disconnection within the circuit or at the patient connection.

---

5. Perform volume, flow, and pressure calibration on a ventilator for quality control purposes (Code: IIB3b) [Difficulty: An]

Follow the manufacturer's guidelines for quality control procedures on mechanical ventilators. The microprocessor ventilators usually have a software package that performs self-diagnostic tests on the unit. If a problem is found it is displayed on the monitor. Obviously the ventilator should deliver the volume, flow, and pressure that is set on the control. Do not use a ventilator that fails a quality control check.

6. Humidification equipment
a. Obtain the necessary equipment for the procedure (Code: IIA1b) [Difficulty: An]

The general discussion of humidification equipment was presented in Chapters 7 and 14. See the figures there and the general discussion for set-ups in ventilator and CPAP breathing circuits. Both heated humidifiers and heat and moisture exchangers are used with pediatric patients.

Heated passover-type humidifiers systems are preferred with neonates.

b. Put the equipment together, make sure that it works properly, and identify any problems with it (Code: IIB1b) [Difficulty: An]

c. Fix any problems with the equipment (Code: IIB2b) [Difficulty: An]

Again, see Chapters 7 and 14 for assembly and troubleshooting of humidification systems. With a cascade-type of passover-type humidifier, the gas temperature is usually maintained close to the neonate's body temperature to maintain a neutral thermal environment. Make sure that the water level is kept in the recommended range to properly humidify the gas.

7. Adequately oxygenate the patient to prevent accidental hypoxemia before and after suctioning, changing the ventilator circuit, or performing other procedures during which the patient is disconnected from the ventilator (Code: IIB4c) [Difficulty: An]

Chapter 12 discusses the suctioning procedure and steps that should be taken to prevent hypoxemia during suctioning. Children younger than 6 months of age should have their oxygen percentage increased by 10% to 20% for the procedure.

MODULE C   **Neonatal assessment**

Refer to Chapter 1 or earlier in this chapter for a detailed discussion on neonatal assessment. Some additional discussion is presented here.

1. Note the patient's subjective response to mechanical ventilation (Code: IIIA1c) [Difficulty: An]

An infant who is attempting to exhale when the IMV breath is being delivered is said to be "bucking" or "fighting" the ventilator. This problem is almost unavoidable because the IMV breaths cannot be synchronized on the majority of neonatal ventilators. If the asynchrony between the infant's efforts and the ventilator are too great, there is an increased risk of hypoxemia and barotrauma or volutrauma. Carefully evaluate the patient to determine if the patient is breathing rapidly because of pain or improper adjustment of the ventilator. Make sure that the flow, rate, pressure limit, and so forth are correctly set for the patient's condition. Sedation or paralysis should be considered only after all other causes of asynchrony have been ruled out.

Antianxiety agents are not typically used with neonates. Morphine sulfate or other opiates are typically used for pain but other less powerful medications may also be tried. If the patient must be paralyzed, pancuronium (Pavulon), atracurium (Tracrium), and vecuronium (Nor-curon) are commonly used. Remember that these paralyzing agents have no effect on the patient's ability to feel pain or to be afraid of what is happening. Pain medications must be given as necessary. As the neonate improves, consideration must be given as to the best weaning method. Specific steps in weaning were discussed earlier with each of the types of common pathologic conditions and the various modes of ventilation. Remember to evaluate your patient's blood gases and vital signs before and after making a change in the ventilator parameters. If the patient's condition deteriorates, the ventilator setting(s) should be placed as before.

The decision to extubate with CPAP therapy and ventilator management is based on the neonate's pathologic condition and was discussed earlier. As a review, if the patient's blood gases and vital signs are acceptable at minimal ventilator support and the endotracheal tube is not needed for a suctioning route, the tube can be removed. Follow-up on blood gases and frequent monitoring of vital signs and breath sounds should be done after extubation. Be prepared to reintubate if the patient's condition deteriorates or a suctioning route is needed.

2. Treat a tension pneumothorax (Code: IIID2) [Difficulty: R, Ap, An]

A chest radiograph and physical examination of the neonate will reveal if abnormal air or fluid is found around the lung(s) or heart. If a patient has a tension pneumothorax, a pleural chest tube *must* be inserted to remove the air and relieve the pressure within the chest. A nontension pneumothorax of greater than 10% is often also treated by inserting a pleural chest tube. A pleural chest tube is also placed to remove blood or other fluid from the pleural space. Chapter 17 has specific information that relates to treating a pneumothorax.

A pneumomediastinum, pneumopericardium, or pneumoperitoneum that puts the patient at risk must also be treated. A chest tube is then inserted into the area where the abnormal air is found. The same chest tube also removes any abnormal collection of fluid. A chest tube is usually placed behind the heart to remove any blood that should leak out after open heart surgery.

3. Measure the volume of air lost through a patient's pleural chest tube (Code: IIIC8b) [Difficulty: Ap, An]

If a neonate is being ventilated on a constant volume ventilator, the amount of air that is lost through the pleural chest tube can be calculated. This is done by subtracting the measured exhaled volume from the measured inhaled volume. For example:

Inspired tidal volume = 40 mL
Exhaled tidal volume = − 30 mL
        10 mL of tidal volume is lost through the pleural chest tube

It is not possible to measure tidal volume when the neonate is ventilated by any other means. In a case like this, it is only possible to make a qualitative judgment on pleural air leak. In other words, if air is seen to bubble out through the pleural drainage system, an air leak is present. When the air stops bubbling, the pleural tear has healed. See Chapter 17 for a complete discussion on pleural drainage systems.

BIBLIOGRAPHY

AARC Clinical Practice Guideline: Application of continuous positive airway pressure to neonates via nasal prongs or nasopharyngeal tube, *Respir Care* 39:817, 1994.

AARC Clinical Practice Guideline: Humidification during mechanical ventilation, *Respir Care* 37:887, 1992.

AARC Clinical Practice Guideline: Neonatal time-triggered, pressure-limited, time-cycled, mechanical ventilation, *Respir Care* 39:808, 1994.

AARC Clinical Practice Guideline: Patient-ventilator system checks, *Respir Care* 37:882, 1992.

AARC Clinical Practice Guideline: Surfactant replacement therapy, *Respir Care* 39:824, 1994.

AARC Clinical Practice Guideline: Ventilator circuit changes, *Respir Care* 39:797, 1994.

Aloan CA, Hill TV: *Respiratory care of the newborn and child*, ed 2, Philadelphia, 1997, JB Lippincott-Raven.

Avery ME et al: Is chronic lung disease in low birth weight infants preventable? A survey of eight centers, *Pediatr* 79:26, 1987.

Barnhart SL, Czervinske MP: *Perinatal and pediatric respiratory care*, Philadelphia, 1995, WB Saunders.

Boros SJ et al: The effect of independent variations in inspiratory-expiratory ratio and end expiratory pressure during mechanical ventilation in hyaline membrane disease: the significance of mean airway pressure, *J Pediatr* 91:794, 1981.

Branson RD, Hess DR, Chatburn RL: *Respiratory care equipment*, ed 2, Philadelphia, 1999, Lippincott Williams & Wilkins.

Burgess WR, Chernick V: *Respiratory therapy in newborn infants and children*, ed 2, New York, 1986, Thieme.

Cairo JM, Pilbeam SP: *Mosby's respiratory care equipment*, ed 6, St Louis, 1999, Mosby.

Carlo WA, Martin RJ: Principles of neonatal assisted ventilation, *Pediatr Clin North Am* 33:221, 1986.

Cavanagh K: High frequency ventilation of infants: an analysis of the literature, *Respir Care* 35:815, 1990.

Chang DW: *Clinical application of mechanical ventilation*, ed 2, Albany, 2001, Delmar.

Chatburn RL: High frequency ventilation: a report on a state of the art symposium, *Respir Care* 29:839, 1984.

Chatburn RL: Principles and practice of neonatal and pediatric mechanical ventilation, *Respir Care* 36:569, 1991.

Chatburn RL, Lough MD: Mechanical ventilation. In Lough MD, Doershuk CF, Stern RC, editors: *Pediatric respiratory therapy*, ed 3, St Louis, 1985, Mosby.

Chatburn RL, Waldemar AC, Lough MD. Clinical algorithm for pressure-limited ventilation of neonates with respiratory distress syndrome, *Respir Care* 281579, 1983.

Coghill CH et al: Neonatal and pediatric high-frequency ventilation: principles and practice, *Respir Care* 36:596, 1991.

Gagnon C, Simoes J: The management of the mechanically ventilated infant receiving pancuronium bromide (Pavulon), *Neonatal Network*, pp 20-24, Dec 1985.

Goldberg RN, Bancalari E: Bronchopulmonary dysplasia: clinical presentation and the role of mechanical ventilation, *Respir Care* 31:591, 1986.

Goldberg RN, Bancalari E: Therapeutic approaches to the infant with bronchopulmonary dysplasia, *Respir Care* 36:613, 1991.

Goldsmith JP, Karotkin EH: *Assisted ventilation of the neonate*, ed 2, Philadelphia, 1996, WB Saunders.

Hess DR, Kacmarek RM: *Essentials of mechanical ventilation*, New York, 1996, McGraw-Hill.

HIFI Study Group: High-frequency oscillatory ventilation compared with conventional mechanical ventilation in the treatment of respiratory failure in preterm infants, *N Engl J Med* 320:88, 1989.

Jobe A: Surfactant treatment for respiratory distress syndrome, *Respir Care* 31:467, 1986.

Koff PB, Eitzman DV, Neu J: *Neonatal and pediatric respiratory care*, ed 2, St Louis, 1993, Mosby.

MacIntyre NR, Branson RD: *Mechanical ventilation*, Philadelphia, 2001, WB Saunders.

Milner AD, Hoskyns EW: High frequency positive pressure ventilation in neonates, *Arch Dis Child* 64:1, 1989.

Miyagawa CI: Sedation of the mechanically ventilated patient in the intensive care unit, *Respir Care* 32:792, 1987.

Nicks JJ, Becker MA: High-frequency ventilation of the newborn: past, present, and future, *Respir Ther* 4(4), 1991.

Pilbeam SP: *Mechanical ventilation: physiological and clinical applications*, ed 3, St Louis, 1998, Mosby.

Schmidt JM: Nitric oxide therapy in neonates: adding to the arsenal, *Respir Ther* 7:37, 1994.

Smith I: The impact of surfactant on neonatal intensive care unit management, *Respir Ther* 4(4):22-26, 1991.

Spear ML, Spitzer AR, Fox WW: Hyperventilation therapy for persistent pulmonary hypertension of the newborn, *Perinatol/Neonat* 9:27, 1985.

Tobin MJ: What should the clinician do when a patient "fights the ventilator"? *Respir Care* 36:395, 1991.

Whitaker K: *Comprehensive perinatal and pediatric respiratory care*, ed 3, Albany, NY, 1997, Delmar.

White GC: *Equipment theory for respiratory care*, ed 3, Albany, NY, 1999, Delmar.

SELF-STUDY QUESTIONS

1. The neonate less than 72-hours old with pulmonary problems should have its PaO_2 kept in the _____ range on the lowest inspired oxygen level.
   A. 40-45 torr
   B. 45-50 torr
   C. 60-70 torr
   D. 80-90 torr

2. If CPAP is administered through an endotracheal tube the child should be extubated when the CPAP pressure is:
   A. 0-2 cm water
   B. 2-3 cm water
   C. 4-6 cm water
   D. 6-8 cm water

3. If you observe that your patient has apnea spells leading to bradycardia, you should:
   A. Start CPAP.
   B. Start mechanical ventilation.
   C. Start an aerosolized bronchodilator.
   D. End CPAP.

4. The time to switch a patient from CPAP to mechanical ventilation is indicated by:
   I. CPAP of 8 to 10 cm water with a resulting PaO_2 of less than 50 torr
   II. F_IO_2 of 0.8 or more resulting in a PaO_2 of less than 50 torr
   III. $PaCO_2$ of greater than 60 torr
   A. I
   B. II
   C. I and II
   D. I, II, and III

5. Identify the rationale for the use of pressure limiting or "square wave ventilation":
   I. It increases the $PaCO_2$.
   II. It reduces the peak pressure.
   III. It decreases the PaO_2.
   IV. It increases the patient's oxygenation.
   V. There is no change in the patient's $PaCO_2$.
   A. I, II, and III
   B. I and III
   C. I, II, and IV
   D. II, IV, and V

6. Given the following choices, which would you select to decrease the $PaCO_2$ in a neonate on a standard, pressure-limited type ventilator?
   I. Increase the inspired oxygen.
   II. Decrease the pressure limit if it has been reached.
   III. Increase the respiratory rate.
   IV. Increase the flow if the pressure limit has not been reached.
   V. Increase the pressure limit if it has been reached.
   A. I
   B. II
   C. III, IV, and V
   D. II and III

7. Hyperventilation is recommended in which of the following types of patients?
   A. Meconium aspiration
   B. PPHN
   C. RDS
   D. Infant with normal lung compliance

8. Increasing the pressure limit on the ventilator increases the patient's risk of:
   A. ROP
   B. Oxygen toxicity
   C. Pneumothorax
   D. Tracheoesophageal fistula

9. You are taking care of a newborn who has aspirated meconium. You would recommend which of the following ventilator settings:
   A. I:E of 1:2
   B. I:E of 2:1
   C. I:E of 1:4
   D. I:E of 1:1

10. Given the following choices, which would you select to increase the PaO_2 in a neonate on a standard pressure-limited type ventilator?
    I. Increase inspiratory time.
    II. Increase the pressure limit if it is reached.
    III. Decrease flow.
    IV. Increase PEEP.
    V. Decrease the IMV rate.
    A. I and V
    B. II and III
    C. III and IV
    D. I, II, and IV

11. If you increase PEEP without increasing the pressure limit by the same amount, the patient's:
    A. Minute volume will increase.
    B. Tidal volume will decrease.
    C. $PaCO_2$ will decrease.
    D. Tidal volume will increase.

12. You are working with a neonate who has PPHN. He has right upper chest and left thigh transcutaneous oxygen monitors in place. His PaO_2 by umbilical artery catheter is 60 torr on 40% oxygen on the ventilator. His $PtcO_2$ at both sites is 55 torr. The nurse suctions his endotracheal tube and calls you over when the thigh $PtcO_2$ alarm sounds. You notice that even though he is back on the ventilator, his thigh reading remains at 30 torr while his shoulder $PtcO_2$ has returned to 55 torr. The most likely problem is:
    A. The thigh monitor should be placed on the right thigh.
    B. The shoulder monitor needs recalibrating.
    C. His ductus arteriosus has opened.
    D. The patient has developed a pneumothorax.

13. All of the following are indications for HFV *except*:
    A. Cleft palate before surgical correction
    B. PPHN
    C. RDS unresponsive to conventional ventilation
    D. Mechanical ventilation patient with unresolved pneumothorax

14. A 20-kg (44-lb) child is admitted with bilateral pneumonia and will be intubated and have mechanical ventilation initiated. What type of ventilator should be selected?
    A. Volume-cycled ventilator
    B. TPTV ventilator
    C. Noninvasive positive pressure ventilator
    D. HFV

15. A premature newborn is becoming progressively more hypoxic and tachypneic despite being in an oxyhood with 50% oxygen. The decision is made to begin CPAP. What initial pressure should the respiratory therapist recommend?
    A. 0-2 cm water
    B. 2-3 cm water
    C. 4-5 cm water
    D. 6-0 cm water

Answer Key

1. **C.** Rationale: A PaO_2 in the range of 60 to 70 torr is adequate for a newborn infant. Less would result in unnecessary hypoxemia. A higher value is not needed. See Table 15-1 for all blood gas recommendations.

2. **B.** Rationale: Extubation is performed with a CPAP level of 2 cm water because this small amount of pressure is used

to maintain the neonate's normal FRC. A lower CPAP pressure while intubated would result in loss of FRC and possibly hypoxemia. If a higher CPAP level is needed to treat a clinical problem, the patient should not be extubated.

3. **B.** Rationale: CPAP does not provide ventilation to support a patient with apnea spells. Mechanical ventilation is indicated to support the patient's breathing when apnea spells leading to bradycardia are present. An aerosolized bronchodilator does not affect a patient in a way that corrects apnea.

4. **D.** Rationale: All three listed items are indications to change from CPAP to mechanical ventilation. A neonatal patient who is receiving 8 to 10 cm water CPAP and 80% oxygen and who is still hypoxemic should have mechanical ventilation started.

5. **D.** Rationale: Pressure limited "square wave ventilation" is widely accepted as the standard way to ventilate the majority of neonatal patients because it: (1) limits the peak pressure to a predetermined safe level, (2) increases the patient's oxygenation by maintaining the peak pressure for the duration of the inspiratory time, and (3) can be adjusted without affecting the patient's carbon dioxide level.

6. **C.** Rationale: Increasing the respiratory rate increases the patient's minute ventilation and lowers the carbon dioxide level. If the patient's preset pressure limit is not reached during inspiration, the tidal volume is not maximized. Increasing the flow so that the pressure limit is reached increases the patient's tidal volume. If the ventilator pressure limit has been reached, the tidal volume can be increased by further raising the pressure limit. Increasing the tidal volume increases the patient's minute ventilation and lowers the carbon dioxide level.

7. **B.** Rationale: It has been clinically shown that hyperventilation of the patient with PPHN causes pulmonary vasodilation. This improves the patient's condition by allowing more blood to pass through the pulmonary circulation to be oxygenated. Hyperventilation has not been shown to improve the other listed conditions.

8. **C.** Rationale: Increasing the pressure limit on the ventilator increases the patient's tidal volume. This increased pressure and tidal volume can increase the risk of lung tissues being torn. This can result in a pneumothorax or other types of barotrauma or volutrauma. ROP is a complex condition related to prematurity and frequent swings in the patient's arterial blood oxygen and carbon dioxide levels. Oxygen toxicity is the related to the patient inhaling a high percentage of oxygen for a prolonged period of time. A tracheoesophageal fistula can be the result of a developmental defect or caused by tissue damage from an endotracheal tube and nasogastric tube.

9. **C.** Rationale: When meconium is aspirated, it causes a serious airway obstruction problem. Because of this, addi-tional time is needed for the patient's tidal volume to be exhaled. Therefore select the longest expiratory time possible.

10. **D.** Rationale: Increased inspiratory time keeps the alveoli open longer to improve oxygenation. If the pressure limit is increased, a larger tidal volume will be delivered and oxygenation will be improved. Additional PEEP increases the patient's FRC and improves oxygenation. If flow is decreased the tidal volume will be decreased. This results in the oxygen level dropping. Decreasing the ventilator's IMV rate decreases the patient's minute volume. This results in the oxygen level dropping.

11. **B.** Rationale: The patient's tidal volume is determined by the difference between the pressure limit and PEEP level. If the PEEP is increased without increasing the pressure limit, the difference between them decreases and the tidal volume decreases. See Fig. 15-8. Minute volume decreases, not increases, if the difference between the pressure limit and PEEP level is decreased. The patient's $PaCO_2$ increases, not decreases, if the tidal volume and minute volume decrease. Tidal volume decreases, not increases, when the difference between pressure limit and PEEP decreases.

12. **C.** Rationale: The described patient oxygen values best fit what is found when the patient has a patent ductus arteriosus. When this condition is present, the patient's preductus oxygen values are higher than the postductus oxygen values. Postductal oxygen values are the same in either thigh or leg. A consistent shoulder transcutaneous oxygen monitor value before and after suctioning indicates that the monitor is functioning properly. If the patient has a pneumothorax, all of the patient's oxygen monitoring sites would show a decreased value.

13. **A.** Rationale: An oral or nasal endotracheal tube is inserted into a patient's airway before a cleft palate is surgically repaired; a standard neonatal ventilator is used if needed. There is no special reason to use HFV. Patients with all of the other clinical situations have been shown to benefit by HFV.

14. **A.** Rationale: A 20-kg (44-lb) child is large enough to be ventilated on a standard volume-cycled ventilator. There is no indication specifically for noninvasive positive pressure ventilation (NPPV). Because the patient has bilateral pneumonia it is likely that an endotracheal tube is needed for suctioning purposes. Although a TPTV-type ventilator can be used, it does not provide a constant tidal volume as a volume-cycled ventilator does. There is no indication specifically for an HFV.

15. **C.** Rationale: It is common clinical practice to begin CPAP at 4 to 5 cm water pressure. Less than this is not likely to improve the patient's condition significantly. An initial CPAP of 6 to 8 cm water may not be needed to improve oxygenation and may result in cardiopulmonary complications. It is safer to start at 4 to 5 cm water, assess the patient, and determine if more CPAP is needed.

16 Home Care and Pulmonary Rehabilitation

A review of the most recent Written Registry Examinations has shown an average of four (4%) questions on home care and/or pulmonary rehabilitation issues.

MODULE A   Patient and family teaching

1. Describe and teach the planned therapeutic goals to the patient and his or her family to achieve optimal therapeutic outcomes (Code: IIIE2b) [Difficulty: An]

Determining the patient's ideal therapeutic goals is best done in a team approach. The patient's physician, nurse, and respiratory therapist should work together. The first consideration should be the patient's diagnosis. Next, determine if the patient's condition is permanent, improving, or worsening. Objective information such as arterial blood gas results, pulmonary function testing results, chest radiographs, sputum production, and vital signs must be evaluated. The patient cannot be expected to do more than he or she is physically capable. It is also important to evaluate the patient's mental state. Is he or she emotionally ready to go home and be taught about self-care or start a rehabilitation program? Each patient's therapeutic goals must be individualized. If the patient is not physically or emotionally ready to take care of himself or herself, the family or a paid care provider is needed.

The patient and family must understand the therapeutic goals and how they are to be achieved. Effective teaching methods include the following:

a. Speak at the patient's and family's level of understanding. Medical language usually reserved for peer discussions is not understandable to people without a medical background. Yet using overly simple explanations can be insulting to someone who is intelligent and/or well educated. In either case, the important information will not be perceived as intended. Give the patient written instructions as needed.
b. Frequently ask the patient and family whether they have any questions and then answer them.
c. Have the patient and family explain back to you in their own words how they understand what you just described.
d. Have the patient and family demonstrate back to you all procedures and techniques.
e. Reteach anything that is misunderstood.
f. Retest the patient and family as needed.
g. Document in the patient's chart what has been instructed.

2. Counsel the patient and family about the importance of smoking cessation (Code: IIIE2b) [Difficulty: An]

Despite denials by the cigarette manufacturers, there is absolute proof that smoking causes emphysema, chronic bronchitis, lung cancer, and heart disease. These conditions occur in the smoker who directly inhales the smoke as well as the nonsmoking spouse and children from second-hand smoke. Asthmatics often find that their bronchospasm is worsened when they inhale tobacco smoke. Obviously it is important that any patient with a smoking-related cardiopulmonary disease cease smoking. The patient's family must also stop smoking. Continued exposure to tobacco smoke harms the patient.

Because the nicotine found in tobacco is highly addictive, many patients find that they cannot stop smoking without suffering from withdrawal symptoms such as agitation and craving for a cigarette. To aid in stopping smoking it is often helpful to meet with a group of people who are also trying to stop. This group support helps the patient feel less alone in his or her efforts to stop smoking. The patient's physician also must be involved in this process.

If the patient has been unable to stop smoking because of withdrawal symptoms, it is likely that he or she is addicted to nicotine. A nicotine replacement system that allows gradual withdrawal greatly aids in smoking cessation. Although no smoking cessation plan works in every case, the highest percentage of patients are able to stop smoking if they have a combination of psychologic support and a gradual reduction in nicotine.

At the current time, there are several well-established nicotine replacement and reduction systems. All are available without prescription. Nicotine polacrilex (Nicorette) is a gum that is chewed by the patient to release a dose of nicotine. Nicotine transdermal patches are a second nicotine reduction system. Prostep, Nicoderm, and Habitrol are three brands of patch that, when placed onto the skin, allow a set amount of nicotine to be absorbed. With these systems, the patient starts with a relatively high dose of the drug and over a period of weeks goes through a series of patches with less and less nicotine. It is critical that the patient not smoke while using one of these systems. Patients who continue to smoke run the risk of a nicotine overdose, which increases the risk of a myocardial infarction.

A third option is taking the drug Zyban (bupropion HCl). It was originally found helpful in the care of patients suffering depression and also acts to alter the brain's chemistry so that nicotine craving is reduced. A physician must prescribe it.

Some patients experience problems with nicotine replacement and reduction systems. The transdermal patch can cause skin irritation. If this happens, the patch should be moved to another site. Some patients report insomnia or strange dreams while taking replacement nicotine at night. Patients with this problem should remove the patch before sleeping.

EXAM HINT

Most past examinations have had a question related to recommending a nicotine replacement system to a patient wishing to stop smoking or possible side effects of the nicotine system.

---

3. Counsel the patient and family about disease management (Code: IIIE2b) [Difficulty: An]

The respiratory therapist should have a solid understanding of the pathophysiology of the commonly found cardiopulmonary and cardiovascular conditions. This includes, but is not limited to asthma, emphysema, chronic bronchitis, pneumonia, pulmonary fibrosis, cystic fibrosis, right and left heart failure, stroke, and neuromuscular diseases. Be prepared to teach the patient and family about the patient's disease, its cause, and its medical management.

MODULE B **Home respiratory care services**

1. Interview the patient to determine what his or her home environment is like (Code: IB6c) [Difficulty: An]

The home environment is an important consideration in discharge planning with the patient and family. Barriers to the patient's mobility and complete recovery must be identified so that they can be eliminated or minimized. Ideally, the patient's home environment is determined by visiting the patient's home; however, the following questions can also be asked in the hospital:

a. How many floors does your home have?
b. Do you have to go up a set of stairs to get into your home?
c. Is your bedroom on the main floor?
d. If your bedroom is upstairs, can it be relocated to a room on the main floor?
e. If your bedroom were relocated to the main floor, would it be easy for you to get to a bathroom and the kitchen?
f. Does anyone who lives with you smoke?
g. Is there anything else in or around your home that puts smoke or dust into the air?

The answers to these types of questions may lead to other questions about the patient's home environment. Think of the patient's disease or condition and the answers

that are given to determine a discharge plan that minimizes any inconveniences or barriers.

2. Interview the patient to determine what his or her family and social life is like (Code: IB6c) [Difficulty: An]

The patient's family and social life is an important consideration in discharge planning with the patient and family. Whether the patient is an adult or a child, it is important to know about his or her home life. Probably no one knows more about the patient or cares more about his or her well being than the immediate family. Very close friends can assist the family or even replace a nonexistent one. The following questions can be asked of an adult patient and family:

a. Is your spouse able to help you at home?
b. Do you have other family members who can help you at home?
c. Are there neighbors or family friends who can help you at home?
d. Do you belong to any clubs or church? Can you get to them?
e. Do you garden, have a pet, or have any hobbies at your home?

The following questions can be asked of the family of a minor child:

a. Do both parents live at home? If not, with whom does the child live? Do both parents care for the child?
b. Are there any siblings who can help care for the child?
c. Do you have other family members who can help you care for the child at home?
d. Are there neighbors or family friends who can help you care for the child at home?
e. Does the child belong to any clubs or church? Can you get the child to them? Can they help you care for the child at home?
f. Can you get the child to and from school?

The answers to these types of questions may lead you to think of other questions about the patient's family and social life. Think of the patient's disease or condition and the answers that are given to determine a discharge plan that minimizes any disturbances in family life.

3. Interview the patient to determine his or her nutritional status (Code: IB6c) [Difficulty: An]

The patient's nutritional status is an important part of the patient's background. Patients who have been ill for more than a few days should be suspected of suffering from malnutrition and/or dehydration to some degree. The longer they have been ill and not eating and drinking, the more they are malnourished and dehydrated. Ask the following questions of the patient or family:

a. How long have you been sick?
b. Were you able to eat and drink normally before you became sick?

c. How long has it been since you were able to drink normally? Do you feel thirsty now?

d. How long has it been since you were able to eat normally? Do you feel hungry now?

e. Is it more difficult to cough out your secretions now than before you became sick?

4. Examine the patient's home and recommend how it can be modified to ensure safety and meet infection control standards (Code: IIIE2c) [Difficulty: An]

Evaluate the following aspects of the patient's home environment:

a. Does the patient live alone or have a spouse or companion to help provide care? Make sure that telephone numbers to relatives, helpful neighbors, the patient's physician, ambulance service, local hospital, pharmacy, and any other support services are posted by each telephone.

b. Make sure that all respiratory care equipment is cleaned (see Chapter 2 for suggestions on methods of disinfection) and functioning properly.

c. Check that home oxygen systems are working properly. If the patient has an oxygen concentrator, make sure that the filters are cleaned and that the alarms are set and working. Make sure that an oxygen cylinder, regulator, and oxygen delivery system are working properly as a backup system if the oxygen concentrator fails.

d. Have the patient centrally locate all necessary items for daily living. The patient should avoid unnecessary stair climbing. It might be recommended that the patient convert the living room, if it is located near the kitchen and bathroom, into a bedroom. Clothing can be modified with Velcro fasteners, snaps, or zippers if the patient cannot use buttons easily. Shoes can be put on more easily with a long-handled shoehorn. Avoid shoes with laces. A long-handled comb or brush makes grooming easier.

e. The kitchen should be modified so that all commonly used equipment is on the counter. Everyday dishes, utensils, and foods should be placed so that they can be easily reached in cabinets and drawers within an arm's reach. The patient should not have to bend over, stoop down, or climb onto a footstool to get anything that is needed.

f. The bathroom may need to have handholds added to the walls by the toilet and shower or tub for extra security when using these facilities. A shower chair can be added so that the patient can sit while bathing. A hand-held shower head might make bathing easier.

g. Check the home for airborne irritants. Smoking by the patient or anyone else in the home must be stopped. The patient should avoid contact with other forms of indoor pollution such as aerosol sprays, paints, varnishes, dust, and so forth. A high-efficiency particulate air (HEPA) filtration system is best for removing indoor

airborne pollutants and irritants. Indoor kerosene-fueled space heaters should not be used because they release carbon monoxide.

h. The patient should avoid contact with any known allergens, people who smoke, or substances to which he or she has a bad reaction.

5. Monitor and maintain all respiratory care equipment used in the home (Code: IIIC2a) [Difficulty: R, Ap, An]

Home care equipment is essentially the same as that found in any hospital. The same types of equipment problems can occur in the patient's home as in the hospital. Those who wish to learn more about specific brands of home care equipment are referred to the several excellent books that discuss respiratory care equipment or the manufacturer's literature. Review, if necessary, the respiratory care procedures presented in this or other respiratory care books because they can be performed in the home care setting as well as in the hospital.

EXAM HINT

Past examinations have included a question related to home respiratory care equipment. Examples include: (1) Recommendation of the use of an oxygen-conserving nasal cannula and oxygen concentrator for the economical delivery of low flow oxygen. (2) Recommendation of the maintenance of an oxygen concentrator (cleaning its filters) and the use of a back-up source of oxygen (switching to an oxygen cylinder) when an oxygen concentrator fails. (3) Provision of telephone instructions to a home care patient whose nasal cannula has no flow through it. This includes having the patient place the cannula under water to check for bubbling, tightening all tubing connections, confirming that gas is flowing from the oxygen concentrator, or replacing a defective cannula.

---

6. Apnea monitoring
a. Perform apnea monitoring (Code: IB9g) [Difficulty: An]

Apnea monitoring is indicated in an infant who has documented periods of apnea of prematurity resulting from an immature central nervous system. This condition is most commonly seen in infants less than 35 weeks' gestational age. The usual monitoring guidelines include apneic periods that last longer than 20 seconds and are associated with bradycardia with a heart rate of less than 100 beats per minute. Hypoxemia is often demonstrated by cyanosis, pallor, or documented desaturation through pulse oximetry. In addition, the infant may show marked limpness, choking, or gagging. Other conditions such as intracranial hemorrhage, patent ductus arteriosus, upper airway obstruction, hypermagnesemia, infection, maternal narcotic agents, and so forth should be ruled out before apnea of prematurity is confirmed. If this is the infant's problem, it is usually outgrown by the time the infant is 40

BOX 16-1 Guidelines for Starting and Stopping Home Apnea Monitoring

INDICATIONS TO START HOME APNEA MONITORING

Infant has had one or more apparent life-threatening apnea events.

Infant is preterm and symptomatic of apnea.

Infant is a sibling of two or more SIDS victims.

Infant has central nervous system-based hypoventilation.

INDICATIONS TO STOP HOME APNEA MONITORING

Two to three months have passed without a significant number of alarms.

Two to three months have passed without an apnea episode.

Infant can tolerate stress of illnesses (e.g., nasopharyngitis) or immunizations (e.g., diptheria-tetanus-pertussis [DPT]) without apnea episodes.

weeks' postconceptional age. Home apnea monitoring is not indicated in normal infants, preterm infants without symptoms of apnea, or to test for sudden infant death syndrome (SIDS). See Box 16-1 for guidelines on starting and stopping home apnea monitoring.

Apnea monitors currently in use sense respiratory efforts through the changing electrical impedance measured through the chest wall as the infant breathes. Impedance is resistance to the flow of electricity through the skin and other organs. The monitor sends out a small, constant electrical current that results in a voltage across the two electrodes on the infant's chest. As the infant breathes and the chest wall expands and contracts there is a resulting change in voltage. This fluctuation is measured and interpreted as inhalation and exhalation. Similarly, smaller voltage changes are measured with each heart beat. This is measured and interpreted as the heart rate.

The following are desirable features on a home apnea monitor: (1) ability to store and display events for later analysis, (2) identification of breathing patterns and apnea periods, (3) identification of heart rate patterns, (4) estimation of tidal volume, and (5) identification of hypoxemia by pulse oximetry. Setting up a home apnea monitor involves placing the electrodes properly on the infant's chest, turning on the monitor, and setting the proper high and low limits for the alarms.

Two electrodes are usually placed where there is the greatest amount of movement during breathing. Most often, this is on the infant's upper chest between the nipples and armpits (see Fig. 16-1). With older infants the electrodes might have to be placed on the sides over the lower ribs. Occasionally one electrode is placed on the chest and the other on the infant's abdomen. Some monitoring systems require that a Velcro belt be placed around the infant over the electrodes to keep them in place. (Obviously this works only if both electrodes are on the chest.) Other systems make use of electrodes with an

adhesive. In either case, for best results the infant's chest should be washed with mild soap and water and dried before the electrodes are placed. This results in the best electrical conduction. Do not use baby oils, lotions, or powders over the electrode sites. Attach the lead wires to the electrodes. These connect to the patient cable that is then connected to the monitor. Occasionally static electricity causes some interference with the signal. A third chest electrode is then added to act as a ground wire.

The monitor should be plugged into a working electrical outlet and turned on. Set the unit to charge the internal battery so that it can be made portable for later use. Confirm that the infant's respiratory and heart rates are being sensed and displayed. If pulse oximetry is a feature on the unit, the probe should be properly placed on the infant and an SpO_2 value should be displayed. Set the high and low alarm values according to the physician's orders or established protocols. For example:

1. Set the apnea alarm to trigger after 20 seconds.
2. Set the low heart rate alarm to trigger if the heart rate is less than 100 beats per minute.
3. If available, set the pulse oximeter alarm to trigger if the SpO_2 drops below 90%.
4. If available, set the high heart rate alarm to trigger if the heart rate is greater than 150 beats per minute.

Multiple alarms provide for a greater margin of patient safety. They also indicate what physiologically deteriorates first in the infant. These backup alarm systems are important because the apnea monitor senses chest wall movement, not air movement. It is possible for the infant to have an upper airway obstruction and continue to make breathing attempts; therefore the apnea monitor will not alarm because the chest wall is moving. The bradycardia or desaturation alarms will signal that the infant is in trouble.

It is critically important that the parent(s) know about the infant's medical condition. They need to understand how the monitor functions and what to do if the alarms go off. They should demonstrate their knowledge of the monitor's functions and be given written instructions on it. The parents should not be more than 10 seconds away from the infant at any time, which means that the infant will not be apneic for more than 30 seconds (20 seconds alarm delay and 10 seconds for the parents to respond). The parents must know how to give tactile stimulation to the infant, use the manual resuscitator, call for emergency help, and perform infant cardiopulmonary resuscitation.

b. Interpret apnea monitoring results (Code: IB10g) [Difficulty: An]

Alarm situations fall into two basic categories: patient alarms and equipment alarms. Patient alarms mean that the infant is either apneic, has a heart rate below or above an acceptable level, or is desaturated. One, any two, or all three alarms may be triggered. Other than the audible alarm, a visual alarm flashes to show the problem(s), and

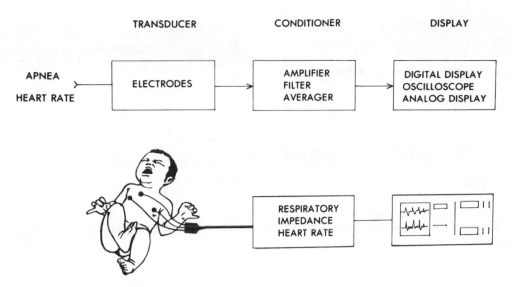

Fig. 16-1 Block diagram for impedance apnea and heart rate monitor. (From Lough MD. In Lough MD, Williams TJ, Rawson JE, editors: *Newborn respiratory care,* St Louis, 1979, Mosby.)

the recording device keeps track of the events. The parents should be instructed to first care for the infant, then, when the infant is back to normal, the alarms can be reset.

There are three types of equipment alarms: electrode or lead problem, low battery, or monitor failure. The unit should have different visual and audible alarms for equipment failure so that the family does not mistakenly think that the infant is in trouble. An electrode or lead problem alarm usually occurs because the electrode came off of the infant or the lead became disconnected. The family should be taught how to fix these types of problems. A low battery alarm indicates that there is not much time left for the monitor to function on battery power. The family should be instructed to plug the monitor into a functioning electrical outlet and the unit should be set to recharge the battery. A monitor failure alarm indicates a serious internal problem with the monitor. It is not functioning properly and should not be used. The family should be instructed to observe the infant continuously and call the home care company for a replacement monitor.

Apnea monitors in current use record and store the alarm situations discussed previously. The information can usually be downloaded into a computer for a visual display of breathing and heart rate patterns, equipment problems, and the dates and times of their occurrences. The therapist or physician should review all this data to determine what kind of problems the patient had.

c. Maintain apnea monitors (Code: IIIE2a) [Difficulty: R, Ap, An]

There is little to maintain on an apnea monitor. Make sure that the battery is recharging properly, test that the

audible and visual alarms go off when an alarm limit is reached, and confirm that the high and low alarm limits are set properly.

The monitor is usually cleaned by wiping it off with a soft cloth that has been dampened. A mild detergent may be added. Do *not* use water, alcohol, or solvents to clean the unit because the electronic components may be damaged. Use another soft cloth to dry off the monitor. The lead wires and patient cable are cleaned in the same way. Follow the manufacturer's guidelines for caring for or replacing the skin electrodes. Typically, permanent electrodes are washed in mild soap and water daily and then rinsed and dried. Alcohol should not be used on them. Disposable electrodes are usually discarded after 2 or 3 days. If an electrode belt is used to hold the electrodes on the infant's chest, it should be washed and dried according to the manufacturer's guidelines.

MODULE C Pulmonary rehabilitation

1. Interview the patient to determine how much exercise he or she can tolerate and how active the patient is on a daily basis (Code: IB6b) [Difficulty: An]

The following subject areas and questions will help you to further determine the patient's exercise tolerance and activities of daily living (ADL):

Personal grooming

a. Do you get short of breath when dressing?

b. What is the most difficult part of dressing?

c. Are you able to wash your hair regularly?

d. Are you (men) able to shave regularly?

e. Does using extra oxygen help you to do these things without getting as short of breath?

In-home activities

a. Can you go up and down stairs without getting short of breath?

b. Can you walk through your home without getting short of breath?

c. Can you cook or prepare nutritious meals?

d. Does using extra oxygen help you to do these things without getting as short of breath?

Out-of-home activities

a. Can you go shopping without getting short of breath?

b. What clubs, church, and so forth do you attend regularly?

c. Can you do yard or garden work?

d. Do you have a pet dog that you walk through the neighborhood?

e. Does using extra oxygen help you to do these things without getting as short of breath?

The patient with chronic and severe cardiopulmonary disease will tell you of a very restricted and limited lifestyle. Extra oxygen may have only a limited benefit. The patient with chronic, but moderate, cardiopulmonary disease is able to live a somewhat limited but full lifestyle. Extra oxygen may help greatly at times when the patient becomes short of breath. The otherwise healthy patient who has an acute cardiopulmonary disease should tell of a previously full and enjoyable lifestyle. Extra oxygen may be needed now but hopefully not upon recovery.

2. Begin a graded exercise program and monitor the patient's progress (Code: IIIE2e) [Difficulty: R, Ap, An]

The patient's physical condition must be evaluated before designing an exercise program. Besides chronic obstructive pulmonary disease (COPD), the patient may have other conditions that further limit his or her ability to safely participate in a rehabilitation program. See Box 16-2 for the suggested parameters to assess. If the patient is too ill or too limited in ability, he or she should not be placed into a rehabilitation program.

Although the patient's physical condition is the most important thing to evaluate from a safety point of view, other aspects of his or her life must also be looked into. These include a nutritional evaluation, a psychosocial evaluation, and a vocational evaluation. Because these areas are beyond the scope of practice of most respiratory therapists, the physician must call in other experts. In addition, any patient who is still smoking must be enrolled in a smoking cessation program.

Similar to preparing a patient for home care, all the patient's physical condition information must be evaluated. Each patient must have an individualized program and be physically and emotionally prepared to begin the rehabilitation program. As discussed next, the patient is placed into either an open- or closed-end program format.

BOX 16-2	Patient Evaluation Before Starting a Pulmonary Rehabilitation Program

History
Complete physical examination
Chest radiograph
Resting diagnostic electrocardiogram
Complete blood count
Serum electrolytes
Urinalysis
Arterial blood gases
Theophylline level
Sputum analysis
Pulmonary function tests
  Spirometry
  Lung volume study
  Diffusion capacity
  Before and after bronchodilator study
Pulmonary stress test including:
  Electrocardiogram
  Blood pressure
  Heart rate
  Respiratory rate
  Pulse oximetry
  Maximum ventilation
  Oxygen consumption
  Carbon dioxide production
  Respiratory quotient

(See Chapter 4 for information on pulmonary function testing and Chapter 17 for information on cardiopulmonary stress testing.)

The starting and ending points of the program are determined based on the patient's physical condition, heart rate target, and stress test results.

A graded exercise program is an individually structured sequence of events that is designed to increase safely the patient's exercise tolerance. It is a critical component of any pulmonary rehabilitation program. In 1942, the Council of Rehabilitation defined rehabilitation "as the restoration of the individual to the fullest medical, mental, emotional, social, and vocational potential of which he/she is capable." In 1974, The American College of Chest Physicians' Committee on Pulmonary Rehabilitation adopted the following:

Pulmonary rehabilitation may be defined as an art of medical practice wherein an individually tailored, multidisciplinary program is formulated which through accurate diagnosis, therapy, emotional support, and education, stabilizes or reverses both the physio- and psychopathology of pulmonary diseases and attempts to return the patient the *highest possible functional capacity* [italics added] allowed by his pulmonary handicap and overall life situation.

It further states: "In the broadest sense, pulmonary rehabilitation means providing good, comprehensive respiratory care for patients with pulmonary disease."

The patient with pulmonary disease who is inactive

BOX 16-3	Effects of Inactivity

METABOLISM

Decreased metabolic rate, decreased protein catabolism, negative nitrogen balance, decubitus ulcers, imbalance of cellular electrolytes, and gastrointestinal hypomotility

PSYCHOSOCIAL

Decreased learning ability, decreased motivation to learn, decreased retention of new material, decreased problem-solving ability, exaggerated or inappropriate emotional reactions, perceptual and motor changes, and increased somatic concerns

RESPIRATORY SYSTEM

Decreased movement of secretions, decreased use of respiratory muscles, and development of microatelectasis and infection

MUSCULAR SYSTEM

Loss of normal muscle tone, decreased muscle efficiency, increased local muscle oxygen consumption, rapid onset of fatigue, and contracture

CARDIOPULMONARY SYSTEM

Decreased cardiac output, venous stasis, thromboembolism, and pulmonary emboli

SKELETAL SYSTEM

Osteoporosis, reabsorption of calcium from the bone, and increased incidence of compression fractures

From May DF: *Rehabilitation and continuity of care in pulmonary disease,* St Louis, 1991, Mosby.

because of his or her condition experiences a slow deterioration in overall body function. It is well known that physical activity is important for general health. Box 16-3 lists the effects of inactivity.

The remainder of this discussion focuses on how to start a patient in a graded exercise program and monitor his or her progress through it. (Note that the education of the patient about normal and abnormal lung function, respiratory care procedures, medications, and so forth is addressed in earlier sections of this book and in other textbooks dedicated solely to pulmonary rehabilitation.)

1. Benefits of an exercise program

The benefits of the exercise program must be stressed to the patient to gain his or her acceptance of it. If the patient does not believe that the program will make his or her life better, it will not be followed. In 1981, the American Thoracic Society Executive Committee adopted the following as principle objectives of pulmonary rehabilitation:

1. To control and alleviate as much as possible the symptoms and pathologic complications of respiratory ailments.
2. To teach the patient how to achieve optimal capability for carrying out his or her activities of daily living.

Most authors agree with the following general therapeutic goals:

1. The primary goal is to increase the patient's functional ability as much as possible. This can best be determined by finding out what the patient wants to be able to do with his or her life on a daily basis. From this list of ADLs, a series of short- and long-term goals can be developed. One of the primary short-term goals should be that the patient feels better. He or she should be able to control or reduce any symptoms. This alone improves the patient's quality of life. Make sure that the patient's goals are realistic and can be reached. The family must be involved with any major decision making. Often it is helpful to break a large goal down into several smaller tasks so that the patient and family receive frequent positive feedback.
2. Improve the patient's self-image. This should follow when goal number one is reached. The patient should experience less anxiety and depression and also feel better about himself or herself.
3. Increase the patient's ability to exercise. This may depend on the level of the patient's disability. In general, the worse the patient's lung disease is, the less able the patient is to increase his or her exercise level.
4. Decrease the frequency and length of any hospitalizations.
5. Prolong the patient's life by the proper use of oxygen and other respiratory care modalities.

Note that the benefits did not list an improvement in the patient's cardiopulmonary condition. Numerous studies have documented that pathologic changes seen in COPD do *not* improve despite the patient being in a rehabilitation program. It is important that the therapist correct any misunderstanding of this.

EXAM HINT

Past examinations have included one or two questions related to identifying the goals and/or benefits of a pulmonary rehabilitation program.

2. Individualized graded exercise program

The program format and features may vary considerably. Minimally, the patient's physician should specify four parts to the exercise prescription: mode, intensity, duration, and frequency. The following program formats and suggestions are typical of what might be ordered.

3. Program format

There are two basic types of formats. Each has its own advantages and disadvantages depending on what the patient's limitations and preferences may be. The *open-end format* allows the patient to enter and progress through the program at his or her own pace. Because each patient's goals are individualized, the time of their accomplishment is relatively unimportant as long as progress is being made. The program facilitator (often a respiratory therapist) acts as a coordinator. This may include making sure that educational materials are available for the patient, exercise equipment is available, and the patient's questions are answered. The patient may stay in the program until the last goal is achieved. The advantages of this program are that it is self-directed and can be adjusted if the patient has a schedule conflict. The disadvantage of this program is that there is no group support or involvement with other people who have COPD.

The *closed-end format* involves the program facilitator setting up a formal schedule of educational topics and exercise sessions. These group events commonly last from 1 to 3 hours and may occur from one to three times per week. The whole program can vary in length from 8 to 16 weeks depending on the content. These events are attended by a group of patients who share a common problem and have common goals to cope with it. One major advantage of this program is that most patients do better when they have peers to call on for emotional support. The facilitator will probably find that it is easier to schedule speakers when a sure time frame can be set. The disadvantages of this program relate to the loss of individual goals and attention. If a patient misses a session, he or she will have to wait for the topic to be repeated at the next program. If the group is too large, the facilitator may not have time to help a patient with an individual goal.

4. Strength training

Many patients are so weak from years of relative inactivity that they must regain muscle strength before working on increased endurance. The specific muscle groups that need strengthening can be determined by physical examination. In general, the large muscle groups of the legs and arms and inspiratory muscles must be strengthened.

Before beginning strength training, the patient must perform calisthenics for about 10 minutes as a "warm up." It is important to stretch the muscles and joints and increase circulation before starting more vigorous activity. See Fig. 16-2, groups 1 to 7, for a series of progressively more demanding calisthenic exercises. All patients should at least be able to perform the calisthenics shown in groups 1 and 2 for a warm up. The patient must focus on breath control (pursed-lips breathing) during the warm-up period to avoid dyspnea.

Arm and leg strengthening can be done in a variety of ways for about 10 minutes. Typically, a 1- or 2-lb weight is used. Barbell weights can be held as the arms are moved to the back, front, sides, and overhead to strengthen the arms, shoulders, and chest and back muscles. Ankle weights can be strapped on. The legs are then moved to the back, front, sides, and the legs lifted with knees bent. Or the initial

calisthenics can be repeated with added weight. The abdominal muscles can be strengthened by having the patient lie on his or her back and placing a 2-lb weight on the abdomen. The patient then concentrates on maintaining breath control against the added weight.

Inspiratory muscle strengthening is done in two ways. First, the patient is told to take in a deep sigh and hold it for a brief time. This both stretches the rib cage and increases the work load of the primary and secondary inspiratory muscles. The deep sigh should be repeated several times. Second, the patient uses a specific inspiratory muscle training device. The PFLEX device is popular because it is inexpensive and can be gradually adjusted to increase the work load as the patient improves.

Finally, the patient should spend about 10 minutes in "cool-down" activities. This may involve more light calisthenics or slow walking. The cool-down period allows

---

BOX 16-4   Guidelines for Strength and Endurance Training

STRENGTH TRAINING

This involves a low number of repetitions of a high-intensity activity, such as lifting weights.

Warm-up period involving calisthenics for about 10 minutes

The following strengthening program should last about 10 minutes:
  a. Three sets of 10 to 15 repetitions of an activity
  b. Each set is followed by a rest period of a few minutes
  c. The patient should work at 85% to 90% of the maximum capacity of the muscles being exercised

Cool-down period involving calisthenics for about 10 minutes.

The patient should exercise every other day; there should be a rest day between the exercise days.

This program may precede or be done simultaneously with an endurance program.

It takes 4 to 8 weeks for improved strength to be realized.

ENDURANCE TRAINING

This involves a high number of repetitions of a relatively low-intensity activity, such as walking.

Warm-up period involving calisthenics for about 10 minutes

The patient should do the following:
  a. Exercise continuously for about 20 to 30 minutes
  b. Exercise at a level that results in the target heart rate being maintained

Cool-down period involving calisthenics for about 10 minutes

The patient should exercise every other day; there should be a rest day between the exercise days.

This program may follow or be done simultaneously with a strength program.

It takes 4 to 8 weeks for improved endurance to be realized.

Modified from May DF: *Rehabilitation and continuity of care in pulmonary disease,* St Louis, 1991, Mosby.

Group 1 Exercises

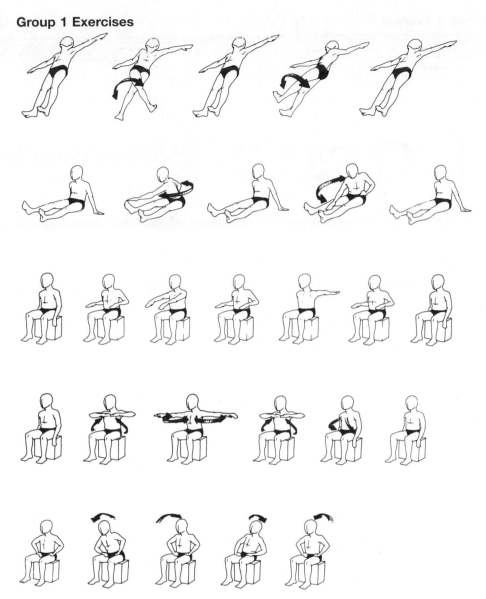

Fig. 16-2   Modified calisthenic exercises. In all groups, the figure to the left is the starting point. The figures to the right show the sequence of steps in the exercise. The patient can adjust the pace of exercises to either increase or decrease the energy that is spent. In general, most patients choose 10 to 15 repetitions per minute. Exercises shown in groups 1 and 2 are useful during the warm-up period of either a strength or endurance program. Exercises shown in groups 3 and 4 are more demanding and can be used for muscle reconditioning by many patients in an endurance program. The most demanding exercises are those shown in groups 5, 6, and 7. Patients with only moderate disability may be able to progress to this level for further muscle conditioning. (From May DF: *Rehabilitation and continuity of care in pulmonary disease,* St Louis, 1991, Mosby.)

(Continued)

the body to return to a slower metabolic rate while still maintaining good circulation to the arms and legs. This helps to eliminate any lactic acid that might have built up in the muscles during the more vigorous exercise. Increased lactic acid may cause some muscle aches after exercise. Inform the patient that there may be some muscle soreness the next day. It can be relieved by taking an antiinflamma-

tory medication such as aspirin if the physician approves. See Box 16-4 for specific guidelines for a strength training program.

It is helpful, but not necessary, for the patient to have access to professional body building equipment found in many gymnasiums. In addition, a physical therapist is helpful in designing a training program.

Group 2 Exercises

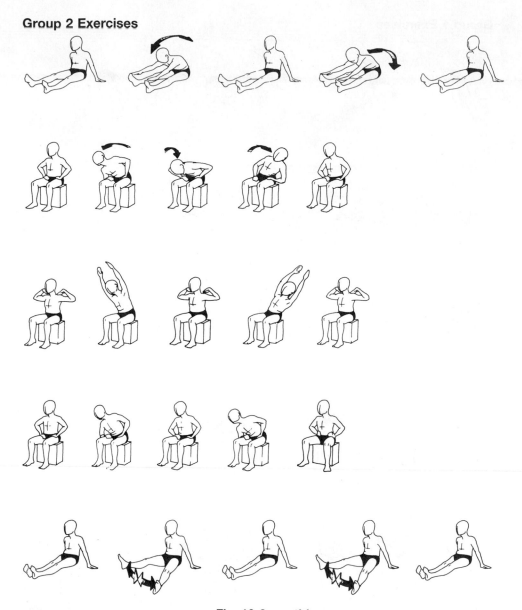

Fig. 16-2, cont'd

5. Endurance training

Endurance training is designed to build up the patient's stamina to perform ADLs. It does this by improving the functioning of the patient's cardiopulmonary and cardiovascular systems. When these systems are functioning better, they can meet the patient's need for increased oxygen delivery to and carbon dioxide removal from exercising muscles.

Endurance training must be preceded by the patient performing calisthenics for about 10 minutes as a warm up. Just as in strength training, it is important to stretch the muscles and joints and increase circulation before starting more vigorous activity. See Fig. 16-2, groups 1 through 7, for a series of progressively more demanding calisthenic exercises. All patients should be able to at least perform the calisthenics shown in groups 1 and 2 for a warm up.

Patients who can perform the activities shown in groups 3 and 4 gain some endurance training as well. Some very debilitated patients may not be able to perform at this higher level. Some less-debilitated patients will eventually be able to advance to the highest levels. The patient must focus on breath control (pursed-lips breathing) during the warm-up period to avoid dyspnea.

The actual endurance exercise that is selected must meet the patient's needs. He or she can walk, use a treadmill, ride a bicycle ergometer, swim, or do a combination of these. The method that is selected must be both practical and fun for the patient. For this reason, walking is usually the main activity; however, the upper body should not be ignored. An arm ergometer, rowing machine, or barbell weights can be used for upper-body endurance.

Group 3 Exercises

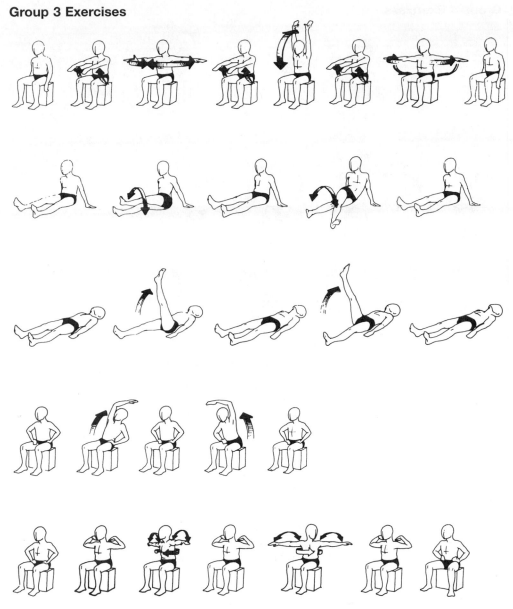

Fig. 16-2, cont'd

A key concept of the endurance program is that the patient must exercise at a level great enough to raise the heart rate to a predetermined level. The increased heart rate reflects the increased metabolic rate and work being performed by the patient. The target heart rate must be maintained for 20 to 30 minutes to have any muscle training effect. Exercising at a lower heart (and metabolic) rate is not as beneficial. Exercising at a higher heart rate may be dangerous to the patient. Karvonen's formula is used to determine the target heart rate for endurance training:

Target heart rate (HR) = [% intensity (maximum HR −
resting HR)] + resting HR

In which:

Target HR = the target heart rate for the exercise period

% intensity = 60% to 80%

Maximum HR = maximum HR determined by either of the following formulas:

   (a) Maximum HR = 220 − age of the patient

   (b) Maximum HR = 210 − (age of the patient × 0.65)

Resting HR = the patient's resting heart rate

Example. Determine the target heart rate for a 50-year-old patient (of either sex) who is enrolled in an endurance training program. The patient has a resting heart

Group 4 Exercises

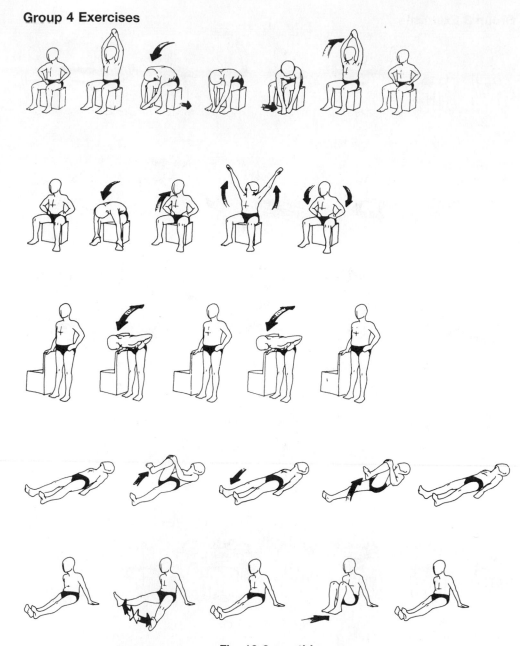

Fig. 16-2, cont'd

rate of 80 beats per minute. The patient's maximum heart rate is 170 (220 − 50 for the patient's age = 170).

Target HR = [% intensity (maximum HR ×

resting HR)] + resting HR

Lowest target HR = [0.60 (170 − 80)] + 80
= [0.60 (90)] + 80
= [54] + 80
= 134 beats per minute

Highest target HR = [0.80 (170 − 80)] + 80
= [0.80 (90)] + 80
= [72] + 80
= 152 beats per minute

The range of target heart rates for this patient is 134 to 152 beats per minute. The patient must monitor his or her heart rate during the exercise period to make sure that it stays within this range. This is most easily accomplished by feeling the radial or carotid pulse and counting heartbeats for a 15-second period, then multiplying by four to find the heart rate for 1 minute.

Finally, as in strength training, the patient should spend about 10 minutes in "cool-down" activities. This may involve light calisthenics or slow walking. As discussed earlier, the cool-down period allows the body to return to a slower metabolic rate while still maintaining good circula-

Group 5 Exercises

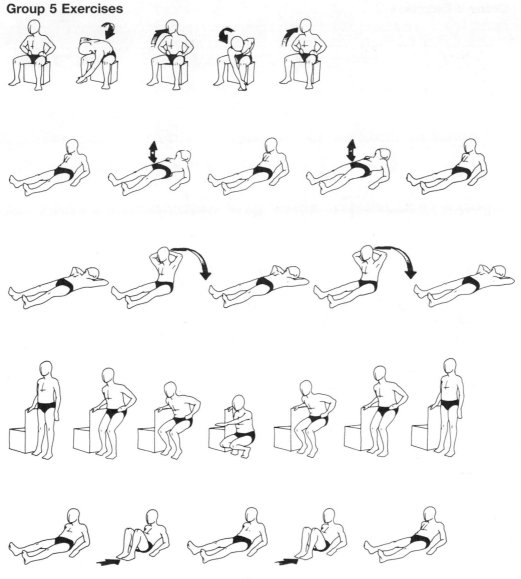

Fig. 16-2, cont'd

tion to the arms and legs. This helps to eliminate any lactic acid that may have built up in the muscles during the endurance exercise. See Box 16-4 for specific guidelines for an endurance training program.

6. Assessment of the patient's progress in the program

The following indicate that the patient is making progress:

1. The patient subjectively feels that he or she is doing as well as can be expected. The patient is motivated to try new things.
2. Symptoms are reduced or at least under control.
3. Cardiopulmonary function tests and blood gases show improvement. Even a slowing in the patient's former rapid rate of decline is a good sign.
4. The patient reports an increase in the distance that can be walked at his or her own pace.
5. The patient reports an increase in the 6-minute or 12-minute walk distance. The 6-minute or 12-minute walk is a measurement of how far a person can maximally walk in the given time period.

The following indicate that the patient's health is deteriorating:

1. He or she subjectively feels worse. The patient is afraid to try new things.
2. Symptoms are worse. The patient feels dyspneic at less exertion than before.
3. The sputum has changed. It may be thick and harder to cough out or have changed color to yellow or green. The patient may be coughing out more than before or less if it cannot be brought up.

Group 6 Exercises

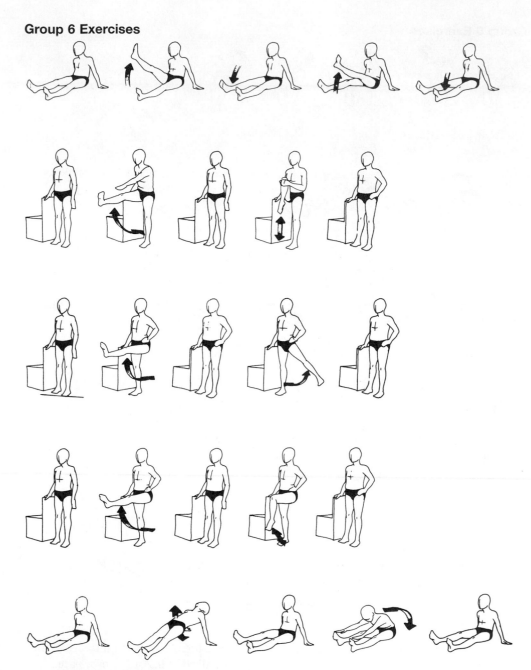

Fig. 16-2, cont'd

4. Cardiopulmonary function tests and blood gases are worse. The patient may need more oxygen, an aerosolized bronchodilator, or other cardiopulmonary medications.

5. The patient cannot walk or perform as much work as before without having the symptoms worsen.

MODULE D   Respiratory care plan

1. Participate in the development of the respiratory care plan (e.g., case management, development and applica-

tion of protocols, disease management education) (Code: IC4) [Difficulty: An]

Respiratory care protocols may be used at home as well as in the hospital. An oxygen therapy protocol can be implemented that uses the patient's pulse oximetry values to adjust the oxygen percentage or flow up or down. For example, keep the patient's SpO_2 less than 95% but greater than 85%. A second protocol may be using inhaled sympathomimetic bronchodilators based on the patient's peak flow results.

The patient's physical condition must be evaluated before designing a home care or rehabilitation program.

Group 7 Exercises

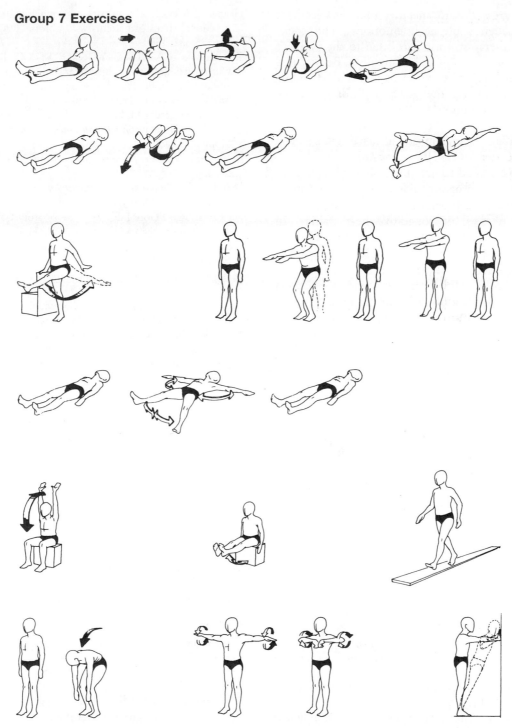

Fig. 16-2, cont'd

Besides the primary diagnosis, the patient may have other conditions that further limit his or her ability to participate safely. If the patient is too ill or too limited in ability, he or she should not be placed into a home care or rehabilitation program.

Although the patient's physical condition is the most important thing to evaluate from a safety point of view, other aspects of his or her life must also be looked into.

These include a nutritional evaluation, a psychosocial evaluation, and a vocational evaluation. Because these areas are beyond the scope of practice of most respiratory therapists, the physician must call in other experts.

Be prepared to evaluate the patient's condition and make suggestions for changing goals, methods, and so forth. The therapist must have a thorough understanding of the patient's condition and individual goals to evaluate his or her progress toward meeting them. Objectively consider the patient's physical, emotional, and social condition. The therapist must also listen to the patient's subjective opinion about his or her situation. Be prepared to make recommendations to the patient and attending physician for modifying the goals depending on the patient's changing condition.

2. Conduct patient education and disease management programs (Code: IIIE2f) [Difficulty: An]

The therapist should be able to implement a patient's disease management program. For example, the patient may have a home care program to manage emphysema, asthma, cystic fibrosis, or congestive heart failure. In addition, the therapist should monitor the patient's compliance to the program. For example, is the patient faithfully following the smoking cessation program or has he or she "cheated"? Is the patient following the asthma control program by monitoring his or her peak flow and adjusting inhaled medications according to the physician's order?

BIBLIOGRAPHY

AARC Clinical Practice Guideline: Oxygen therapy in the home or extended care facility, *Respir Care* 37:918, 1992.

Bell CW et al: *Home care and rehabilitation in respiratory medicine*, Philadelphia, 1984, JB Lippincott.

Belman MJ, Wasserman K: Exercise training and testing in patients with chronic obstructive pulmonary disease, *Basics Respir Dis* 10(2), 1981.

Branson RD, Hess DR, Chatburn RL, *Respiratory care equipment*, ed 2, Philadelphia, 1999, Lippincott Williams & Wilkins.

Christopher KL: At-home administration of oxygen. In Kacmarek RM, Stoller JK, editors: *Current respiratory care*, Toronto, 1988, BC Decker.

Connors G, Hilling L, editors: *American Association of Cardiovascular and Pulmonary Rehabilitation: guidelines for pulmonary rehabilitation programs*, Champaign, IL, 1993, Human Kinetics.

Dunlevy CL: Patient education and health promotion. In Scanlan CL, Wilkins RL, Stoller JK, editors: *Egan's fundamentals of respiratory care*, ed 7, St Louis, 1999, Mosby.

Edge RS: Infection control. In Barnes TA, editor: *Respiratory care practice*, St Louis, 1988, Mosby.

Eubanks DH, Bone RC: *Comprehensive respiratory care*, ed 2, St Louis, 1990, Mosby.

Gilmartin M: Transition from the intensive care unit to home: patient selection and discharge planning, *Respir Care* 39:456, 1994.

Hodgkin JE: Home care and pulmonary rehabilitation. In Kacmarek RM, Stoller JK, editors: *Current respiratory care*, Toronto, 1988, BC Decker.

Hodgkin JE, Celli BR, Connors GL: *Pulmonary rehabilitation: guides to success*, ed. 3, Philadelphia, 2000, Lippincott Williams & Wilkins.

Hodgkin JE, Connors GA: Pulmonary rehabilitation. In Burton GG, Hodgkin JE, Ward JJ, editors: *Respiratory care: a guide to clinical practice*, ed 4, Philadelphia, 1997, JB Lippincott.

Holden DA et al: The impact of a rehabilitation program on functional status of patients with chronic lung disease, *Respir Care* 35:332, 1990.

Kwiatkowski CA, Tougher-Decker R, O'Sullivan-Maillet J: Nutritional aspects of health and disease. In Scanlan CL, Wilkins RL, Stoller JK, editors: *Egan's fundamentals of respiratory care*, ed 7, St Louis, 1999, Mosby.

Lewis ML, Hagarty EM, Lawlor B: Home respiratory care. In Fink JB, Hunt GE, editors: *Clinical practice in respiratory care*, 1999, Lippincott Williams & Wilkins.

Lucas J et al: *Home respiratory care*, Norwalk, CN, 1988, Appleton & Lange.

May DF: *Rehabilitation and continuity of care in pulmonary disease*, St Louis, 1991, Mosby.

McInturff SL, O'Donohue WJ Jr: Respiratory Care in the Home and Alternate Sites. In Burton GG, Hodgkin JE, Ward JJ, editors: *Respiratory care: a guide to clinical practice*, ed 4, Philadelphia, 1997, JB Lippincott.

McPherson SP: *Respiratory therapy equipment*, ed 4, St Louis, 1990, Mosby.

Mulligan SC et al: Clinical and pharmacokinetic properties of a transdermal nicotine patch, *Clin Pharmacol Ther* 47:331, 1990.

Nett LM: The physician's role in smoking cessation, *Chest Suppl* 97(2):28s, 1990.

Petty TL: Pulmonary rehabilitation: better living with new technology, *Respir Care* 30:98, 1985.

Petty TL, Nett LM: *Enjoying life with emphysema*, Philadelphia, 1987, Lea & Febiger.

Pulmonary rehabilitation: official American Thoracic Society statement, *Am Rev Respir Dis* 124:663, 1981.

Rennard SI, Daughton D: Transdermal nicotine for smoking cessation, *Respir Care* 38:290, 1993.

Scanlan CL, Heuer A, Wyka KA: Respiratory care in alternate sites. In Scanlan CL, Wilkins RL, Stoller JK, editors: *Egan's fundamentals of respiratory care*, ed 7, St Louis, 1999, Mosby.

Sobush D, Dunning M, McDonald K: Exercise prescription components for respiratory muscle training: past, present, and future, *Respir Care* 30:34, 1985.

Taylor C, Lillis C, LeMond P: *Fundamentals of nursing: the art and science of nursing care*, ed 2, Philadelphia, 1993, JB Lippincott.

White GC: *Equipment theory for respiratory care*, ed 3, Albany, NY, 1999, Delmar.

Wyka KA, Myslinski MJ: Cardiopulmonary rehabilitation. In Scanlan CL, Wilkins RL, Stoller JK, editors: *Egan's fundamentals of respiratory care*, ed 7, St Louis, 1999, Mosby.

SELF-STUDY QUESTIONS

1. The therapeutic goals of a rehabilitation program include all the following *except*:
   A. Decreased hospitalizations
   B. Reversal of lung disease
   C. Increase the patient's energy level
   D. Increase the patient's ability to perform ADL

2. A home care patient calls to say that he cannot feel any oxygen coming out of the nasal cannula. Also, the oxygen concentrator is making odd cycling noises. What should the respiratory therapist recommend?
   A. Reset the circuit breaker on the concentrator and call back in an hour.

B. Switch the cannula to a liquid oxygen system at a higher flow rate than the concentrator.

C. Switch the cannula to an oxygen cylinder at the same flow rate as the concentrator.

D. Disassemble the concentrator and clean out the air filter.

3. An open-end format exercise program should be recommended to a patient who has an unpredictable work and social schedule because of the following:

   I. Members of the exercise group can offer support to each other.

   II. It is self-directed by the patient.

   III. The facilitator can easily plan group activities.

   IV. The patient can adjust the schedule of activities if necessary.

   A. II and IV only

   B. I and III only

   C. IV only

   D. II and III only

4. All of the following are indications for monitoring infant apnea at home *except:*

   A. Surgically repaired cleft palate

   B. Apnea periods lasting 25 seconds

   C. Two older siblings died of SIDS

   D. Premature infant with apnea periods and bradycardia

5. The components of a strength training program include:

   I. Cool-down period

   II. Strengthening exercises performed daily

   III. Warm-up period

   IV. Strengthening exercises performed every other day

   V. Exercises performed for 20 to 30 minutes continuously

   A. I and II only

   B. III, IV, and V only

   C. II, III, and V only

   D. I, III, and IV only

6. You are supervising a patient who is participating in an endurance training rehabilitation program. Her target heart rate is between 130 and 150 beats per minute. She is exercising on a bicycle ergometer and her heart rate is 167 beats per minute. What would you advise her to do?

   A. Exercise only until she begins to perspire

   B. Continue exercising if she feels that she can handle the workload

   C. Exercise a maximum of 10 minutes each day

   D. Slow down on the ergometer until her heart rate drops to the target level

7. Home apnea monitoring can usually be stopped when all the following conditions exist *except:*

   A. The infant has gone 30 days without an apnea episode.

   B. The infant has had a DPT immunization without any consequences.

   C. Three months have passed without any alarms sounding.

   D. Two months have passed without an apnea episode.

8. A pulmonary rehabilitation patient is ordered to perform a 12-minute walk to improve her endurance. The patient should be instructed to:

   A. Ride a bicycle ergometer for 12 minutes and note the distance pedaled.

   B. Walk as quickly as possible for 6 minutes and double the distance covered.

   C. Walk as far as possible in 12 minutes and note the distance.

   D. Walk as far as possible in 3 minutes and multiply the distance by four.

9. The respiratory therapist is working with a group of COPD patients who need to begin a pulmonary rehabilitation program. A closed-end program would be best for the group for all of the following reasons *except:*

   A. Group members can offer emotional support to each other.

   B. The program facilitator can direct group activities.

   C. Learning activities can be optimally sequenced.

   D. Each patient can easily adjust activities if a scheduling conflict arises.

10. A COPD patient who is trying to quit smoking is using a nicotine patch. He complains of skin irritation on his arm where the patch is placed and difficulty sleeping. The respiratory therapist should recommend the following:

    I. Apply a topical cortisone cream to the irritated skin.

    II. Move the patch to another area.

    III. Take a sleeping pill.

    IV. Remove the patch before going to bed.

    V. Drink a beer or a glass of wine before going to bed.

    A. IV and V only

    B. II and IV only

    C. I, III, and IV only

    D. I, II, IV, and V only

11. A patient receiving public aid is being discharged. The physician has ordered 2 L/min of home oxygen as needed for shortness of breath. Which of the following should be set up in the home?

    A. A bank of H tanks and simple oxygen mask

    B. Liquid oxygen system with air entrainment mask

    C. Oxygen concentrator with oxygen-conserving cannula

    D. A portable, shoulder bag oxygen tank and a regular nasal cannula

12. A 50-year-old patient with COPD is a participant in an exercise program. Which of the following are expected benefits of the program?

    I. Improved pulmonary function studies

    II. Increased strength

    III. More exercise tolerance

    IV. Reversal of lung disease

    A. I and II only

    B. II and III only

    C. I, II, and III only

    D. I, II, III, and IV

Answer Key

1. **B.** Rationale: Research has shown that lung disease cannot be reversed by a patient attending a rehabilitation program. However, a rehabilitation program can be expected to decrease a patient's number of hospitalizations, increase the patient's energy level, and increase the patient's ability to perform ADLs. These are all worthy goals that will improve the quality of the patient's life.

2. **C.** Rationale: The oxygen concentrator has failed. The patient should switch the cannula to an oxygen cylinder at the same flow rate as the concentrator. This delivers the

needed oxygen supply to the patient until the therapist can repair the unit. It is not the patient's responsibility to perform equipment repairs such as resetting the circuit breaker on the concentrator or disassembling the concentrator to clean out the air filter. In addition, the patient should not have to run the risk of not having the ordered oxygen while waiting an hour to call the therapist back for an equipment update or to ask for further assistance. The patient should not be told to increase the flow of oxygen through a liquid oxygen system above that which has been ordered by the physician through the concentrator.

3. **A.** Rationale: An open-end exercise program offers these two advantages: (1) It is self-directed by the patient. (2) The patient can adjust the schedule of activities if necessary. A closed-end exercise program offers these two advantages: (1) Members of the exercise group can offer support to each other. (2) The facilitator can easily plan group activities.

4. **A.** Rationale: A surgically repaired cleft palate has no connection with infant apnea. Apnea periods lasting 25 seconds, death of two or more older siblings from sudden infant death syndrome (SIDS), and a premature infant with apnea periods and bradycardia are all serious enough situations that apnea monitoring is indicated. See Box 16-1 if needed.

5. **D.** Rationale: These three steps are needed in a strengthening program: (1) Warm-up period. (2) Strengthening exercises performed every other day. (3) Cool-down period after the strengthening exercises. Strengthening exercises should not be performed daily because the muscles that have been worked need a day to recover before exercising again. Endurance exercises should be performed for 20 to 30 minutes continuously, *not* strengthening exercises.

6. **D.** Rationale: It would be safer to have the patient slow down on the ergometer until her heart rate drops to the target level. The patient's target heart rate range is based on the her age and physical conditioning. If the patient exercised only until she began to perspire she would probably not gain any exercise benefit. As previously stated, the target heart rate range is based on the patient's age and physical conditioning. She should not continue exercising at this elevated heart rate even if she feels that she can handle the workload. The patient gains little benefit from exercising for a maximum of 10 minutes each day. Current guidelines dictate that a person should exercise for 20 to 30 continuous minutes.

7. **A.** Rationale: Current guidelines dictate that an infant must go at least 2 to 3 months without an apnea episode, *not* 30 days without an apnea episode to discontinue apnea monitoring. An infant can have apnea monitoring stopped if the other listed options are met. See Box 16-1 if necessary.

8. **C.** Rationale: A 12-minute walk test requires that the patient walk as far as possible in 12 minutes and note the distance. It is hoped that as the patient's conditioning improves, her distance walked will increase. The patient must walk rather than ride a bicycle ergometer for 12 minutes. It is improper in a 12-minute walk test to walk as quickly as possible for 6 minutes and double the distance covered. It is improper in a 12-minute walk test to walk as far as possible in 3 minutes and multiply the distance by four. The test requires the patient to walk continuously and cover the greatest distance possible in 12 minutes.

9. **D.** Rationale: It is only in an open-end format rehabilitation program that each patient can easily adjust activities if a scheduling conflict arises. In a closed-end format rehabilitation program, all group members do the same thing at the same time. This way they can offer emotional support to each other and the program facilitator can direct group activities and optimally sequence learning activities.

10. **B.** Rationale: Moving the patch to another area of skin allows the irritated area to heal. Removing the patch before going to bed removes the stimulating nicotine that has been preventing sleep. A physician should make the recommendation to apply a topical cortisone cream to the irritated skin, not a respiratory therapist. Only a physician should make the recommendation that the patient take a sleeping pill. Although a patient may choose to drink a beer or a glass of wine before going to bed to help induce sleep, the respiratory therapist should not make this recommendation. If nicotine is preventing the patient from sleeping at night, it is best to remove the patch. Sleeping pills and alcohol can probably be avoided if the nicotine patch is removed at night.

11. **C.** Rationale: An oxygen concentrator and oxygen-conserving cannula economically provides the necessary oxygen to the patient. A bank of H tanks is expensive to set up and takes up more space than a concentrator. In addition, a nasal cannula is preferred over a simple oxygen mask to deliver 2 L/min of oxygen to a patient going home. A liquid oxygen system is more expensive to set up than a concentrator for a patient who will be using the system only during periods of shortness of breath. In addition, an air entrainment mask order must specify the patient's oxygen percentage (24%, 28%, and so on). A portable oxygen tank does not provide a long enough duration of flow to the cannula if the patient has prolonged shortness of breath. Also, an oxygen-conserving cannula is more economical than a regular cannula.

12. **B.** Rationale: Studies have shown that patients who complete a rehabilitation program can expect benefits of increased strength and more exercise tolerance. Unfortunately, the patient cannot expect to experience clinically significant improvement in pulmonary function studies. This is because the lung damage COPD patients have is not reversible.

17 | Special Procedures

A review of the most recent Written Registry Examinations has shown an average of seven questions (7% of the examination) that deal with the following special procedures.

MODULE A	Participate in air or land patient transportation (Code: IIID3) [Difficulty: R, Ap, An]

Be prepared to perform all the respiratory care practices and procedures that have been described in this and other texts during patient transport. It is extremely important that all equipment and supplies be accounted for before leaving the hospital. Obviously, once under way, there is no way to obtain something that was forgotten. To help ensure that this does not happen, it is wise to have a checklist of everything that may be needed. In addition, all equipment must be checked for proper function. Calculate the duration of the oxygen cylinders at expected liter flows. Make sure that batteries and light bulbs work and have spare batteries and light bulbs.

If mechanical ventilation will be needed, bring a unit that is lightweight and portable, has solid state circuitry, and can be powered by both alternating current (AC) and direct current (DC) from batteries. If the ventilator will be used for helicopter or unpressurized cabin fixed-wing aircraft, it must be able to deliver an intermittent mandatory ventilation (IMV)/synchronous intermittent mandatory ventilation (SIMV) mode through a demand valve rather than through a reservoir system. The ventilator controls should not be adversely affected by changes in atmospheric pressure during assent and landing.

EXAM HINT

There is usually one question on the examination that deals with the effects of increased altitude when flying in a unpressurized helicopter or airplane. Remember that as altitude increases, barometric pressure (P_B) decreases. Decreased barometric pressure directly leads to a decrease in the alveolar pressure of oxygen (PAO_2) that results in a decrease in the patient's arterial pressure of oxygen (PaO_2). In addition, as barometric pressure decreases at increased altitude, gases within the patient (stomach and intestine, pneumothorax, and lung) expand. Also, the air within the endotracheal tube cuff expands and the delivered tidal volume increases. This requires adjustments in the ventilator settings. Later, when the aircraft descends to land, the increased barometric pressure results in a decrease in the tidal volume and the patient's internal gas volumes. Be prepared to adjust the ventilator again.

MODULE B	Assist the physician who is performing the following procedures

1. Conscious sedation (Code: IIIE1l) [Difficulty: R, Ap, An]

The phrase *conscious sedation* refers to the administration of a sedative agent that calms a patient during a medical procedure (for example cardioversion or bronchoscopy) but does not cause the patient to lose consciousness. The sedated patient is still able to cooperate and follow commands during the procedure. Typically, the patient has no memory of the procedure after it is completed.

Medications in the benzodiazepine group are preferred for conscious sedation and are given intravenously. Currently midazolam (Versed) is preferred but diazepam (Valium) is also commonly used. When the patient's procedure is completed, these medications can be reversed by intravenous flumazenil (Romazicon). There is more discussion of these and other sedative agents in Chapter 8, Pharmacology.

The respiratory therapist must be prepared for the possibility of the patient being overdosed with a sedative agent. This may result in a decreased respiratory rate and tidal volume or apnea. The patient's breathing, pulse oximetry values, heart rate, blood pressure, and electrocardiogram (ECG) must be monitored. The therapist must be prepared to administer supplemental oxygen or begin bag-mask ventilation if needed.

2. Insertion of lines for invasive monitoring (Code: IIIE1k) [Difficulty: R, Ap, An]

Chapter 5, Advanced Cardiopulmonary Monitoring, contains discussions on the set up and troubleshooting of central venous, arterial, and pulmonary artery lines. Review the chapter if needed.

Each hospital or physician may have a prescribed method to perform catheter insertion. The general steps are listed here:

1. Inform the patient of the procedure and have him or her sign the medical release form if time permits.
2. Have a sedative or pain-relieving agent administered if needed.

3. If necessary, shave all body hair from the insertion site.

4. Put on a sterile mask, cap, gown, and gloves according to protocol.

5. Disinfect the insertion site with an iodine (Betadine) soaked sterile 4- x 4-inch gauze pad. Place the pad at the center of the insertion site and move the pad in a widening spiral away from the center. Repeat with a second sterile gauze pad. Let the iodine dry.

6. Protect the area around the insertion site with a sterile fenestrated surgical drape.

7. Prepare the sterile field with the scalpel, supplies, and so forth. Have a local anesthetic such as lidocaine (Xylocaine) available in a syringe with needle. The physician injects this into the insertion site.

8. Assist the physician into his or her sterile mask, cap, gown, and gloves.

9. Get the properly sized catheter for the procedure or patient.

10. Assist the physician with the procedure as needed. This may include connecting the catheter to the tubing system, flushing the catheter and tubing system, and inflating the balloon on a pulmonary artery catheter.

11. Make any adjustments in the patient's respiratory care equipment as needed.

12. Dispose of any used supplies and so forth after the procedure is completed.

13. Tend to the patient's comfort.

3. Cardioversion (Code: IIIE1h) [Difficulty: An]

Cardioversion (or countershock) refers to deliberately sending a direct current (DC) electrical shock through the patient's heart. Its purpose is to suppress an abnormal heartbeat so that the normal pacemaker at the sinoatrial (SA) node takes over. This is accomplished if a great enough electrical current is sent through the chest wall to cause the depolarization of a critical mass of myocardial cells. After this, the SA node should take over as the pacemaker, provided that the heart muscle is oxygenated and not too acidotic. There are two different types of cardioversion: defibrillation (also called unsynchronized cardioversion) and synchronized cardioversion. Both were introduced in Chapter 10 for the treatment of specific arrhythmias.

Defibrillation is performed in an emergency situation. Patients who need to be defibrillated include those in ventricular fibrillation or ventricular tachycardia when they are pulseless, unresponsive, or hypotensive or have pulmonary edema. Because the fastest possible action is needed, no attempt is made to synchronize the defibrillation shock with the heart's rhythm. While cardiopulmonary resuscitation (CPR) is being performed, the defibrillator unit is prepared. The defibrillating paddles (large positive and negative electrodes) are placed on the patient's right anterior and left lateral chest wall. The physician or other qualified person (respiratory therapist, registered nurse, or paramedic) performing the defibrillation should call out, "Stand clear." All other medical personnel should stand back from the patient and the bed and not touch anything that is electrically grounded. When the buttons on the paddles are pushed, the shock is administered. If successful, the patient's heartbeat returns to normal sinus rhythm. If the initial shock is unsuccessful, CPR is continued. The defibrillator is then recharged for another attempt as quickly as possible. Box 17-1 shows the sequence of increasingly more powerful countershocks that can be given.

Synchronized cardioversion is similar in some ways to defibrillation. An electrical shock is sent by two paddles through the heart to suppress paroxysmal atrial tachycardia, atrial flutter, atrial fibrillation, or hemodynamically stable ventricular tachycardia so that the SA node takes over. Its major difference from defibrillation is that the electrical shock is administered automatically by the

---

BOX 17-1   Wattage Used in Synchronous Cardioversion and Defibrillation

SYNCHRONIZED CARDIOVERSION OF AN INFANT
0.5-1.0 J (watt-seconds) per kg
Stepwise increases in energy should be used if the initial shock fails to convert the rhythm.

SYNCHRONIZED CARDIOVERSION OF AN ADULT
Atrial flutter and paroxysmal atrial tachycardia:
50-100 J
Stepwise increases in energy should be used if the initial shock fails to convert the rhythm: 200, 300, 360.
Atrial fibrillation:
100 J
Stepwise increases in energy should be used if the initial shock fails to convert the rhythm: 200, 300, 360.
Ventricular tachycardia with a regular form and rate with or without a pulse:
100 J
Stepwise increases in energy should be used if the initial shock fails to convert the rhythm: 200, 300, 360.
Ventricular tachycardia with an irregular form and rate:
200 J
Stepwise increases in energy should be used if the initial shock fails to convert the rhythm: 300, 360.

DEFIBRILLATION
Infant:
2 J/kg
4 J/kg for second and succeeding attempts
Adult:
200 J on first attempt
200-300 J on second attempt
Up to 360 J on third and succeeding attempts

J, Joules. 1 Joule = 1 watt-second of power

defibrillator after an R wave is recognized by the ECG monitor. The ECG electrodes must be in place and the best lead (often lead II) selected to show a clear, strong, upright R wave. The defibrillator unit is set for synchronized cardioversion. The physician holds the paddles on the patient's right anterior and left lateral chest wall. When the discharge buttons are pushed on the paddles, the shock is sent after the next R wave and is identified by the ECG monitor.

Cardioversion is not considered an emergency; however, it is performed as quickly as possible so that the patient does not stay in the abnormal rhythm any longer than necessary. Synchronized cardioversion is performed only if medical treatment with antiarrhythmia drugs or carotid artery massage have no effect. Because these patients are usually conscious, they should be sedated with diazepam (Valium), midazolam (Versed), or a similar medication. Patients who are hypotensive or already unconscious should not be sedated.

The respiratory therapist's role in cardioversion may include:

a. Making sure that the ECG electrodes are properly positioned for either monitoring or diagnosing the rhythm, as the physician requires.

b. Making sure that the ECG monitor and electrocardiograph are working properly.

c. Making sure that the ECG lead that results in a strong R wave is selected; usually the R wave is upright in lead II.

d. Charging the defibrillator to the power level ordered by the physician.

e. Adding the electrode cream to the electrode paddles to decrease the skin's resistance to electricity.

f. Being prepared to keep a patent airway, manually ventilate the patient, or begin chest compressions, if necessary.

4. Bronchoscopy

a. Recommend a bronchoscopy procedure to get additional information on the patient's condition (Code: IA2b) [Difficulty: An]

Bronchoscopy is a procedure that involves looking directly into the patient's tracheobronchial airways. The physician can perform a number of diagnostic and therapeutic tasks under direct vision. (See Box 17-2 for uses, limitations, and risks of bronchoscopy.)

b. Select a bronchoscope for the planned procedure (Code: IIA1u) [Difficulty: An]

The rigid bronchoscope is a straight, hollow, stainless steel tube (see Fig. 17-1). It has a distal light source so that the airway can be seen and a side port for providing oxygen or mechanical ventilation to the patient. The right and left mainstem bronchi can be observed by passing a mirror through the main channel. A hook or net can be passed through the main channel into the trachea or either bronchus to remove a foreign body. The rigid broncho-scope is preferred for the treatment of massive hemoptysis or to remove a foreign body.

Flexible fiberoptic bronchoscopy (FFB) uses a smaller diameter flexible tube with two sets of fiberoptic bundles that shine light into the airway and allow viewing of the airway. It has gained wide popularity because it is better tolerated by the patient and allows for better visualization and collection of specimens from smaller bronchi (Figs. 17-2 and 17-3). The adult bronchoscopy tube is about 5 to 6 mm outer diameter (OD) and the pediatric tube is about 3 mm OD. The small diameter and ability to guide the catheter allow the operator to look into the bronchus to each lung segment (segmental bronchi). The fiberoptic bronchoscope is preferred over the rigid one when the patient is being mechanically ventilated or has disease or trauma to the skull, jaw, or cervical spine. As shown in Fig. 17-2, a photo connection allows the assistant to either take still photographs of pulmonary anatomy or videotape the entire procedure.

A limitation of the pediatric unit is that there is no channel outlet for suctioning purposes. This is because of its small size. If a patient has an obstructing bronchial tumor, a special laser fiberoptic bronchoscope is used to burn away part of it. This enables the patient to breathe more easily but this procedure is not a cure for the cancer.

c. Put the fiberoptic bronchoscope together, make sure that it works properly, and identify any problems (Code: IIB1s) [Difficulty: R, Ap]

The fiberoptic bronchoscope comes preassembled (see Fig. 17-2 for its primary features). If photographing or videotaping is planned, the camera must be attached at the photo connection. Have a central or portable suctioning system set up with suctioning tubing. In addition, the following steps must be used to check for proper functioning:

1. Make sure the light source shines through to the distal end of the bronchoscope.

2. Look through the eyepiece. Point the distal end of the bronchoscope at a close object and adjust the lens to bring it into focus.

3. Adjust the thumb control to bend the distal tip.

4. Pass biopsy forceps or brush through the channel port to the outlet.

5. Make sure the suctioning tubing connects to the channel port.

d. Fix any problems with the equipment (Code: IIB2t) [Difficulty: R, Ap]

If the light source does not work, you must check the manufacturer's equipment manual to help determine if the problem could be something simple such as a burned out light bulb or a more serious problem. Similarly, problems with the camera equipment can be resolved by checking the manufacturer's equipment manual.

BOX 17-2   Uses, Limitations, and Risks of Bronchoscopy

RIGID BRONCHOSCOPY
Diagnostic use:
  Biopsy of tumors within the main airway
Therapeutic uses:
  Treatment of massive hemoptysis by cold-saline lavage or
    placement of a Fogarty catheter to occlude the airway
  Removal of foreign body in infants and small children
  Aspiration of inspissated secretions and mucous plugs
Limitations:
  Cannot be used for observing or treating problems beyond
    the left or right mainstem bronchus
  Cannot be used with patients with disease or trauma of the
    cervical spine who cannot hyperextend their neck
  Cannot be used with patients with disease or trauma of the
    jaw who cannot open their mouth wide enough to pass
    the tube

FIBEROPTIC BRONCHOSCOPY
Diagnostic uses:
  Search for the origin of a positive sputum cytology
  Evaluate lung lesions and perform transbronchial biopsy
    of lung tissue (should be done only under fluoroscopic
    control)
  Stage lung cancer preoperatively
  Investigate unexplained hemoptysis, unexplained cough,
    localized wheeze, or stridor
  Search for the cause of unexplained paralysis of a vocal cord
    or hemidiaphragm
  Search for the cause of superior vena cava syndrome,
    chylothorax, or unexplained pleural effusion
  Assess airway patency and investigate suspected bronchial tear
    or other injury after thoracic trauma

Investigate a suspected tracheoesophageal fistula
Investigate problems related to an endotracheal tube such
    as tracheal damage, airway obstruction, or tube placement
Obtain mucus for identification of pathogens
Investigate suspected injury secondary to inhaled superheated
    gas and smoke from an enclosed fire
Investigate suspected injury secondary to the aspiration of
    gastric contents
Perform bronchoalveolar lavage
Therapeutic uses:
  Remove secretions or mucous plugs that cannot be cleared
    by other methods
  Remove small foreign bodies
  Remove abnormal endobronchial tissue or foreign material
    by forceps or laser techniques
Increased risks related to rigid or fiberoptic bronchoscopy:
  Recent myocardial infarction or unstable angina
  Unstable cardiac arrhythmia
  Partial tracheal obstruction
  Unstable bronchial asthma
  Severe hypoxemia
  Hypercarbia
  Pulmonary hypertension (risk of hemorrhage after
    biopsy)
  Bleeding disorder (risk of hemorrhage after biopsy)
  Lung abscess (airway may be flooded with purulent
    material)
  Pulmonary infection from contaminated equipment
  Pneumothorax from transbronchial biopsy
  Respiratory failure requiring mechanical ventilation of the
    patient

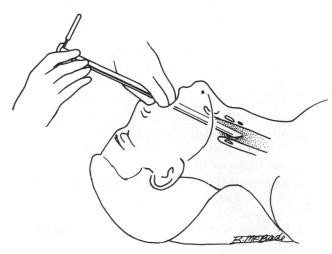

Fig. 17-1   Rigid tub bronchoscope being inserted into patient's trachea. Note how head and neck must be hyperextended. (From Simmons KF. In Scanlan CL, Spearman CB, Sheldon RL, editors: *Egan's fundamentals of respiratory care,* ed 5, St Louis, 1990, Mosby.)

Failure to pass a biopsy forceps or brush through the channel port probably means that there is an obstruction such as dried blood or tissue. Try applying suction through the channel port to clear out the debris. It may also be helpful to squirt sterile distilled water from a syringe through the channel. Try suctioning again or pushing the biopsy forceps through the channel. If alternating suction, instilling water, and pushing the forceps through the channel does not dislodge the debris, the unit cannot be used. Try soaking the bronchoscope in water to soften the debris before repeating the above processes. If the channel cannot be cleared the unit must be sent back to the manufacturer for repairs.

e. Assist with the bronchoscopy procedure (Code: IIIE1a) [Difficulty: An]

Typical duties of the respiratory therapist during bronchoscopy may include the following:
  1. Inform the patient of the procedure and have him or her sign the medical release form.

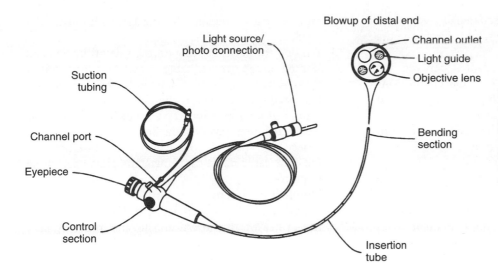

Fig. 17-2 Flexible fiberoptic bronchoscopy with its components and special features. (From Simmons KF. In Scanlan CL, Spearman CB, Sheldon RL, editors: *Egan's fundamentals of respiratory care,* ed 5, St Louis, 1990, Mosby.)

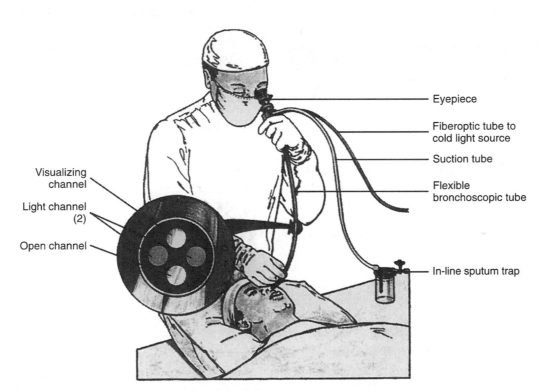

Fig. 17-3 Flexible fiberoptic bronchoscopy procedure being performed on patient. (From Williams SF, Thompson JM: *Respiratory disorders,* St Louis, 1990, Mosby.)

2. Have a sedative such as midazolam (Versed) or (diazepam) Valium administered if needed.
3. Nebulize a topical anesthetic, such as 4% lidocaine (Xylocaine), to the airway.
4. Check the fiberoptic unit for proper function: working light source, working thumb control to flexible tip, working adjustable eyepiece focus, patency of the suction and biopsy channel.
5. Check the functioning of the biopsy brush and forceps.
6. Set up and monitor the patient's ECG.
7. Monitor the patient's vital signs.
8. Place and monitor the pulse oximeter on the patient.
9. Administer oxygen via a nasal catheter or the suction and biopsy channel on the unit.
10. Collect all suctioned material or other specimens for culture and sensitivity.
11. Perform biopsies and brushings for cytology.
12. Operate any photographic equipment.

13. If the patient is being mechanically ventilated during fiberoptic bronchoscopy, perform the following:
    a. Place a bronchoscopy adapter between the endotracheal tube and Y of the circuit. This keeps a seal around the bronchoscopy tube to minimize any drop in tidal volume.
    b. Watch for an increase in the peak pressure from the increased resistance caused by the bronchoscopy tube.
    c. Be prepared to make adjustments in inspired oxygen, rate, flow, and tidal volume.
    d. Be prepared to switch from conventional volume ventilation to high frequency jet ventilation if needed.
14. Tend to the patient's comfort.
15. Use a glutaraldehyde disinfecting solution (Cidex) on the equipment between patients.

▶ EXAM HINT

There is usually one question on the examination that asks about indications for bronchoscopy or hazards related to the procedure.

---

5. Management of pleural disorders

a. Assist with the thoracentesis procedure (Code: IIIE1b) [Question difficulty: An]

Thoracentesis (also called thoracocentesis) is the surgical puncture of the chest wall and pleural space with a needle to aspirate pleural fluid for therapeutic or diagnostic purposes.

Thoracentesis is performed as a therapeutic procedure to remove air or fluid that has accumulated in the pleural space and is causing the patient pain, dyspnea, and/or hypoxemia. Thoracentesis is also performed as a diagnostic procedure to get a fluid sample for analysis to diagnose the cause of a pleural effusion. Pleural fluid may be a *transudate* that results from congestive heart failure, cirrhosis, nephrotic syndrome, or hypoproteinemia. Pleural fluid may also be an *exudate* that results most often from inflammatory, infectious, or neoplastic diseases of the pleura or lung. Other causes of an exudate include pulmonary infarction, chest trauma, drug hypersensitivity, and collagen vascular disease.

The respiratory therapist may be responsible for preparing the patient, disinfecting the puncture site, setting up the sterile field around it, and preparing the equipment and supplies. Each hospital or physician may have a prescribed way of doing this. The general steps listed here apply to a thoracentesis procedure and a percutaneous needle biopsy of the pleura and lung (described later):

1. Inform the patient of the procedure and have him or her sign the medical release form if time permits.

2. Have a sedative or pain-relieving agent administered if needed.
3. Position the patient sitting on the side of the bed and leaning on the overbed table as shown in Fig. 17-4; or the patient may straddle a chair and rest his or her arms and head on the back of the chair. The patient who cannot sit up is positioned on his or her side with the unaffected lung down on the bed.
4. If necessary, shave all body hair from the insertion site.
5. Put on a sterile mask, cap, gown, and gloves according to protocol.
6. Disinfect the insertion site with an iodine (Betadine) soaked sterile 4- x 4-inch gauze pad. Place the pad at the center of the insertion site and move it in a widening spiral away from the center. This step should be repeated with a second sterile gauze pad. Let the iodine dry.
7. Protect the area around the insertion site with a sterile fenestrated surgical drape.
8. Prepare the sterile field with needed supplies such as 1% lidocaine (Xylocaine) and a variety of needles and syringes. Note: A Curity Thoracentesis Tray or other prepackaged tray contains the supplies that are used most commonly.
9. Assist the physician into his or her sterile mask, cap, gown, and gloves.
10. Assist the physician with the procedure as described later.
11. Make any adjustments in the patient's respiratory care equipment as needed.
12. Dispose of any used supplies and so forth after the procedure is completed.
13. Tend to the patient's comfort.

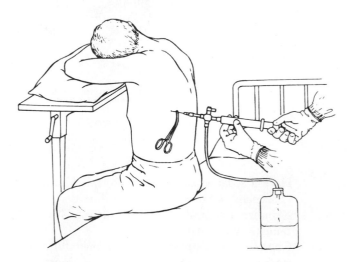

Fig. 17-4 Technique for thoracentesis. Patient sits up leaning on overbed table. Pleural fluid is withdrawn through needle by syringe and then directed into collection jar. (From Anderson HL, Bartlett RH. In Burton GG, Hodgkin JE, Ward JJ, editors: *Respiratory care: a guide to clinical practice,* ed 3, Philadelphia, 1991, JB Lippincott.)

1. General steps in the removal of pleural fluid:

1. Check the patient's chest radiograph for the location of the pleural fluid (or targeted tissue for a needle biopsy) and its relationship to the ribs and other tissues.
2. Tell the patient to not move or cough during the procedure to avoid accidental needle damage to the pleura or lung.
3. The physician anesthetizes the thoracentesis site as shown in Fig. 17-5, *A* and *B.*
4. The physician inserts a large gauge needle (often 16 gauge) with attached 50-mL syringe into the pleural fluid (see Fig. 17-5, *C*). (A cutting needle is used during a needle aspiration of pleural or lung tissue.)
5. The sample is then aspirated. If there is more than 50 mL of pleural fluid, the two-way valve or three-way stopcock, rubber hose, and collection tube are assembled to remove the fluid (see Fig. 17-4).
6. The needle is removed and a bandage is placed over the puncture site.
7. Place the patient with the unaffected side down on the bed for 1 hour.
8. Observe the patient for dizziness, cyanosis, and changes in heart rate and/or respiratory rate. Auscultate for diminished breath sounds over the affected lung as a sign of pneumothorax. The physician should order a chest radiograph to check for pneumothorax. (See

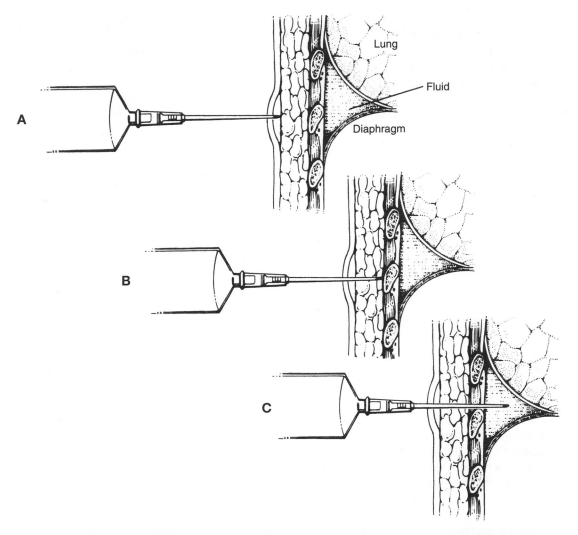

Fig. 17-5   Anesthetizing needle insertion site and performing thoracentesis. **A,** 25-gauge needle is used to inject lidocaine (Xylocaine) into thoracentesis puncture site until skin is raised. **B,** 22-gauge needle is used to inject lidocaine into periosteum of rib and surrounding tissues. The properly anesthetized patient should feel no pain during thoracentesis. **C,** 22- or larger-gauge aspirating needle is pushed through numbed tissues, over top edge of rib, and into pleural space. Fluid sample can now be aspirated. (From Martin L: *Pulmonary physiology in clinical practice: the essentials for patient care and evaluation,* St Louis, 1987, Mosby.)

BOX 17-3	Common Complications of a Thoracentesis

Infection
Hemothorax
Subcutaneous emphysema
Air embolism
Pneumothorax
Sudden mediastinal shift from removal of a large amount of pleural fluid (usually greater than 1500 mL in an adult)
Unstable vital signs from the sudden mediastinal shift
Pulmonary edema from the sudden reexpansion of the lung and mediastinal shift

BOX 17-4	Indications for the Insertion of a Chest Tube

PLEURAL SPACE (See Fig. 17-6, **D**.)
Tension pneumothorax
Greater than a 10% to 20% simple pneumothorax
Hemothorax
Empyema
Pleural effusion
Chylothorax

MEDIASTINAL SPACE
Free air
Free blood or other fluid

PERICARDIAL SPACE (See Fig. 17-7.)
Cardiac tamponade
Pneumopericardium

Box 17-3 for the commonly seen complications of a thoracentesis or needle biopsy.)

9. Evaluate the gross appearance of the fluid that has been removed. Transudative fluid may be clear, serous, or light yellow. Opalescent, pearly white fluid probably indicates chyle in the pleural cavity (chylothorax). Chyle is lymphatic fluid that backs up into the pleural cavity when the thoracic duct is blocked. Sanguineous or serosanguineous (red) fluid is probably bloody. If the patient has a lung infection and empyema, the fluid will be thick and puslike with a foul odor. Send the collected sample to the laboratory for analysis.

b. Assist with percutaneous needle aspiration biopsies of the lung (Code: IIIE1f) [Difficulty: R, Ap, An]

Percutaneous aspiration of pleural tissue or lung tissue involves the insertion of a cutting needle through the chest wall into the target tissue(s) and the removal of a tissue sample. The general procedure for a needle aspiration is described previously in the description of a thoracentesis procedure.

A pleural biopsy is indicated when exudative fluid is found during a thoracentesis procedure. The cause may be an infection, including tuberculosis, or a lung tumor. In addition, a pleural biopsy is indicated when a chest radiograph shows a pleural tumor or unexplained pleural thickening. A cutting needle is inserted into the parietal pleura to withdraw a specimen for analysis.

A lung biopsy is indicated when a chest radiograph or computed tomography (CT) scan indicates pulmonary parenchymal disease. A tissue sample is needed to determine if the cause is lung cancer, granuloma, infection, or sarcoidosis. A cutting needle is inserted through the parietal and visceral pleura to withdraw a specimen of suspicious lung tissue for analysis.

c. Treat a tension pneumothorax (Code: IIID2) [Difficulty: R, Ap, An]

In an emergency when the patient has a tension pneumothorax and rapidly worsening vital signs, the pleural air must be rapidly removed from the chest. This is done by placing a large-bore needle (16 gauge or larger) through the second or third intercostal space in the midclavicular line of the affected lung. The intrapleural air leaves the chest allowing the lung to expand. A pleural chest tube is then inserted for a long-term solution to the problem.

d. Assist with the insertion of chest tubes (Code: IIIE1j) [Difficulty: R, Ap, An]

A chest tube (also called tube thoracostomy) may be inserted into either one or both pleural spaces around the lungs, the mediastinal space, or pericardial space around the heart. This procedure is indicated when air and/or fluid in any of these spaces interferes with normal lung or heart function. Box 17-4 lists the indications for the insertion of a chest tube.

General steps in inserting a pleural chest tube follow:
1. Check the patient's chest radiograph for the location of the air or fluid in the pleural space and its relationship to the ribs and other tissues.
2. Prepare the patient as described in the thoracentesis procedure. The patient is usually positioned to lie on his or her back or with the lung of the unaffected side down on the bed.
3. The physician anesthetizes the tube insertion site as shown in Fig. 17-5, *A* and *B*.
4. The physician creates an opening into the patient's chest wall to place the chest tube (see Fig. 17-6). A tube to remove *air* is placed into one of two places and then advanced toward the apex of the lung. With a midclavicular approach, the tube is placed over the top edge of a rib into the second to fourth intercostal space. With a midaxillary approach (preferred site), the tube is placed over the top edge of a rib into the fourth to sixth intercostal space. A tube to remove *fluid* is placed over the top edge of the rib into the sixth to eighth intercostal space. It is inserted at the midaxillary line

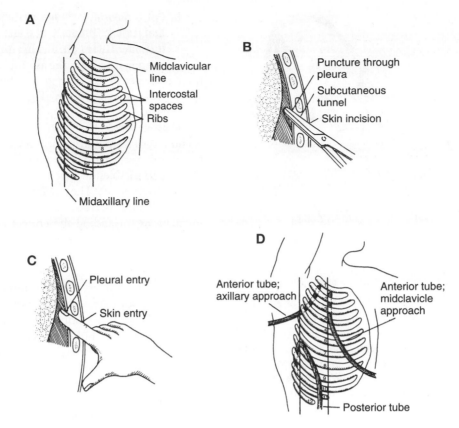

Fig. 17-6 Technique for inserting pleural chest tube. **A,** Anatomical landmarks. **B,** Dissecting through tissues with hemostat. **C,** Using finger to widen opening and ensure that lung has not been punctured. **D,** Proper tube placement. Air is removed by tube that is placed toward apex of lung. Fluid is removed by tube placed toward the posterior base of lung. (Modified from Anderson HL, Bartlett RH. In Burton GG, Hodgkin JE, Ward JJ, editors: *Respiratory care: a guide to clinical practice,* ed 3, Philadelphia, 1991, JB Lippincott.)

and advanced toward the posterior base of the lung. Mediastinal or pericardial tubes are placed via an opening below the xiphoid process and placed posterior to the heart (see Fig. 17-7). This is most commonly done during open heart surgery.

5. The tube is secured by sutures and/or a 4- x 4-inch gauze pad and bandage.
6. The other end of the tube is connected to the drainage system (discussed later).
7. Place the patient with his or her back against the bed or with the unaffected side down on the bed. The physician may want the head of the bed elevated or flat.
8. Observe the patient for dizziness, cyanosis, and changes in heart rate and respiratory rate. (See Box 17-3 for the most commonly seen complications.)

EXAM HINT

Every past examination has had at least one question that relates to identifying a patient having a tension pneumothorax, requiring the insertion of a large-bore needle, or a pleural chest tube. Know the indications of a tension pneumothorax, including sudden deterioration of vital signs and hypoxemia, decreased breath sounds over the affected lung, decreased chest wall movement over the affected lung, hyperresonant percussion note over the affected lung, and shift of the mediastinal structures away from the affected lung.

6. **Pleural drainage system**
   a. **Select a pleural drainage system (Code: IIA1r) [Difficulty: An]**

   Modern drainage systems consist of either three or four chambers or sections designed to regulate the vacuum level, hold any drained fluids, prevent any outside air from entering the patient's thorax, and act as a pressure relief valve in case the vacuum regulator should fail. Argyle and Pleurovac are two well-known manufacturers. The systems for draining the pleural space are discussed here, but the principles are the same for draining the mediastinal and pericardial spaces.

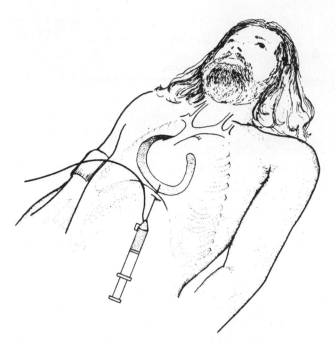

Fig. 17-7 Pericardiocentesis with needle and syringe. Pericardial or mediastinal chest tube is also inserted by substernal approach. (From Sproul CW, Mullanney PJ, editors: *Emergency care: assessment and interventions,* St Louis, 1974, Mosby.)

b. Put a pleural drainage system together, make sure that it works properly, and identify any problems with it (Code: IIB1r) [Difficulty: An]

Refer to Fig. 17-8 for the assembly and operation of the three-chamber drainage system. The four-chamber drainage system is shown in Fig. 17-9 and is discussed concurrently.

Vacuum level. The operation of the wall or central vacuum systems was discussed in Chapter 12. It is common practice to set a partial vacuum of −15 to −20 cm water pressure to the pleural space.

Suction control. The suction control chamber is dry when the unit is unpacked. Follow the manufacturer's instructions for adding the correct amount of water. The proper water level is generally 15 to 20 cm high and results in that level of vacuum being applied to the patient's pleural space.

It is normal to have room air drawn into the opening on top and bubbling through the water column. This corresponds to bottle or chamber C in Fig. 17-9. The constant air bubbling causes the water level to gradually drop from evaporation. Water must be added occasionally.

Water seal. The water-seal chamber, which corresponds to chamber B in Fig. 17-9, is a safety feature. It is dry when unpacked. Follow the manufacturer's directions as to the

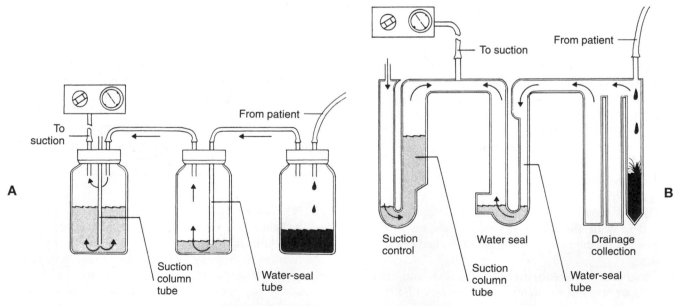

Fig. 17-8 Three-chamber pleural drainage systems. **A,** Homemade three-chamber drainage system. Depth that suction column tube is placed under water determines the level of vacuum applied against patient's pleural space. **B,** Schematic drawing of modern manufactured three-chamber drainage system. (From Shapiro BA, Kacmarek RM, Cane RD et al: *Clinical application of respiratory care,* ed 4, St Louis, 1991, Mosby.)

amount of water to add. Typically, the water-seal tube should have about 2 cm of water in it for any patient air to bubble through. As indicated by the arrows, it is designed to permit air to leave the patient's chest cavity. (Air will also be seen bubbling through when fluid enters the drainage collection chamber and displaces some of its air.) However, room air cannot be drawn "backward" through the water to enter the chest if the vacuum fails or is disconnected.

The water-seal chamber must be checked regularly to see if there is any air bubbling through from the patient's chest. If so, the patient has an active air leak. If the chest tube has been placed into the pleural space, it shows that the patient has an unhealed pneumothorax or bronchopleural fistula. If the chest tube has been placed into the mediastinum or pericardium, it indicates that air is leaking through a tear in the lung structures to these areas. When the air leak stops, it indicates that the tissues have healed over the tear.

Drainage collection. The drainage collection chamber, which corresponds to bottle or chamber A in Fig. 17-9, is designed to hold any fluid that is removed from the pleural space. It is divided into several sections that are marked off for volume measurement. The volume that has accumulated in the chamber should be recorded each hour. A sudden, significant increase in the amount of drainage should be called to the physician's attention. This is especially important if the patient is losing blood. Note the color of the drainage. Blood is obviously red, chyle is white, pus from an empyema is yellow or green, and pleural effusion fluid is a straw yellow color. The whole drainage system must be replaced when the drainage collection chamber becomes filled.

Pressure relief valve on the four-chamber system. This additional chamber is a safety feature and is seen on four-chamber systems such as those shown in Fig. 17-9, chamber D. Its purpose is to act as an escape route for any gas leaking from the patient if the vacuum system is accidentally turned off or disconnected. Without the relief valve, air pressure from a pneumothorax may increase to a dangerous level. Instead, the air and pressure are released. In three-chamber systems, the pressure has to build up to the point that water in the suction control chamber "geysers" out before the pressure is relieved.

c. Fix any problems with the pleural drainage system (Code: IIB2r) [Difficulty: An]

A number of problems can occur with chest drainage systems. The practitioner must understand how the systems are designed to work and how to recognize and correct the situation. See Table 17-1 for examples of problems and their correction. Fig. 17-10 lists important considerations when assessing the patient on chest drainage.

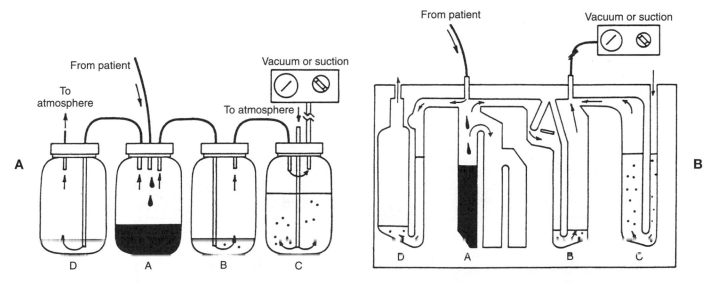

Fig. 17-9 Four-chamber pleural drainage systems. **A,** Homemade four-chamber drainage system. Depth that suction column tube in chamber C is placed under water determines level of vacuum that will be applied against patient's pleural space. **B,** Schematic drawing of modern manufactured four-chamber drainage system. Fourth chamber acts to vent high-pressure air if vacuum should be turned off or malfunction. (From Pilbeam SP, Deshpande VM: *Curr Rev Respir Ther* 5:151, 1983.)

TABLE 17-1 Troubleshooting Problems With Chest Drainage Systems

Problem	Corrective action
Drainage system is cracked open or drainage tubing is permanently disconnected from the drainage system	If the patient has a leaking pneumothorax: Leave the tube open to room air so the pleural air can be vented out. As quickly as possible, place the distal end of tubing into a glass of water to create a water seal. If the patient does not have a leaking pneumothorax, clamp the distal end of the tube to prevent room air from being drawn into the pleural space. In either case attach the tube to a new drainage system as soon as possible.
No bubbling through the suction control chamber	Increase the vacuum pressure. Correct any leak in the system.
Water is spouting out of the suction control chamber (3-bottle system)	Turn on the vacuum. Remove obstruction inside tubing between vacuum and drainage system.
Air leak through the water seal chamber	Check the patient for a pneumothorax; report a new air leak to the physician. Check for a leaking seal between the drainage tube and the patient's chest. Check for a hole in the drainage tube, a loose connection between the tube and the drainage system, or if a fenestration in the tubing has pulled out of the chest wall.
Fluid has filled a dependent loop in the tubing	Drape the tubing so that there are no loops or kinks.
No change in drainage	Check for loops or kinks in tube. Milk the tube to remove any clots. No action if drainage has ceased.
Drainage collection chamber is full	Prepare another unit, clamp the tube while making the exchange, and unclamp the tube after the new unit is functioning.

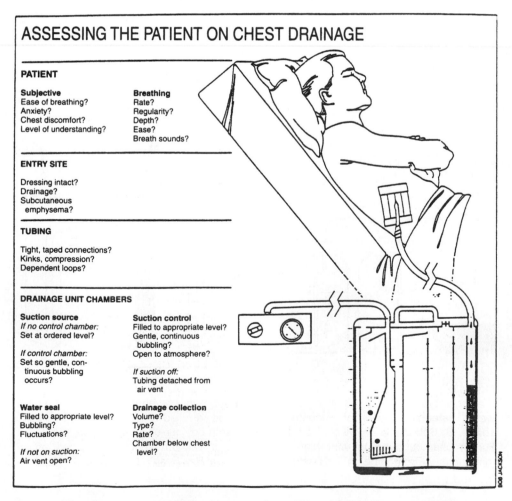

Fig. 17-10 Assessing patient on chest drainage. (From Erickson RA: *Nursing* 89, 19:47, 1989.)

EXAM HINT

Remember that a pleural drainage system is operating properly when air leaking from a pneumothorax is seen bubbling through the water seal. Most examinations have a question concerning this or some other aspect of managing a patient with a pleural drainage system.

7. Intubation (Code: IIIE1i) [Difficulty: An]

The procedure for a therapist performing oral endotracheal intubation was discussed in Chapter 11. The following discussion is limited to assisting an anesthesiologist or other trained physician in performing a nasal endotracheal intubation. Most commonly, the respiratory therapist is the assistant. See Box 17-5 for indications and contraindications and Box 17-6 for complications of nasal endotracheal intubation. There are two different procedures for passing an endotracheal tube by the nasal route: blind nasotracheal intubation and direct vision nasotracheal intubation.

Blind nasotracheal intubation. Be prepared to assist in blind nasotracheal intubation by positioning the patient properly, providing supplemental oxygen or manual ventilation to the patient, and getting and preparing the endotracheal tube or other equipment. A stylet is not indicated. Often, the physician orders the patient to be prepared by having 1% phenylephrine sprayed into the nares. This medication constricts the blood vessels, which dilates the nasal passages, making intubation easier and also reducing the risk of bleeding. Often, 4% lidocaine (Xylocaine) is sprayed into the nares for its local anesthetic effect. The distal end of the endotracheal tube is usually also covered with sterile lidocaine ointment.

This procedure is done without the aid of a laryngoscope to visualize the patient's anatomy and expose the trachea. The general procedure is to place the patient in the sniffer's position, advance the tube to the oropharynx, and then continue to advance it on inspiration only. Changing the patient's head position, feeling for air movement through the tube or pressure over the larynx, or pulling on the tongue may be needed to help guide the tube into the trachea.

In addition, there are several different devices that can aid in this intubation. The physician may choose to place a so-called *trigger tube* into the patient. This special endotracheal tube has a wire placed into it along the inside curve to the tip (see Fig. 11-23). The wire is pulled when the tube is near the larynx to bend the tip more anterior to aim it into the trachea. A *lighted stylet* can be passed through the tube so that the light source is at the distal tip. The light shines through the skin over the larynx. When this is seen, the tube is advanced and the stylet is removed. A *fiberoptic bronchoscope* can be placed through the tube and guided into the patient's trachea. The tube is then advanced and the bronchoscope removed. Another choice is the *intuba-*

BOX 17-5 Indications and Contraindications for Nasal Endotracheal Intubation

GENERAL INDICATIONS FOR ENDOTRACHEAL INTUBATION
Provide a secure, patent airway
Provide a route for mechanical ventilation
Prevent aspiration of stomach or mouth contents
Provide a route for suctioning the lungs
General anesthesia

INDICATIONS FOR NASAL INTUBATION
Patient has a cervical spine abnormality or injury
Use of muscle relaxants may cause a complete loss of the airway
Limited movement of the cervical spine or mandible
Lower facial injury or surgery

CONTRAINDICATIONS FOR NASAL INTUBATION
Basilar skull fracture
Nasal tumors
Deviated nasal septum
Severe coagulation disorder

BOX 17-6 Complications of Nasal Endotracheal Intubation

GENERAL COMPLICATIONS
Reflex laryngospasm
Perforation of the esophagus or pharynx
Esophageal intubation
Bronchial intubation
Reflex bradycardia
Tachycardia or other arrhythmias from hypoxemia
Hypotension
Bronchospasm
Aspiration of tooth, blood, gastric contents, laryngoscope bulb
Laceration of pharynx or larynx
Nosocomial infection
Vocal cord injury
Laryngeal or tracheal injury from the tube or the excessive cuff pressure
Mucosal bleeding
Trauma to the larynx during an attempted blind intubation
Sinusitis

COMPLICATIONS AFTER EXTUBATION
Reflex laryngospasm
Aspiration of stomach contents or oral secretions
Sore throat
Hoarseness
Laryngeal edema (postintubation croup)
Subcutaneous or mediastinal emphysema

tion guide. This is a stylet with a flexible tip that can be bent by the physician through a proximal handle (see Fig. 17-11). The intubation guide is passed through and beyond the distal end of the endotracheal tube. When the guide is in the oropharynx, the tip can be bent in an anterior direction and directed into the trachea. The tube is then advanced over the guide and into the trachea. The guide is then removed.

Direct vision nasotracheal intubation. The respiratory therapist assists with direct vision nasotracheal intubation and prepares the patient and endotracheal tube as with blind endotracheal intubation. This procedure is different from the previous procedure in that intubation equipment is used to visualize the patient's anatomy and see the glottis. Prepare a laryngoscope handle, the physician's choice of either a straight or curved blade, and Magill forceps.

The lubricated tube is advanced to the oropharynx. The laryngoscope blade is then placed into the mouth and used to expose the glottis. The Magill forceps is then placed into the mouth. It is used to grasp the endotracheal tube and guide it into the trachea (see Fig. 17-12). Care must be taken not to place the pinchers over the cuff to avoid tearing it.

With either method, the tube must be properly positioned so that the cuff is in the trachea beyond the vocal cords (see Fig. 17-13). The cuff is then inflated, its pressure adjusted to a safe level, the tube secured in place by tape, and an radiograph taken of the chest and neck.

8. Tracheostomy (Code: IIIE1d) [Difficulty: An]

A *tracheostomy* is a surgical opening in the anterior tracheal wall. The opening is usually placed below the cricoid cartilage and through the second, third, or fourth ring of tracheal cartilage (Fig. 17-14, *A*). The term *tracheotomy* is used to describe the surgical procedure itself (the two terms are often used interchangeably).

Commonly, the tracheostomy is created in the operating room under sterile conditions. When the respiratory therapist is called to assist, it is usually because of a patient emergency. The emergency situation commonly involves an upper airway obstruction such as facial trauma or surgery in which an endotracheal tube cannot be placed by either the oral or nasal route. Because of time constraints, the full sterile technique may be skipped over in favor of a clean technique. The physician's preference and the situation itself dictates how the procedure is performed. The respiratory therapist may also be called to

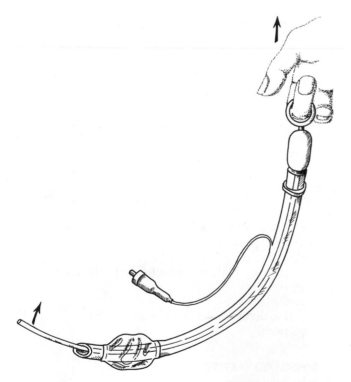

Fig. 17-11 Intubation guide stylet. Flexible tip can be guided by pulling or pushing on ring attached to wire running to distal end. Once the end of the guide is directed into trachea the endotracheal tube is slipped over it. After intubation the guide is withdrawn. (Modified from Heffner JE: *Respir Manage* 19(3), 1989.)

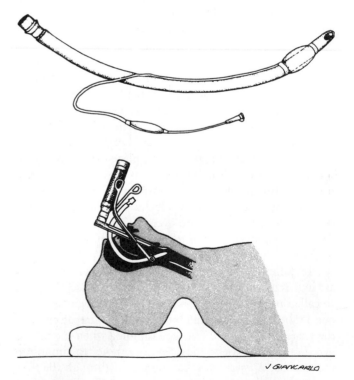

Fig. 17-12 Direct vision nasotracheal intubation. Note that Magill forceps and laryngoscope and blade are both used. Magill forceps is used to grasp tip of endotracheal tube and pull it anterior into trachea. (From Shapiro BA, Harrison RA, Cane RD: *Clinical application of respiratory care,* ed 4, St Louis, 1991, Mosby.)

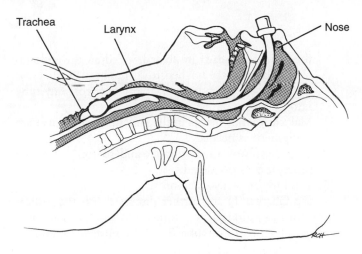

Fig. 17-13 Properly placed nasotracheal tube. (From Shapiro BA, Harrison RA, Cane RD: *Clinical application of respiratory care,* ed 4, St Louis, 1991, Mosby.)

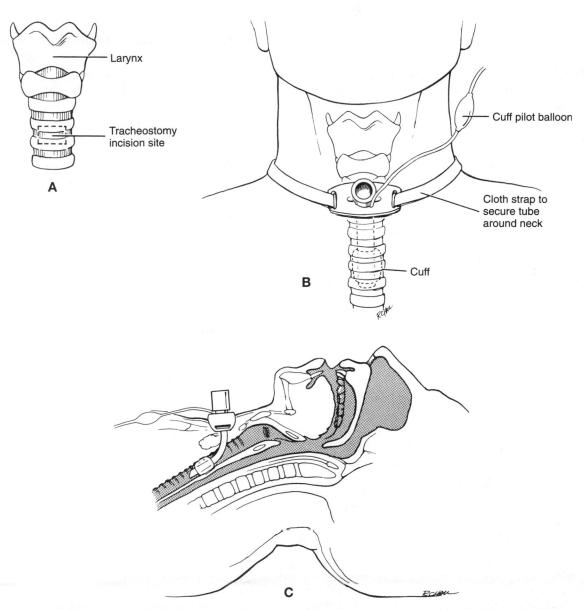

Fig. 17-14 Anatomy of larynx and insertion of tracheostomy tube. **A,** Close-up of larynx and tracheostomy incision site. **B,** Anterior cut-away view of tracheostomy tube after its insertion. **C,** Lateral cut-away view of tracheostomy tube after its insertion. (From Eubanks DH, Bone RC: *Comprehensive respiratory care: a learning system,* ed 2, St Louis, 1990, Mosby.)

assist in the procedure when the patient is already intubated. Usually this involves an unstable patient who requires long-term mechanical ventilation. Because of the patient's critical condition, the physician makes the decision to perform the tracheostomy at the bedside rather than in the operating room. The respiratory therapist may be responsible for preparing the patient, disinfecting the tracheostomy site, setting up the sterile field around the site, and setting up the equipment and supplies. Each hospital or physician may have a prescribed way that this is done. The general steps are listed here:

1. Inform the patient of the procedure and have him or her sign the medical release form if time permits.
2. Have a sedative or pain-relieving agent administered if needed.
3. If necessary, shave the insertion site clear of body hair.
4. Put on a sterile mask, cap, gown, and gloves according to protocol.
5. Disinfect the insertion site with an iodine (Betadine) soaked sterile 4- x 4-inch gauze pad. Place the pad at the center of the insertion site and move it in a widening spiral away from the center. This step should be repeated with a second sterile gauze pad. Let the iodine dry.
6. Protect the area around the insertion site with a sterile fenestrated surgical drape.
7. Prepare the sterile field with the tracheostomy tube, scalpel, supplies, and so forth. Have a local anesthetic such as lidocaine (Xylocaine) available in a syringe with needle. The physician injects this into the insertion site.
8. Assist the physician into his or her sterile mask, cap, gown, and gloves.
9. Get the properly sized tracheostomy tube (see Table 11-1).
10. Assist the physician with the procedure as needed. If

the patient is already intubated, withdraw the endotracheal tube after the tracheostomy has been created and the physician is ready to place the tracheostomy tube into the opening.

11. Make any adjustments in the patient's respiratory care equipment as needed.
12. Dispose of any used supplies and so forth after the procedure is completed.
13. Tend to the patient's comfort.

See Chapter 11 for further discussion on the indications for the various airway routes and when to routinely change a tracheostomy tube. Table 17-2 lists the common complications of a tracheostomy.

9. Transtracheal aspiration (Code: IIIE1c) [Difficulty: R, Ap, An]

Transtracheal aspiration is a procedure in which a large-bore needle is inserted through the cricothyroid membrane. A catheter is then passed through the needle and advanced into the trachea where a sputum sample is aspirated (see Figs. 17-14 and 17-15). The purpose of this

TABLE 17-2	Common Complications of a Tracheostomy
Complication	**Approximate time of onset**
Bleeding	During and after surgery for up to 24 hours; if possible, do not replace the first tube for 2 to 3 days
Pneumothorax	During the procedure
Infection of the stoma or lungs	Usually seen after second day
Subcutaneous or mediastinal emphysema	May be seen during the procedure or at any later time

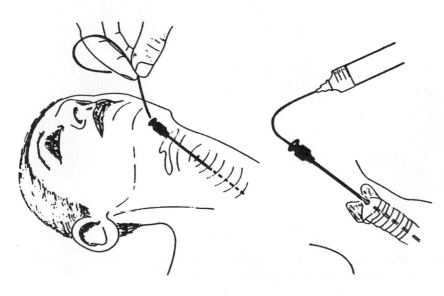

Fig. 17-15 Procedure for transtracheal aspiration. (From Couperus JJ, Elder H. In Burton GG, Hodgkin JE, editors: *Respiratory care: a guide to clinical practice,* ed 2, Philadelphia, 1984, JB Lippincott.)

procedure is to obtain a sputum sample that is uncontaminated by oral flora. Samples gotten by the patient coughing up sputum or through nasotracheal suctioning or bronchoscopy are usually contaminated by upper airway organisms. Transtracheal aspiration is quite safe but does have possible complications of infection, bleeding, and subcutaneous emphysema.

The respiratory therapist may be responsible for preparing the patient, disinfecting the puncture site, setting up the sterile field around it, and preparing the equipment and supplies. Each hospital or physician may have a prescribed way of doing this. The general steps are listed here:

1. Inform the patient of the procedure and have him or her sign the medical release form.
2. Have a sedative or pain-relieving agent administered if needed.
3. Position the patient properly. Usually this means the patient lies on his or her back with the neck hyperextended into the sniff position.
4. If necessary, shave all body hair from the insertion site.
5. Put on a sterile mask, cap, gown, and gloves according to protocol.
6. Disinfect the insertion site with an iodine (Betadine) soaked sterile 4- x 4-inch gauze pad. Place the pad at the center of the insertion site and move it in a widening spiral away from the center. This step should be repeated with a second sterile gauze pad. Let the iodine dry.
7. Protect the area around the insertion site with a sterile fenestrated surgical drape.
8. Prepare the sterile field with these supplies:
   a. Local anesthetic such as 1% lidocaine (Xylocaine) available in a 5-mL syringe with a 25-gauge 5/8-inch needle. The physician injects some of the lidocaine into the skin.
   b. A 14-gauge 3-inch needle available for inserting through the cricothyroid membrane into the larynx.
   c. Catheter small enough to pass through the 14-gauge needle for removing the mucous sample.
   d. A 10-mL syringe for collecting the mucous sample.
   e. A 10-mL syringe with sterile, preservative-free saline for instillation into the trachea if needed.
   f. Sterile 2- x 2-inch gauze pads and adhesive bandage.
9. Assist the physician into his or her sterile mask, cap, gown, and gloves.
10. Assist the physician with the procedure as needed.
11. Make any adjustments in the patient's respiratory care equipment as needed.
12. Dispose of any used supplies and so forth after the procedure is completed.
13. Tend to the patient's comfort.

General steps in the transtracheal aspiration procedure follow:

1. Check the patient's upper airway and/or chest radiograph as indicated.
2. Prepare the patient as described earlier.
3. The physician anesthetizes the needle insertion site.
4. The physician inserts the needle in alignment with the trachea.
5. Insert the catheter through the needle into the trachea. If possible, do not allow the patient to cough.
6. Attach the syringe to the catheter and apply vacuum to obtain a sample of mucus. If the secretions are too viscous to be aspirated, a 2- to 5-mL bolus of sterile, preservative-free saline may be instilled into the trachea through the catheter. This should make the aspiration easier.
7. Withdraw the catheter and needle.
8. Apply the gauze pad and/or bandage to the insertion site.
9. Observe the patient for bleeding, subcutaneous emphysema, cyanosis, and changes in heart rate and/or respiratory rate.
10. Send the collected sample to the laboratory for analysis.

10. Stress testing

a. Review the patient's chart for information on any metabolic studies (Code: IA1i) [Difficulty: R, Ap, An]

A metabolic study is performed to evaluate a patient's oxygen consumption in 1 minute ($\dot{V}O_2$) and carbon dioxide production in 1 minute ($\dot{V}CO_2$) as part of a general nutritional assessment. The bedside testing procedure is called *indirect calorimetry* and involves collecting the patient's exhaled gases to send them through a rapid O_2 analyzer and CO_2 analyzer. In a normal person, the cellular metabolic processes, lung function, and cardiovascular function are working properly. As can be seen in Fig. 17-16, this results in a cellular respiratory quotient (RQ) of 0.80 and a resulting respiratory exchange ratio (R) measured at the lung of 0.80. This indicates normal oxygen consumption and carbon dioxide production. The calculation is shown later.

Sick patients often have an R value of greater than 0.80. This can be the result of the patient's diet. However, in many sick patients, the high R value is because of the inability of the lungs to remove carbon dioxide (many COPD patients) or insufficient oxygen delivery to the tissues. Tissue hypoxia results in anaerobic metabolism with resulting lactic acid production. This lactic acid, in turn, converts to excessive carbon dioxide. Even a normal person can have an increased R value during heavy

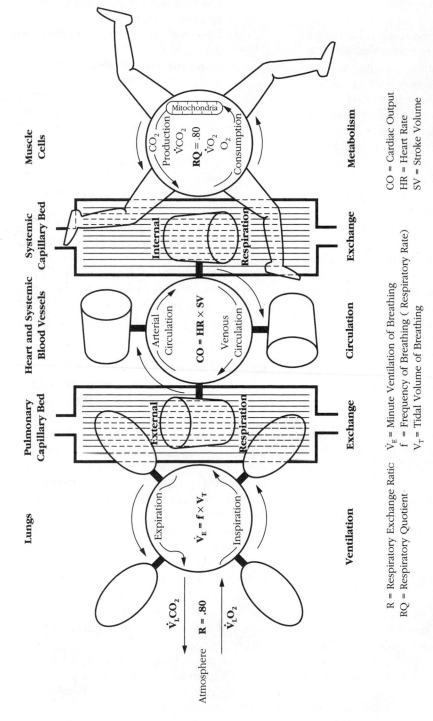

Fig. 17-16 Representation of the interconnected relationships between the pulmonary system, cardiovascular system, and tissues of the body to show the processes of oxygen delivery and consumption and carbon dioxide production and exhalation. Note how the relationship of oxygen consumption and carbon dioxide production in the mitochondria of cells results in the respiratory quotient (RQ) of .80 and the intake of oxygen and the exhalation of carbon dioxide by the lungs results in matching respiratory exchange ratio (R) of .80. This allows indirect calorimetry to be used to evaluate a patient's metabolism at rest and during exercise to assess the pulmonary system, cardiovascular system, and muscle function. (From *Pulmonary Function Testing and Cardiopulmonary Stress Testing,* 2nd ed., by V.C. Madama © 1998. Reprinted with permission of Delmar a division of Thomson Learning. Fax: 800 730-2215.)

exercise. This is discussed later in conjunction with stress testing.

b. Recommend a cardiopulmonary stress test to get additional information on the patient's condition (Code: IA2h) [Difficulty: R, Ap, An]

Stress testing is performed to determine a patient's exercise limits. The limiting factor(s) to exercise tell much about a patient's medical condition. Box 17-7 lists the indications for stress testing.

Before starting a stress test, the patient's chart should be reviewed for information on any previous stress testing. It is important to know the type of testing that was performed, how the patient tolerated it, and what caused the patient to stop the test. Review the physician's evaluation of the test results and the patient's diagnosis.

c. Assist with a cardiopulmonary stress test (Code: IIIE1e) [Difficulty: R, Ap, An]

Stress testing is the intentional exercising of the patient to the point of exhaustion or physiologic deterioration when the test must be stopped because the patient cannot continue. Because of this, the procedure is inherently risky to the patient. It is imperative that the patient be carefully evaluated before, during, and after the procedure. An informed consent statement must be signed by the patient before beginning. A physician should be present during the test along with the therapist and possibly a nurse.

Despite the risks involved in the procedure, a stress test is an important diagnostic or clinical evaluation tool for many patients. Box 17-8 lists the steps in the patient work-up before testing can be safely performed. Box 17-9 lists the contraindications to exercise testing. Patients with any of these problems are too ill to be jeopardized by the procedure.

1. Commonly measured patient parameters specific to exercise testing

Metabolic equivalent of basal metabolic rate. A person who is sleeping or totally relaxed is consuming the

---

BOX 17-7   Indications for Exercise Testing

Evaluation of nonspecific dyspnea on exertion
Evaluation of the patient's ventilatory response to increased work
Evaluation of the patient's need for supplemental oxygen
Serial testing of the patient to help in evaluating the response to therapy, medication, smoking cessation, or a rehabilitation program
To determine the presence and/or nature of ventilatory limits to exercise, such as decreased flows, increased or decreased lung volumes, and/or decreased diffusing capacity
To determine the presence and/or nature of cardiovascular limits to exercise, such as heart rate, cardiac output, arrhythmias, blood pressure, and/or angina pectoris
To determine the presence and/or nature of muscular limits to exercise such as general deconditioning or decreased local perfusion
Preoperative assessment for a lung resection or transplantation
Assessment for the degree of impairment for disability evaluation
Assess an apparently healthy adult more than 40 years old before starting a vigorous exercise program

---

BOX 17-8   Patient Evaluation Before Testing

History of acute or chronic illness leading to the need for stress testing
General physical examination
Resting 12-lead ECG to exclude unexpected cardiac disease
Chest radiograph
Laboratory studies for complete blood count and serum electrolytes
Spirometry with measurement of flows, all lung volumes and capacities, and maximum voluntary ventilation
Carbon monoxide diffusing capacity
Pulse oximetry or arterial blood gases for PaO_2
Before and after bronchodilator spirometry studies if the patient is using an inhaled B_2 medication or has a history of exercise-induced asthma

---

BOX 17-9   Contraindications to Exercise Testing

Arterial blood gases:
    PaO_2 less than 50 torr when breathing room air
    SpO_2 less than 85% when breathing room air
Pulmonary:
    Severe pulmonary hypertension
    Recent pulmonary embolism
    Untreated or unstable asthma
    $FEV_{1.0}$ less than 30% of predicted
Cardiovascular:
    Myocardial infarction within the last 4 weeks
    Dissecting thoracic or abdominal aortic aneurysm
    Dissecting ventricular aneurysm
    Thrombophlebitis
    Systemic embolism
    Uncontrolled hypertension
    Unstable angina pectoris
    Second-degree or third-degree heart block
    Atrial arrhythmias with a rapid ventricular response
    Frequent premature ventricular contractions or other life-threatening ventricular arrhythmias
    Congestive heart failure with pulmonary edema
    Severe aortic stenosis
    Acute pericarditis
    Resting diastolic blood pressure greater than 110 mm Hg or resting systolic blood pressure greater than 200 mm Hg
Neuromuscular disorders that prevent or limit the testing
Orthopedic disorders that prevent or limit the testing

minimum number of calories and least amount of oxygen to stay alive. The minimum amount of carbon dioxide is being produced as a waste product of metabolism. He or she is said to be at basal metabolic rate (BMR). At BMR, a person consumes about 3.5 mL of oxygen/kg of body weight/min. Multiplying this value by the person's body weight produces the metabolic equivalent of basal metabolic rate for oxygen, or MET as it is abbreviated. The average adult at BMR consumes about 250 mL of oxygen/min and produces about 200 mL of carbon dioxide/min. Obviously, the more active a person is, the more calories and oxygen are consumed and the more carbon dioxide is produced. Often a person's exercise limit is quantified in terms of how many METs he or she can perform. For example, light household cleaning might be 2 METs of exercise and competitive swimming might be 8 to10 METs of exercise.

Respiratory quotient and respiratory exchange ratio. RQ is the ratio, at the cellular level, of the amount of carbon dioxide produced in 1 minute to the amount of oxygen consumed in 1 minute. It must be readily apparent that it is impossible to directly measure the RQ because it looks at cellular metabolism; however, the same gases can be easily measured in the lungs. Respiratory exchange ratio (R or RER) is the ratio, at the alveolar level, of the amount of carbon dioxide produced in 1 minute to the amount of oxygen consumed in 1 minute. The volume of these two gases is determined through indirect calorimetry, as discussed previously. Using the oxygen consumption and carbon dioxide volumes discussed earlier, the R (or RQ) of a resting adult is calculated as:

$$R = \frac{\dot{V}CO_2}{\dot{V}O_2} = \frac{200 \text{ mL } CO_2}{250 \text{ mL } O_2} = 0.80$$

The R value (and RQ) of 0.80 remains quite steady during light to moderate exercise. (See Fig. 17-16.) A normal person can quite easily increase the amount of oxygen consumed and eliminate the extra carbon dioxide produced during exercise. This is what is seen during aerobic metabolism when all body systems are functioning smoothly. It is only during heavy exercise that the body has difficulty coping and must eventually stop.

Maximum oxygen consumption and maximum carbon dioxide production. The maximum oxygen consumption ($\dot{V}O_{2 \text{ max}}$) is the highest oxygen consumption a person can attain. Men have a greater capacity for oxygen consumption than women, and both sexes have a natural decline with age. The oxygen consumption at less than a maximum level is recorded as the volume in milliliters of oxygen used in a minute and abbreviated as $\dot{V}O_2$. The maximum carbon dioxide production ($\dot{V}CO_{2 \text{ max}}$) is the highest carbon dioxide production attainable by a person. The carbon dioxide production at less than a maximum level is recorded as the volume in milliliters of CO_2

produced in 1 minute and abbreviated as $\dot{V}CO_2$. Healthy, athletic people can increase their $\dot{V}O_2$ and $\dot{V}CO_2$ by 8 to 10 times their basal metabolic rate.

Anaerobic threshold. Anaerobic threshold (AT) is the highest oxygen consumption attainable during exercise, above which a sustained lactic acidosis occurs. When an exercising patient hits the AT, he or she demonstrates a sudden increase in respiratory rate and tidal volume (minute volume). This is an attempt by the patient to blow off the sudden increase in carbon dioxide production that occurs as a result of anaerobic metabolism from the inability to get enough oxygen to the exercising muscles.

If the patient's oxygen consumption and carbon dioxide production values are graphed out during heavy exercise when AT is reached, the patient has a respiratory exchange ratio of 1.0. This indicates equal values for both gases. An R value of 1.0 is reached in most people during heavy exercise at about 50% to 60% of the $\dot{V}O_{2 \text{ max}}$. At this exercise level, insufficient oxygen reaches the muscles resulting in the formation of lactic acid. This then converts to additional carbon dioxide until the level of CO_2 production equals (or exceeds) the level of oxygen consumption. Most healthy people can continue to exercise vigorously for a short time with an R value of 1.1 to 1.2 until they must stop. Older persons or patients with cardiopulmonary disease are rarely intentionally stressed to the AT.

Maximum heart rate. The maximum heart rate (HR_{max}) is the highest heart rate that a person should be able to achieve. Either of the following prediction equations for maximum heart rate in beats per minute can be used (the standard deviation for these formulas is ±10 to 15 beats per minute):

HR_{max} for males and females = 210 − (0.65 × age in years)

HR_{max} for males and females = 220 − (age in years)

Because it is obviously hazardous to exercise anyone to his or her maximum heart rate for a prolonged time, a lower target heart rate is usually calculated. Initially, a target heart rate of 60 to 70% of maximum is often used. Later, as the patient becomes better conditioned, the target heart rate may be raised.

There are many other concepts and formulas that may be studied by the student who wishes to learn more and become more skilled in performing and interpreting stress tests.

Exercise equipment. Whether the patient is exercising on a treadmill or a bicycle, it is necessary to perform indirect calorimetry by analyzing the patient's exhaled gases for oxygen and carbon dioxide. There are two different types of systems for this. One uses a mixing chamber from which the patient's gases are periodically analyzed. The other is a breath-by-breath system that samples and analyzes each exhaled breath (see Fig. 17-17). The measured patient parameters in both systems usually

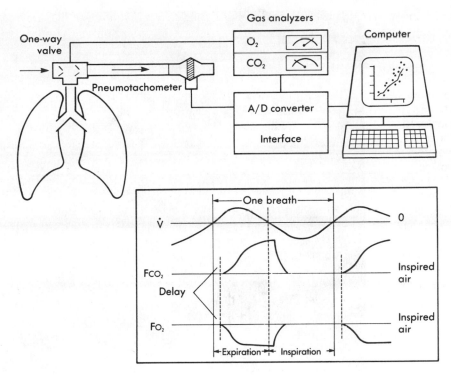

Fig. 17-17 Schematic drawing of the breath-by-breath system for gas analysis during exercise testing. Gas is taken continuously from sampling port. The gas sample in combination with the pneumotachometer information are integrated by the computer to yield data on average mixes of exhaled oxygen (F_EO_2) and carbon dioxide (F_ECO_2), respiratory rate, tidal volume, minute volume, $\dot{V}O_2$, $\dot{V}CO_2$, and respiratory quotient. The insert shows a single breath. During inspiration, the oxygen percentage increases and carbon dioxide percentage decreases. During expiration, oxygen percentage decreases and carbon dioxide percentage increases. There is an unavoidable delay as gas flows to the analyzer to determine the gas concentrations and sends data to the computer for display. Information that is displayed will still be on a breath-by-breath basis but not synchronized with the patient's real-time breathing efforts. (From Ruppel G: *Manual of pulmonary function testing*, ed 7, St Louis, 1998, Mosby.)

include: (a) fraction of exhaled oxygen (F_EO_2), (b) fraction of exhaled carbon dioxide (F_ECO_2), (c) respiratory rate, (d) exhaled gas temperature, (e) exhaled volume, and (f) time from the start of the test.

Treadmill. The treadmill is a motorized, continuously looped belt combined with a ramp. The belt's speed may be adjusted from the stopped position to 1.5 to 10 miles per hour (great enough to exhaust a trained runner). The ramp may be adjusted from flat (0% grade) to sloped (30% grade) (great enough to require the patient to run to keep from falling off the back). There is a railing for the patient to hold if necessary. Commonly, there is also an emergency button that the patient can hit to stop the unit. Adjunct equipment is nearby for monitoring the ECG, exhaled gases, and so forth (Fig. 17-18). The treadmill has an advantage over the bicycle ergometer in that it trains the patient's muscles that are needed for walking. This is an important practical consideration for most patients. However, it is more difficult to quantitate the exercise test results from a treadmill compared with a bicycle because the patient's stride and mechanics of walking vary as the speed increases.

Bicycle ergometer. The bicycle ergometer is a stationary cycle with seat, handle bars, and electronics for calculating distance, effort, and so forth. The electromechanical units as shown in Fig. 17-19 have electronic brakes to increase the patient's workload. Although less practical in training muscles for everyday tasks such as walking, the ergometer allows for easier workload adjustments and calculation of the exercise test results. Other exercise methods such as an arm ergometer or a rowing machine are rarely performed on patients.

2. Exercise protocols

There are a number of exercise protocols that may be followed. Basically, they fall into one of the two following test categories and may be performed on either a treadmill or a bicycle ergometer.

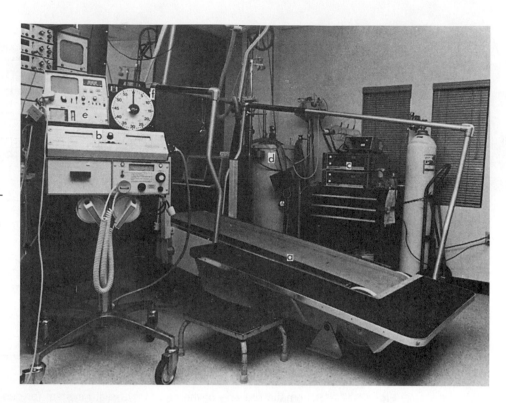

Fig. 17-18 *A,* Typical treadmill setup for an exercise test. Additional equipment includes: *B,* treadmill controls for speed and slope. *C,* rapid analyzers for oxygen and carbon dioxide (metabolic cart). *D,* Tissot spirometer for measuring exhaled volume during test. *E,* Electrocardiogram monitor with recorder. *F,* Electric timer for test. (From Ruppel G: *Manual of pulmonary function testing,* ed 5, St Louis, 1991, Mosby.)

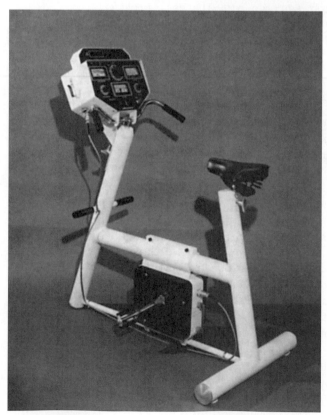

Fig. 17-19 Electromechanical bicycle ergometer with controls for electronic braking, pedaling resistance, test timer, meters for pedaling frequency in revolutions per minute (RPM), and external workload in watts. (From Warren E. Collings, Braintree, Mass.)

Progressive multistage test. This test is designed to examine the effects of rapidly increasing workloads on the cardiopulmonary system. A steady state may or may not be reached because the goals are to trend the measured exercise parameters and find the maximum workload. The following parameters are measured: maximum oxygen consumption, maximum carbon dioxide production, maximum minute ventilation, and maximum heart rate. This is a less exhausting test than the steady state and may be repeated if necessary. This test may be used for its own purposes or to establish maximum workloads before having the patient perform the steady state test.

Patients with known or suspected cardiac disease use a version of the progressive multistage test called the Modified Bruce Protocol. Its goal is to rapidly increase the patient's workload until a target heart rate of 85% of predicted is reached. To do this, the speed and angle of the treadmill are increased every 3 minutes until the target heart rate is reached or the patient feels the need to stop.

Steady state test. This test is designed to measure cardiopulmonary parameters under steady metabolic conditions. Commonly, these levels are 50% and 75% of the predicted maximum oxygen consumption. The following parameters are measured: oxygen consumption, carbon dioxide production, minute ventilation, and heart rate. This is a more exhausting test than the progressive multistage test because it takes longer. It usually is not repeated the same day. General steps in the procedure follow:

1. Explain the procedure to the patient. Answer any

questions. Show the patient how to stop the test in case of an emergency. Develop a hand signal system so that the patient can approve an increase in workload (thumb up) or warn you of the need to stop the test (thumb down).

2. Set up the following monitoring equipment on the patient:
   a. ECG with chest leads placed as usual and limb leads moved to the shoulder areas and lower abdominal areas
   b. Pulse oximetry monitor for SpO_2 or (rarely) arterial line for monitoring PaO_2, other blood gas values, and continuous blood pressure
   c. Arm cuff and sphygmomanometer for automatic or manual blood pressure monitoring if an arterial line is not inserted
   d. Mouthpiece with one-way valves or head hood to gather exhaled gases for analysis

3. Have the patient breathe normally through the system and take a set of baseline parameters. Tell the patient to warm up on the equipment by exercising at a low level (approximately 25% of $\dot{V}O_{2max}$). Take a set of parameters. Note: Steps 4, 5, and 6 are for the steady state test. With the progressive multistage test, the patient exercises at a given level for only a few minutes before moving to a higher work level.

4. Begin the test by having the patient exercise at a predetermined moderate level (approximately 50% of $\dot{V}O_{2max}$) for 5 to 8 minutes. Take a set of parameters in the last 1 to 2 minutes.

5. Increase the workload (approximately 75% of $\dot{V}O_{2max}$) and have the patient exercise at it for 5 to 8 minutes. Take a set of parameters in the last 1 to 2 minutes. Alternatively, the patient may be given a short rest period or low exercise period between the steps of increased workload.

6. Repeat step 5, if necessary, at a higher workload until the patient is exhausted or cannot continue because of one of the conditions listed in Box 17-10.

7. Have the patient exercise at a low level for several minutes during a cool down or recovery period. It is important to monitor the patient during the recovery period because a sudden drop in blood pressure and fainting are known to occur when exercise stops too quickly. Note how long it takes for the patient to return to baseline conditions.

Interpret the results from the procedure. Normal physiologic changes follow:

a. Tidal volume, respiratory rate, and minute volume: All patients find the combination of tidal volume and respiratory rate that allows the most efficient ventilation. Patients with normal lungs increase their tidal volume to about 60% of their vital capacity. They then increase the respiratory rate to produce the maximum ventilation possible. Patients with obstructive airways

---

BOX 17-10 — Indications for Stopping an Exercise Test

ARTERIAL BLOOD GASES
PaO_2 decreasing to less than 55 torr
Acidosis with or without a rise in the $PaCO_2$
SpO_2 less than 83% or >4 less than the baseline value

PULMONARY
Exercise-induced bronchospasm
Severe dyspnea

CARDIOVASCULAR
20 mm Hg fall in systolic blood pressure below the baseline value
Systolic blood pressure greater than 250 mm Hg
Diastolic blood pressure greater than 120 mm Hg
Onset of angina pectoris
Frequent premature ventricular contractions (PVCs)
Ventricular tachycardia
ST segment depression or elevation of more than 1 mm
Onset of second-degree or third-degree heart block
Onset of left or right bundle branch block

EQUIPMENT
Monitoring equipment failure
Unavailability of CPR equipment and defibrillator

MISCELLANEOUS
Request by patient, lightheadedness, mental confusion, or headache
Muscle cramping
Nausea or vomiting
Sweating and pallor
Cyanosis

---

disease are flow limited and cannot increase their respiratory rate adequately. They attempt to raise their tidal volume to increase minute volume but must stop exercising earlier than predicted. Patients with restrictive lung disease cannot increase their tidal volume as expected. Instead, they increase their respiratory rate to raise their minute volume. They too must stop exercising earlier than predicted.

b. Heart rate, stroke volume, and cardiac output: At low and moderate workloads the stroke volume increases from about 80 mL to 110 mL in healthy adults. Increases in heart rate account for the rest of the increase in cardiac output from low to heavy exercise. The heart rate increases are almost parallel with the increases in $\dot{V}O_2$ (see Fig. 17-20). A patient with a diseased left ventricle or heart block is unable to increase cardiac output sufficiently when exercising and must stop earlier than predicted.

c. Oxygen consumption, carbon dioxide production, and RQ: Both the oxygen consumption and carbon dioxide

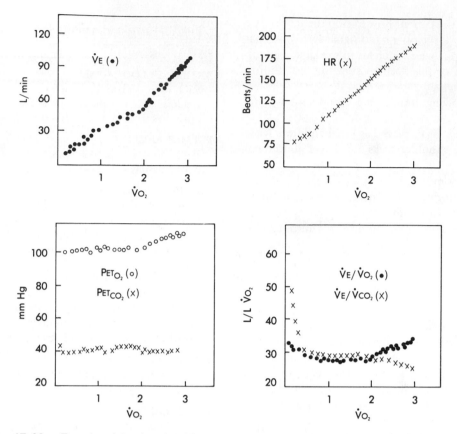

Fig. 17-20 Exercise data showing 30-second averages from normal adult subject. Heart rate (HR) increases linearly as workload is increased and is not the limiting factor in this exercise test. The other three graphic displays show that the anaerobic threshold (AT) occurs at 2 L/min of $\dot{V}O_2$. The following key points should be noted: (a) minute volume ($\dot{V}_E$) increases sharply at AT, (b) end-tidal carbon dioxide ($P_{ET}CO_2$) and the ventilatory equivalent for carbon dioxide ($\dot{V}_E/\dot{V}CO_2$) both decrease at AT, which shows the disproportionate increase in CO_2 production secondary to lactic acid formation, and (c) end-tidal oxygen ($P_{ET}O_2$) and ventilatory equivalent for oxygen ($\dot{V}_E/\dot{V}O_2$) both increase at AT. (From Ruppel G: *Manual of pulmonary function testing,* ed 7, St Louis, 1998, Mosby.)

production increase linearly with low and moderate exercise. The RQ remains about 0.80 or increase slightly. As the patient exercises at levels closer and closer to the $\dot{V}O_{2max}$, the muscles are progressively starved for oxygen. This results in local anaerobic metabolism with lactic acid production. Lactic acid in turn converts to carbon dioxide. Because of this added CO_2, the respiratory center is stimulated to increase ventilation even more than expected. Eventually, this fails to keep up with the increased production and the CO_2 level increases. The AT is identified when oxygen consumption equals carbon dioxide production and the RQ reaches 1.0.

d. Blood gases and pH: PaO_2, $PaCO_2$, and pH remain stable in the normal ranges during low and moderate exercise. The cardiopulmonary system is able to deliver adequate oxygen to the tissues and remove sufficient carbon dioxide to keep the body functioning properly. However, at high levels of work, a lactic acid buildup

occurs and a progressive metabolic acidosis is seen. This forces the patient to decrease the exercise level. Some may need to stop. Patients with cardiopulmonary disease are not able to exercise heavily because they can provide only very limited increases of oxygen to the muscles or eliminate the extra carbon dioxide produced during even moderate exercise. Fig. 17-20 shows the parameter changes seen as a healthy individual exercises from a low to a maximal level.

3. Limitations because of abnormal physiology

Patients who are forced to stop exercising at a lower than predicted workload probably fall into one of the following three broad categories. Box 17-10 lists conditions that require that the stress test be stopped. Table 17-3 lists parameters that help in differentiating between deconditioned muscles, pulmonary limitations, or cardiac limitations as the reason that exercise had to be stopped.

Deconditioned muscles. Normal, healthy people are

TABLE 17-3 Exercise Intolerance: Differentiating Between Heart Disease, Lung Disease, and Deconditioned Muscles

Parameter	Heart disease	Lung disease	Deconditioned muscles
$\dot{V}O_{2max}$	D	D	D
Heart rate reserve	D	I	I
Breathing reserve	N	D	N
Exercise PaO_2 or SpO_2	N	D	N
$\dot{V}O_2$ at anaerobic threshold	D	N	D
$\dot{V}O_2$/heart rate	D	N	N
Exercise $P(A-a)O_2$	N	I	N
Exercise V_D/V_T	N	I	N
Exercise electrocardiogram	Abnormal	Normal	Normal
Common chief complaint	Chest pain	Dyspnea Bronchospasm	Leg fatigue or cramps

D, Decreased; *I*, increased; *N*, normal.
(Based on a table in Sue D: Exercise testing and the patient with cardiopulmonary disease. In Goldman AL, editor: *Problems in pulmonary disease*, 2(1), 1986.)

quite commonly seen in this category. They are deconditioned from lack of exercise. These people are able to do quite well in a training program if there are no underlying cardiopulmonary limitations.

Pulmonary limitations. As discussed earlier, patients with obstructive airways disease or restrictive lung disease have limited ventilatory reserve. This limits their exercise tolerance even if they have a normal cardiovascular system. If the limitation is caused by bronchospasm, this may be treated by inhaling a bronchodilator before exercising. These patients may also be able to increase their exercise tolerance if given supplemental oxygen to prevent desaturation.

Cardiovascular limitations. Patients with a damaged or diseased left ventricle, heart block, exercise-induced angina because of coronary artery disease, hypertension, and so forth are unable to exercise to expected levels. Medical or surgical intervention may enable them to increase their work level.

MODULE C Sleep disordered breathing

1. Respiratory inductive plethysmography
a. Perform respiratory inductive plethysmography (Code: IB9g) [Difficulty: [An]

Respiratory inductive plethysmography (RIP) is a noninvasive way to monitor a patient's tidal volume, respiratory rate, I:E ratio, and chest and abdominal movements during breathing. RIP is performed by placing two sets of Teflon-insulated coils of wire around a patient's chest and abdomen. See Fig. 17-21. These coils of wire are connected to oscillators that monitor the change in electrical resistance (impedance) as the wire coils are stretched and relaxed during breathing ef-

forts. The unit should be calibrated by having the patient tidal volume breathe and then breathe a larger volume as the two electrical impedances are measured. When properly calibrated, RIP can provide useful information on the patient's breathing as part of a sleep study or apnea study.

b. Interpret the results of respiratory inductive plethysmography (Code: IB10g) [Difficulty: An]

Normally, when a person breathes, the chest and abdominal areas expand and contract at the same time during inspiration and exhalation. There are two breathing abnormalities that can be easily identified with RIP. First, the patient's chest and abdominal areas do not move in synchrony as they should. This is called thoracoabdominal dyssynchrony. The more common term of "see-saw" breathing is also used to describe the chest and abdomen moving in opposite directions during breathing. The second situation involves the patient making breathing efforts without any air entering the lungs. The chest and abdomen are seen to move in synchrony but because of an upper airway obstruction problem the throat is closed off and the patient cannot inhale. This is found with obstructive sleep apnea.

2. Sleep studies
a. Review the results of previous sleep studies (Code: IA1i) [Difficulty: R, Ap, An]

Before starting the current sleep study, it is important to check the patient's chart for information on any previous studies. If a sleep study was done previously, check the results for data related to the patient's tolerance of the test, the physician's interpretation of the test results, and any treatment. For example, was the patient diagnosed with obstructive, central, or mixed apnea? Was the patient

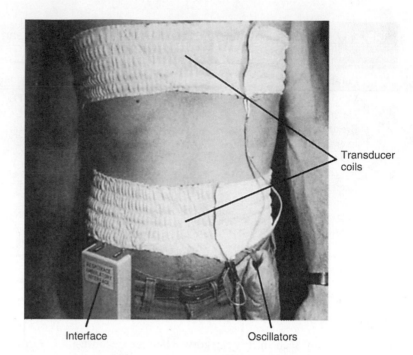

Fig. 17-21 Placement of transducer coils in elastic bands around chest and abdominal area for respiratory inductive plethysmography. (From Ruppel G: *Manual of pulmonary function testing,* ed 6, 1994, Mosby.)

with obstructive sleep apnea fitted with a continuous positive airway pressure (CPAP) mask?

b. Perform a sleep study (Code: IB9g and IC1f) [Difficulty: R, Ap, An] or assist a physician in a sleep study (Code: IIIE1g) [Difficulty: R, Ap, An]

A sleep study (cardiopulmonary sleep study or *polysomnogram*) is performed to determine if the patient has sleep apnea or sleep-disordered breathing. Furthermore, it can help to determine the type of disorder and follow the patient's response to treatment. See Box 17-11 for the indications for a cardiopulmonary sleep study. The cardiopulmonary sleep study is important but only as part of the patient's work-up for a diagnosis. The following are usually performed before the sleep study:

1. History of the problem from both the patient's and the bed partner's viewpoint
2. Physical examination including neck, upper airway, blood pressure, heart rate, and respiratory rate and pattern
3. Arterial blood gases
4. Hemoglobin
5. Thyroid function
6. Chest and upper airway radiographs; may include a CT scan of the upper airway if obstructive sleep apnea is suspected
7. ECG

The following physiologic parameters are usually measured during a cardiopulmonary sleep study:

1. Sleep stages through an electroencephalogram (EEG) recording of brain wave activity and electro-oculogram recording of eye movements
2. Inspiratory and expiratory airflow by nasal thermis-

BOX 17-11   Indications for a Cardiopulmonary Sleep Study

Patient with COPD whose awake PaO_2 is greater than 55 torr but who has pulmonary hypertension, right heart failure (cor pulmonale), or polycythemia

Patient whose awake PaO_2 is less than 55 torr without continuous supplemental oxygen and who must have the proper oxygen flow rate set for sleeping at night. Overnight sleep ear oximetry should be performed.

Patient with restrictive ventilatory impairment secondary to chest wall or neuromuscular disturbances who also has chronic hypoventilation, polycythemia, pulmonary hypertension, disturbed sleep, morning headaches, or daytime somnolence and fatigue

Patient with awake $PaCO_2$ greater than 45 torr who also has polycythemia, pulmonary hypertension, disturbed sleep, morning headaches, or daytime somnolence and fatigue

Patient with snoring, obesity, and other symptoms indicating disturbed sleep pattern

Patient with excessive daytime sleepiness or sleep maintenance insomnia

Patient with nocturnal cyclic bradytachyarrhythmias, atrioventricular conduction abnormalities while asleep, or increased abnormal ventricular beats compared to when awake

---

tor, pneumotachometer, or end-tidal carbon dioxide analyzer

3. Inspiratory and expiratory effort by RIP (some may prefer to have the patient swallow a transducer to measure esophageal pressure changes)
4. Oxygen saturation by ear or bridge of nose

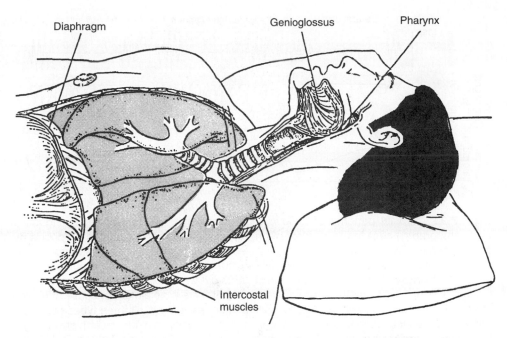

Fig. 17-22   Obstructive sleep apnea. These patients often obstruct when lying supine and genioglossus muscle of the tongue fails to oppose the negative force on the airway during inspiration. (From Des Jardins TL: *Clinical manifestations of respiratory disease,* ed 2, St Louis, 1990, Mosby.)

oximetry; finger oximetry not recommended because of patient movement
5. Body position related to normal and abnormal breathing patterns
6. Periodic arm and leg movements
7. ECG for monitoring heart rate and arrhythmias

The respiratory therapist may be responsible for preparing the patient and setting up the equipment and supplies. Each hospital or physician may have a prescribed way of doing this. The general steps are listed here:
1. Inform the patient of the procedure and have him or her sign the medical release form.
2. Attach the monitoring leads and equipment to the patient.
3. Calibrate the equipment and make sure that it is working properly.
4. Record the patient's parameters during the course of a 6-hour or longer sleep period. The patient may also be video- and audiorecorded during the sleep period.
5. Make any adjustments in the patient's respiratory care equipment as needed.
6. Dispose of any used supplies and so forth after the procedure is completed.
7. Tend to the patient's comfort.

c. Interpret the results of a sleep study (Code: IC2g) [Difficulty: R, Ap, An]

Apnea is the cessation of breathing for 10 seconds or longer. For a diagnosis of sleep apnea to be made, the patient must experience at least 30 apneic periods during 6 hours of sleep. The EEG tracing should confirm that the apnea periods occur during both of the major sleep stages. The first stage is called nonrapid eye movement (non-REM) sleep and starts soon after the person loses consciousness. The second stage is called rapid eye movement (REM) sleep and follows the non-REM stage. Normally, people cycle through both stages about every 1 to 1½ hours during the night. This normal cycle of sleep is important for both mental and physical health. People with disturbed sleep do not dream as they should and are not physically rested when they rise for the day.

Obstructive sleep apnea. Obstructive sleep apnea results when the patient's upper airway is obstructed despite continued breathing efforts (Figs. 17-22 and 17-23). Patients with this problem often exhibit the following symptoms: loud snoring (reported by the bed partner), morning headache, excessive daytime sleepiness, depression or other personality changes, decreased intellectual ability, sexual dysfunction, bed wetting (nocturnal enuresis), and/or abnormal limb movements during sleep.

Obstructive sleep apnea is associated with the following: middle age men, obesity, short neck, hypothyroidism, testosterone administration, myotonic dystrophy, temporomandibular joint disease (TMJ disease), narrowed upper airway from excessive pharyngeal tissue, enlarged tongue (macroglossia), enlarged tonsils or adenoids, deviated nasal septum, recessed jaw (micrognathia), goiter, laryngeal

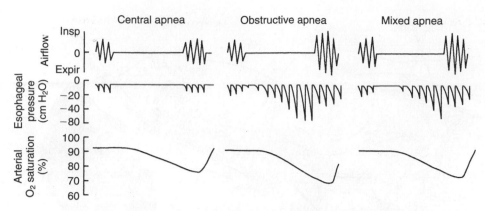

Fig. 17-23 Typical patterns of airflow, esophageal pressure (or respiratory inductive plethysmography) showing respiratory effort, and arterial oxygen saturation produced by central, obstructive, and mixed sleep apnea. Central apnea shows lack of respiratory effort resulting in no airflow. Obstructive apnea shows continued respiratory effort but no airflow because of airway obstruction. Mixed apnea starts out with initial lack of respiratory effort (central apnea). Later, breathing efforts are made but there is no airflow because of airway obstruction (obstructive apnea). Arterial desaturation results from all three types of apnea. When desaturation becomes great enough and the carbon dioxide level high enough, the patient (hopefully) awakens enough to breathe again. (From Des Jardins TL: *Clinical manifestations and assessment of respiratory disease,* ed 3, St Louis, 1995, Mosby.)

stenosis or web, or pharyngeal neoplasm. Management of patients with obstructive sleep apnea may include any of the following:

1. Weight reduction
2. Sleeping on either side or the abdomen; do not sleep in the supine position
3. CPAP mask or BiPAP mask
4. Surgery to open the airway: mandibular advancement, palatopharyngoplasty, or tracheostomy
5. Medication with protriptyline (Triptil, Vivactil) to decrease REM sleep when most obstructive episodes occur
6. Having the patient wear a tongue-retaining device to prevent it from obstructing the pharynx
7. Having the patient wear a neck collar to keep the head and neck aligned with the body

Central sleep apnea. Central sleep apnea is diagnosed when the respiratory center of the medulla fails to signal the respiratory muscles for breathing to occur. The patient makes no respiratory effort and there is no air movement (see Fig. 17-23). Patients with this problem often exhibit these symptoms or traits: normal weight; mild snoring; insomnia; and lesser levels of daytime sleepiness, depression, or sexual dysfunction than the obstructive sleep apnea patient.

Central sleep apnea is associated with the following: primary alveolar (idiopathic) hypoventilation (Ondine's curse), muscular dystrophy, bilateral cervical cordotomy, bulbar poliomyelitis, encephalitis, brain stem infarction or neoplasm, spinal surgery, and hypothyroidism. Manage-

ment of patients with central sleep apnea may include the following:

1. Negative pressure ventilation for sleeping
2. Intubation or tracheostomy and positive pressure ventilation if the patient has acute ventilatory failure
3. Phrenic nerve pacemaker

Mixed sleep apnea. Mixed sleep apnea is diagnosed when the patient shows evidence of both central and obstructive apnea. It is usually found that the patient first stops all breathing efforts (central apnea). After a period of time, the patient makes attempts to breathe but cannot because the upper airway is blocked (obstructive apnea) (see Fig. 17-23). Patients with mixed sleep apnea may show a variety of symptoms and traits from those listed earlier. Clinical management may include any of the treatments mentioned that prove to be effective.

Whatever the cause of the sleep apnea, it must be treated. If left to continue its pathologic course, the patient may develop a number of problems such as pulmonary hypertension, cor pulmonale, polycythemia, cardiac arrhythmias, and even unexplained nocturnal death. Minimally, the patient's personal, family, and social life suffers.

✎ EXAM HINT

Know how to differentiate between the findings that indicate which type of sleep apnea problem the patient has. Signs and symptoms of obstructive sleep apnea have been tested before.

MODULE D | Mass spectrometry

1. Perform mass spectrometry (Code: IB9a) [Difficulty: An]

A mass spectrometer is an instrument used to determine the masses of positively charged ions (cations). The device offers the most sophisticated and accurate way to quickly determine the composition of respiratory gases. Because of the expense of the instrument, it is typically used to sequentially monitor several patients receiving mechanical ventilation in operating rooms or in the intensive care unit. A sample of exhaled patient gases is directed into the unit. The gases are then ionized. A magnetic field accelerates and deflects each gas based on its mass. For example, the less massive gases, such as helium, do not travel as far as more massive gases, such as carbon dioxide. Each gas strikes a collector plate that generates an electric signal that is proportional to the amount of the gas (percentage) found in the patient sample.

2. Interpret the results of mass spectrometry (Code: IB10a) [Difficulty: An]

The results from mass spectrometry should be very accurate as long as each sampled gas has a unique mass, including oxygen, nitrogen, carbon dioxide, water vapor, helium, nitric oxide, and the anesthetic gases such as ethrane and halothane. However, most mass spectrometers cannot separate out two gases with the same mass. For example, nitrous oxide (often used with anesthesia) and carbon dioxide both have a mass of 44 and carbon monoxide and nitrogen both have a mass of 28. Instead, an analyzer that is specific to each of these gases must be used to determine the percentage of each found in an exhaled patient sample.

MODULE E | Respiratory care plan

1. Review the interdisciplinary patient and family care plan (Code: IC3c) [Difficulty: An]

2. Participate in the development of the respiratory care plan [e.g., case management, development and application of protocols, disease management education] (Code: IC4) [Difficulty: An]

Some discussion on pathophysiology was presented with each of the preceding procedures. Further reading is recommended. Review the discussion with each of the preceding procedures and previous chapters in this book if needed.

Be prepared to work with other members of the health care team to determine the patient's care plan. Based on the patient's progress or failure to meet the plan's objectives, be prepared to make recommendations on how the care plan should be modified.

MODULE F | Quality assurance

1. Perform respiratory care quality assurance procedures (Code: IC3a) [Difficulty: An]

2. Develop a quality assurance program (Code: IC3b) [Difficulty: An]

The broad concept of quality assurance can be viewed as a personal and departmental philosophy that ensures constant improvement in production and service. There are a number of ways to approach the subject. A key to quality assurance is understanding what the respiratory care department should do for the patients, the physicians, the nurses, and other allied health professionals, as well as for the hospital. Once these objectives are determined, the quality assurance program can be instituted. Minimally, the following can be done:

1. Make sure that all respiratory care equipment is working properly or, if malfunctioning, is repaired.
2. Audit the patient's medical records to find out if all ordered services were performed. If not, find out why.
3. Communicate with patients during their hospitalization and after discharge to find out their impressions of the care they received.
4. Communicate with the physicians, nurses, and so forth to find out if their needs for optimizing patient care are being met.
5. Work with the hospital administration to find ways to contain unnecessary costs, expand into new areas as opportunities arise, and so forth.

BIBLIOGRAPHY

AARC Clinical Practice Guideline: Exercise testing for evaluation of hypoxemia and/or desaturation, *Respir Care* 37:907, 1992.

AARC Clinical Practice Guideline: Fiberoptic bronchoscopy assisting, *Respir Care* 38:1173, 1993.

AARC Clinical Practice Guideline: Management of airway emergencies, *Respir Care* 40:749, 1995.

AARC Clinical Practice Guideline: Polysomnography, *Respir Care* 40:1236, 1995.

Anderson HL, Bartlett RH: Respiratory care of the surgical patient. In Burton GG, Hodgkin JE, Ward JJ, editors: *Respiratory care: a guide to clinical practice*, ed 3, Philadelphia, 1991, JB Lippincott.

Arand DL, Bonnet MH: Sleep-disordered breathing. In Burton GC, Hodgkin JE, Ward JJ, editors: *Respiratory care: a guide to clinical practice*, ed 4, Philadelphia, Lippincott Raven, 1997.

Barnes TA, editor: *Core textbook of respiratory care practice*, ed 2, St Louis, 1994, Mosby.

Branson RD, Hess DR, Chatburn RL, editors: *Respiratory care equipment*, ed 2, Philadelphia, 1999, Lippincott Williams & Wilkins.

Brutinel WM, Cortese DA: Fiberoptic bronchoscopy. In Burton GC, Hodgkin JE, Ward JJ, editors: *Respiratory care: a guide to clinical practice*, ed 4, Philadelphia, 1997, Lippincott-Raven.

Cairo JM: Assessment of physiologic function. In Cairo JM, Pilbeam SP, editors: *Mosby's respiratory care equipment,* ed 6, St Louis, 1999, Mosby.

Cairo JM: Sleep diagnostics. In Cairo JM, Pilbeam SP, editors: *Mosby's respiratory care equipment,* ed 6, St Louis, 1999, Mosby.

Chadha TS et al: Noninvasive monitoring of breathing patterns during wakefulness and sleep, *Respir Ther* 27-40, May/June 1985.

Chavis AD, Grum CM: Fiberoptic bronchoscopy with mechanical ventilation, *Choices Respir Manage* 21:4, 1991.

Chavis AD, Grum CM: Pulmonary procedures during mechanical ventilation, *Choices Respir Manage* 21:29, 1991.

Coppolo DP et al: A role for the respiratory therapist in flexible fiberoptic bronchoscopy, *Respir Care* 30:323, 1985.

Curity Thoracentesis Tray (package insert), Kendall Hospital Products, Boston, MA.

Decker MJ, Smith BL, Strohl KP: Center-based vs. patient-based diagnosis and therapy of sleep- related respiratory disorders and role of the respiratory care practitioner, *Respir Care* 39:390, 1994.

Deshpande VM, Pilbeam SP, Dixon RJ: *A comprehensive review in respiratory care,* East Norwalk, Conn, 1988, Appleton & Lange.

Des Jardins TL: *Clinical manifestations of respiratory disease,* ed 3, St Louis, 1997, Mosby.

Downey R III, Dexter JR: Assessment of sleep and breathing. In Wilkins RL, Krider SJ, Sheldon RJ, editors: *Clinical assessment in respiratory care,* ed 3, St Louis, 1995, Mosby.

Erickson RA: Chest drainage. I, *Nursing89* 19:37, 1989.

Erickson RA: Chest drainage. II, *Nursing89* 19:47, 1989.

Eubanks DH, Bone RC: *Comprehensive respiratory care: a learning system,* ed 2, St Louis, 1990, Mosby.

Garay SM: Therapeutic options for obstructive sleep apnea, *Respir Manage* 17:11, 1987.

Guidelines for fiberoptic bronchoscopy, *ATS News* 12:14, 1986.

Homedco Home Infant Monitoring Guidelines, Homedco, Fountain View, Calif.

Howard TP: Foreign body extraction by means of combined rigid and flexible bronchoscopy: a case report, *Respir Care* 33:786, 1988.

Indications and standards for cardiopulmonary sleep studies, *Am Rev Respir Dis* 139:559, 1989.

Johnson MD: Noninvasive monitoring. In Aloan CA, Hill TV, editors: *Respiratory care of the newborn and child,* ed 2, Philadelphia, 1997, Lippincott-Raven.

Lough MD: Newborn respiratory care procedures. In Lough MD, Williams TJ, Rawson JE, editors: *Newborn respiratory care,* St Louis, 1979, Mosby.

Madama VC: *Pulmonary function testing and cardiopulmonary stress testing,* ed 2, Albany, NY, 1998, Delmar.

Mathewson HS: Drug therapy for obstructive sleep apnea, *Respir Care* 31:717, 1986.

Mims BC: You *can* manage chest tubes confidently, *RN* 48:39, 1985.

Mishoe SC: The diagnosis and treatment of sleep apnea syndrome, *Respir Care* 32:183, 1987.

Peters RM: Chest trauma. In Moser KM, Spragg RG, editors: *Respiratory emergencies,* ed 2, St Louis, 1982, Mosby.

Phillipson EA: Breathing disorders during sleep, *Basics Respir Dis* 7:1, 1979.

Plevak DJ, Ward JJ, Airway management. In Burton GC, Hodgkin JE, Ward JJ, editors: *Respiratory care: a guide to clinical practice,* ed 4, Philadelphia, 1997, Lippincott-Raven.

Podnos SD, Chappell TR: Hemoptysis: a clinical update, *Respir Care* 30(11):977-985, 1985.

Rapaport DM: Techniques for administering nasal CPAP, *Respir Manage* 17:17, 1987.

Ruppel G: *Manual of pulmonary function testing,* ed 6, St Louis, 1994, Mosby.

Shapiro BA et al: *Clinical application of respiratory care,* ed 4, St Louis, 1991, Mosby.

Strollo PJ Jr, Fernandes KS: Disorders of sleep. In Scanlan CL, Wilkins RL, Stoller JK, editors: *Egan's fundamentals of respiratory care,* ed 7, St Louis, 1999, Mosby.

Whitaker K: *Comprehensive perinatal & pediatric respiratory care,* ed 2, Albany, NY, 1997, Delmar.

Williams SF, Thompson JM: *Respiratory disorders,* St Louis, 1990, Mosby.

SELF-STUDY QUESTIONS

1. The best way to obtain a sample of mucus that contains only those organisms from the lower respiratory tract would be:
   A. Bronchoscopy
   B. Oropharyngeal suctioning
   C. Nasotracheal suctioning
   D. Transtracheal aspiration

2. All the following should be done when preparing to helicopter transport an adult patient requiring mechanical ventilation *except:*
   A. Select a heated cascade-type humidification system.
   B. Calculate the duration of the oxygen cylinder that will be used.
   C. Select a ventilator that uses a demand valve IMV system rather than one with an external reservoir IMV system.
   D. Select a lightweight and portable ventilator.

3. A patient was found to have a $\dot{V}O_2$ of 2000 mL and a $\dot{V}CO_2$ of 1700 mL during an exercise test. Calculate her respiratory exchange ratio (R).
   A. 0 .85
   B. 1.18
   C. 2000
   D. 3700

4. Your patient is performing an exercise test and has the following signs and symptoms: systolic blood pressure of 260 mm Hg, cyanosis, headache, and dizziness. Which of the following would you recommend?
   A. Continue the test until the patient's R value hits 1.1.
   B. Stop the test.
   C. Continue the test until the patient complains of shortness of breath.
   D. Continue the test at a lower work level.

5. A patient is performing a stress test. Which of the following R values would confirm that the patient has reached the AT?
   A. 0.8
   B. 0.9
   C. 1.0
   D. 1.1

6. Calculate the maximum heart rate for a 55-year-old woman who is about to undergo a stress test.
   A. 55/min
   B. 174/min
   C. 265/min
   D. 275/min

7. What would be expected of a patient's ventilation efforts during light exercise that progresses to moderate exercise?
   A. It decreases as $\dot{V}O_2$ increases.
   B. It decreases as carbon dioxide production increases.
   C. It increases as workload levels increase.
   D. It remains constant in normal subjects as workload levels increase.

8. As a respiratory therapist you are assisting with biopsy procedures of a suspected left lung tumor in a 50-year-old patient. The patient is intubated and receiving mechanical ventilation. A transtracheal lung biopsy is performed via bronchoscopy and a percutaneous needle biopsy of the lung is also performed. After the procedures are completed the peak pressure on the ventilator is noted to be markedly higher. What could cause this situation?
   I. Pneumothorax
   II. Bronchospasm
   III. Congestive heart failure
   IV. Intrapleural hemorrhage
   A. I only
   B. I and II only
   C. II, III, and IV only
   D. I, II, and IV only

9. A 60-year-old patient with a smoking history and recurrent bouts of left lung pneumonia has a persistent chest radiograph shadow in the left lower lobe area. Despite 2 days of postural drainage with percussion and incentive spirometry, the haziness has not cleared. What should be recommended next?
   A. Nebulize a bronchodilator medication.
   B. Rigid tube bronchoscopy.
   C. Flexible fiberoptic bronchoscopy.
   D. Nebulize hypertonic saline to induce a cough.

10. Which of the following conditions is first treated by placing a large-bore needle at the midclavicular line through the second or third intercostal space?
    A. 5% pneumothorax
    B. Pleural effusion
    C. Hemothorax
    D. Tension pneumothorax

11. Which of the following should the respiratory therapist evaluate to determine if a patient's chest drainage system is functioning properly and removing pleural air?
    A. Fluid is present in the collection chamber.
    B. The vacuum level is set at −15 cm water.
    C. Air is bubbling in the water seal chamber.
    D. Air is bubbling in the suction control chamber.

12. An intubated patient receiving mechanical ventilation will be transported from Chicago to Denver by an airplane with an unpressurized cabin. A pressure-cycled transport ventilator will be used. The patient should be monitored for all of the following during the flight.
    I. Increased cuff volume

II. Decreased tidal volume
III. Hypoxemia
IV. Increased tidal volume
V. Fluid retention
A. I, III, and IV only
B. II, III, and V only
C. II and III only
D. I and IV only

13. A mechanically ventilated patient is having a central venous line inserted by the subclavian vein route. He coughs vigorously. Within a minute the peak pressure on the ventilator increases significantly and the SpO_2 value is progressively dropping. Chest percussion demonstrates a hyperresonant sound over the right side of the chest and breath sounds are diminished on the right side. What is the most important thing to do at this time?
    A. Complete the insertion of the CVP line.
    B. Insert a pleural chest tube on the right side.
    C. Get a chest radiograph.
    D. Compare the peak and plateau pressures on the ventilator.

14. A conscious adult patient with atrial fibrillation is being prepared for synchronous cardioversion. Which of the following should be recommended?
    I. Administer midazolam (Versed) before starting.
    II. Administer flumazenil (Romazicon) before starting.
    III. Charge the defibrillator to 100 J.
    IV. Charge the defibrillator to 360 J.
    V. Set the ECG machine to lead II.
    VI. Have a manual resuscitator on standby.
    A. II and III only
    B. I, II, and IV only
    C. I, III, and V only
    D. I, III, V, and VI only

15. While performing a sleep study, the respiratory therapist noticed the following information: the RIP reading indicates chest and abdominal movement, the nasal thermistor shows no air movement, and the patient's pulse oximeter value drops to 85%. After 35 seconds the patient snores loudly, rolls on his side, and resumes normal breathing. What best describes the patient's problem?
    A. Central sleep apnea
    B. Airway obstruction
    C. Cheyne-Stokes respiration
    D. Hyperventilation

16. All of the following may be done by a respiratory therapist during a tracheostomy procedure *except*:
    A. Insert the tracheostomy tube into the new stoma.
    B. Disinfect the surgical site.
    C. Check for proper functioning of the tracheostomy tube.
    D. Withdraw the endotracheal tube when the stoma is ready for the tracheostomy tube.

17. A respiratory therapist is assisting an anesthesiologist in a direct vision nasotracheal intubation of a patient. All of the following equipment will be needed *except*:
    A. Magill forceps
    B. Laryngoscope handle with blade
    C. Sterile, water-soluble lubricant
    D. Lubricated stylet.

Answer Key

1. **D.** Rationale: Transtracheal aspiration involves the introduction of a sterile catheter into the patient's trachea. By doing this, any upper airway contaminants are bypassed and the mucous sample would only contain organisms from the patient's lower airway. Because a bronchoscope passes through either the patient's nasal or oral airway, it is likely to be contaminated with upper airway organisms that are carried into the lower airways. Oropharyngeal suctioning involves suctioning saliva from the mouth or throat or mucus coughed into the throat. This mixture of saliva and mucus (sputum) would be contaminated with upper airway organisms. Nasotracheal suctioning involves passing a suction catheter through the patient's nasopharynx into the trachea. This contaminates the lower airway with upper airway organisms. In clinical practice, a bronchoscopy or nasotracheal suctioning specimen are often analyzed for lower airway organisms when transtracheal aspiration is inappropriate. However, strictly speaking, only a transtracheal suctioning specimen would be uncontaminated with upper airway organisms.

2. **A.** Rationale: A heated cascade-type humidification system is inappropriate because the water will splash through the ventilator circuit and into the patient because of the constant motion during transport. A heat and moisture exchanger should be used instead. The oxygen cylinder duration should be calculated to be sure that it lasts long enough for the trip. A demand valve IMV system should be chosen because it is not affected by altitude changes. A lightweight and portable ventilator is needed because the helicopter has a weight limit for equipment and passengers and the chosen ventilator should be designed to tolerate the rough motion that can occur during a transport.

3. **A.** Rationale: The R is calculated by placing the patient's $\dot{V}O_2$ and $\dot{V}CO_2$ values into the following equation:

$$R = \frac{\dot{V}CO_2}{\dot{V}O_2} = \frac{1700 \text{ mL}}{2000 \text{ mL}} = .85$$

4. **B.** Rationale: The test should be stopped because the patient's signs and symptoms indicate that he is not tolerating the procedure. See Box 17-10 for a complete listing of the indications to stop an exercise test. A healthy person who does not have dangerous signs and symptoms may tolerate a respiratory exchange ratio of 1:1 for a short time; this patient should not be pushed to this point. This patient has several signs and symptoms showing intolerance and does not need to be pushed to complain of shortness of breath. Although the patient may tolerate the stress test at a lower work level, it is safer to stop the test and evaluate the patient.

5. **C.** Rationale: When indirect calorimetry is used to evaluate a patient's oxygen consumption and carbon dioxide production during a stress test, the AT is confirmed by a R of 1.0. See the calculation in the question 3 rationale. Before the R value hits 1.0 the patient dramatically increases his or her tidal volume and respiratory rate when the tissues are hypoxic and anaerobic metabolism occurs.

6. **B.** Rationale: Maximum heart rate can be calculated by two different equations. Both are shown here for this 55-year-old patient. The first equation was used for this question.

(1) HR_{max} for males and females $= 210 - (0.65 \times \text{age in years})$
$= 210 - (0.65 \times 55)$
$= 210 - (35.75)$
$= 174.25$. Round off to the nearest whole number for a maximum heart rate of 174/min.

(2) HR_{max} for males and females $= 220 - (\text{age in years})$
$= 220 - (55)$
$= 165$.

According to this alternate equation, the patient's maximum heart rate would be 165/min.

7. **C.** Rationale: Normally, as a person progressively exercises more vigorously, his or her ventilation efforts (larger tidal volume and faster respiratory rate) increase proportionately. This is because the exercising muscles produce more carbon dioxide and require more oxygen. A decreasing or constant ventilation effort at increasing workload levels is abnormal. The patient would soon have to stop exercising. Decreasing ventilation when carbon dioxide production increases results in a respiratory acidosis. This would be markedly abnormal and cause the person to quickly stop exercising.

8. **D.** Rationale: Needle aspiration of lung tissue requires piercing the chest wall and visceral and parietal pleura of the lung to get to the suspected tumor. This procedure can result in an air leak into the pleural space (pneumothorax) and bleeding into the pleural space (intrapleural hemorrhage). Bronchospasm can result from piercing the tracheal wall during the transtracheal lung biopsy. Each of these conditions can result in a increase in the patient's peak pressure. (Pneumothorax and intrapleural hemorrhage also increases the plateau pressure on the ventilator.) Congestive heart failure causes pulmonary edema. This results in an increased plateau pressure and, as a result, an increased peak pressure. However, it is unlikely that these two diagnostic procedures would cause congestive heart failure.

9. **C.** Rationale: A flexible fiberoptic bronchoscopy is indicated for two reasons. First, the patient has a history of smoking and recurrent bouts of pneumonia of the left lung. Second, other treatment procedures have failed to produce improvement in the patient's chest radiograph. These things should make one suspicious of a lung tumor. It is very doubtful that nebulizing a bronchodilator medication or hypertonic saline will make any difference in this patient's condition. There is no indication of bronchospasm or retained secretions. A rigid tube bronchoscope cannot be used to look into the left lower lobe bronchus because it is not flexible. It can be used only to view the trachea and right and left mainstem bronchi.

10. **D.** Rationale: A tension pneumothorax can be immediately treated by placing a large-bore (often 16 gauge) needle through the second or third intercostal space at the midclavicular line on the affected side. Later, a pleural chest tube should be inserted. Although a 5% pneumothorax is abnormal, it is probably not life threatening. Sometimes the patient is given supplemental oxygen as needed and monitored. The pneumothorax gas may be reabsorbed into the tissues and no other treatment may be necessary. A pleural effusion or hemothorax requires a thoracentesis

procedure to remove the fluid. This would probably be done through the lower area of the patient's back because the fluid is gravity dependent. See Fig. 17-4.

11. **C.** Rationale: If air is seen to bubble in the water seal chamber, it is known that there is vacuum applied to the drainage system and the patient has pleural air (pneumothorax) that is being removed. The presence of fluid in the collection chamber confirms that the patient has pleural fluid that is being removed. It does not confirm that pleural air is being removed. A vacuum level of −15 cm water is normal and should result in air being seen to bubble in the suction control chamber. However, it does not confirm that pleural air is being removed. See Figs. 17-8 and 17-9.

12. **A.** Rationale: According to Boyle's law, pressure and volume are inversely proportional. Therefore as barometric pressure decreases at increased altitude, the volume of gas in the patient's endotracheal tube cuff increases and the tidal volume increases. Despite the increased tidal volume, the patient is likely to become hypoxic because the alveolar pressure of oxygen (P_AO_2) drops and therefore the arterial pressure of oxygen (PaO_2) drops as the barometric pressure decreases. The patient's tidal volume should be monitored and adjusted during the flight and pulse oximetry value should be monitored to look for hypoxemia and the need to increase the inspired oxygen percentage. There is no link between fluid retention and change in barometric pressure.

13. **B.** Rationale: All of the stated signs point to a tension pneumothorax. Because the patient's condition is rapidly deteriorating, it is most important to insert a pleural chest tube on the right side. Because it is very likely that the CVP needle pierced the lung and caused the pneumothorax, the procedure should be stopped at this time. Although a chest radiograph is indicated if the patient's condition were stable, getting one now will unnecessarily delay inserting the needed chest tube. There is nothing of clinical value to be gained at this time by comparing the peak and plateau pressures on the ventilator. They will both increase because of the tension pneumothorax. This information only reinforces the previous signs and doing this procedure now delays the needed chest tube.

14. **D.** Rationale: Before a conscious patient undergoes a cardioversion procedure he or she should be given a sedative.

The drug midazolam (Versed) is given intravenously for conscious sedation. The proper initial power setting for the first attempt at cardioversion of an adult patient with atrial fibrillation is 100 J. See Box 17-1. Set the ECG machine to lead II so that an upright R wave is detected by the unit. On occasion, the medication midazolam and shock from the cardioversion can cause a patient to temporarily stop breathing. For this reason the respiratory therapist should have a manual resuscitator on standby and be ready to assist the patient's breathing. The drug flumazenil (Romazicon) is given intravenously *after* the procedure is finished to reverse the sedating effect of the midazolam. A defibrillator charge of 360 J is the maximum used to defibrillate a patient. It is far too high for a first attempt at cardioversion. See Box 17-1.

15. **B.** Rationale: The lack of air movement and related hypoxemia while making respiratory efforts documents that the patient has an airway obstruction problem. If the patient had central sleep apnea he would have stopped making breathing efforts during the time when no air was moving. Cheyne-Stokes respiration is identified by cyclical increasing and decreasing of tidal volume breaths. There may or may not be short periods of apnea between the cycles. Hyperventilation can be documented only by a decreased arterial carbon dioxide level.

16. **A.** Rationale: The surgeon should insert the first tracheostomy tube into the stoma in case there is a problem. A respiratory therapist may replace a tracheostomy tube after the stoma is well established. The therapist may assist with the procedure by disinfecting the surgical site, checking the tube cuff, and withdrawing the endotracheal tube when the surgeon has created the stoma and is ready to insert the tracheostomy tube.

17. **D.** Rationale: A stylet (lubricated or not) is not put through an endotracheal tube during a nasotracheal intubation procedure. This is because the tube should be kept flexible to follow the natural contours of the patient's airway anatomy. A stylet makes the endotracheal tube stiff and causes damage to the nasal passage. A Magill forceps is used to lift the tip of the tube for insertion into the trachea. A laryngoscope handle with blade are used as during an oral intubation procedure. See Fig. 17-12. The tip of the endotracheal tube is lubricated so that it slides easily through the patient's nasal passage.

INDEX